Recent Advances in
HEMATOLOGY-5

Recent Advances in
HEMATOLOGY-5

Editors

Vandana Puri
MD(Pathology) DNB(Pathology) DM(Hematopathology) MNAMS
Professor
Department of Pathology
Lady Hardinge Medical College
New Delhi, India

Jasmita Dass
MD(Pathology) DM(Hematopathology)
Associate Professor
Department of Hematology
All India Institute of Medical Sciences
New Delhi, India

Brig Tathagata Chatterjee
MD(Pathology) PGT(Oncopathology) DM(Hematopathology) FNAMS FUICC
Senior Professor Hematology and Pathology
Department of Hematology/IHBT
ESIC Medical College and Hospital
Faridabad, Haryana, India

Forewords

Renu Saxena
Sunita Sharma

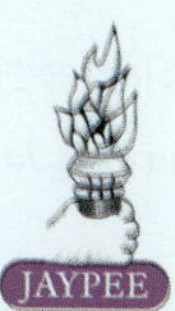

JAYPEE BROTHERS MEDICAL PUBLISHERS
The Health Sciences Publisher
New Delhi | London

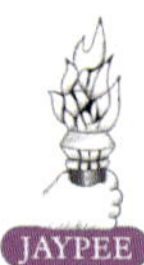

Jaypee Brothers Medical Publishers (P) Ltd

Headquarters
EMCA House, 23/23-B
Ansari Road, Daryaganj
New Delhi 110 002, India
Landline: +91-11-23272143, +91-11-23272703
+91-11-23282021, +91-11-23245672
e-mail: jaypee@jaypeebrothers.com

Corporate Office
4838/24, Ansari Road, Daryaganj
New Delhi 110 002, India
Phone: +91-11-43574357
Fax: +91-11-43574314
e-mail: jaypee@jaypeebrothers.com

Overseas Office
JP Medical Ltd.
83, Victoria Street, London
SW1H 0HW (UK)
Phone: +44-20 3170 8910
e-mail: info@jpmedpub.com

EU GPSR Authorised Representative
Logos Europe, 9 rue Nicolas Poussin
17000, La Rochelle, France
Phone: +33 (0) 6 67 93 73 78
e-mail: contact@logoseurope.eu

Website: www.jaypeebrothers.com
Website: www.jaypeedigital.com

Inquiries for bulk sales may be solicited at: jaypee@jaypeebrothers.com

Recent Advances in Hematology-5* / *Vandana Puri, Jasmita Dass, Tathagata Chatterjee

First Edition: **2026**

ISBN: 978-93-6616-832-6

Printed in India at Sterling Graphics Pvt. Ltd.

DEDICATED TO

My parents; my loving soulmate, Dr Shakti Tiwari; and my wonderful children, Arsh and Amaira, for their unconditional love and support. To my teachers and students, whose inspiration continues to guide and motivate me.

—Vandana Puri

My mother Dr Reva Dass for being a pillar in my life and her unconditional support. My thanks go to all my teachers who were instrumental in shaping my career and students for challenging and inspiring me.

—Jasmita Dass

My wife Sonali Jha Chatterjee for her constant encouragement and support throughout the project and to my amazing daughters Malavika and Nayanika for inspiring me.

—Tathagata Chatterjee

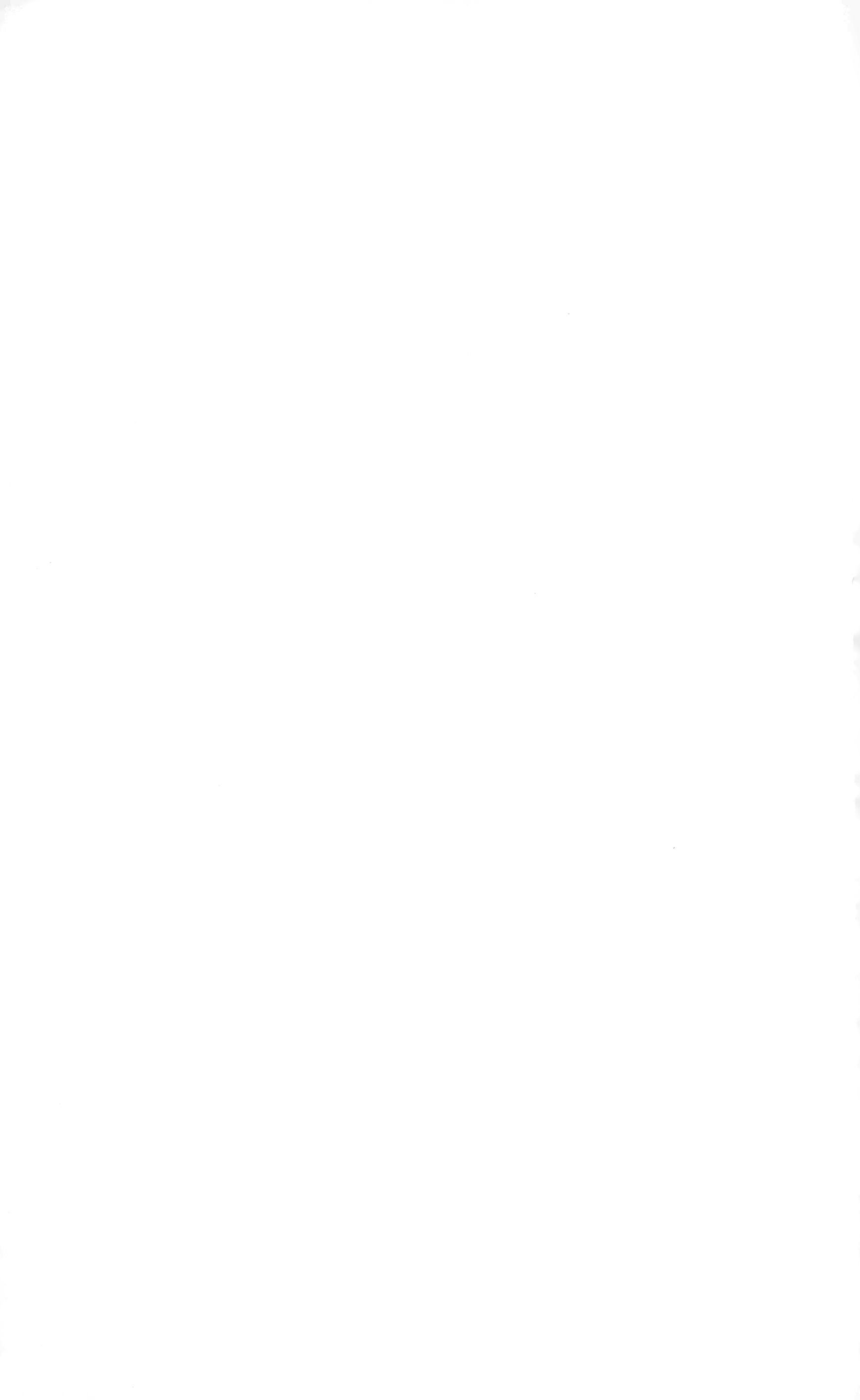

CONTRIBUTORS

Aastha Gupta MBBS MD DM(Hematopathology)
Additional Director and Head
Department of Hematopathology
Fortis Memorial Research Institute
Gurugram, Haryana, India

Abhishek Purohit DM(Hematopathology)
Additional Professor
Department of Pathology
All India Institute of Medical Sciences
Jodhpur, Rajasthan, India

Aditya Kumar Gupta MBBS MD FNB MAMS Fellowship Pediatric Oncology (Sydney, Australia)
Additional Professor
Division of Pediatric Oncology
Department of Pediatrics
All India Institute of Medical Sciences
New Delhi, India

Anamika Bakliwal MD DM
Consultant
Department of Hemato-Oncology and Bone Marrow Transplantation
BLK-Max Super Speciality Hospital
New Delhi, India

Ananthvikas Jayaram MBBS DCP MD(Pathology)
Pathologist
Department of Pathology
Neuberg Anand Reference Laboratory
Bengaluru, Karnataka, India

Anil Handoo MD Post-Doctoral Fellowship (PDF) (Kings College Hospital, London, UK)
Principal Director and Head
Department of Hospital Lab Services
Max Healthcare Institute Limited
BLK-MAX Super Speciality Hospital
New Delhi, India

Anil Kumar Gupta MD
Professor
Department of Pathology
NC Medical College
Panipat, Haryana, India

Anita Chopra MD(Pathology) DM(Hematopathology)
Professor
Department of Laboratory Oncology
All India Institute of Medical Sciences
New Delhi, India

Ankur Ahuja MD DM(Hematopathology)
Professor
Department of Pathology
Armed Forces Medical College
Pune, Maharashtra, India

Anumeha Chaturvedi MBBS DNB(Pathology) PDF(Hematopathology)
Consultant
Department of Hematopathology
Homi Bhabha Cancer Hospital and Research Centre
Visakhapatnam, Andhra Pradesh, India

Asish Rath MD(Pathology) DM(Hematopathology)
Consultant
Department of Laboratory Hematology
Tata Medical Center
Kolkata, West Bengal, India

Balamurugan Thirunavukkarasu MD DM FRCPath
Assistant Professor
Department of Pathology
All India Institute of Medical Sciences
New Delhi, India

Lt Col (Dr) Barun Kumar Chakrabarty MD DNB(Pathology) PDF Cytogenetics(TMCK)
Associate Professor
Department of Pathology
Armed Forces Medical College
Pune, Maharashtra, India

Bipin Prakash Kulkarni PhD Postdoc
Scientist E
Department of Hemostasis and Thrombosis
ICMR – National Institute of Immunohaematology
Mumbai, Maharashtra, India

Devasis Panda MD(Pathology)
Senior Consultant
Department of Hematopathology
Rajiv Gandhi Cancer Institute and Research Centre
New Delhi, India

Dinesh Bhurani MD DM FRCPA
Director
Department of Hemato-oncology and Bone Marrow Transplantation
Rajiv Gandhi Cancer Institute and Research Centre
New Delhi, India

Dinesh Chandra MD(Pathology) DM(Hematopathology)
Additional Professor
Department of Hematology (Lab)
Sanjay Gandhi Postgraduate Institute of Medical Sciences
Lucknow, Uttar Pradesh, India

Gadha Krishna Leons MSc
Student and Senior Research Fellow
Department of Laboratory Oncology
All India Institute of Medical Sciences
New Delhi, India

Ganesh Kumar V MBBS MD DNB DM
Associate Professor
Department of Hematology
All India Institute of Medical Sciences
New Delhi, India

Gaurav Chhabra MBBS MD
Additional Professor
Department of Pathology and Laboratory Medicine
All India Institute of Medical Sciences
Bhubaneswar, Odisha, India

Ghazala Sabereen MSc Microbiology-CSIR SRF
Department of Hematology
Sanjay Gandhi Postgraduate Institute of Medical Sciences
Lucknow, Uttar Pradesh, India

Gurleen Oberoi MD DM DNB MNAMS
Senior Consultant
Department of Hematology
Medanta – The Medicity
Gurugram, Haryana, India

Gurpreet Kaur MD(Pathology) DM(Hematopathology)
Professor, Department of Pathology
Armed Forces Medical College
Pune, Maharashtra, India

Harish Chandra MD FUICC
Professor
Department of Pathology and Laboratory Medicine
All India Institute of Medical Sciences
Rishikesh, Uttarakhand, India

Himil Parikh MD DM(Hematopathology)
Consultant Hematopathologist
Department of Hematology
HOC Vedanta
Ahmedabad, Gujarat, India

Jagdish Prasad Meena MBBS MD
Additional Professor
Division of Pediatric Oncology
Department of Pediatrics
All India Institute of Medical Sciences
New Delhi, India

Jasmina Ahluwalia MBBS MD
Professor
Department of Hematology
Postgraduate Institute of Medical Education and Research
Chandigarh, India

Jasmita Dass MD(Pathology) DM(Hematopathology)
Associate Professor
Department of Hematology
All India Institute of Medical Sciences
New Delhi, India

Kailash Chander Aggarwal MD
Professor and Head
Department of Pediatrics
NC Medical College
Panipat, Haryana, India

Kaniyappan Nambiar MBBS MD DM
Assistant Professor
Department of Pathology
Jawaharlal Institute of Postgraduate Medical Education and Research
Puducherry, India

Kanwaljeet Singh MBBS MD(Pathology)
Trained in Molecular Biology
Professor
Department of Pathology
Command Hospital Eastern Command
Kolkata, West Bengal, India

Khaliqur Rahman MD(Pathology) MNAMS
Professor
Department of Hematology
Sanjay Gandhi Postgraduate Institute of Medical Sciences
Lucknow, Uttar Pradesh, India

Manisha Rajan Madkaikar MD(Medicine)
Director
Department of Pediatric Immunology
ICMR – National Institute of Immunohaematology
Mumbai, Maharashtra, India

Manish Kumar Singh MD(Pathology)
Associate Professor
Department of Hematology
Sanjay Gandhi Postgraduate Institute of Medical Sciences
Lucknow, Uttar Pradesh, India

Manu Jamwal PhD
Scientist/Project Manager
Department of Hematology
Postgraduate Institute of Medical Education and Research
Chandigarh, India

Man Updesh Singh Sachdeva MD DNB(Pathology)
Professor
Department of Hematology
Postgraduate Institute of Medical Education and Research
Chandigarh, India

Mayur Parihar MD PDF - Cytogenetics
Senior Consultant
Department of Cytogenetics, Molecular Pathology and Lab Hematology
Tata Medical Center
Kolkata, West Bengal, India

Mohd Rizwan Shaikh MD DrNB
Assistant Professor
Department of Clinical Hematology
Seth GS Medical College and KEM Hospital
Mumbai, Maharashtra, India

Mrinalini Kotru MD DNB MNAMS DM(Hematopathology) (AIIMS, Delhi)
Director-Professor
Department of Pathology
UCMS and GTBH, New Delhi, India

Mukesh Desai MD(Pediatrics)
Professor
Department of Immunology
BJ Wadia Hospital for Children
Mumbai, Maharashtra, India

Mukul Aggarwal MBBS MD PDCC DM PGDHM
Associate Professor
Department of Hematology
All India Institute of Medical Sciences
New Delhi, India

Narasimhapriyan Kannan MD DM
Fellow Molecular Hemato-oncology
Department of Hematopathology
Advance Centre for Treatment Research and Education in Cancer (ACTREC)
Tata Memorial Centre
Chennai, Tamil Nadu, India

Narender Kumar MBBS MD
Professor
Department of Hematology
Postgraduate Institute of Medical Education and Research
Chandigarh, India

Narender Tejwani DM(Hematopathology)
Senior Consultant
Department of Hematopathology
Rajiv Gandhi Cancer Institute and Research Centre
New Delhi, India

Nikesh Krishna Kawankar MSc(Applied Biology) PG-DMLT
Technical Officer 'A'
Department of Hemostasis and Thrombosis
ICMR – National Institute of Immunohaematology
Mumbai, Maharashtra, India

Nikhil Patkar MD DNB
Clinician Scientist and Professor
Department of Hematopathology
Advance Centre for Treatment Research and Education in Cancer (ACTREC)
Tata Memorial Centre
Navi Mumbai, Maharashtra, India

Papagudi Subramanian MBBS MD(Pathology)
Head
Department of Hematopathology
Advanced Centre for Treatment, Research and Education in Cancer (ACTREC), Tata Memorial Centre
Navi Mumbai, Maharashtra, India

P Lalita Jyotsna MBBS MD(Pathology)
Professor
Department of Pathology
Lady Hardinge Medical College
New Delhi, India

Prabhu Manivannan MD DNB DM(Hematopathology) MNAMS
Additional Professor
Department of Pathology
Jawaharlal Institute of Postgraduate Medical Education and Research
Puducherry, India

Prakhar Gupta MD(Pathology) PDCC(Hematoapthology) PDF(Molecular Pathology)
Consultant
Department of Molecular Pathology
Tata Medical Center
Kolkata, West Bengal, India

Prashant Sharma MD DNB DM
Professor
Department of Hematology
Postgraduate Institute of Medical Education and Research
Chandigarh, India

Prateek Bhatia MD(Pathology) DNB SCYMi(ASCP, USA) DipRCPath(Hematology-UK) PGDHM
Additional Professor
Department of Pediatrics
Postgraduate Institute of Medical Education and Research
Chandigarh, India

Praveen Sharma MBBS MD DNB DM
Associate Professor
Department of Hematology
Postgraduate Institute of Medical Education and Research
Chandigarh, India

Preeti Tripathi MD(Pathology) DM(Hematopathology)
Professor of Hematopathology
Department of Laboratory Sciences and Molecular Medicine
Army Hospital Research and Referral
New Delhi, India

Prerna Arora DM(Hematopathology) (AIIMS, ND) MD DNB(Pathology)
Professor
Department of Pathology (Hematology Section), Maulana Azad Medical College and Associated LN Hospitals
New Delhi, India

Priyanka Mishra MD(Pathology) DM(Hematopathology)
Professor of Hematopathology
Department of Laboratory Sciences and Molecular Medicine
Army Hospital Research and Referral
New Delhi, India

Rahul Naithani MD DM FRCP(Edinburgh)
Chief
Department of Hematology and Bone Marrow Transplant
Artemis Hospital
Gurugram, Haryana, India

Rakhee Kar MBBS MD DNB DM
Professor and Head
Department of Pathology
Jawaharlal Institute of Postgraduate Medical Education and Research
Puducherry, India

Col Dr Rama Hariharan MD(Pathology) DM(Hematopathology)
Associate Professor
Department of Lab Sciences and Molecular Diagnostics
Command Hospital
Lucknow, Uttar Pradesh, India

Reena Das MD DNB(Pathology)
Professor and Head
Department of Hematology
Postgraduate Institute of Medical Education and Research
Chandigarh, India

Renjith Mathew Verghese MD(Medicine) DM(Clinical Hematology)
Assistant Professor
Department of Medicine
Command Hospital Southern Command
Pune, Maharashtra, India

Renu Saxena MD FNAMS
Senior Director
Department of Hematology and Pathology
Medanta – The Medicity
Gurugram, Haryana, India

Richa Chauhan DM(Hematopathology)
Assistant Professor
Department of Hematology
All India Institute of Medical Sciences
New Delhi, India

Richa Juneja DM(Hematopathology)
Associate Professor
Department of Pathology
All India Institute of Medical Sciences
Nagpur, Maharashtra, India

Roopam Deka DM(Hematopathology)
Assistant Professor
Department of Pathology
All India Institute of Medical Sciences
Guwahati, Assam, India

Ruchi Gupta MD(Pathology)
Professor
Department of Hematology
Sanjay Gandhi Postgraduate Institute of Medical Sciences
Lucknow, Uttar Pradesh, India

Sangeeta Pahuja MBBS MD(Pathology) DNB
Professor and Head
Department of Immunohematology and Blood Transfusion
Lady Hardinge Medical College
New Delhi, India

Sanjeev Kumar Gupta MD DNB DM(Hematopathology)
Professor
Department of Laboratory Oncology
All India Institute of Medical Sciences
New Delhi, India

Sanjeev Kumar Sharma MD DM
Director
Department of Hemato-Oncology and Bone Marrow Transplantation
BLK-Max Super Speciality Hospital
New Delhi, India

Sarika Singh Postgraduation with Research Fellowship in Hemato-Oncopathology
Professor
Department of Pathology
Maulana Azad Medical College
New Delhi, India

Sarjana Tiwari MBBS MD DM(Hematopathology)
Consultant, Hematopathology and Molecular and Molecular Biology
Department of Hematopathology
Max Super Speciality Hospital
Lajpat Nagar II, Patparganj
New Delhi, India

Satyam Arora MBBS MD
Additional Professor
Department of Immunohematology and Blood Transfusion
Post Graduate Institute of Child Health
Noida, Uttar Pradesh, India

Saumyaranjan Mallick MD
Professor, Department of Pathology
All India Institute of Medical Sciences
New Delhi, India

Shailaja Shukla MBBS MD(Pathology)
Director Professor
Department of Pathology
Lady Hardinge Medical College
New Delhi, India

Shamee Shastry MBBD MD
Professor
Department of Immunohematology and Blood Transfusion
Kasturba Medical College, Manipal
Manipal, Karnataka, India

Sharda Dilip Shanbhag MSc(Applied Biology) PG-DMLT
Technical Officer 'B'
Department of Hemostasis and Thrombosis
ICMR – National Institute of Immunohaematology
Mumbai, Maharashtra, India

Shivangi Harankhedkar MD DM PDF
In-charge and Head
Department of Molecular Diagnostics and Research
IMS and SUM Hospital
Bhubaneswar, Odisha, India

Sreejesh Sreedharanunni MBBS MD DNB DM
Additional Professor
Department of Hematology
Postgraduate Institute of Medical Education and Research
Chandigarh, India

Sujata Raychaudhuri MD(Pathology) DCP MAMS
Professor
Department of Pathology
Post Graduate Institute of Medical Sciences and Research
New Delhi, India

Sujay Ramaprasad MBBS MD(Pathology)
Pathologist and Medical Director
Department of Pathology
Neuberg Anand Reference Laboratory
Bengaluru, Karnataka, India

Sumeet Gujral MD
Professor and Pathologist (Honorary Consultant)
Department of Pathology
Tata Memorial Hospital
Mumbai, Maharashtra, India

Sumeet Mirgh MD DM
Associate Professor
Department of Medical Oncology Adult Hematolymphoid and BMT Division
Advanced Centre for Treatment, Research and Education in Cancer (ACTREC), Tata Memorial Centre
Mumbai, Maharashtra, India

Sunita Sharma MBBS MD(Pathology)
Director General of Health Services
Department of Directorate General of Health Services
Ministry of Health and Family Welfare
Noida, Uttar Pradesh, India

Surabhi Jain MD DNB
PhD Scholar
Department of Pathology
All India Institute of Medical Sciences
New Delhi, India

Sweta Rajpal MBBS MD(Pathology) DM(Hematopathology) PDF Molecular Hemato-oncopathology
Associate Professor
Department of Hematopathology
Advanced Centre for Treatment, Research and Education in Cancer (ACTREC), Tata Memorial Centre
Navi Mumbai, Maharashtra, India

Swetha Palla MD DM
Medical Research Associate
Department of Pediatrics
Postgraduate Institute of Medical Education and Research
Chandigarh, India

Tanishq Khatavkar MD
Department of Hematopathology
Advance Centre for Treatment Research and Education in Cancer (ACTREC)
Tata Memorial Centre
Mumbai, Maharashtra, India

Brig Tathagata Chatterjee
MD(Pathology) PGT(Oncopathology) DM(Hematopathology) FNAMS FUICC
Senior Professor Hematology and Pathology
Department of Hematology/IHBT
ESIC Medical College and Hospital
Faridabad, Haryana, India

Umair Ahmed Nazir Ahmed Bargir
MBBS DCP
Scientist C (Medical)
Department of Pediatric Immunology
ICMR – National Institute of Immunohaematology
Mumbai, Maharashtra, India

Vandana Puri MD(Pathology) DNB(Pathology) DM(Hematopathology) MNAMS
Professor
Department of Pathology
Lady Hardinge Medical College
New Delhi, India

Vijay Kumar MD(Pathology) (PGI CHD) DNB(Pathology) MNAMS
Professor and Head
Hematology and Clinical Pathology Unit
Department of Pathology
ABVIMS and Dr RML Hospital
New Delhi, India

Vikram Singh MBBS MD(Pathology) DM(Histopathology)
Associate Professor
Department of Pathology
Armed Forces Medical College
Pune, Maharashtra, India

FOREWORD

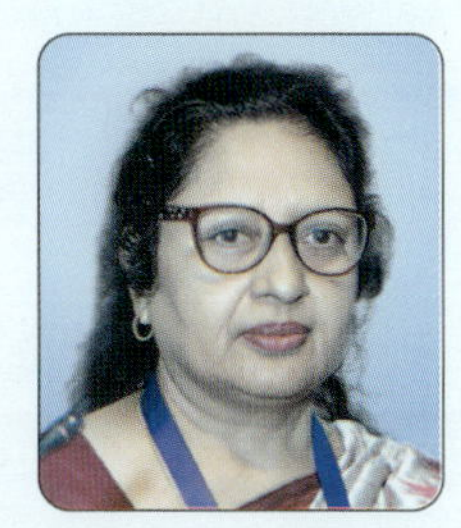

"*Recent Advances in Hematology-5*" is a comprehensive and up-to-date guide that explores the evolving landscape of hematology. It is designed to meet the needs of both newcomers entering this dynamic specialty and experienced clinicians seeking to enhance their knowledge in hematology. Covering the latest developments, evidence-based approaches, and cutting-edge research, this book serves as an invaluable resource for anyone involved in the study and practice of hematology.

Authored by leading experts, each chapter blends a wealth of clinical experience with a strong commitment to education, ensuring that the content is both informative and highly relevant to patient care. The book provides in-depth coverage of a broad spectrum of topics, from benign blood disorders to the complexities of hematologic malignancies and coagulation disorders. Additionally, it emphasizes a multidisciplinary approach, incorporating insights from genetics, pathology, and modern therapeutic advances, including immunotherapy and targeted treatments.

In an era of rapid technological advancements, this text offers both a solid theoretical foundation and practical guidance to help navigate the complexities of hematology. Whether engaging with the material for the first time or revisiting key concepts, readers will gain a deeper understanding of blood disorders and their management, empowering them to make meaningful contributions to patient care.

The editors have meticulously curated state-of-the-art topics, ranging from fundamental hematology to the latest innovations, ensuring comprehensive coverage of the field. This book serves as an essential reference for residents, faculty members, and specialists in pathology, hematopathology, pediatrics, internal medicine, and transfusion medicine who seek the most up-to-date knowledge in hematology.

Renu Saxena MD FNAMS
Senior Director
Path and Lab Medicine and Head, Hematopathology
Medanta – The Medicity
Gurugram, Haryana, India
Former Professor and Head
Department of Hematology
All India Institute of Medical Sciences
New Delhi, India

FOREWORD

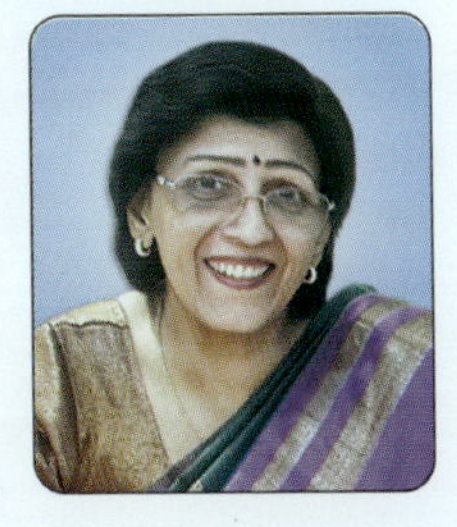

"*Recent Advances in Hematology-5*" is a comprehensive yet accessible update that spans the breadth of hematology—from benign disorders to malignancies and coagulation abnormalities. Authored by experts, it integrates the latest research, evidence-based practices, and innovations like immunotherapy and targeted treatments. Designed for medical students, residents, and specialists in hematology, pathology, internal medicine, pediatrics, and transfusion medicine, the book emphasizes a multidisciplinary approach and clinical relevance. It serves as both a foundational text and an advanced reference, reflecting current trends and future directions in hematology.

Sunita Sharma MD(Pathology)
Director General of Health Services (DGHS)
Ministry of Health and Family Welfare
Government of India

PREFACE

"*Recent Advances in Hematology-5*" is a reflection of the dynamic and ever-evolving nature of hematology as a medical specialty. With rapid developments in molecular diagnostics, targeted therapies, and immunomodulatory approaches, the field continues to transform the way we understand and manage hematologic diseases.

This book aims to serve as a comprehensive yet accessible resource for medical students, postgraduate trainees, practicing clinicians, and laboratory scientists. It presents up-to-date insights into both benign and malignant hematologic disorders, integrating recent guidelines, breakthrough research, and practical clinical applications. Special emphasis has been placed on topics such as myeloid and lymphoid neoplasms, advances in coagulation and transfusion medicine, and the growing impact of personalized medicine and genomics.

The contributions of dedicated experts and specialists in various subfields have enriched the content of this volume. Their experience and clarity ensure that each chapter offers both depth and relevance to everyday clinical practice.

We hope this book will not only enhance knowledge but also inspire curiosity and critical thinking among readers. As hematology continues to evolve, it is our collective responsibility to stay updated and adapt in order to offer the best possible care to our patients.

We are grateful to all contributors, reviewers, and mentors who have supported this endeavor. Their expertise and encouragement have been invaluable in bringing this project to fruition.

Vandana Puri
Jasmita Dass
Tathagata Chatterjee

ACKNOWLEDGMENTS

First, we would like to express our eternal gratitude to the blessings of Almighty God. We thank our parents for their blessings, everlasting love, and support. We wish to sincerely thank our teachers and faculty for being the source of our inspiration and knowledge and who helped us to achieve a lot in our personal and professional lives.

We gratefully acknowledge all the contributing authors for their invaluable efforts in crafting the individual chapters of *"Recent Advances in Hematology-5"*. Each chapter reflects the depth of their clinical experience, academic rigor, and thoughtful analysis of current developments in the field. The diversity of perspectives and the high standard of scholarship presented in this volume are a testament to their dedication and collaboration. Their timely contributions, attention to detail, and commitment to advancing hematology education have been instrumental in shaping this book into a comprehensive and authoritative resource.

We are especially thankful to the patients and their families, who have been our greatest teachers. Their experiences, resilience, and trust continue to guide our understanding and advance our practice.

Our special thanks go to Mr Sabyasachi Hazra [Director (PG and PNR Content)], Ms Sadhna Rajan (Development Editor), and the entire team of M/s Jaypee Medical Publishers and Distributors Pvt Ltd, New Delhi, India, for their wholehearted support in the publication of this book. We have no words to describe the role, efforts, inputs, and initiatives.

Vandana Puri
Jasmita Dass
Tathagata Chatterjee

CONTENTS

CHAPTER 1

Molecular Diagnosis of Inherited Hemolytic Anemias Beyond Thalassemia

Prashant Sharma, Manu Jamwal

ABSTRACT

Inherited hemolytic and dyserythropoietic anemias [hereditary hemolytic anemias (HHAs)] encompass a heterogeneous group of disorders involving defects in red cell membrane proteins, metabolic enzymes, and erythroid development. Traditional diagnostic algorithms relied on clinical features and stepwise laboratory tests, but recent advances in molecular diagnostics have transformed the diagnostic approach. Next-generation sequencing (NGS)—including targeted gene panels, whole-exome sequencing (WES), and copy number analysis—now enable precise identification of pathogenic variants in diverse HHAs, particularly in atypical or overlapping phenotypes.

Hereditary membranopathies and channelopathies, such as spherocytosis, elliptocytosis, and stomatocytosis, are linked to mutations in structural (*ANK1*, *SPTA1*, *SLC4A1*) or ion-channel genes (*PIEZO1*, *KCNN4*). Enzymopathies, especially the common glucose-6-phosphate dehydrogenase (G6PD) and PK deficiencies, are amenable to enzyme activity assay-based diagnoses, but rarer ones and ambiguous cases frequently require molecular confirmation. Congenital dyserythropoietic anemias (CDAs), are best diagnosed through NGS in conjunction with the marrow morphology and other tests like the flow cytometric eosin-5′-maleimide (EMA)-binding assay for CDA type II.

Molecular findings not only confirm diagnosis but also inform therapeutic decisions (e.g., mitapivat in PK deficiency, avoiding splenectomy in *PIEZO1* mutations) and facilitate genetic counseling. Variant interpretation based on the American College of Medical Genetics and Genomics (ACMG) guidelines, supported by functional data and bioinformatics tools, is essential for clinical relevance. As diagnostic technologies evolve, integrated genomic approaches are becoming central to modern hematology practice.

INTRODUCTION

Hemolytic anemias (HAs) are characterized by shortened red blood cell (RBC) survival, and may be inherited or acquired. The inherited or hereditary HAs (HHAs) encompass a diverse group of disorders affecting erythrocytic membrane proteins, enzymatic pathways, heme and globin synthesis, and erythroid proliferation, differentiation and kinetics **(Table 1)**. HHAs with mainly peripheral blood destruction of RBCs (the traditional HHAs) typically show reticulocytosis, while those with predominantly intramedullary death (for e.g., CDAs or thalassemias) show inappropriately low reticulocyte counts for the degree of anemia **(Table 2)**.

Despite their pathogenetic diversity, the clinical phenotypes of HHAs overlap extensively with each other **(Table 3)**. Hemogram, peripheral blood, and bone marrow findings and biochemical parameters too are often not sufficiently discriminatory, and are moreover often impacted by recent blood transfusions.

TABLE 1: Classification and key laboratory features of the hereditary hemolytic anemias.

Category	Disorder	Pathophysiology	Key laboratory features
Membrane cytoskeletal defects	Hereditary spherocytosis (HS)	Defective α/β spectrin, ankyrin, band 3 or protein 4.2 → RBC membrane instability	Spherocytes, ↑ incubated osmotic fragility, ↓ EMA binding, ↑ MCHC
	Hereditary elliptocytosis (HE)	Defective spectrin dimer self-association	Elliptocytes, normal EMA binding, ↑ osmotic fragility (severe cases)
	Hereditary pyropoikilocytosis (HPP)	Severe spectrin mutation → extreme RBC fragmentation	RBC fragments, micro-spherocytes, ↓ EMA binding, ↑ thermal sensitivity
Membrane channel abnormalities	Overhydrated hereditary stomatocytosis	Altered membrane cation permeability: RHAG abnormalities	↑ MCV, ↓ MCHC, Stomatocytes, ↑ Osmotic fragility
	Cryohydrocytosis	SLC4A1 (Band 3) abnormalities	Similar to OHSt, cold-induced swelling
	Dehydrated hereditary stomatocytosis (DHSt)	RBC dehydration due to K+ efflux: PIEZO1, KCNN4 abnormalities	↑ MCHC, ↓ Osmotic fragility, Target cells, Splenomegaly
	Syndromic stomatocytic disorders	Stomatin-deficient cryohydrocytosis with mental retardation, seizures and hepatosplenomegaly; Phytosterolemia (Mediterranean stomatocytosis with macrothrombocytopenia); DHSt with perinatal edema and/or pseudohyperkalemia	
Enzyme deficiencies	G6PD deficiency	↓ G6PD enzyme → ↓ NADPH → oxidative stress	Bite cells, Heinz bodies, ↓G6PD levels (avoid testing during acute crisis)
	Pyruvate kinase (PK) deficiency	Impaired glycolysis → ↓ ATP → RBC rigidity	Echinocytes, ↑ 2,3-DPG, normal osmotic fragility, ↓ PK activity
	Other rare enzyme defects	Deficiencies in hexokinase, phosphoglycerate kinase, glucose-6-phosphate isomerase, etc.	Varies by enzyme deficiency

Continued

Continued

Category	Disorder	Pathophysiology	Key laboratory features
Hemoglobin disorders	Sickle cell disease (SCD)	HbS polymerization → RBC sickling → hemolysis and vaso-occlusion	Sickle cells, target cells, Hb electrophoresis: HbS predominant
	Thalassemias (α and β), other variant hemoglobins (E, D-Punjab, C, Lepore, etc.)	Defective globin synthesis → imbalance and RBC destruction	HPLC or Hb electrophoresis show abnormal fraction. Confirm by a 2nd technique
	Unstable hemoglobin variants	Mutations → unstable hemoglobin → precipitation and hemolysis	Heinz bodies, bite cells, heat/isopropanolol stability tests. Hb HPLC or electrophoresis may be normal or abnormal

(EMA: eosin-5′-maleimide; G6PD: glucose-6-phosphate dehydrogenase; HPLC: high performance cation-exchange chromatography; MCHC: mean corpuscular hemoglobin concentration; OHSt: overhydrated hereditary stomatocytosis; RBC: red blood cell; RHAG: Rh-associated glycoprotein)

TABLE 2: Classification and key laboratory features of the congenital dyserythropoietic anemias (CDA).

CDA type, gene	Protein function (inheritance)	Salient laboratory and morphological findings
Relatively more common forms of CDA		
CDA I *CDAN1* (most common), *C15orf41*	Codanin-1 (chromatin assembly), C15orf41 (DNA replication) (autosomal recessive)	• Macrocytic anemia • *Ineffective erythropoiesis:* Binuclear erythroblasts, chromatin bridges between erythroblasts • *Electron microscopy (EM):* Abnormal Swiss cheese heterochromatin • Elevated sTfR, EPO • Interferon-α responsive in some cases
CDA II (HEMPAS) *SEC23B*	Golgi trafficking (COP II vesicle formation) (autosomal recessive)	• Normocytic/mild macrocytic anemia • Double membrane-bound erythroblasts • Positive acidified serum lysis test (HEMPAS test) • *Increased band 3 glycosylation*: Low eosin-5′-maleimide fluorescence • *EM:* Endoplasmic reticulum (ER) dilation, vesicular changes
CDA III *KIF23* or *RACGAP1*	Kinesin family member (cytokinesis) (autosomal dominant *KIF23* or autosomal recessive *RACGAP1*)	• Mild anemia, macrocytosis • Gigantoblasts and multinucleated erythroblasts • Retinal abnormalities, monoclonal gammopathy in some cases

Continued

Continued

CDA type, gene	Protein function (inheritance)	Salient laboratory and morphological findings
CDA IV *KLF1*	Erythroid transcription factor (autosomal dominant)	• Mild-to-severe anemia • High HbF; increased bilirubin • Dysplastic erythropoiesis
Rarer forms of CDA		
XR-CDA (X-linked dyserythropoietic anemia with thrombocyto-penia) *GATA1*	Erythroid/megakaryocytic transcription factor (X-linked)	• Moderate anemia, thrombocytopenia • Dyserythropoiesis + thrombocytopenia • Low reticulocyte count • Platelet dysfunction
CDA with spasticity and cerebellar hypoplasia *C15orf41* (homozygous loss)	DNA replication factor (autosomal recessive)	• CDA I-like erythroid changes • Severe neurological features • Early onset developmental delay
Majeed syndrome *LPIN2*	Regulates lipid metabolism and inflammation via the NLRP3 inflammasome pathway (autosomal recessive)	• Chronic recurrent multifocal osteomyelitis; neutrophilic dermatosis • Mild-to-moderate anemia (dyserythropoietic changes on BM) • Elevated inflammatory markers (ESR, CRP)

(CRP: C-reactive protein; ESR: erythrocyte sedimentation rate; EPO: erythropoietin; sTfR: soluble transferrin receptor; HEMPAS: hereditary erythroblastic multinuclearity with positive acidified serum lysis test)

TABLE 3: Common helpful nonmolecular diagnostic features of inherited hemolytic anemias (HAs).

Feature	Comment
Positive family history	Suggests inherited nature and in some cases, the disorder [for e.g., hereditary spherocytosis is mostly autosomal dominant, glucose-6-phosphate dehydrogenase (G6PD) deficiency is X-linked recessive, most other enzymopathies are autosomal recessive]
Splenomegaly, gallstones, extramedullary hematopoiesis	Suggestive clinical/imaging features, especially if gallstones at a young age
Anemia	May range from virtually asymptomatic to being transfusion-dependent to sustain life. The well-compensated patients tend to have high reticulocyte counts and markedly hyperplastic erythropoiesis
Reticulocytosis	• An extremely useful, technically simple, and economical laboratory marker of hemolysis that provides an estimate of erythropoietic activity of the bone marrow. May however by affected by recent transfusions, parvoviral aplastic crisis, secondary folate deficiency, etc. • A normal range or inappropriately-low reticulocyte count (for the degree of anemia) is a feature of most thalassemias and the dyserythropoietic anemias

Continued

Continued

Feature	Comment
Polychromasia, circulating nucleated RBCs	Relatively nonspecific, often may not correlate with the reticulocyte count
Other specific peripheral smear abnormalities	Inexpensive and often very helpful in guiding investigations. Should be done as a first-line steps in all anemias. Skilled interpretation requires knowledge of the clinical background as well as awareness of pitfalls and sensitivity issues
Bone marrow abnormalities	Erythroid hyperplasia and increased iron stores are nonspecific. Bone marrow evaluation is typically not required in the work-up of inherited HAs, and patients with anemia and reticulocytosis are mostly diagnosed on peripheral blood investigations rather than marrow findings
Elevated lactate dehydrogenase	Lactate dehydrogenase (LDH) is an important oxido-reductive enzyme that catalyzes the reversible conversion of lactate to pyruvate with the reduction of NAD+ to NADH. Nonspecific for hemolysis. Levels increase due to increased erythropoietic activity as well as release of RBC cytosolic contents into plasma
Unconjugated/ indirect hyperbilirubinemia	Due to increased breakdown of heme in the reticuloendothelial system
Reduced haptoglobin	Haptoglobin binds free hemoglobin; especially low or undetectable in intravascular hemolysis
Hemoglobinemia and hemoglobinuria	Signify intravascular hemolysis, renal damage may occur
Increased urinary urobilinogen	Not frequently used in laboratory practice
Hemosiderinuria	Indicates chronic intravascular hemolysis (of at least 7–10 days duration)

Hence, traditional diagnostic approaches have been complex, focusing on step-wise algorithmic testing using multiple first-line and confirmatory tests, with molecular diagnosis being used only sparingly in specific situations. These approaches aimed to be economical by avoiding unnecessary testing but were time consuming.

MOLECULAR DIAGNOSTIC APPROACH TO THE INHERITED HEMOLYTIC ANEMIAS

Diagnosis of inherited HAs that lack typical clinical/peripheral blood presentations may be challenging as there is no single diagnostic test or even a small panel of simple tests. As a first step, focused clinical information including age/sex/transfusion history, duration of symptoms, and the clinical presentation are vital to selecting the optimal diagnostic strategy. Family history, including ethnicity also guides the laboratory workup. Physical examination findings should include features of anemia, the presence of jaundice, spleen and liver sizes, and any relevant dysmorphic features or any non-hematological manifestations.

Laboratory tests for HHAs were previously often done in two stages—an initial routine laboratory evaluation followed by specialized tests for confirmation of a diagnosis or exclusion of differential diagnoses. In recent years, carefully performed and accurately interpreted molecular genetic tests have acquired a level of sophistication sufficient for them to become confirmatory tests in many settings.

MOLECULAR PATHOPHYSIOLOGY OF INHERITED HEMOLYTIC ANEMIAS

Red Blood Cell Membranopathies

Genetic mutations causing hereditary erythrocyte membrane disorders occur in genes encoding integral transmembrane or cytoskeletal proteins of erythrocytes. The main consequences of these genetic alterations are decreased RBC deformability and a shortened red cell survival. Mutations in various genes are implicated, including those encoding:

- *Cytoskeletal proteins:* Spectrin (α and β subunits encoded by *SPTA1* and *SPTB*), ankyrin-1 (*ANK1*), protein 4.2 (*EPB42*), and protein 4.1 (*EPB41*): Mutations disrupt the structural organization of the RBC membrane.
- *Transmembrane proteins:* Band 3 (*SLC4A1*), Rh-associated glycoprotein (*RHAG*), glucose transporter 1 (*SLC2A1*), the mechanosensitive ion channel coded for by *PIEZO1*, and the Gardos channel (*KCNN4*): Mutations affect both structural integrity and transport functions of the RBC membrane.

Disease-wise, the mutations are:

- *Hereditary spherocytosis (HS):* Mutations in the genes of the ankyrin complex (*ANK1*, *SPTB*, and *SLC4A1*) weaken the vertical interaction between the cytoskeleton and the phospholipid bilayer, reducing erythrocyte elasticity and deformability.
    - *ANK1* mutations are a major cause of both dominant and recessive HS. Truncating mutations (nonsense, frameshift, and splice site) in *ANK1* are typically associated with HS. While most *ANK1* mutations are autosomal dominant, autosomal recessive, and *de novo* mutations also occur.
    - *SPTB* mutations account for 15–30% of HS cases and are usually dominant, with *de novo* mutations also described.
    - Mutations in *SLC4A1* (band 3) are responsible for 20–35% of HS mutations and are dominantly inherited. Notably, missense mutations in *SLC4A1* can also cause overhydrated stomatocytosis by converting band 3 into a cation channel.
    - *SPTA1* (<5%) and *EPB42* (<5%) mutations are less common in HS and are inherited recessively. Homozygous and compound heterozygous mutations in *SPTA1* can cause significant morbidity. Common polymorphic modifiers such as α-LeLY and α-LePRA alleles of *SPTA1* can influence the expression of HS. Compound heterozygosity involving these low-expression alleles and other *SPTA1* variants can lead to autosomal recessive HS or hereditary pyropoikilocytosis (HPP).

- *Hereditary elliptocytosis (HE) and HPP:* These are now considered part of a continuous spectrum with shared genetic etiologies, primarily involving mutations in *SPTA1*, *SPTB*, and *EPB41*:
  - HPP often results from homozygous or compound heterozygous mutations affecting the α-β heterodimer self-association site, leading to a weakened RBC membrane and more severe hemolytic anemia.

Red Blood Cell Channelopathies

- *Hereditary stomatocytosis (HSt):* This group of disorders is characterized by an inability to regulate RBC cation homeostasis.
  - *Dehydrated hereditary stomatocytosis (DHSt)/hereditary xerocytosis (HX):* Gain-of-function mutations in *PIEZO1* are a common cause. These mutations alter the kinetics of the PIEZO1 channel. Mutations in the Gardos channel gene *KCNN4* can also cause HX.
  - *Overhydrated hereditary stomatocytosis (OHSt):* Mutations in *RHAG*, encoding an ammonium/carbon dioxide channel, lead to increased intracellular water content. The *RHAG* mutation F65S has been reported in association with OHSt.
  - Mutations in *SLC4A1* that convert band 3 into a cation channel can also cause stomatocytosis. Stomatin-deficient cryohydrocytosis is associated with recessive mutations in *SLC2A1*, encoding the glucose transporter GLUT1, leading to sodium and potassium leakage.
  - Gardos channelopathy can be caused by *KCNN4* mutations.
  - *Familial pseudohyperkalemia:* Mutations in the *ABCB6* gene cause this condition.
- Sitosterolemia (or Mediterranean stomatocytosis with macrothrombocytopenia) is caused by mutations in the *ABCG5* or *ABCG8* genes that are responsible for transporting sterols, including plant sterols. These mutations lead to increased intestinal absorption and decreased biliary excretion of plant sterols, resulting in their accumulation in the blood and tissues.

Erythrocytic Enzymopathies

Table 4 gives an overview of the genetic and clinical features of the red cell enzyme deficiencies:

Challenges in ascribing genetic bases to RBC membranopathies and channelopathies are:

- *Variable expressivity and genetic heterogeneity:* The molecular genetics of erythrocyte membrane disorders highlight the difficulty in establishing a strict phenotype-genotype correlation.
- Different mutations in the same gene (allelic heterogeneity) or mutations in different genes (genetic heterogeneity) can lead to similar phenotypes, and conversely, different mutations in the same gene can result in variable clinical expressivity.
- *Oligogenic inheritance:* Studies using next-generation sequencing (NGS) have revealed that at least 3% of inherited diseases, including RBC membrane defects, are oligogenic, i.e., a coinheritance of multiple disease genotypes

TABLE 4: Genetic and clinical overview of the red cell enzymopathies.

Enzyme deficiency	Pathway	Gene	Chromo-some	Inheritance	Key features
Glucose-6-phosphate dehydrogenase (G6PD)	Hexose mo-nophosphate (HMP) shunt	*G6PD*	Xq28	X-linked recessive	Episodic hemolysis, triggered by infections, drugs (e.g., sulfa), fava beans; PBF: bite cells, Heinz bodies
Pyruvate kinase (PK)	Glycolysis	*PKLR*	1q21	Autosomal recessive	Chronic hemolytic anemia, jaundice, splenomegaly
Hexokinase (HK)	Glycolysis	*HK1*	10q22	Autosomal recessive	Mild-to-moderate hemolytic anemia; decreased ATP generation
Phosphofructo-kinase (PFK, Tarui disease)	Glycolysis	*PFKM*	12q13	Autosomal recessive	Exercise intolerance, hemolysis; myopathy with muscle cramps
Triosephosphate isomerase (TPI)	Glycolysis	*TPI1*	12p13	Autosomal recessive	Severe hemolytic anemia, develop-mental delay, often fatal in infancy
Aldolase A deficiency	Glycolysis	*ALDOA*	16q22	Autosomal recessive	Hemolytic anemia with myopathy
Glyceraldehyde-3-phosphate dehydrogenase (GAPDH)	Glycolysis	*GAPDH*	12p13	Autosomal recessive	Very rare; hemolytic anemia, neurologic findings
Phosphoglycerate kinase (PGK)	Glycolysis	*PGK1*	Xq13	X-linked recessive	Hemolytic anemia ± myopathy, mental retardation
Red cell enolase (ENO1)	Glycolysis	*ENO1*	1p36	Autosomal recessive	Very rare; hemolysis with neurologic symptoms
Lactate dehydro-genase A (LDHA)	Glycolysis	*LDHA*	11p15	Autosomal recessive	Exercise-induced hemolysis, myopathy
Glucose phosphate isomerase (GPI)	Glycolysis	*GPI*	19q13	Autosomal recessive	Moderate hemolytic anemia; neurologic involvement
Adenylate kinase (AK1)	Purine metabolism	*AK1*	9q34	Autosomal recessive	Hemolytic anemia, developmental delay
Pyrimidine 5′-nucleotidase (P5′N)	Nucleotide metabolism	*NT5C3A*	7p15	Autosomal recessive	Basophilic stippling; chronic hemolysis; accumulation of pyrimidine nucleotides

Continued

Continued

Enzyme deficiency	Pathway	Gene	Chromo-some	Inheritance	Key features
Glutathione synthetase deficiency	Glutathione metabolism	*GSS*	20q11	Autosomal recessive	Hemolysis, metabolic acidosis, neurologic signs
Glutamate-cysteine ligase (GCL)	Glutathione metabolism	*GCLC/ GCLM*	6p12/ 1p22	Autosomal recessive	Rare; hemolytic anemia, oxidative stress sensitivity
Glutathione reductase deficiency	Glutathione metabolism	*GSR*	8p21	Autosomal recessive	Hemolysis under oxidative stress
Glutathione peroxidase deficiency	Glutathione metabolism	*GPX1, GPX4*	3p21, 19p13	Variable	Rare; oxidative stress-induced hemolysis
Red cell adenosine deaminase (ADA)	Purine salvage pathway	*ADA*	20q13	Autosomal recessive	Combined immuno-deficiency + hemo-lysis in rare cases
Ribose-phosphate pyrophosphokinase (PRPP synthetase) overactivity	Nucleotide synthesis	*PRPS1*	Xq22	X-linked	Gout, uric acid overproduction, occasional hemolysis

contributes to the wide variability in disease manifestations. Complex interactions between low-expression alleles and other pathogenic variants also influence the phenotype.

DIAGNOSTIC IMPLICATIONS

Identifying the specific genetic mutation is crucial for accurate diagnosis. NGS technologies, particularly targeted NGS panels, have become essential tools for the molecular diagnosis of hereditary HAs, including membranopathies. These panels typically include genes encoding RBC membrane proteins and enzymes. The transition from single-gene Sanger sequencing to NGS has allowed for the simultaneous analysis of multiple genes and the identification of novel mutations. In cases where t-NGS is nondiagnostic, whole-exome sequencing (WES) or whole-genome sequencing (WGS) may be considered. Understanding the specific genetic mutation can also have implications for treatment decisions, such as whether splenectomy is appropriate or if specific therapies targeting the underlying defect are available or in development. Genetic counseling is also important for family members.

Molecular diagnostic tests broadly fall into two categories—those designed to detect (1) small nucleotide changes—such as point mutations, small insertions, and deletions—and (2) larger structural variations in DNA copy number, including deletions and duplications typically exceeding 1 kilobase in size. For identifying small sequence variants, sequencing methods such as Sanger sequencing and NGS are the techniques of choice. In contrast, large copy number alterations are more challenging to detect using conventional sequencing platforms. These are more effectively identified using targeted approaches such as gap-polymerase chain reaction (PCR) and multiplex ligation-dependent probe amplification (MLPA). Although NGS has the potential to detect copy number variations (CNVs), its current application in this context is limited due to high costs and the need for advanced bioinformatic analysis. As a result, its use for this purpose is largely confined to research settings at present.

Sanger sequencing is a well-established technique, particularly for germline disorders, including HHAs. Sanger sequencing may provide a cost-effective approach in a gene-by-gene investigation. As such, this technique is widely used for variant Hbs and nondeletional thalassemias, since a limited number of genes needs to be examined.

Sanger sequencing is most effective when the gene of interest is known in advance, and when a limited number of specific variants are suspected. This approach is time-consuming and cost-inefficient for conditions with high genetic heterogeneity, where multiple genes may be involved. In such scenarios, targeted NGS panels, WES, or WGS offer more comprehensive and efficient alternatives. These methods enable simultaneous analysis of multiple genes and are particularly valuable in diagnosing complex or genetically diverse conditions.

NGS has been in clinical use for over a decade, with its diagnostic value well-established across various genetic disorders. Depending on the breadth of genomic coverage and the number of genes analyzed, NGS can be categorized into targeted NGS (t-NGS), WES, and WGS. Each of these approaches offers distinct advantages and limitations, which should be considered when selecting the appropriate testing strategy **(Box 1)**. An example of a gene panel (in use at the authors' institution) is given in **Table 5**.

BOX 1: Molecular diagnostic approaches in hereditary hemolytic anemias (HHAs).

Single-gene testing:

- ARMS-PCR, PCR-RFLP, and reverse dot-blot PCRs for specific point mutations and very small indels
- Gap-PCR for larger deletions
- Sanger sequencing for detection of any mutation in a specific gene/region

Next-generation sequencing (NGS) panels:

- Targeted NGS panels for genes already known to be implicated in hemolytic or dyserythropoietic anemia
- *Advantages over traditional methods:* High-throughput, time and labor saving, cost per base sequenced is lower

Whole-exome sequencing (WES)/whole-genome sequencing (WGS):

- Applications in complex or undiagnosed cases undiagnosed by gene panel sequencing
- Detection of novel variants
- More voluminous data, complex analysis

Copy number variation (CNV) analysis: Gap-PCR, MLPA, and array CGH for detecting large deletions/duplications

RNA sequencing and functional genomics:

- Role of transcriptomics in diagnosing splicing mutations
- Functional validation using patient-derived models

(ARMS-PCR: amplification refractory mutation system-polymerase chain reaction; CGH: comparative genomic hybridization; MLPA: multiplex ligation-dependent probe amplification; RFLP: restriction fragment length polymorphism)

TABLE 5: An example of a comprehensive targeted next-generation sequencing (NGS) panel for inherited disorders of red cells and erythropoiesis. This panel also combines genes for familial erythrocytosis and the sideroblastic anemias for diagnostic efficiency.

Red cell membranopathies and channelopathies	*ANK1, SPTB, SPTA1, SLC4A1, EPB42, EPB41, GYPA, GYPC, RHAG, PIEZO1, KCNN4, SLC2A1, ABCB6, STOM, DMTN, ADD2, ABCG5, ABCG8, ABCG2, CD59*
Hemoglobinopathies	*HBA1, HBA2, HBB, HBD, HBG1, HBG2, SUPT5H, ATRX, NPRL3*
Enzymopathies	*G6PD, PKLR, GPI, PGK1, AK1, HK1, NT5C3A, TPI1, GSS, GCLC, PFKM, PFKL, ALDOA, ADA, MTRR, GPX1, GSR*
Congenital dyserythropoietic anemias	*CDAN1, C15orf41, SEC23B, KLF1, RACGAP1, GATA1, KIF23, VPS4A, MTR, LPIN2*
Sideroblastic anemias	*ALAS2, SLC25A38, YARS2, GLRX5, HSPA9, SF3B1, PUS1, TMPRSS6*
Unconjugated hyperbilirubinemia	*UGT1A1, OATP1, MRP2*
Familial erythrocytosis	*JAK2, EPOR, VHL, EGLN1 (PHD2), EPAS1 (HIF2A), EPO, SH2B3 (LNK), CALR, BPGM*
Others	*CYB5R3, HMOX1, PIGA*

PHENOTYPE MODIFIERS IN HEREDITARY HEMOLYTIC ANEMIAS

These include genetic and nongenetic factors. The clinical manifestations of HHAs can range from asymptomatic to life-threatening, influenced by both genetic and nongenetic factors.

Genetic Modifiers

- Low-expression genetic variants. They affect the high inter- and intrafamilial phenotypic variability of erythrocyte structural defects. They should be evaluated in suspected HS, HE or HPP, alongside other *SPTA1* variants. These common pathogenic modifiers such as α-LeLY and α-LePRA are found in >1% of the general population, and lead to low expression of the *SPTA1* gene. While α-LeLY is typically included in most t-NGS panels, the α-LePRA variant (c.4339-99C > T) falls outside the ±10 base pair intronic boundaries flanking exons that are routinely included. It may also be inadvertently excluded during bioinformatics filtering. Therefore, specific consideration should be given to its inclusion. The α-LePRA is often coinherited with the α-Bughill allele [a missense variant, p.(Ala970Asp)], which is reliably detected by standard t-NGS panels. This coinheritance allows indirect confirmation of α-LePRA using alternative molecular approaches.
- Gilbert syndrome. *UGT1A1* partial deficiency is common and causes disproportionate unconjugated hyperbilirubinemia.
- G6PD deficiency and α and β thalassemia trait. These are very commonly coinherited and can worsen the anemia in HHAs.

Nongenetic Modifiers

- Inherited or acquired modifiers of iron status may dramatically affect the phenotype in dehydrated hereditary stomatocytosis.
- Folic acid supplementation is important especially during infectious or surgical episodes to prevent secondary megaloblastosis.
- Confounding factors such as other hemolytic disorders (autoimmune hemolytic anemia, alloimmunization in patients receiving transfusions, and paroxysmal nocturnal hemoglobinuria), bone marrow, renal or hepatic diseases, including Parvovirus B19 infection, nutrient deficiencies or extra-hematological signs/symptoms may pose difficulties in the diagnosis of HHAs.

VARIANT INTERPRETATION AND REPORTING

- Classification of variants in inherited disorders is done using the American College of Medical Genetics and Genomics (ACMG) guidelines.
- Functional impact prediction tools such as polymorphism phenotyping (PolyPhen), sorting intolerant from tolerant (SIFT), combined annotation-dependent depletion (CADD), etc., can help predict variant impact *in silico*.
- Websites such as varsome.com and franklin.genoox.com apply several of the earlier mentioned predictive tools simultaneously, greatly helping variant classification.
- Integrating molecular findings with clinical and laboratory data is vital to overcoming challenges in interpretation of variants of uncertain significance (VUSs).

Some likely upcoming advances in molecular diagnostics of these disorders are listed in **Box 2**.

GENOTYPE-FIRST VERSUS PHENOTYPE-FIRST APPROACH

The "genotype-first" approach in genetic disorders refers to a strategy where molecular or genomic data (especially DNA sequence variants) are analyzed first, and only then correlated with clinical features (phenotype), as opposed to the traditional "phenotype-first" method where a clinical diagnosis is made initially and then genetic testing is used to confirm or refine it **(Table 6)**.

BOX 2: Recent advances in molecular diagnostics.

- *Third-generation sequencing (Oxford Nanopore and Pacific Biosciences)*: Long-read sequencing for structural variations
- *CRISPR-based diagnostic approaches*: Emerging role in variant detection
- *Multiomics approaches*: Integration of genomics, transcriptomics, proteomics, and metabolomics
- *Machine learning and AI in molecular hematology*:
  - AI-driven variant classification
  - Predictive modeling for phenotype-genotype correlations

TABLE 6: Genotype-first approach contrasted with a phenotype-first approach.

Feature	Phenotype-first	Genotype-first
Starting point	Clinical signs and symptoms	Genetic variant
Application	Traditional diagnostics, syndromic disorders	Gene discovery, variant interpretation
Strengths	Leverages deeper clinical insight, develops diagnostic skills without relying on tests that may not be easily available	Unbiased, detects atypical or subtle phenotypes, may save time
Limitations	May miss atypical cases or variable expressivity; usually more time-consuming	May overinterpret variants of uncertain significance (VUS); usually more expensive; requires skilled molecular genetic testing setup; reference genomes should represent the patient's ethnicity

Take Home Points

- Next-generation sequencing has revolutionized the diagnosis of HHAs, enabling the identification of pathogenic variants in both classical and atypical cases, often replacing complex multistep diagnostic workflows.
- Inherited membranopathies and channelopathies result from mutations in structural and transport proteins of the red cell, including *ANK1*, *SPTA1*, *SPTB*, *EPB42*, *SLC4A1*, *PIEZO1*, and *KCNN4*, with variable expressivity and phenotypic overlap.
- Erythrocytic enzymopathies such as G6PD, PK, and glucose phosphate isomerase (GPI) deficiencies have characteristic clinical and morphological features, but require molecular confirmation for definitive diagnosis and identification of rare variants.
- Congenital dyserythropoietic anemias are best diagnosed by targeted NGS panels, especially in settings with overlapping morphologic features and normal reticulocyte counts despite anemia.
- Molecular diagnostics guide critical management decisions, such as avoiding splenectomy in PIEZO1/KCNN4-related stomatocytosis and identifying candidates for mitapivat therapy in PK deficiency.
- Genetic heterogeneity and modifiers, including low-expression alleles (e.g., α-LeLY, α-LePRA in *SPTA1*), significantly influence disease severity and presentation, underscoring the importance of integrated interpretation.
- Copy number variations and complex inheritance (e.g., oligogenic inheritance) are increasingly recognized in HHAs and require complementary molecular techniques like MLPA or long-read sequencing.
- Standardized variant classification using ACMG criteria and integration of clinical, laboratory, and bioinformatic data are essential for the interpretation of VUSs and for enabling genetic counseling.

Case-related Multiple Choice Questions

Q1: Regarding molecular diagnostics in hereditary hemolytic anemias (HHAs), which of the following statements are TRUE?

A. Targeted NGS panels can detect both single nucleotide variants and large structural variations
B. Whole exome sequencing (WES) is useful when targeted NGS panels are nondiagnostic
C. MLPA is effective in identifying large deletions in genes like *HBA1*
D. Gap-PCR is suitable for detecting small nucleotide substitutions

Correct answers: B, C

Q2: Which of the following are correctly matched enzyme deficiencies and their associated features?

A. G6PD deficiency—Heinz bodies and bite cells
B. Pyruvate kinase deficiency—decreased ATP and echinocytosis
C. Triosephosphate isomerase deficiency—exercise-induced hemolysis without neurologic findings
D. Pyrimidine 5′-nucleotidase deficiency—basophilic stippling and chronic hemolysis

Correct answers: A, B, D

Q3: Which of the following genetic mutations are implicated in hereditary stomatocytosis or related channelopathies?

A. *PIEZO1*—dehydrated hereditary stomatocytosis (DHSt)
B. *SPTB*—overhydrated hereditary stomatocytosis
C. *KCNN4*—Gardos channelopathy
D. *RHAG*—overhydrated hereditary stomatocytosis

Correct answers: A, C, D

Q4: In congenital dyserythropoietic anemias (CDAs), which of the following associations are CORRECT?

A. CDA II (HEMPAS)—*SEC23B* mutations and decreased band 3 glycosylation
B. CDA I—*KLF1* mutations and interferon-α responsiveness
C. CDA III—*KIF23* mutations and retinal abnormalities
D. XR-CDA—*GATA1* mutation with thrombocytopenia

Correct answers: A, C, D

SUGGESTED READINGS

1. Agarwal AM, McMurty V, Clayton AL, Bolia A, Reading NS, Mani C, et al. Clinical utility of targeted next-generation sequencing panel in routine diagnosis of hereditary hemolytic anemia: A national reference laboratory experience. Eur J Haematol. 2023;110(6):688-95.
2. Agarwal AM, Rets AV. Molecular diagnosis of hereditary hemolytic anemias: Recent updates. Int J Lab Hematol. 2023;45 (Suppl 2):79-86.
3. Chueh HW, Shim YJ, Jung HL, Kim N, Hwang SM, Kim M, et al.; Red Blood Cell Disorder Working Party of the Korean Society of Hematology. Current status of molecular diagnosis of hereditary hemolytic anemia in Korea. J Korean Med Sci. 2024;39(18):e162.
4. Fermo E, Vercellati C, Bianchi P. Screening tools for hereditary hemolytic anemia: new concepts and strategies. Expert Rev Hematol. 2021;14(3):281-92.
5. Risinger M, Emberesh M, Kalfa TA. Rare hereditary hemolytic anemias: diagnostic approach and considerations in management. Hematol Oncol Clin North Am. 2019;33(3):373-92.
6. Jamwal M, Aggarwal A, Palodhi A, Sharma P, Bansal D, Trehan A, et al. Next-Generation Sequencing-Based Diagnosis of Unexplained Inherited Hemolytic Anemias Reveals Wide Genetic and Phenotypic Heterogeneity. J Mol Diagn. 2020;22(4):579-90.

CHAPTER 2

Recent Advances in the Prognostication of Chronic Lymphocytic Leukemia and Multiple Myeloma

Gurleen Oberoi, Renu Saxena

ABSTRACT

Recent advancements in the prognostication of chronic lymphocytic leukemia (CLL) and multiple myeloma (MM) have significantly improved risk stratification and patient management. These developments stem from enhanced molecular understanding and the discovery of novel biomarkers. For CLL, traditional staging systems have been complemented by new genetic markers, including IGHV mutational status and TP53 aberrations, guiding personalized treatment strategies. Minimal residual disease (MRD) and circulating tumor DNA (ctDNA) are emerging as crucial biomarkers for evaluating therapeutic efficacy. In MM, traditional staging methods such as the Durie-Salmon and the International Staging System (ISS) are being integrated with cytogenetic abnormalities to refine risk assessment. The Revised International Staging System (R-ISS) incorporates additional biomarkers and imaging techniques, while advancements in AI-driven models are paving the way for dynamic prognostication and personalized treatment approaches. Thus, by amalgamating traditional risk assessments with emerging biomarkers and genetic insights, we can stratify patients now more effectively, enhancing treatment outcomes, especially within high-risk populations.

INTRODUCTION

The prognostication of chronic lymphocytic leukemia (CLL) and multiple myeloma (MM) has witnessed significant advancements in recent years. Enhanced understanding of molecular pathogenesis, the discovery of novel biomarkers, and the integration of cutting-edge technologies have collectively refined risk stratification and patient management. This chapter delves into the latest developments in the prognostication of these two diseases, focusing on molecular and genetic markers, risk assessment tools, and the implications of these advancements for personalized treatment.

PROGNOSTICATION IN CHRONIC LYMPHOCYTIC LEUKEMIA

Chronic lymphocytic leukemia is known to have clinical heterogeneity and an unpredictable disease course. Recent years have seen significant advancements in understanding the molecular and genetic underpinnings of CLL, driven by breakthroughs in targeted therapies and novel prognostic markers. These developments emphasize personalized treatment strategies facilitated by robust prognostic tools.

The Rai staging (1975) and Binet staging systems (1981) have been the cornerstone of CLL prognostication. These clinical staging methods rely on physical examination and laboratory findings to categorize the patients into the stages of low, intermediate, and high-risk groups. While these systems remain clinically relevant, they do not account for the molecular heterogeneity of CLL. It has also been seen that the absolute survival estimates reported in the original publications are significantly shorter than expected survival with modern therapies. Before moving to advances, let us interpret the following case scenario.

CASE SCENARIO

A 55-year-old male patient presented with leukocytosis and persistent lymphocytosis. His laboratory results show a WBC count of 23,500/μL with lymphocytosis. Immunophenotyping is consistent with CLL [CD5+, CD19+, CD23+, CD200+ CD20+ (dim)], and his bone marrow biopsy shows hypercellularity with predominance of small lymphocytes. Fluorescence in situ hybridization (FISH) analysis revealed a 17p deletion in 20% of the cells. No deletions on chromosomes 11q, and no trisomy 12 detected.

His β2-microglobulin level is 2.8 mg/L, and his Binet stage is classified as A due to the presence of no significant symptoms and organomegaly. How will you prognosticate this case? For answering this, let us go through current and established prognostic markers.

ADVANCES IN PROGNOSTIC MARKERS

In current clinical practice, testing for *TP53* mutation, del(17p), IGHV mutation status, LDH, and beta-2 microglobulin are now routinely being done for prognostication. Prior to therapy and the start of each new line of treatment, all these tests are repeated. With more and more use of targeted therapies, testing of gene mutations in the B-cell receptor (BCR) and *BCL2* pathways is increasingly being considered. **Table 1** highlights all the prognostic factors used and studied.

Here are the changes in prognostication and shift in the relevance of existing markers in the era of targeted therapies.

IGHV Mutational Status

IGHV is usually evaluated with Sanger sequencing, and *IGHV* genes are considered mutated when a >2% difference in nucleotide sequence in comparison with germline DNA is found. It remains a cornerstone of CLL prognostication and

TABLE 1: Prognostic markers.

Category	Prognostic biomarkers
Serum markers	Thymidine kinase, beta2-microglobulin, lactic dehydrogenase, lymphocyte doubling time, autocrine interleukin-6, copper, free light chains, lipoprotein lipase, c-reaction protein, BAFF, TACI, APRIL, BCMA, EZH2
Immunophenotypic markers	CD38, ZAP70, CD49d, CD26, CD54, CD44, CD52, CD69, CD25, CD5, CD95, CD39, CD11c, CD36, and CD150
IGHV mutation status	Mutated and unmutated CLL
Chromosome aberrations	Del13q, del11q, tri12, del17p, del16q, del19p21, del10q23, total or partial trisomies of chromosomes 3, 8, 18, 19, and duplications in 2p24
Gene mutations	TP53, ATM, NOTCH1, BIRC3, MYD88, SF3B1, FBXWY, POT1, CHD2, RPS15, IKZF3, ZNF292, ZMYM3, ARID1A, PRPN11, COBLL1, LPL, ZAP70
Noncoding RNA and others	MiR-15a, miR-16-1, miR-155, miR-29a, miR-29b, miR-34a, miR-125a, miR-155, miR-181b, I-tRF-GlyCCC

also impacts the choice of therapy; thus, IGHV mutation testing is recommended in pretreatment evaluation of CLL/small lymphocytic lymphoma (SLL).

Patients with unmutated *IGHV* genes typically exhibit shorter lymphocyte doubling time and CD38 overexpression. They have a more aggressive disease and shorter time to treatment initiation than mutated CLL. However, in the era of targeted therapies, the prognostic impact of IGHV status is nuanced. Studies indicate that while unmutated IGHV correlates with inferior outcomes in chemoimmunotherapy, its relevance diminishes in patients treated with BTK inhibitors.

TP53 Aberrations

TP53 mutations and del(17p) are among the most adverse prognostic markers in CLL, predicting resistance to chemoimmunotherapy and poor survival outcomes. Recent guidelines recommend comprehensive testing for TP53 aberrations before initiating therapy with nonchemotherapy-based regimens as the preferred treatment strategy for affected patients.

Chronic Lymphocytic Leukemia International Prognostic Index (2018)

This international prognostic system is the one currently used widely in clinical practices. It combines genetic, biochemical, and clinical parameters and can enable a more targeted management of CLL. Five parameters mentioned in **Table 2** emerged as independent prognostic markers for overall survival (OS), which help in stratifying patients into four Chronic Lymphocytic Leukemia International Prognostic Index (CLL-IPI) categories as mentioned in **Table 3**.

Let us reassess the CLL-IPI in this era of targeted therapies (Langerbeins P et al. 2024).

TABLE 2: Prognostic markers for Chronic Lymphocytic Leukemia International Prognostic Index (CLL-IPI).

Parameters	Points
TP53 status (del17p, TP53 mutations, or both)	4 points
IGHV mutational status (unmutated)	2 points
Scrum beta 2 microglobulin (B2M) concentration (>3.5 mg/L)	2 points
Clinical stage (Binet B-C or Rai I-IV)	1 point
Age (<65 years vs. >65 years)	1 point

TABLE 3: Chronic Lymphocytic Leukemia International Prognostic Index (CLL-IPI) categories.

CLL-IPI category	Risk score	Treatment recommendations	5 years overall survival ($p < 0.001$)
Low risk	0–1	Do not treat	93%
Intermediate risk	2–3	Do not treat unless the disease is highly symptomatic	79%
High risk	4–6	Treat unless the patient is asymptomatic	63%
Very high risk	7–10	If the decision is made to treat, use novel agents or treatment in a clinical trial rather than chemotherapy	23%

While the CLL-IPI remains a valuable tool, its applicability in the context of targeted therapies is evolving. This study, published in 2024, highlighted the improved outcomes of targeted therapy over chemoimmunotherapy. The limitations found are as follows:

- Though CLL-IPI is found to retain its prognostic importance in predicting progression-free survival (PFS) on treatment with targeted therapy, reduced predictive power for OS in patients treated with BTK inhibitors or venetoclax-based regimens is found.
- Inability to account for dynamic changes in disease biology during therapy.

In the era of targeted therapies, its applicability can be improved by incorporating novel markers such as MRD status and circulating tumor DNA (ctDNA) into existing models and by developing therapy-specific prognostic tools to enhance clinical decision-making.

International Prognostic Score for Early-stage CLL (2020)

Chronic lymphocytic leukemia can have a very variable course. It can present in a very indolent form, with some patients remaining asymptomatic for years, while others progress more rapidly.

The International Prognostic Score for Early-Stage CLL (IPS-E), designed for asymptomatic, early-stage CLL patients, predicts the likelihood of requiring treatment within 5 years of diagnosis of early-stage CLL/SLL utilizing routine clinical and laboratory variables. This model uses three parameters:

1. Unmutated *IGHV* genes
2. Absolute lymphocyte count (≥15 × 10^9/L)
3. Elevated beta-2 microglobulin levels

It stratifies patients into low-, intermediate-, and high-risk groups and facilitates informed decisions regarding monitoring and treatment initiation.

Emerging Biomarkers (Still Under Research to be Included in Prognostication Models)

Minimal Residual Disease

Minimal residual disease has emerged as a pivotal biomarker for assessing treatment efficacy and predicting long-term outcomes. MRD negativity is associated with prolonged PFS and OS, particularly in patients receiving venetoclax-based regimens.

Genetic Markers

Studies have identified a few additional genetic abnormalities influencing CLL prognosis:

- *NOTCH1 mutations*: Associated with aggressive disease and increased risk of Richter transformation, *NOTCH1* mutations are associated with unmutated IGHV. ~4 to 13% of CLL/SLL patients can be associated with NOTCH1 mutation. NOTCH1 mutations are virtually mutually exclusive with *SF3B1* mutations. Poor response to anti-CD20 therapies can be predicted by assessing NOTCH1 mutation.
- *BIRC3 mutations*: BIRC3 negatively regulates apoptosis and plays a key role in the NF-κB pathway. Its mutation is indicative of shorter PFS and poor response to conventional treatments.
- *SF3B1 mutations*: It is found in 15–18% of CLL/SLL patients and is linked to adverse outcomes and resistance to certain therapies.

It is to be noted that above discussed mutations are not usually performed inCLL/SLL routinely, and the value of these mutations in prognostication is still controversial. Further studies and trials are needed to establish their importance.

BTK, PLCg2, and BCL2 Mutations

BTK is a key component of the BCR signaling pathway, which plays a critical role in CLL/SLL. PLCγ2 is another critical protein in the BCR pathway. BTK inhibitors, such as ibrutinib, are one of the main targeted therapies for CLL/SLL, and they work by blocking the BCR pathway. BCL2 is an antiapoptotic protein that helps CLL cells survive by inhibiting cell death. Venetoclax, an oral BCL2 inhibitor, is a newer targeted therapy used in CLL/SLL, and it is often combined with other agents such as rituximab. These mutations can lead to *resistance* to these targeted therapies, they are not routinely tested at diagnosis, as such mutations typically emerge during the course of treatment, especially after relapse or progression. These mutations may impact subsequent treatment choices, as patients with resistant mutations may need alternative therapies (e.g., acalabrutinib, which is less prone to the C481S mutation).

Cytogenetic Abnormalities

Fluorescence in situ hybridization identifies chromosomal abnormalities such as deletions in 13q (favorable prognosis) and 11q or 17p (poor prognosis). Complex karyotypes with major structural abnormalities predict poor response to chemoimmunotherapy when complex karyotypes.

Circulating Tumor DNA

The analysis of ctDNA offers a noninvasive method for monitoring tumor burden and detecting resistance mutations. This approach is particularly valuable in tracking clonal evolution during targeted therapy.

Epigenetic Markers and MicroRNAs

MicroRNAs (miRNAs) are small noncoding RNAs which regulates gene expression. Epigenetic alterations, such as DNA methylation and miRNAs (e.g., miR-155 and miR-29), have been implicated in disease progression and treatment resistance. These markers can complement genetic analyses and enhance risk stratification.

Impact of Targeted Therapies on Prognostication

The advent of targeted therapies has transformed CLL management, necessitating a re-evaluation of prognostic markers.

- *BTK inhibitors (ibrutinib and acalabrutinib)*: High-risk patients, such as those with TP53 aberrations, are now achieving improved outcomes with BTK inhibitors. But cases of IGHV status and del(17p) are less predictive in patients receiving these agents.
- *BCL-2 inhibitors (venetoclax)*: Venetoclax-based regimens, particularly when combined with obinutuzumab, achieve high rates of MRD negativity. Dynamic monitoring of MRD is essential to guide treatment duration and detect early relapses in such cases.
- *CD20 monoclonal antibodies*: The integration of obinutuzumab with targeted therapies enhances depth of response, particularly in MRD-negative cases.

The recommendations and prognostic relevance for genomic biomarkers in CLL patients treated with targeted therapies are shown in **Table 4**.

These recent updates, the evolving nature of disease biology and treatment responses, highlight the necessity for dynamic prognostication.

Coming back to our case, the overall prognosis is usually assessed using the CLL-IPI nowadays. So in this case, the patient's age of 55 years, β2-microglobulin level of <3.5 mg/L, and Binet stage (A) due to no significant symptoms/organomegaly are the favorable parameters and chromosomal abnormalities (17p deletion). But his unmutated IGHV status, combined with the presence of the *17p deletion*, places him in a high-risk category. The unmutated IGHV is associated with a more **(Fig. 1)** aggressive disease course, and the 17p deletion in particular is one of the most significant adverse prognostic factors in CLL, as it is often linked to poor treatment responses. The *17p deletion* further worsens his prognosis, indicating that his disease may be more resistant to chemotherapy and other therapies. Therefore, based on these factors, this patient would be classified into

TABLE 4: Genomic biomarkers in chronic lymphocytic leukemia (CLL) patients treated with targeted therapies.

Biomarker	Recommended by guidelines	Prognostic significance	
		BTKi ± anti-CD20 monoclonal antibodies	Venetoclax-based
IGHV unmutated status	Yes	Probable	Yes
del(17p)/*TP53* abnormalities	Yes	Yes (ibrutinib)	Yes
Gene mutations other than *TP53*	No	Uncertain	Uncertain
Complex karyotype	In clinical trials	Yes (ibrutinib)	Yes
Measurable residual disease	In clinical trials	Uncertain	Yes
Gene mutations for resistance	No	Uncertain	Uncertain

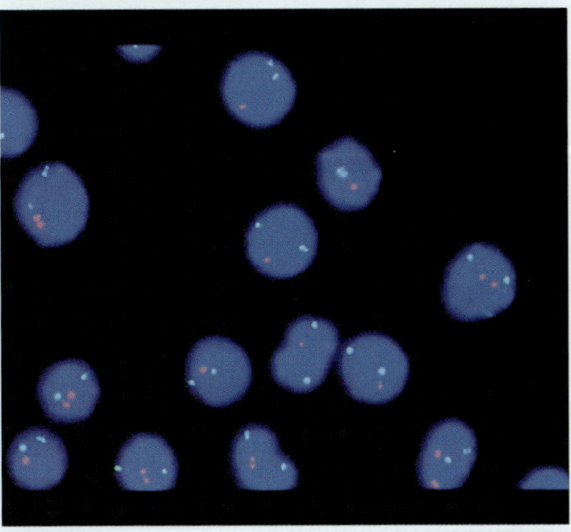

FIG. 1: Interphase nuclei showing one red and one green signal pattern using TP53/ATM dual color probe, indicating positive for *TP53* gene deletion in 20% of cells.

the *high-risk* group on the CLL-IPI, indicating a poorer OS and shorter time to treatment.

PROGNOSTICATION IN MULTIPLE MYELOMA

Multiple myeloma exhibits a highly variable disease course, with some patients experiencing rapid progression and organ dysfunction, while others have a more indolent form of the disease.

The prognosis of patients with MM is dependent on four factors:

1. *Disease staging*: This is done by staging systems that classify the myeloma patients into various risk categories and help in evaluating the disease severity. Staging systems such as the Durie-Salmon staging system (1975) and the International Staging System (ISS) (2005) have been a cornerstone;

however, they do not take into consideration the crucial genetic factors. Now Revised International Staging System (R-ISS) is being preferred.

2. *Patient characteristics*: This includes patient-related parameters such as age, general health, and underlying medical conditions that influence the overall prognosis and response to treatment. These factors can significantly impact how a patient tolerates treatment and their survival outcomes.
3. *Disease characteristics*: The underlying biological characteristics of the disease, including the presence of aggressive features such as plasmablastic morphology, high plasma cell turnover, increased circulating plasma cells, extramedullary disease, plasma cell immunophenotype, and specific genetic mutations. These factors can greatly affect the course of the disease and how it responds to therapy.
4. *Availability and response to therapy*: Access to the therapy and response is another key determinant of prognosis. With the advent of novel agents such as proteasome inhibitors (bortezomib), immunomodulatory drugs (lenalidomide), and monoclonal antibodies (daratumumab), significantly improved outcomes are being observed, but still, those with high-risk disease biology may respond less favorably to standard therapies.

Along with established parameters of prognosis, there has been a lot of new development in the prognostication of MM. With the routine inclusion of molecular testing along with the advent of numerous of new treatment modalities and targeted therapies, there has been a dynamic shift in prognostication. Let us understand prognostication and its advances through the following case.

CASE SCENARIO

A 59-year-old female presented to the clinic with complaints of persistent fatigue, weakness, and generalized malaise. She had been experiencing progressive pallor and backache for the past several months. On examination, the patient appeared pale with no organomegaly.

Investigations: CBC showed normocytic normochromic anemia with rouleaux formation.

Serum albumin was 3.3 g/dL, and serum beta-2 microglobulin (β2M) was 6.2 mg/L.

Serum protein electrophoresis (SPEP) showed an M band, found to be IgG kappa on immunofixation electrophoresis (IFE). Magnetic resonance imaging (MRI) of the spine reveals multiple lytic lesions in the lumbar and thoracic vertebrae. Bone marrow examination showed 45% clonal plasma cells. Following are the cytogenetic/FISH abnormalities:

- *CKS1B(1q21)*: 1q gain—positive in 96% of cells
- *Monosomy 13*: Positive in 97% of cells
- *IgH(14q32) gene rearrangement*: Positive in 92% of cells
- *FGFR3::IgH: t(4;14)*: Positive in 92% of cells
- She was negative for trisomies and del(17p), del(1p), t(11;14), t(14;16), t(14;20), and t(6;14).

In which category would you put her in the current risk stratification? To understand and answer this, let us go through the advances in prognostication.

■ ADVANCES IN PROGNOSTICATION OF MULTIPLE MYELOMA

Cytogenetic and Molecular Markers

Chromosomal Abnormalities

Fluorescent in situ hybridization is the preferred technique as it can detect specific chromosomal abnormalities at the molecular level. The most favored method for detecting cytogenetic abnormalities in MM is interphase FISH on bone marrow plasma cells. Two FISH techniques used are interphase FISH on purified plasma cells *and* light chain-restricted plasma cell cytoplasmic immunoglobulin-enhanced FISH. These techniques improve the sensitivity of detecting abnormalities in plasma cells and help distinguish them from other cell types in the marrow. ~25% of MM patients can have high-risk genetic abnormalities (mentioned in **Table 5**), and with standard therapy, these patients have a shortened median survival. These high-risk abnormalities are also included in (R-ISS). On the other hand, deletion 13 and hypodiploidy on

TABLE 5: Updated mSMART 3.0 (Mayo stratification for Myeloma and Risk Adapted Therapy 3.0) (2024).

Risk groups	Percentage of newly diagnosed patients with the abnormality
Standard risk	
• Trisomies • t(11;14) (most common) • t(6;14)	60%
High risk	
• *High-risk genetic abnormalities*: ○ t(4;14) ○ t(14:16) ○ t(14;20) ○ del(17p) ○ gain(1q) ○ del(1p) ○ *Double-hit myeloma*: Any 2 ○ High-risk factors ○ *Triple-hit myeloma*: Any 3 or more high-risk factors • RISS stage 3 • High plasma cell S-phased • *GEP*: High-risk signature	40%

Note: The presence of concurrent trisomies may ameliorate the high-risk effect.

detection by conventional cytogenetic abnormalities are suggested to have an adverse prognosis; however, they are not considered independent predictors when detected by FISH. Trisomies of odd-numbered chromosomes lead to hyperdiploidy, which is widely accepted to have a favorable outcome.

Chromosome 1 abnormalities: These are shown to have shorter survival. Most common abnormalities are 1q gain (gain of 3 copies), 1q amplification (addition of 4 or more copies), and 1p deletion, and 1q21 aberrations are associated with poor prognosis and progression. *The second revision of the* ISS *(R2-*ISS*)* has incorporated 1q gain/amplification.

Gene Expression Profiling

Gene expression profiling (GEP) studies have identified high-risk gene signatures, such as the proliferation index, which predicts aggressive disease.

Mutational Landscape

On the basis of the coordinates of the translocation breakpoints in the *NSD2* gene, subsets of MM with t(4;14) are identified, which can be detected by next-generation sequencing (NGS). In studies, it has been shown that these subsets, which differed by breakpoint location, have different median OS and were divided into late disruption, no disruption, and early disruption. NGS has revealed recurrent mutations in genes such as *KRAS*, *NRAS*, *BRAF*, and *TP53*, which influence disease progression and treatment resistance. Identification of clonal evolution and detection of MRD is now enabled by NGS.

Revised International Staging System (Palumbo et al. 2015)

The R-ISS is currently the favored staging system for MM, replacing the earlier used systems, including Durie-Salmon, the International Staging System (ISS), and the International Myeloma Working Group (IMWG)-2014 staging system. The R-ISS combines the ISS with cytogenetic abnormalities and lactate dehydrogenase (LDH) levels to provide a more comprehensive risk stratification tool. Patients are classified into three stages **(Table 6)** with significantly different OS and PFS in 5 years.

TABLE 6: Stages of R-ISS for myeloma.

Stages	Criteria
I	• Serum albumin ≥3.5 g/dL • Serum beta-2-microglobulin <3.5 mg/L • No high-risk cytogenetics, standard-risk cytogenetics • Normal serum lactate dehydrogenase level
II	*Intermediate features*: Not fitting stage I or III
III	*Both of the following*: • Serum beta-2-microglobulin >5.5 mg/L • High-risk cytogenetics [t(4;14), t(14;16), or del(17p)] or elevated serum lactate dehydrogenase level

The second revision of the ISS *(R2-ISS) (2022)* incorporates 1q gain/amplification to provide better risk stratification of patients with intermediate-risk disease. Unlike the R-ISS, t(14;16) is not included in the R2-ISS.

Role of Advanced Imaging

Modern imaging modalities, including positron emission tomography (PET)-computed tomography (CT) and MRI, have enhanced the detection of skeletal and extramedullary disease, improving risk assessment. Advances in PET imaging have allowed for more sensitive detection of MRD, which is a critical predictor of relapse in MM. PET-CT can detect low-level disease that would not be visible with conventional imaging, thus enabling clinicians to stratify patients more accurately according to their risk of relapse. While 18F-FDG PET is the most commonly used tracer, recent studies have explored the use of immuno-PET and other tracers [e.g., 18F-fluorodeoxyuridine (18F-FUDR) or 11C-methionine PET] to target myeloma-specific markers. These radiotracers may offer enhanced sensitivity in detecting minimal disease, especially in cases of extramedullary or early-stage disease. Patients with *higher* maximum standardized uptake value (SUVmax) in their PET-CT scans tend to have more aggressive disease and poorer response to therapy.

Emerging Biomarkers

The following are being researched to be included in mainstream prognostication and risk stratification systems:

- *Minimal residual disease*: In MM, the detection of MRD has emerged as a crucial prognostic factor in recent years. Studies have shown that achieving MRD-negative status after treatment is strongly associated with longer PFS and OS, offering a more precise measure of treatment success than traditional metrics such as complete response. Therefore, MRD monitoring is increasingly being integrated into clinical practice, offering a more personalized approach to patient care. MRD assessment is particularly valuable in identifying high-risk subgroups that may not achieve MRD negativity even after intensive therapy. For instance, patients with high-risk cytogenetic abnormalities [e.g., del(17p), t(4;14)] might remain MRD-positive despite initial responses to treatment, suggesting the need for more aggressive or novel treatment approaches. Recent studies have shown that patients who achieve sustained MRD-negative status after induction therapy can safely discontinue maintenance therapy without a high risk of relapse, offering a potential strategy for reducing treatment burden and side effects. As MRD testing becomes more routine, standardization of methodologies is crucial.
- *Immunophenotypic markers*: Markers such as CD28, CD56, CD38, CD138, and SLAMF7 are being investigated for their prognostic and therapeutic implications. *SLAMF7* targeting could lead to improved survival outcomes in patients with specific immune profiles. Some studies have suggested that *CD56-negative MM* cells are associated with *more aggressive disease, increased relapse risk*, and *reduced response to therapy.* Research is ongoing to better

understand the prognostic significance of these markers and their ability to predict responses to new therapies.

- *MiRNAs* (e.g., *miR-15a*) are being investigated for their role in MM progression and poor prognosis. Combining biomarkers offers a more comprehensive risk profile, enhancing personalized treatment. Biomarkers such as miRNAs and ctDNA may become standard tools for monitoring MRD, guiding clinical decisions about treatment intensification or de-escalation.
- *ctDNA*: ctDNA analysis provides a noninvasive method for monitoring tumor burden, detecting emerging resistance mutations, MRD, and disease relapse.

Impact of Novel Therapies

The introduction of proteasome inhibitors (e.g., bortezomib), immunomodulatory drugs (e.g., lenalidomide), and monoclonal antibodies (e.g., daratumumab) has redefined treatment paradigms. Prognostic models now incorporate the impact of these agents, as they have significantly improved outcomes even in high-risk patients.

After going through this part, let us prognosticate our case now.

Our patient had a high β2-microglobulin level (6.2 mg/L), low serum albumin (3.3 g/dL), and high-risk cytogenetic abnormalities, including monosomy 13, 1q21 gain, and t(4;14) **(Figs. 2A to C)**. Based on the findings, this 59-year-old female with MM is classified into the high-risk group according to the R-ISS.

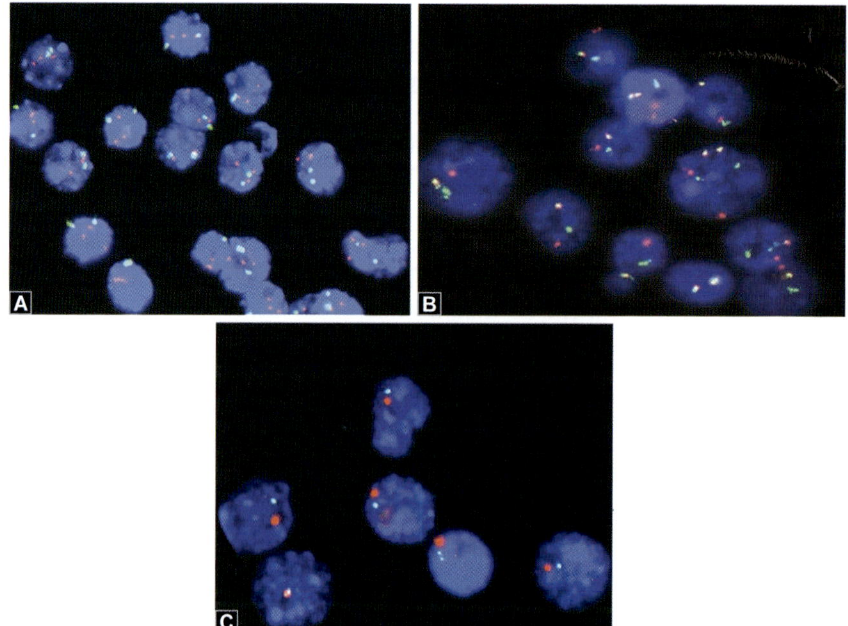

FIGS. 2A TO C: (A) Interphase nuclei using 1p/1q locus-specific identifier (LSI) probe indicating positive for 1q gain; (B) Interphase nuclei showing one fusion (yellow), one red one green signal pattern using t(4;14) *FGFR3::IGH* DF probe indicating positive for t(4;14); (C) Interphase nuclei showing one red and one absent signal pattern using LSI probe indicating positive monosomy 13.

These factors indicate a higher tumor burden, aggressive disease, and poor prognosis. The combination of these markers suggests a shorter OS and poor treatment response, necessitating aggressive therapy, including combination chemotherapy and possibly stem cell transplantation.

FUTURE DIRECTIONS FOR CHRONIC LYMPHOCYTIC LEUKEMIA AND MULTIPLE MYELOMA PROGNOSTICATION

- *Multi-omics integration*: Genomics, transcriptomics, proteomics, and metabolomics can be used in a combined way to provide a holistic view of disease biology, thus enabling more nuanced risk stratification and developing more precise prognostic models.
- *Dynamic risk stratification*: Continuous monitoring of disease markers to account for clonal evolution and treatment responses. These are dynamic in the sense that they incorporate treatment-induced changes, such as clonal evolution and MRD status, which are critical for maintaining prognostic accuracy over time.
- *Artificial intelligence (AI) and machine learning (ML)*: AI algorithms are being developed to analyze complex datasets, identify novel prognostic patterns, and predict treatment responses, thus holding the potential to revolutionize risk assessment in CLL and MM. *AI and ML* models leverage complex clinical, laboratory, and genetic data and identify hidden patterns for personalized predictions of MM progression, relapse, and minimal residual disease. *These models* offer an innovative approach to overcoming these challenges by analyzing large-scale, multidimensional datasets to predict disease progression more accurately and in real time.
- *Bayesian joint models for dynamic prognostication (2024)*: Bayesian joint models combine longitudinal data (e.g., repeated measurements of biomarkers and imaging findings) and time-to-event data (e.g., PFS and OS) within a unified framework. This approach allows for the simultaneous modeling of multiple outcomes and their interdependence, making it particularly useful for dynamic prognostication, where clinicians need to adjust predictions over time based on ongoing clinical and laboratory data. They integrate longitudinal data from multiple biomarkers and account for time-dependent changes, enhancing dynamic prognostication. These models are particularly useful for assessing disease progression and therapy response over time. Bayesian models enhance predictions for progression risk and survival, especially for patients undergoing multiple lines of therapy, as they allow for continuous updating of prognostic risk based on ongoing biomarker changes. Bayesian models are increasingly used in clinical settings to assess patient outcomes with high-risk MM and CLL, adjusting treatment based on biomarker trends.
- *Conditional survival analysis*: An important statistical method that adjusts survival at specific time points and allows clinicians to refine treatment plans based on the changing landscape of prognostic factors. High-risk

chromosomal abnormalities have less impact over time for patients who achieve remission. CS has become essential in refining prognosis, especially for patients undergoing autologous stem cell transplantation (ASCT) or novel therapies. CS models are now used to recalculate prognosis during remission phases, ensuring individualized management in long-term disease control.

- *Personalized medicine*: Now, leveraging prognostic insights to tailor therapy for individual patients based on individual risk profiles and molecular characteristics is the way to go.

Take Home Points

- Prognostication in CLL and MM has advanced significantly, driven by molecular discoveries and technological innovations.
- The integration of genetic, epigenetic, and clinical markers into comprehensive risk stratification tools has improved patient outcomes and enabled personalized treatment approaches.
- Future directions involve multi-omics integration and AI models to further refine prognostic accuracy and individualize patient care.
- Ongoing research and the development of novel biomarkers hold the promise of further refining prognostic models, ultimately enhancing the care of patients with these complex hematologic malignancies such as the R-ISS for MM prioritizes a comprehensive understanding of disease characteristics for better outcomes.

SUGGESTED READINGS

1. Urso A, Martino EA, Cuneo A, Gentile M, Rigolin GM. Chronic Lymphocytic Leukemia: Prognostic Factors in the Era of Novel Drugs. Cancers. 2024;16:2732.
2. Condoluci A, Terzi di Bergamo L, Langerbeins P, Hoechstetter MA, Herling CD, De Paoli L, et al. International prognostic score for asymptomatic early-stage chronic lymphocytic leukemia. Blood. 2020;135(21):1859-69.
3. Langerbeins P, Giza A, Robrecht S, Cramer P, von Tresckow J, Al-Sawaf O, et al. Reassessing the chronic lymphocytic leukemia International Prognostic Index in the era of targeted therapies. Blood. 2024;143(25):2588-98.
4. Hallek M, Cheson BD, Catovsky D, Caligaris-Cappio F, Dighiero G, Döhner H, et al. iwCLL guidelines for diagnosis, indications for treatment, response assessment, and supportive management of CLL. Blood. 2018;131(25):2745-60.
5. Mejia Saldarriaga M, Darwiche W, Jayabalan D, Monge J, Rosenbaum C, Pearse RN, et al. Advances in the molecular characterization of multiple myeloma and mechanism of therapeutic resistance. Front Oncol. 2022;12:1020011.
6. Guo P, Wang Y, He H, Chen D, Liu J, Qiang W, et al. Elevated serum levels of soluble B-cell maturation antigen as a prognostic biomarker for multiple myeloma. Clin Exp Immunol. 2024;217(3):221-32.
7. Kumar S, Rajkumar SV. Multiple myeloma: 2024 update on diagnosis, risk-stratification, and management. Blood Cancer J. 2024;12(4):41.

CHAPTER 3

WHO 2022 Update of the Classification of MDS and MPN: Practical Algorithms for Diagnosis

Richa Chauhan, Abhishek Purohit

ABSTRACT

The objective of this chapter is to highlight the changes in the latest WHO-HAEM5 classification of myelodysplastic neoplasm (MDS) and myeloproliferative neoplasms (MPNs). The current classification takes into account the "precursor" myeloid proliferations along with overt MDS and MPNs. Increased technical sensitivity and methological advancement has enabled inclusion of well-defined molecular myeloid neoplasms and omission of "provisional" categories. Though pan-India advances in molecular testing is already underway, the role of morphology can not be overlooked as the initial step in evaluation. Molecular findings go-hand-in-hand with morphology and red-flags or diagnostic features in tandem can guide to the correct diagnosis. Herein, we have attempted to concisely present the updates with real life case studies for the readers.

INTRODUCTION

Extensive information on genomics in myeloid neoplasms has revamped the World Health Organization (WHO) classification of hematolymphoid neoplasms. Decades after myelodysplastic syndromes, henceforth "neoplasm" (MDS) was recognized as a premalignant state for acute myeloid leukemia (AML), "*myeloid precursor lesions*" called *clonal hematopoiesis (CH)* were introduced in the latest edition to describe clonal outgrowth of the hematopoietic stem cells (HSCs) regardless of its cause. *Age-related clonal hematopoiesis (ARCH)* is CH in the aging population without quantification or defined gene alteration. *Clonal hematopoiesis of indeterminate potential (CHIP)* and *clonal cytopenia of undetermined significance (CCUS)* are shown in **Flowchart 1**. (1) These premalignant lesions for myeloid neoplasms are also associated with a higher risk of a range of nonhematological diseases such as atherosclerotic cardiovascular disorders and autoinflammatory states. Various environmental, immune,

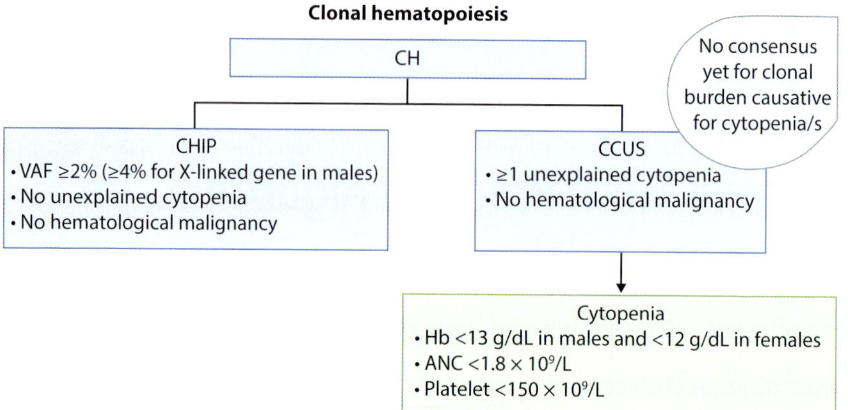

FLOWCHART 1: CH is seen in myeloid malignancy associated genes in healthy individuals. Any unexplained cytopenia in CH will qualify for CCUS.

(ANC: absolute neutrophil count; CCUS: clonal cytopenia of undetermined significance; CH: clonal hematopoiesis; CHIP: clonal hematopoiesis of indeterminate potential; Hb: Hemoglobin; VAF: variant allele frequency)

and ethnic factors contribute to the 10–40% prevalence of CHIP in the elderly. (2) These myeloid precursor lesions are enumerated in **Table 1**. This chapter discusses the changes in myeloid neoplasms in the fifth edition of the WHO and practical algorithms for diagnosis in the Indian setting.

CASE VIGNETTES

- *Case 1*: An 82-year-old male diagnosed with chronic immune thrombocytopenia (ITP) on and off thrombopoietin receptor (TPO-R) agonists, with a prior workup for bicytopenia nearly 10 years ago attributed the symptoms to romiplostim-induced marrow fibrosis (MF). Cytogenetics and fluorescence in situ hybridization (FISH) were negative till 7 years back. However, these investigations were not performed until now, when he presented with dyspnea on exertion, weight loss, pallor, and splenomegaly on examination and circulating blasts reported from a private laboratory. Hemoglobin (Hb) 98 g/L, total leucocyte count (TLC) 5.4 × 10^9/L, platelets 52 × 10^9/L, circulating blasts 7%, 5 nucleated red cells (nRBCs)/100 WBCs were found on hemogram. Bone marrow (BM) was hemodiluted, and BM biopsy showed diffuse MF grade 3 reticulin fibrosis with an interstitial increase in blasts (17%), increased myeloid-to-erythroid (M:E) ratio, and megaloblastic erythroid maturation. A diagnosis of *MDS with increased blasts and fibrosis (MDS-F)* was rendered based on cytogenetics and next-generation sequencing (NGS) report, revealing 46XY+8 and mutation in *TP53* with a variant allele frequency (VAF) of 47%.
- *Case 2*: A 35-year-old male was evaluated for fatigability and recurrent blood transfusions. His evaluation revealed pancytopenia, absolute neutrophil count (ANC) 350/µL, with a hypocellular (overall cellularity ~10%) bone marrow, and 15% erythroid dyspoiesis without increased blasts. Immunohistochemistry with CD34 and CD117 showed 03% blasts without abnormal localization.

Serum lactate dehydrogenase (LDH) was normal, and no paroxysmal nocturnal hemoglobinuria (PNH) clone was detected. His conventional karyotype was 46XY. A diagnosis of severe aplastic anemia was rendered, and he showed a response to immunosuppressive therapy after which an allogeneic stem cell transplant with his 10/10 match sibling was planned. Meanwhile, the NGS showed a *DDX41* pathogenic variant with a VAF of 54%. With a final diagnosis of hypoplastic MDS (hMDS), Sanger sequencing of the potential sibling donor for *DDX4*1 was suggested to evaluate the germline variant of *DDX41* gene and to avoid transplant from such a donor.

- *Case 3*: A 71-year-old female with suspected chronic myeloid leukemia (CML) based on moderate splenomegaly and hemogram showed Hb 89 g/L, TLC 65.94 × 10^9/L, platelets 45 × 10^9/L showed 01% blasts, 02% basophils, and myeloid bulge. Bone marrow was hypercellular with M:E 5.8:1, a prominent left shift in granulocytic series, 01% blasts, and no dysgranulopoiesis. There was significant dysmegakaryopoiesis. A provisional CML versus myelodysplastic/myeloproliferative neoplasm (MDS/MPN) diagnosis was kept, and a molecular workup was advised. *BCR::ABL1* and *JAK2* mutations were negative. NGS revealed *ASXL1* and *SF3B1* gene mutations. Finally diagnosed as atypical CML (now MDS/MPN with neutrophilia) and treated with hydroxyurea. She developed an undiagnosed fever during the COVID-19 lockdown and succumbed to her illness.
- *Case 4*: A 62-year-old female with constitutional symptoms, requirement of blood transfusions, massive splenomegaly, Hb 10.9 g/L, TLC 11.4 × 10^9/L, platelets 312 × 10^9/L was diagnosed as overt-primary myelofibrosis (Ph-negative MPN) in 2014 until polymerase chain reaction (PCR)-based MPN reflex testing for *JAK2p.V617F, CALR,* and *MPL* mutations was available in laboratory in 2016, that were all negative. She was stable on hydroxyurea, allopurinol, and aspirin till 2019 when she presented with worsening symptoms and a high TLC of 90.25 × 10^9/L. This time, NGS testing revealed deletion insertion mutation in exon 10 of *MPL,* c.1543_1544delinsAA (p.Trp515Lys), along with an *ASXL1* mutation.

WHO 2022 PRECURSOR MYELOID LESIONS AND CLASSIFICATION FOR MDS

Table 1 lists the WHO HAEM5 classification for myeloid precursor lesions and defines myelodysplastic neoplasms (MDS). **Table 2** shows the WHO-HAEM5 classification of MDS.

WHO 2022 MPN CLASSIFICATION

The main types of MPN are largely similar to the prior edition and are shown in **Table 3**. Initial diagnostic evaluation of MPN still depends on the close correlation between clinical features, molecular diagnostics, and usually morphologic evaluation of a trephine bone marrow biopsy. Most MPN patients are diagnosed in a chronic phase (CP), which may progress into a blast phase (BP) associated with accumulating secondary cytogenetic and/or molecular aberrations.

TABLE 1: Myeloid precursor lesions and myelodysplastic neoplasm.

Entity		Cytopenia	Dysplasia	Mutation/VAF	Gene specificity
CH and associated abnormalities	CH	No	No	≥2% (≥4% for X in males)	List of 54 gene alterations in WHO 2022, most are associated with myeloid malignancies
	ARCH (CH in the aging population)	No	No	No cut-off	No specific gene association
	CHIP	No	No	≥2% (≥4% for X in males)	Genes associated with myeloid malignancy
	CCUS (CH + cytopenia)	Yes*	No	≥2% (≥4% for X in males)	Driver genes associated with CH
ICUS		Yes* (persistent for 4 months)	No	No	No association with driver mutations
MDS	CH + cytopenia + dysplasia	≥1*, Cut-off of cytopenia may be waivered if definite dysplasia and molecular mutation are present. Thrombocytosis is permissible in MDS-5q	Yes, ≥1 lineage	Yes, either chromosomal aberrancy or myeloid gene pathogenic variation qualifying for CH	Genetic alterations at the chromosomal level or in the driver genes specific to MDS

*Cut-offs Hb <13 g/dL (male), <12 g/dL (female), ANC < 1.8×10^9/L, patelets < 150×10^9/L.

(ANC: absolute neutrophil count; CCUS: clonal cytopenia of undetermined significance; CH: clonal hematopoiesis; ICUS: idiopathic cytopenia of unknown significance; MDS: myelodysplastic syndromes)

TABLE 2: WHO 2022 classification of MDS.

Entity		Blasts	Cytogenetics	Molecular findings	2016 WHO category
MDS with a defining genetic abnormality					
MDS with low blasts and 5q deletion (MDS-5q)	Thrombocytosis is permissible	<5% in bone marrow (BM) and <2% in peripheral blood (PB)	5q deletion alone except 7/7q-	Any except multihit *TP53*; may harbor *SF3B1*	*MDS with 5q deletion*
MDS with low blasts and *SF3B1* mutation (MDS-SF3B1)	No thrombo-cytosis	<5% in BM and <2% in PB	5q-/-7/7q- / complex karyotype/AML-defining genetic abnormality should be excluded	• SF3B1 mutation (VAF ≥ 10%) and ring sideroblast (RS) ≥ 5% • If SF3B1 wild then ≥15% RS in BM for nomenclature of MDS-RS • Exclude multi-hit *TP53*, AML defining genetic abnormality and MDS/MPN (*JAK2, CALR,* and *MPL* mutations)	*MDS with single lineage dysplasia or multilineage dysplasia (SLD/MLD) with RS*
MDS with biallelic *TP53* inactivation (MDS-*biTP53*)		<20% in BM and PB	Usually complex	≥2 *TP53* mutations, or 1 mutation with evidence of copy-number loss or copy-neutral loss (LOH)	*Did not exist in 2016*
MDS, morphologically defined					
MDS with low blasts (MDS-LB)		<5% in BM and <2% in PB	Any	Any except multihit *TP53* or *SF3B1*	*MDS-SLD/MLD*
MDS, hypoplastic (hMDS)		<5% in BM and <2% in PB	Any	Any except multihit *TP53* or *SF3B1*	*The provisional entity in 2016*
MDS with increased blasts (MDS-IB)	MDS-IB1	5–9% in BM and 2–4% in PB	Any	Any except multihit *TP53* or *SF3B1*	*MDS-excess blasts-1*
	MDS-IB2	10–19% in BM and/or 5–19% in PB or Auer rods	Any	Any except multi-hit *TP53* or *SF3B1*	*MDS-excess blasts-1*
	MDS with fibrosis (MDS-F)	5–19% in BM and/or 2–19% in PB	Any	Any except multihit *TP53* or *SF3B1*	*Provisional entity*

TABLE 3: MPN classification of WHO HAEM5.

Entity	Diagnostic criteria		Requirement for diagnosis
Chronic neutrophilic leukemia (CNL)	• TLC > 25 × 10^9/L; neutrophils and band forms >80% of the WBCs • Neutrophil precursors <10%; rare blasts; monocytes < 10% of WBCs; no dysgranulopoiesis • Hypercellular BM; neutrophil granulocytes increased; blasts <5% • Diagnostic criteria for other myeloid neoplasms are not met • Presence of CSF3Rp.T618I or another CSF3R activating mutation or persistent neutrophilia (>3 months), splenomegaly, and no identifiable cause of reactive neutrophilia		All four criteria
Polycythemia vera (PV)	*Major criteria*[a]: • *High hemoglobin*: >16.5 g/dL in men and >16.0 g/dL in women; or high hematocrit of >49% in men and >48% in women • BM biopsy showing age-adjusted hypercellularity with panmyelosis, including prominent erythroid, granulocytic, and an increase in pleomorphic, mature megakaryocytes without atypia • Presence of JAK2V617F or JAK2 exon 12 mutation	*Minor criteria:* Subnormal serum erythropoietin level	Either all three major criteria or The first two major criteria plus the minor criterion
Essential thrombocythemia (ET)	*Major criteria:* • Platelet count > 450 × 10^9/L • BM biopsy showing proliferation mainly of the megakaryocytic lineage, with increased numbers of enlarged, mature megakaryocytes with hyperlobulated nuclei; no significant increase or left shift in neutrophil granulopoiesis or erythropoiesis; very rarely a minor (grade 1) increase in reticulin fibers	*Minor criteria:* Presence of clonal marker or exclusion of reactive thrombocytosis	Either all the major criteria or The first three major criteria plus a minor criterion

Continued

Continued

Entity	Diagnostic criteria		Requirement for diagnosis
	• Diagnostic criteria for other myeloid neoplasms are not met • *JAK2*, *CALR*, or *MPL* mutation		
Primary myelofibrosis (PMF)-early/prefibrotic stage (pre-PMF)	*Major criteria:* • BM biopsy showing megakaryocytic proliferation and atypia, BM fibrosis grade, increased age-adjusted BM cellularity, granulocytic proliferation, and (often) decreased erythropoiesis • *JAK2*, *CALR*, or *MPL* mutation or presence of another clonal marker or absence of reactive BM reticulin fibrosis • Diagnostic criteria for other myeloid neoplasms are not met	*Minor criteria:* • Anemia not attributed to a comorbid condition • Leukocytosis $>11 \times 10^9$/L • Palpable splenomegaly • Elevated lactate dehydrogenase level	All three major criteria and at least one minor criterion confirmed in two consecutive determinations
PMF, overt fibrotic stage	*Major criteria:* • BM biopsy showing megakaryocytic proliferation and atypia, accompanied by reticulin and/or collagen fibrosis grades 2 or 3 • *JAK2*, *CALR*, *MPL* mutation, or presence of another clonal marker or absence of reactive myelofibrosis • Diagnostic criteria for other myeloid neoplasms are not met	*Minor criteria:* • Anemia not attributed to a comorbid condition • Leukocytosis $>11 \times 10^9$/L • Palpable splenomegaly • Elevated lactate dehydrogenase level • Leukoerythroblastosis	
Chronic eosinophilic leukemia	*Essential criteria:*[b] Hypereosinophilia is defined as peripheral blood eosinophilia $> 1.5 \times 10^9$/L on at least two occasions over 4 weeks; not meeting diagnostic criteria for other myeloid or lymphoid neoplasms		

Continued

Continued

Entity	Diagnostic criteria		Requirement for diagnosis
Juvenile myelomonocytic leukemia (JMML)[c]	*Clinical, hematological, and laboratory criteria (all are required):* • Peripheral blood monocytosis > 1×10^9/L • Blasts and promonocytes are <20% in BM • Clinical evidence of organ infiltration, most commonly splenomegaly • No Ph chromosome or *BCR::ABL1* fusion • No *KMT2A* (*MLL*) gene rearrangement	*Genetic criteria (one criterion is required):* • Mutation in a component or a regulator of the canonical RAS pathway • Noncanonical clonal RAS pathway pathogenic variant or fusions causing activation of genes upstream of the RAS pathways	*Other criteria—if none of the genetic criteria are met, then at least two of the following (in addition to A):* • Increased HbF for age • Myeloid and erythroid precursors on peripheral smear • Thrombocytopenia with hypercellular marrow often shows decreased number of megakaryocytes • Hypersensitivity of myeloid progenitors to GM-CSF
Myeloproliferative neoplasm NOS (unclassifiable)	*All three of the following are required*: • Presence of any one of—(a) clinical and hematological features of MPN, (b) BM hypercellularity and megakaryocytic hyperplasia without dysplasia, and (c) clinical and morphological features can be discrepant • Not meeting criteria of any other MPN, MDS, MDS/MPN, or myeloid/lymphoid neoplasm with eosinophilia and tyrosine kinase gene fusions • Presence of driver mutations such as *JAK2*, *CALR*, or *MPL* mutations or other clonal marker	*Requires absence of both of the following*: • Insufficient clinical data or inadequate BM specimen for accurate evaluation and classification • Recent history of cytotoxic or growth factor therapy, particularly when dysplastic features are seen	

[a] Increased red blood cell (RBC) mass has been removed as a component of major criteria.

[b] Omission of "NOS" from name.

[c] Inclusion of JMML to MPN category.

WHAT CHANGES FOR HEMATOPATHOLOGISTS AND CLINICAL HEMATOLOGISTS?

- *New terminology*: Myelodysplastic neoplasms, now abbreviated as MDS, underscores their neoplastic nature, aligning with their myeloproliferative counterpart MPN.
- *The definition of cytopenias* is now consistent across CCUS, MDS, and MDS/MPN. These are Hb <12 g/dL in females, <13 g/dL in males, ANC <1.8 × 10^9/L for leucopenia, and platelets <150 × 10^9/L, wherein, persistence means >4 months. Also, MDS-NOS is now CCUS. Though the recommended threshold for dysplasia is set at 10% for all three lineages, as before, the number of cytopenia and total number of lineage dysplasia are eliminated. The terminology "low blast count" accounts for ≥1 lineage dysplasia and ≥1 cytopenia/s **(Table 2)**.
- *Emphasis on morphologic and genetic aberrancies*: MDS entities are now grouped as those with defining genetic abnormalities and those that are morphologically defined.
- *New entities:* MDS with *SF3B1* mutation [VAF ≥10% and ≥5% ring sideroblasts (RS)] is a logical entry as most cases with RS show this mutation, which also benefits most with luspatercept as per the COMMANDS trial. The scope of immunosuppressive therapy in hMDS and a subgroup harboring constitutional bone marrow failure cases make this entity unique. Aligning with the prognostic impact, MDS-f and MDSbi*TP53* show the highest blast burden and cytogenetic complexity. In *Case 1*, a monoallelic *TP53* of VAF 47% and MDS with fibrosis will not qualify for MDS*biTP53*. Nevertheless, such cases should be followed to know the significance of single mutations in MDS.
- *Dichotomy*: MDS with low blasts (MDS-LB) and MDS with increased blasts (MDS-IB) have been separated while retaining longstanding cutoffs.
- *Note* that before diagnosing MDS, MPN, or MDS/MPN, defining genetic abnormalities for AML should be excluded. For example, AML with NPM1 mutation, or AML with *RUNX1::RUNX1T1* fusion, can mimic MDS or MDS/MPN when the blast counts are <20%. A provisional morphological impression can be followed up with the final diagnosis once the molecular workup is at hand.
- Defining genetic anomalies for AML if present will trump the morphological impression of MDS, MDS/MPN, or MPN and low blast counts of <20%. Hence, AML PCR reflex testing or NGS results with a rapid turnover help in timely categorization and treatment.
- Vacoulation, E1 enzyme, X-linked, autoinflammatory somatic (VEXAS) is CH with an overlap of autoinflammatory and hematological features and can present as MDS or monoclonal gammopathies. Beck et al. have identified somatic mutations in X-linked UBA1 in genome-wide association studies (GWAS). These disorders have typical vacuolations in erythroid myeloid precursors, bone marrow failure, polychondritis, arthralgia, and thrombosis. So, while assessing bone marrows from elderly males, hematopathologists can document the presence of vacuolations in the absence of reactive causes such as alcoholism, lead, or copper toxicity.

- Mutations leading to complete or almost complete loss of function of the *TP53* gene impart a poor prognosis irrespective of blast count or categorization into MDS or AML. The ICC has thus encompassed all entities with ≥10% blasts and *TP53* mutation (≥10% VAF) as MDS/AML. However, WHO HAEM5 still considers AML with *TP53* only as an unfavorable risk category rather than a separate entity in AML. For MDS, only biallelic *TP53* mutation qualifies for separate MDS categorization. Two or more mutations of the *TP53* gene, complex cytogenetics, or VAF of ≥50% are surrogate markers for biallelic status when copy-number alterations are unavailable (*Case 1*). Patients with a history of cytotoxic therapy or radiation exposure and MDS-f will harbor most of the MDS*biTP53*, hence, checking for exposure history and assessing fibrosis during morphological examination is a good practice.
- Germline predisposition to myeloid neoplasms can present as hypoplastic bone marrow in adulthood. These include *DDX41*-associated myeloid neoplasms, Fanconi anemia, *GATA2* deficiency syndromes, etc. Although these entities can have hypercellular marrow with dysplastic changes in evolution to MDS, hypocellularity causes a dilemma with idiopathic aplastic anemia (*Case 2*). These patients have a significant risk of progression to acute leukemia compared to idiopathic SAA along with extrahematological malignancies. Choosing a matched sibling transplant donor may be difficult if the same likely pathogenic/pathogenic variant is found in the donors.
- The terminology of childhood MDS types is updated. The broad terminology is myelodysplastic neoplasms of childhood and has two subtypes—childhood MDS with low blasts (cMDS-LB) replaces the former term "refractory cytopenia of childhood (RCC)" and childhood MDS with increased blasts. Some cases of cMDS-LB arise from underlying inherited bone marrow failure syndromes such as Fanconi's anemia and dyskeratosis congenita or from genetic germline predisposition syndromes that harbor germline variation in *RUNX1, ETV6, GATA2, SAMD9*, or *SAMD9L* genes.
- The accelerated phase of CML has been removed in the TKI era wherein refined criteria for defining high-risk features are included instead.
- Juvenile myelomonocytic leukemia (JMML) has been placed into the MPN category for decades being included first in MDS and then MDS/MPN. WHO has taken account of blast equivalent promonocytes for blast cutoff and in addition to negativity for *BCR::ABL1, KMT2A* rearrangement should also be absent for essential criteria. Noncanonical clonal RAS pathway pathogenic variants, e.g., *RRAS, RRAS2*, or fusions causing activation of genes upstream of the RAS pathway, such as *ALK, PDGFRB*, and *ROS1* are included as one of the genetic criteria. These gene fusions are usually seen in older patients. Monosomy 7 is no longer required if the genetic criteria are not met. Instead in that case, ≥2 criteria including hypomegakaryocytic thrombocytopenia with or without dysplasia along with elevated HbF, circulating erythroid and myeloid precursors in peripheral blood, hypersensitivity to GM-CSF and STAT5 phosphorylation, are required to be met.
- Minor changes in the classification of classical Ph-negative MPNs include the removal of red cell mass from the major criterion for PV. There are no major

changes in the diagnosis of ET and PMF. However, it is important to distinguish prefibrotic PMF from ET, or PV, as it imparts a poorer prognosis.

- Minor modifications in nonclassical Ph-MPNs such as chronic eosinophilic leukemia (CEL) include the removal of increased blasts as an alternative to clonality, and hence, relaxing the blasts cut-off for inclusion under this poor prognostic entity. Also, the duration for defining the persistence of eosinophilia is reduced from 6 months to 4 weeks.
- Major changes in the MDS/MPN include the change in the terminology of atypical CML to MDS/MPN with neutrophilia (*Case 3* would be recategorized to MDS/MPN with neutrophilia in the post-COVID HAEM5 era). Notably, its molecular biology (*CSF3R* mutation) and disease course match CNL. In the future, we may find Ph-MPNs categorized according to genetic alterations such as those with *CSF3R*, and *JAK2V617F* mutations with the morphological entities as a spectrum of manifestations of those alterations.
- *Sensitive NGS techniques* with improved read depths have a higher pick-up of low mutational burden, especially in triple-negative MPNs (*Case 4*). Hence, NGS testing for myeloid panels including the *MPN* gene panel should be considered for cases where morphology is typical of MPN but *BCR::ABL1* or *JAK2/CALR/MPL* is negative. RNA fusion transcript analysis gives an added advantage of picking up atypical translocations of the *BCR* or *ABL* genes. Some cases may still require FISH with break-apart probes and translocation-specific PCR techniques for future monitoring of disease burden. Interestingly, fusion partner genes qualifying for myeloid/lymphoid neoplasms with tyrosine kinase fusion can be picked up in *BCR::ABL1* negative MPNs.
- The clinicians should not be tempted to rely on the molecular VAF versus blasts cut-off for treatment decisions because the first well-researched classifier is still a good morphological blast count rather than the VAF that may not be standardized across various platforms.
- Risk stratification is better with detailed molecular profiling in MPNs; thus, incorporation into the prognostic scoring models helps in the early identification of transplant candidates. The Mutation-Enhanced International Prognostic Scoring System for Transplant-Age patients (MIPSS-70) considers somatic mutations of high molecular risk (HMR) *ASXL1, SRSF2, EZH2, IDH1, IDH2, U2AF1* p.Q157 in risk scoring and assessment. Leukemic transformation is more common and additional mutations are more frequent in PMF than in ET or PV.

The approach to diagnosis of myeloid neoplasms in adults is charted in **Flowcharts 2A** (approach to diagnosis of MDS) **and B** (approach to diagnosis of MPN).

SUMMARY

A lot of changes based on molecular markers have been incorporated into the new classification of myeloid proliferations in the new WHO HEME5 book. Through this write-up, we have briefly covered the CH and associated lesions that form the base block for all malignant myeloid proliferations. Classification

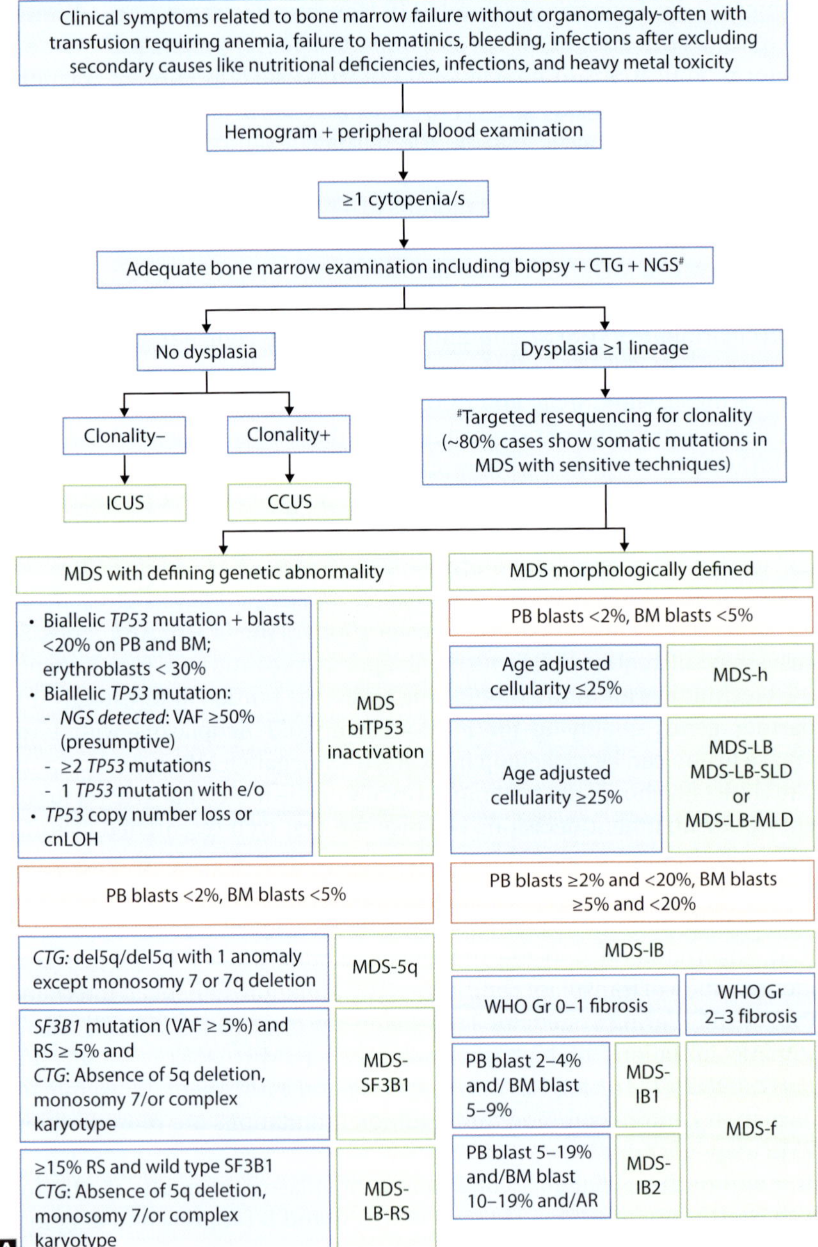

FLOWCHARTS 2A AND B: *Continued*

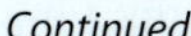

Continued

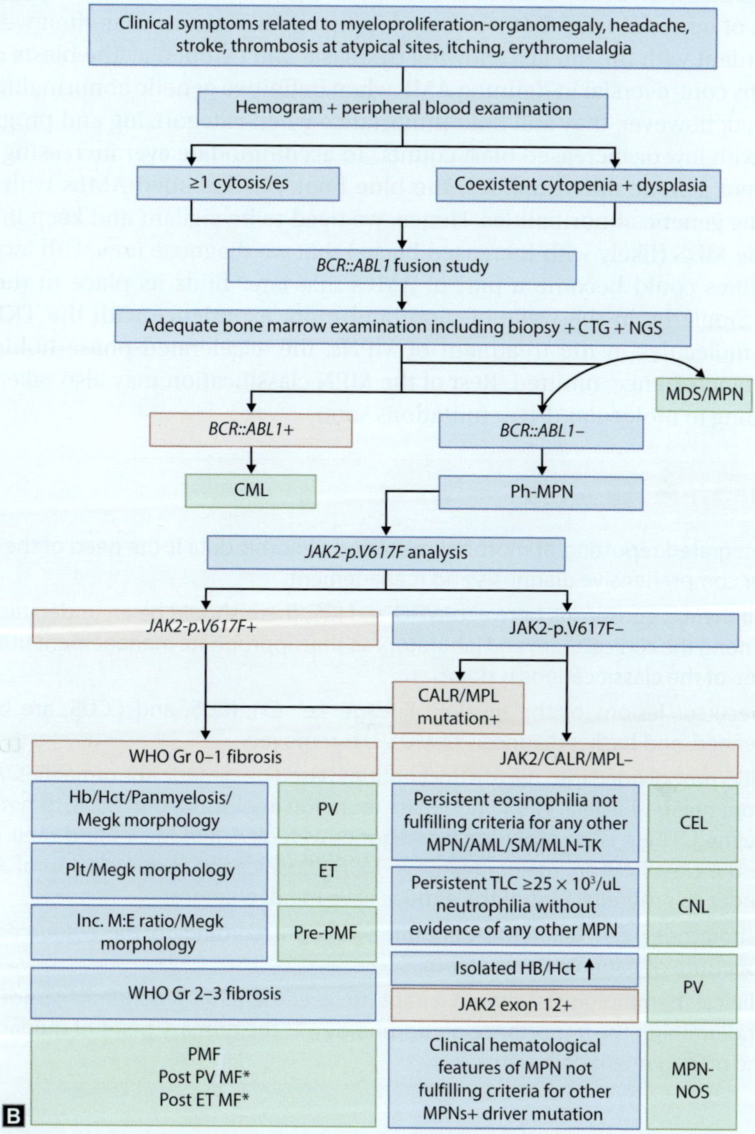

Clinical symptoms related to myeloproliferation-organomegaly, headache, stroke, thrombosis at atypical sites, itching, erythromelalgia

↓

Hemogram + peripheral blood examination

↓

≥1 cytosis/es | Coexistent cytopenia + dysplasia

↓

BCR::ABL1 fusion study

↓

Adequate bone marrow examination including biopsy + CTG + NGS

↓

MDS/MPN

BCR::ABL1+ → CML

BCR::ABL1– → Ph-MPN

↓

JAK2-p.V617F analysis

JAK2-p.V617F+ | JAK2-p.V617F–

CALR/MPL mutation+

WHO Gr 0–1 fibrosis

- Hb/Hct/Panmyelosis/Megk morphology → PV
- Plt/Megk morphology → ET
- Inc. M:E ratio/Megk morphology → Pre-PMF
- WHO Gr 2–3 fibrosis → PMF, Post PV MF*, Post ET MF*

JAK2/CALR/MPL–

- Persistent eosinophilia not fulfilling criteria for any other MPN/AML/SM/MLN-TK → CEL
- Persistent TLC ≥25 × 10^3/uL neutrophilia without evidence of any other MPN → CNL
- Isolated HB/Hct ↑ ; JAK2 exon 12+ → PV
- Clinical hematological features of MPN not fulfilling criteria for other MPNs+ driver mutation → MPN-NOS

B

*Post-ET MF: MF in a known case of ET; Post-PV MF: MF in a known case of PV.

#Targeted resequencing for clonality.

FLOWCHARTS 2A AND B: Cytopenia defined as Hb <12 g/dL in females, <13 g/dL in males, ANC <1.8 × 10^9/L for leucopenia, and platelets <150 × 10^9/L; cytosis defined as Hb >16.5 g/dL in men and >16.0 g/dL in women; or high hematocrit of >49% in men and >48% in women; TLC ≥10 × 10^9/L; platelets ≥450 × 10^9/L.

(CCUS: clonal cytopenia of undetermined significance; CEL: chronic eosinophilic leukemia; CNL: chronic neutrophilic leukemia; CTG: cytogenetics; ET: essential thrombocythemia; ICUS: idiopathic cytopenia of undetermined significance; MDS biTP53: MDS with biallelic TP53 inactivation; MDS: 5q MDS with 5q deletion; MDS: myelodysplastic neoplasm; MDS-f: MDS with fibrosis; MDS-h: MDS-hypoplastic; MDS-IB: MDS with increased blasts; MDS-LB-MLD: MDS with low blasts and multilineage dysplasia; MDS-LB-RS: MDS with low blasts and ring sideroblasts; MDS-LB-SLD: MDS with low blasts and single lineage dysplasia; MDS-SF3B1: MDS with SF3B1 mutation; MPN: myeloproliferative neoplasm; MPN-NOS: MPN-not otherwise specified; NGS: next-generation sequencing; PMF: primary myelofibrosis; Pre-PMF: prefibrotic primary myelofibrosis; PV: polycythemia vera)

of MDS into genetically defined and morphologically defined has simplified the jargon of terminologies that were used in the older versions that often were not concordant with the lineage showing dysplasia and cytopenia. The blasts cut off remains controversial in defining AML when definitive genetic abnormalities are detected; however, they still hold importance when categorizing and prognostic MDS with low or increased blast counts. To accommodate ever increasing list of recurrent genetic abnormalities, the blue book has included AMLs with other defining genetic abnormalities. Hence, we need to be vigilant and keep in mind that the MDS (likely with increased blasts) that we diagnose now with available modalities could become a part of AMLs that later finds its place in the blue book. Similarly, in the wake of more and more experience with the TKIs and small molecules in the treatment of MPNs, the accelerated phase holds little importance, hence, omitted. Rest of the MPN classification may also take shape according to molecular driver mutations soon.

Take Home Points

- Integrated reporting of morphological and genomic data is the need of the hour for comprehensive diagnosis and management.
- Till there is consensus between WHO and ICC, there should be an understanding among the clinical team and laboratory so that appropriate management utilizing one of the classifications is done.
- Precursor lesions of the myeloid lineage, i.e., CH, ICUS, and CCUS, are better defined, and basket diagnosis of MDS-U is removed.
- MDS now divided into two distinct entities based on genetic abnormalities. Apart from del5q-, biallelic TP53 and SF3B1 mutation are included in MDS, genetically defined. There is no provisional categories as h-MDS and MDS-f find their place in the classification. Major change in MPN classification is re-inclusion of JMML under its umbrella. Rest of the entities have minor changes.
- Laboratories can tailor the genomic workup according to the resources and spectrum of patients they cater to.
- Clinical hematologists should adapt to ever-increasing genomic jargon not undermining the importance of morphology as the primary point of guidance in the management of patients.

SUGGESTED READINGS

1. WHO Classification of Tumours Editorial Board. Haematolymphoid tumours. Lyon (France): International Agency for Research on Cancer; 2024. WHO Classification of Tumours Series, 5th edition. vol. 11.
2. Singh J, Li N, Ashrafi E, Phuong Thao LT, Curtis D, Wood EM, et al. Clonal Hematopoiesis of indeterminate potential as a prognostic factor: A systematic review and meta-analysis. Blood Adv. 2024;8(14):3771-84.
3. Platzbecker U, Della Porta MG, Santini V, Zeidan AM, Komrokji RS, Shortt J, et al. Efficacy and safety of luspatercept versus epoetin alfa in erythropoiesis-stimulating agent-naive, transfusion-dependent, lower-risk myelodysplastic syndromes (COMMANDS): interim analysis of a phase 3, open-label, randomised controlled trial. Lancet. 2023;402(10399): 373-85.

4. Beck DB, Bodian DL, Shah V, Mirshahi UL, Kim J, Ding Y, et al. Estimated Prevalence and Clinical Manifestations of UBA1 Variants Associated with VEXAS Syndrome in a Clinical Population. JAMA. 2023;329(4):318-24.
5. Molteni E, Bono E, Gallì A, Elena C, Ferrari J, Fiorelli N, et al. Prevalence and clinical expression of germ line predisposition to myeloid neoplasms in adults with marrow hypocellularity. Blood. 2023;142(7):643-57.
6. Kiladjian J-J. The spectrum of JAK2-positive myeloproliferative neoplasms. Hematology Am Soc Hematol Educ Program. 2012;2012(1):561-6.

CHAPTER 4

Critical Appraisal of WHO and ICC Classification of Acute Myeloid Leukemia

Rama Hariharan, Sujata Raychaudhuri, Tathagata Chatterjee

ABSTRACT

Myeloid neoplasms have undergone significant advancements in molecular pathology and genetics, along with clinicopathological and immunophenotypic characteristics since the introduction of the 4th World Health Organization (WHO) edition in 2008 and its revised edition in 2016.

Improvements in diagnostic modalities such as cytogenetics, next-generation sequencing (NGS), and fluorescent in situ hybridization (FISH) helped unravel several genetic and molecular pathologies forming the basis of the classification of acute myeloid leukemia (AML). Two parallel classification systems emerged in 2022. WHO 5th edition, WHO-HAEM5 (2022) and International Consensus Classification 2022 (ICC 2022). Both systems focus on definitions based on genetics, thereby incorporating changes in the form of inclusion of some newer entities with a refinement of existing diagnostic criteria and recommended ancillary techniques guiding the diagnosis and addressing how the diagnosis can be applied in routine clinical practice. The aim of this chapter is to compare the two classification systems and to highlight and critique their impact on clinical practice.

INTRODUCTION

Acute myeloid leukemia (AML) is a group of genetically distinct disorders that are heterogeneous and is one of the most aggressive hematologic malignancies with an abysmal prognosis and a median survival of <1 year in patients in the intermediate and high-risk groups. The revisions of WHO classifications in 2001, 2008, and the revised edition in 2016 at different points in time have been done considering the results of numerous published research articles and studies with an understanding of ever-evolving disease biology, and these served as international standards. The revised classification of hematolymphoid malignancies published by the WHO in 2022 (WHO-HAEM5) was based on newer research results to refine diagnostic criteria, upgrade previously defined provisional entities, and identify and include newer entities. The International Agency for Research in Cancer (IARC) separated from the clinical advisory committees (CAC) members in WHO 2022, and this eventually led to another classification proposal for hematolymphoid neoplasms in the same year, the ICC 2022.

What is known?

WHO 2022: SUMMARY OF MAJOR CHANGES

Compared to the previous classification, WHO-HAEM 5 has incorporated genetic abnormalities as a criterion, leading to the evolution of two subtypes in AML, namely AML with defining genetic abnormalities (DGA) and AML defined by differentiation. The category of AML with recurrent genetic abnormalities has been replaced by AML with DGA to emphasize the role of genetics. The blast cut-off of 20% is eliminated in AML with DGA based on molecular inputs due to the fact that any of these entities can progress to overt AML eventually . However, in a few subtypes, the 20% blast cut-off is still retained despite the molecular inputs: (i) *AML with BCR::ABL1* to differentiate it from chronic myeloid leukemia in blast phase (CML) and (ii) *AML with CEBPA mutations*. Based on recent research, in ICC, it is concluded that CEBPA in-frame mutations affecting the basic leucine zipper region (bZIP) confer a favorable outcome, irrespective of biallelic or single allele mutation status. Hence, both monoallelic bZIP mutation, smbZIP-CEBPA (single mutations in the basic leucine zipper region) is included in WHO. However, the blast percentage of CEBPA is retained as there is a lack of current evidence to substantiate the reduction of the blast cutoff in this entity; (iii) *AML-MR (AML-myelodysplasia related)* replaces AML-MRC (myelodysplasia-related changes) of WHO-HAEM4 and is also genetically defined. The diagnostic criteria of AML-MRC were based on morphology and a blast cutoff of 20%. However, the WHO 2022 includes eight somatic mutations and updated cytogenetic criteria to characterize AML-MR with DGA. AML-MR also requires documentation of a prior myelodysplastic neoplasm-myelodysplastic syndrome (MDS) or MDS/myeloproliferative neoplasm (MPN) history. In WHO 2022, AML-MR can be subclassified as (a) AML with a prior documented history of MDS or MDS/MPN and (b) AML with at least a single genetic abnormality; (iv) *Another entity* that can be diagnosed irrespective of the blast count and defined by mutations includes *AML with NPM1*. Patients with NPM1-mutated myeloid malignancies with blast percent <20% have a poor prognosis, and they respond well to AML upfront therapy. The variant allele frequency (VAF) can be a prognostic factor. High NPM1 VAF is associated with shortened OS and EFS and has a high risk of noncomplete remission. Low VAF has a high likelihood of complete remission (CR). The significance of NPM1 VAF can also vary depending on the context of other mutations and clinical parameters. A combination of NPM1 plus IDH1 and IDH2 and DNMT3A has a worse prognosis. The prognostic effect of VAF NPM1 is adverse in patients who are treated with hematopoietic stem cell transplantation (HSCT) in first CR. Patients with a prior documented MDS or MDS/MPN with NPM1 show a rapid progression to AML.

Furthermore, AML with DGA where a gene has multiple partners are renamed as follows:

- AML with t(9;11)(p21.3;q23.3); *KMT2A-MLLT3* is now named as AML with *KMT2A* rearrangement.
- AML with inv(3)(q21.3q26.2) or t(3;3)(q21.3;q26.2); *GATA2::MECOM* is known as AML with *MECOM* rearrangement.
- Addition of AML with *NUP98* rearrangement.

In the entity AML with KMT2A rearrangement, there are more than 80 KMT2A fusion partners, of which a few such as MLLT3, AFDN, ELL, and MLLT10 are the most relevant clinically. The identification of the fusion partner would help yield prognostic information and guide disease monitoring.

Some newly added/emerging entities:

- *RUNX1T3(CBFA2T3)::GLIS2*: Rare type of pediatric AML with dismal prognosis. Non-Down syndrome AMKL (non-DS AMLL) expresses a unique RAM phenotype. It is seen in infants and children <5 years of age and comprises 30% non-DS AML in the pediatric population. Cryptic inversion of Chr16 joins GLIS2. Fusion transcript upregulates BMP2 and GATA3, which are downstream targets of Hedgehog signaling and JAKSTAT pathway.
- *KAT6A::CREBBP*: Cryptic insertion in t(8;16). Seen in congenital AML with spontaneous remission
- *FUS::ERG*: Oncofusion protein t(16;21)(p11;q22) high risk adult AML
- *MNX1::ETV6*: Seen in infant AMKL t(7;12)
- *NPM1::MLF*: Nucleophosmin as a molecular chaperone seen in 30% of adult de novo AML with NPM1 mutation. There is NPM1-MLF1 high frequency of FLT-3 ITD involvement with shortened OS and EFS. AML with distinct clinical and prognostic behavior.

The above emerging entities with rare genetic abnormalities in AML do not require 20% blasts, as there is no evidence in the literature to support the percentage of blasts.

A distinct provisional entity of AML with *RUNX1* of WHO-HAEM 4 is excluded in WHO-HAEM5, while ICC 2022 has incorporated it into AML-MR. RUNX1 lacks specificity and has limited clinical significance. It is a transcription factor and has a key role in early differentiation and hematopoiesis and is seen in 6–15% AML cases but is not an independent prognostic factor for survival and does not significantly impact clinical outcome.

Acute myeloid leukemia patients with DGA have clinical implications similar to those with 20% blasts and hence is independent of the blast cutoff of 20%. The previous entity AML-NOS (not otherwise specified) has been replaced by AML with differentiation and included in AML-MR. The cutoff of >20% blasts applies to AML defined by differentiation, where the diagnosis relies on morphologic criteria enabling the categorization by blasts cut off due to lack of recognizable genetic abnormalities and to differentiate it from MDS (renamed as myelodysplastic neoplasms, MDN).

Pure erythroid leukemia (PEL) has been replaced by acute erythroid leukemia (AEL) to maintain similarity in classification and is included in the category of AML defined by differentiation. AEL is a distinct type of AML, characterized by

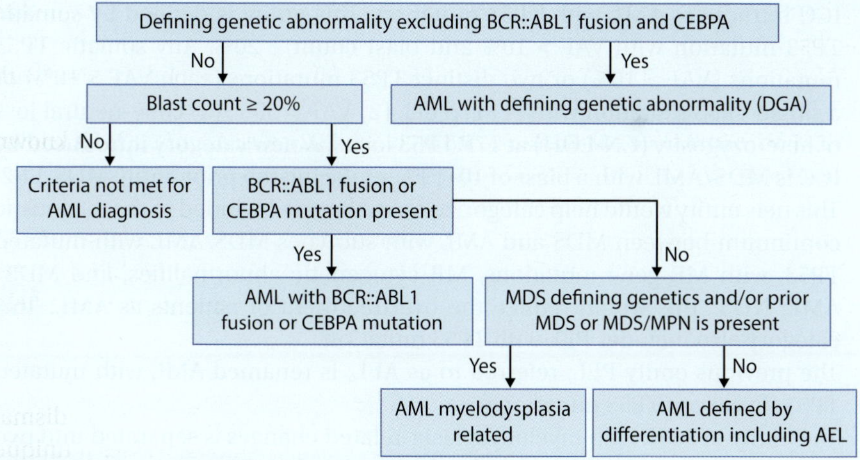

FLOWCHART 1: WHO 2022 AML classification algorithm.

(AEL: acute erythroid leukemia; AML: acute myeloid leukemia; MDS: myelodysplastic syndrome; MPN: myeloproliferative neoplasm)

the arrest of maturation of erythroid cells and neoplastic proliferation of erythroid cells and their precursors along with the presence of biallelic *TP53* alterations. Diagnostic criteria include erythroid predominance, usually ≥80% of bone marrow elements, of which ≥30% are proerythroblasts (or pronormoblasts), the same as WHO-HAEM4. The presence of *TP53* mutations portends aggressive disease and poor patient outcomes.

The basis of the changes in classification structure of WHO 2022 AML strictly lays emphasis on integrating clinical data, morphological parameters, and molecular/genetic abnormalities along with a sound clinicopathological approach. **Flowchart 1** summarizes the WHO 2022 AML classification.

INTERNATIONAL CONSENSUS CLASSIFICATION (ICC) 2022: SUMMARY OF CHANGES

In contrast, the ICC exhibits significant differences in the classification of AML. ICC requires >10% blasts or myeloid blasts in the bone marrow or peripheral blood.

A few prominent changes that have been implemented in ICC are:

- The 20% cutoff for blasts in various subtypes of AML with recurrent genetic abnormalities has been reduced to 10%. Exceptions to this include AML with *BCR::ABL1* which retains the 20% blast cutoff as in WHO 2022. However, many of the previous entities of AML with recurrent genetic abnormalities have been retained with more focus on the genetic basis of classification.
- AML with rearrangements of *MECOM* and *KMT2A* are divided based on their fusion partners as AML with *MLLT3::KMT2A* (or *GATA2::MECOM*) and AML with other *KMT2A* or *MECOM*-r rearrangements.
- Additional category of AML with other rare recurring translocations.
- Single mutation and biallelic CEBPA mutations are included in WHO 2022, while ICC accepts in-frame bZIP CEBPA mutations.

- ICC introduces AML with TP53 mutation. This entity is defined by somatic TP53 mutation with VAF > 10% and blast count ≥ 20%. Any somatic TP53 mutations (VAF > 10%) or two distinct TP53 mutations (each VAF > 10%) or a single TP53 mutation with (1) 17p del, (2) VAF > 50%, (3) copy-neutral loss of heterozygosity (CN-LOH) at 17P TP53 locus. A new category introduced by ICC is MDS/AML with a blast of 10–19%, replacing the prior entity MDS-EB2. This new entity would help categorize cases that are included in the diagnostic continuum between MDS and AML with subtypes MDS/AML with mutated TP53, with MR gene mutations, MR cytogenetic abnormalities, and MDS/AML, NOS. This would reduce the overtreatment of patients as AML. This category also includes PEL with TP53 mutation.
- The previous entity PEL, referred to as AEL, is renamed AML with mutated TP53 (in case of TP53 mutations).
- The entity of AML with myelodysplasia-related changes is separated into two categories: (i) AML with myelodysplasia-related (MR) gene mutations and (ii) AML with myelodysplasia-related cytogenetic abnormalities.
- RUNX1 mutations are no longer a separate entity but are included as myelodysplasia defining in the AML MR.

An algorithm summarizing the ICC 2022 is given in **Flowchart 2**.

A comparison of classification of AML by WHO 2022 and ICC 2022 is summarized in **Table 1**.

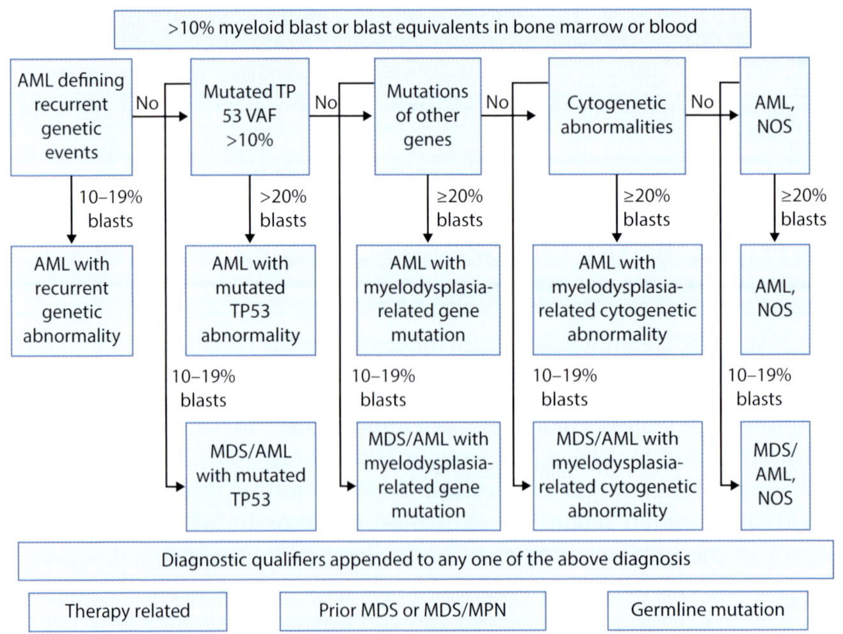

FLOWCHART 2: Algorithm summarizing the ICC 2022.

(AEL: acute erythroid leukemia; AML: acute myeloid leukemia; VAF: variant allele frequency; NOS: not otherwise specified)

Source: https://www.cap.org/member-resources/articles/whats-new-in-aml-classification-who-2022-vs-international-consensus-classification.

TABLE 1: Comparison of WHO 2022 versus ICC 2022.

2017	WHO 2022	ICC 2022
AML with recurrent genetic abnormalities	• AML with defining genetic abnormalities • AML with *RUNX1::RUNX1T1* fusion • AML with *CBFB::MYH11* fusion • Acute promyelocytic leukemia with *PML::RARA* fusion • AML with *KMT2A* rearrangement • AML with *DEK::NUP214* fusion AML with *MECOM* rearrangement • AML with *RBM15::MRTFA* fusion • AML with *BCR::ABL1* fusion* AML with *NUP98* rearrangement AML with other (rare) defined genetic alterations • AML with *NPM1* mutation • AML with *CEBPA* mutation	• AML with recurrent genetic abnormalities • AML with t(8;21)(q22;q22.1)/ *RUNX1::RUNX1T1* • AML with inv(16)(p13.1q22) or t(16;16)(p13.1;q22)/*CBFB::MYH11* • Acute promyelocytic leukemia (APL) with t(15;17)(q24.1;q21.2)/ *PML::RARA*; APL with other *RARA* rearrangements • AML with t(9;11)(p21.3;q23.3)/ *MLLT3::KMT2A*; AML with other *KMT2A* rearrangements • AML with t(6;9)(p22.3;q34.1)/ *DEK::NUP214* AML with inv(3) (q21.3q26.2) or t(3;3)(q21.3;q26.2)/ *GATA2::MECOM* (*EVI1*); AML with other *MECOM* rearrangements • AML with *BCR::ABL1* fusion* • AML with other rare recurring translocations • AML with mutated NPM1 • AML with in-frame bZIP CEBPA mutations AML with mutated TP53 (VAF >10%)
AML not otherwise specified	• AML, defined by differentiation • AML with minimal differentiation • AML without maturation • AML with maturation • Acute myelomonocytic leukemia • Acute monoblastic/monocytic leukemia • Acute erythroid leukemia • Acute megakaryoblastic leukemia • Acute basophilic leukemia	• AML not otherwise specified (NOS) • AML with minimal differentiation • AML without maturation • AML with maturation • Acute myelomonocytic leukemia • Acute monoblastic/monocytic leukemia • Pure erythroid leukemia† • Acute megakaryoblastic leukemia • Acute basophilic leukemia
Blast cutoffs	Blast cutoff eliminated in AML with defining genetic abnormalities (DGA), *except*: • AML with *BCR::ABL1* • AML with *CEBPA* and • AML with defined rare CEBPA and genetic alterations Blast count is ≥ 20% for subtypes without DGA	• ≥10% for all AML with defining recurrent genetic abnormalities (RGA) • ≥ 20% for subtypes without RGA and *TP53* mutated AML or mutations in other genes, cytogenetic abnormalities or AML, NOS

Continued

Continued

2017	WHO 2022	ICC 2022
CEBPA mutation	Bi-allelic *CEBPA* mutations and single mutations sm bZIP-*CEBPA*	In-frame bZIP *CEBPA* (bi- and monoallelic); mutations in TAD domain are not counted
Rearrangements	• AML with *KMT2A* rearrangement • AML with *MECOM* rearrangement	• AML with t(9;11) (p21.3;q23.3)/ *MLLT3::KMT2A*; AML with other *KMT2A* rearrangements • AML with inv(3)(q21.3q26.2) or t(3;3)(q21.3;q26.2)/*GATA2::MECOM* (*EVI1*) AML with other *MECOM* rearrangements
AML with myelodysplasia related changes	*AML-MR defining cytogenetic abnormalities:* • Complex karyotype (≥3 abnormalities) • 5q deletion or loss of 5q due to unbalanced translocation Monosomy 7, 7q deletion, or loss of 7q due to unbalanced translocation • 11q deletion • 12p deletion or loss of 12p due to unbalanced translocation Monosomy 13 or 13q deletion 17p deletion or loss of 17p due to unbalanced translocation isochromosome 17q idic(X)(q13) • *Defining somatic mutations:* WHO *ASXL1, BCOR, EZH2, SF3B1, SRSF2, STAG2, U2AF1, ZRSR2* • Prior history of MDS or MDS/ MPN remains a disease premise • Morphology alone as a diagnostic qualifier eliminated	• *AML with MR cytogenetic abnormalities:* Defining cytogenetic abnormalities ICC complex karyotype (≥3 abnormalities) del(5q)/t(5q)/ add(5q) • Monosomy 7, 7q deletion • Trisomy 8 • del(12p)/t(12p)/add(12p) • Monosomy 17/add(17p) or del(17p) isochromosome 17q idic(X)(q13) del(20q) *AML with MR gene mutations:* • Defining somatic mutations ICC *ASXL1, BCOR, EZH2, SF3B1, SRSF2, STAG2, U2AF1, ZRSR2, RUNX1*‡ • Prior history of MDS or MDS/MPN-disease qualifier but not disease classifier in ICC • Morphology alone as a diagnostic qualifier eliminated
Subtypes eliminated	• AML with RUNX1 mutation • AML, NOS • Therapy-related myeloid neoplasms (now a new entity as secondary myeloid neoplasm)	• AML with RUNX1 mutation • Therapy-related myeloid neoplasms (now diagnostic qualifier rather than classifier)
Additional subtypes	*Secondary myeloid neoplasm (MN):* • MN postcytotoxic therapy • MN associated with germline predisposition • MN associated with Down syndrome	• AML/MDS (blast count 10–19%) • AML with mutated *TP53* is a diagnostic qualifier

*Retains 20% blast in AML with DGA.

†AEL is a type of AML with differentiation.

‡RUNX1 retained in ICC under AML with MR gene mutation.

IMPACT ON CLINICAL PRACTICE

Though there is almost 90% overlap between the two systems, there are discrepancies that will impact the diagnostic criterion and the clinical decisions influencing the targeted therapy. The differences can impact clinical practice as follows:

- *Diagnosis*: Reduction in the blast percent to <20% in WHO and at least 10% in ICC will aid in early diagnosis of AML. Variations in blast percentage thresholds between the two systems and genetic criteria may lead to differences in disease diagnosis, classification, and treatment decisions.
- *Prognosis*: Distinct categorization of genetic mutations, such as TP53, presence DNMT3A, and TET2 provides more precise prognostic information, guiding therapeutic strategies. DNMT3A improves with daunorubicin, while TET mutations can be targeted using hypomethylating agents. A combination of NPM1 plus IDH1 and IDH2 and DNMT3A has a worse prognosis. The prognostic effect of high VAF in NPM1 is adverse in patients treated with HSCT in first CR.
- *Treatment*: Integration of genomic data of distinct AML types by NGS helps to plan the targeted therapies and treatment based on the molecular profile of the disease.

The clinician or the physician must be able to decipher the genetic defect and its impact on treatment.

CONCLUSION

The chapter highlights the significant differences in the two classification systems along with the challenges of reconciling both systems in hematology. This chapter acknowledges the historical precedent of multiple classification systems in hematology, suggesting a potential return to that scenario. Knowledge of both systems with potential convergence toward a single favored approach is crucial for optimal patient care. Some experts believe one system will eventually take precedence and gain wider acceptance.

Take Home Points

- WHO and the ICC updated their definitions of acute myeloid leukemia (AML) in 2022.
- *Focus on genetics*: The new classifications emphasize genetic abnormalities over traditional morphology-based criteria, leading to a more accurate understanding of the disease and its prognosis.
- *Reduced reliance on blast count*: Blast percentage thresholds for AML diagnosis are now more nuanced, with some defining/recurrent genetic abnormalities requiring only any number (WHO) or ≥10% blasts (ICC), while others still need 20%, namely AML with *BCR::ABL1* fusion, AML with *CEBPA* mutations, and AML-myelodysplasia related.

- *New categories*: Both WHO and ICC introduced new categories, like "(MDS)/AML" for cases with 10–19% blasts and with specific genetic features such as TP53 mutations and "AML with recurrent genetic abnormalities" for cases with poor prognosis.
- *Some disagreements remain*: While both classifications share many similarities, there are still minor differences in the criteria for certain categories, which can lead to confusion.
- Overall, the 2023 updates to AML classification bring us closer to a more accurate and unified understanding of this complex disease. However, ongoing efforts are needed to address remaining discrepancies and ensure consistent diagnosis and treatment worldwide.
- The importance of clear communication and collaboration among healthcare professionals to avoid confusion when using the different classification systems.
- The changes in AML classification are expected to have a significant impact on diagnosis, risk stratification, and treatment decisions.

SUGGESTED READINGS

1. Khoury JD, Solary E, Abla O, Akkari Y, Alaggio R, Apperley JF, et al. The 5th edition of the World Health Organization Classification of Haematolymphoid Tumours: Myeloid and Histiocytic/Dendritic Neoplasms. Leukemia. 2022;36(7):1703-19.
2. Huber S, Baer C, Hutter S, Dicker F, Meggendorfer M, Pohlkamp C, et al. AML classification in the year 2023: How to avoid a Babylonian confusion of languages. Leukemia. 2023;37(7):1413-20.
3. Arber DA, Orazi A, Hasserjian RP, Borowitz MJ, Calvo KR, Kvasnicka HM, et al. International Consensus Classification of Myeloid Neoplasms and Acute Leukemias: Integrating morphologic, clinical, and genomic data. Blood. 2022;140(11):1200-28.
4. Zhao D, Zhou Q, Zarif M, Eladl E, Wei C, Atenafu EG, et al. AML with CEBPA mutations: A comparison of ICC and WHO-HAEM5 criteria in patients with 20% or more blasts. Leukemia Res. 2023;134:107376.
5. Park HS, Kim HK, Kim H, Yang Y, Han HS, Lee KH, et al. The new diagnostic criteria for myelodysplasia-related acute myeloid leukemia is useful for predicting clinical outcome: comparison of the 4th and 5th World Health Organization classifications. Annals of Hematology. 2022;101(12):2645-54.
6. Li W. The 5th Edition of the World Health Organization Classification of Hematolymphoid Tumors. Exon Publications eBooks; 2022. pp. 1-21.
7. Weinberg OK, Porwit A, Orazi A, Hasserjian RP, Foucar K, Duncavage EJ, et al. The International Consensus Classification of acute myeloid leukemia. Virchows Archiv. 2023;482(1):27-37.
8. Prassek VV, Rothenberg-Thurley M, Sauerland MC, Herold T, Janke H, Ksienzyk B, et al. Genetics of acute myeloid leukemia in the elderly: Mutation spectrum and clinical impact in intensively treated patients aged 75 years or older. Haematologica. 2018;103(11):1853-61.
9. Su L, Shi YY, Liu ZY, Gao SJ. Acute Myeloid Leukemia with CEBPA Mutations: Current Progress and Future Directions. Front Oncol. 2022;12:806137.
10. Salman H. Comparative Analysis of AML Classification Systems: Evaluating the WHO, ICC, and ELN Frameworks and Their Distinctions. Cancers. 2024;16(16):2915-5.
11. Alonso CM, Llop M, Sargas C, Pedrola L, Panadero J, Hervás D, et al. Clinical Utility of a Next-generation Sequencing Panel for Acute Myeloid Leukemia Diagnostics. J Mol Diagn. 2019;21(2):228-40.

CHAPTER 5

CAR-T Therapy: Managing Toxicity and Long-term Outcome Assessment

Sumeet Mirgh, Mohd Rizwan Shaikh, Dinesh Bhurani

ABSTRACT

Chimeric antigen receptor T-cells (CAR-T) are at the perfect interface of humoral and cellular immunity, as they modify self T-cells and empower them with a unique ability to kill cancer cells. They bypass the need of human leukocyte antigen (HLA) for antigen recognition and are "antigen specific." After infusion, there is rapid expansion of CAR-T cells which expand, reach a peak and then persist. During their expansion, multiple cytokines are released which cause inflammatory manifestations called as "cytokine release syndrome." Cytokine release syndrome (CRS) typically manifests with fever, but can progress to hypotension, and hypoxia as per severity. Along with or shortly after CRS, some patients can develop a constellation of neurological symptoms called immune cell associated neurotoxicity syndrome (ICANS). Other toxicities include cytopenias, B-cell aplasia, and development of second malignancies. With respect to long-term outcomes, approximately 30–40% patients for large B-cell lymphomas and pediatric acute lymphoblastic leukemia (B-ALL) achieve long-term durable remissions. There is debate as to which B-ALL patients should undergo consolidative allogeneic stem-cell transplant after CAR-T. Disease biology, disease burden prior to CAR-T, CAR-T kinetics postinfusion and persistence along with sensitive methods of residual disease detection can help decide whom to "pre-emptively" consolidate with allogeneic stem-cell transplant.

INTRODUCTION

Chimeric antigen receptor T-cells (CAR-T) are the most complex and novel form of cellular therapy. It is the perfect semblance of cellular engineering and medicine. A normal T-cell receptor (TCR) identifies a tumor antigen with the help of human leukocyte antigen (HLA) present on the cancer cells. However, cancer cells are "smart" enough to escape kill by downregulating their HLA. CAR-T cells have a receptor that has a fusion of the antigen-binding domain of the immunoglobulin molecule along with the transmembrane and intracellular domain of a normal TCR. This unique ability enables them to identify any "specific" tumor antigen without the need for HLA. Thus, CAR-T cells are at the unique interface of humoral and cellular immunity, overcoming the limitations of identifying and killing cancer cells **(Fig. 1)**. The durability of response of these CAR-T cells is enhanced by adding multiple costimulatory domains, which increase proliferation and response to repeated exposures to the same antigen.

CHIMERIC ANTIGEN RECEPTOR T-CELL GENERATIONS

Over time, CAR-T cell constructs have evolved to make them more effective. These include first-generation CARs, which contain the CD3ζ intracellular domain responsible for T-cell activation with low cytotoxicity and antitumor efficacy.

Second-generation CARs: It contains CD3ζ and costimulatory domains such as CD28, which enhances T-cell proliferation.

Third-generation CARs: These CAR T-cells have an extracellular antigen-recognizing domain, three intracellular domains, CD3ζ, and two costimulatory domains.

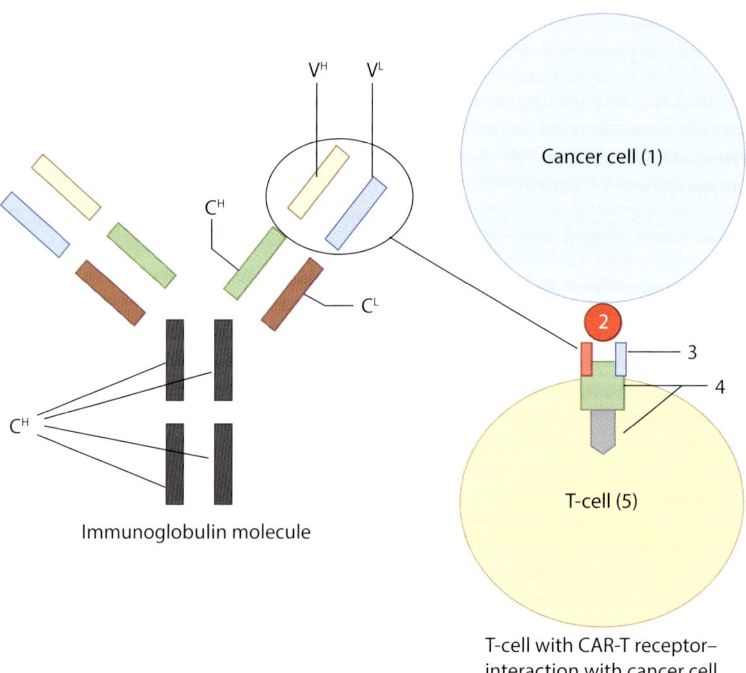

FIG. 1: Complex interaction of cancer cell with T-cell expressing chimeric antigen receptor (CAR). Components (on right side) 1—Cancer cell, 2—Tumor antigen, 3 + 4—CAR T-cell receptor (TCR) (3—extracellular TCR composed of variable domain of heavy and light chains for antigen specificity, 4—CD3 transmembrane and intracellular domain), 5—T-cell; (on left side) immunoglobulin molecule.

(VL: variable portion of light chain; VH: variable portion of heavy chain; CL: constant portion of light chain; CH: constant portion of heavy chain)

Fourth-generation CARs: Also known as T-cell redirected for universal cytokine-mediated killing (TRUCKs), these CAR T-cells are genetically modified to secrete cytokines.

Fifth-generation CARs: These CAR T-cells have an additional truncated cytoplasmic interleukin (IL)-2 receptor β-chain domain. This domain allows drug-dependent switches to control CAR T-cell functions, thus potentially optimizing therapeutic outcomes.

Chimeric Antigen Receptor T-cell Manufacturing

Manufacturing CAR-T cells involves isolating and processing T-cells from a patient's blood, genetically modifying them, and then expanding them.

Steps

- *Collect blood:* Apheresis, or leukapheresis, is used to remove blood from the patient and separate the leukocytes.
- *Isolate T-cells:* The leukocytes are enriched for T-cells using magnetic beads or density-based methods.
- *Activate T-cells:* The T-cells are activated in vitro.
- *Introduce CAR transgene:* A lentiviral or retroviral vector encoding the CAR cassette is used to genetically modify the T-cells.
- *Expand the T-cells:* The T-cells are expanded until the desired therapeutic dose is reached.
- *Formulate:* The final CAR-T cells are formulated.
- *Perform quality control:* The CAR-T cells undergo quality control testing throughout the process.
- *Infuse into patient:* The CAR-T cells are cryopreserved and thawed at the bedside before being infused into the patient.

Six CAR-T products have been approved for use, either for B-lymphoid malignancies or plasma cell dyscrasias **(Table 1)**. In this review, we will cover toxicities and long-term outcomes with CAR-T. Currently approved CAR-T products use the second-generation constructs described earlier.

TOXICITIES

Case 1

A 21-year-old boy, with relapsed B-acute lymphoblastic leukemia (B-ALL) after two prior lines of therapy underwent CD19 CAR-T cell therapy after fludarabine-cyclophosphamide conditioning. Prior to CAR-T, he had morphological disease 12% blasts. On day +4 after infusion, he developed high spiking fever [maximum temperature (T-max) 103°F/39°C)] which was not responding to antipyretics. He did not have any focus of infection, but was started on broad spectrum antibiotics (injection cefoperazone sulbactum and injection amikacin). On day+5, during morning rounds, it was noticed that patient felt fatigued. His pulse volume was low, with blood pressure (BP) readings—90/50–96/56. His usual BP readings in normal health varied between 120/82–130/88 on one antihypertensive

TABLE 1: US-FDA approved CAR-T products with their target antigens, names, and indications.

CAR-T target antigen	CAR-T product	Indication	Approved use in indications
Anti-CD 19	Tisagenlecleucel (*Tisa-cel*)	B-ALL, and B-NHL (DLBCL, follicular lymphoma)	• LBCL after ≥2 lines of therapy (2018) • FL after ≥2 lines of therapy (2022) • R/R B-ALL (2017)
	Axicabtagene ciloleucel (*Axi-cel*)	B-NHL (Both DLBCL and indolent B-NHL)	• LBCL refractory to first-line therapy or relapsing at <12 months of first-line therapy (2022) • Relapsed LBCL after ≥2 lines of therapy (2017) • Relapsed FL after ≥2 lines of therapy (2021)
	Lisocabtagene maraleucel (*Liso-cel*)	B-NHL (Both DLBCL and CLL)	• LBCL refractory to first-line or relapsing at <12 months of first-line therapy or relapsing on first-line therapy and not eligible for HSCT (2022) • Relapsed LBCL after >2 lines of therapy (2021)
	Brexucabtagene autoleucel (*Brexu-cel*)	B-ALL and Mantle cell lymphoma	R/R B-ALL (2021) R/R mantle cell lymphoma (2020)
Anti-BCMA	Idecabtagene vicleucel (*Ida-cel*)	Multiple myeloma (MM)	After ≥4 lines of therapy—R/R multiple myeloma (2021)
	Ciltacabtagene autoleucel (*Cilta-cel*)		After ≥4 lines of therapy—R/R multiple myeloma (2022)

(B-ALL: B-acute lymphoblastic leukemia; BCMA: B-cell maturation antigen; B-NHL: B non-Hodgkin lymphoma; CAR-T: chimeric antigen receptor T-cell; CLL: chronic lymphocytic leukemia; DLBCL: diffuse large B-cell lymphoma; FL: follicular lymphoma; HSCT: hematopoietic stem-cell transplant; LBCL: large B-cell lymphoma; R/R: relapsed-refractory)

drug, i.e., oral amlodipine 5 mg OD. He did not respond to a saline bolus with persistent hypotension. He was treated with intravenous tocilizumab 8 mg/kg. His fever dramatically crashed after tocilizumab, and BP picked up. He did not have subsequent recurrence of fever and marrow studies on day +28 revealed morphological complete remission (CR) with minimal residual disease (MRD) negative status.

The given case highlights the typical scenario of a cardinal toxicity of CAR-T, i.e., cytokine release syndrome (CRS). CRS is a multisystemic inflammatory syndrome due to the release of multiple cytokines [IL-6, IL-2, and Interferon (IFN)-γ], which manifests with fever, with or without chills, as the first sign. Although there are multiple systems for grading its severity, the most widely used grading system is the one recommended by the American Society of

Transplantation and Cellular Therapy (ASTCT). While fever (>38°C) is typically present in grade 1, other signs include hypoxia (*Grade 2:* Low-flow oxygen, i.e., <6 L/min, or *Grade 3:* >6 L/min), hypotension (*Grade 3:* Hypotension needing single vasopressor, *Grade 4*: Needing multiple vasopressors), and tachypnea (needing positive pressure ventilation) which develop as the severity of CRS increases. It typically develops between 2 and 7 days after infusion but can happen as late as 14 days after. Rarely, it can progress to multiorgan dysfunction with hepatic, renal, and cardiac failure.

Can We Predict Cytokine Release Syndrome, before it Develops?

Risk factors for the development of CRS typically include disease burden [nodal burden for lymphoma and/or bone marrow (BM) burden for acute leukemias], poor Eastern Cooperative Oncology Group performance status (ECOG-PS), low baseline platelet counts, increased pretreatment inflammatory markers, need for bridging therapy, need for intensive lymphodepletion, high CAR-T cell doses, high peak levels of CAR-T cells in blood, and type of CAR-T product (grade 3–5 CRS for large B-cell lymphoma—*Liso-cel* 1–2% vs. *Tisa-cel/Axi-cel* 5–15%). Importantly, the kinetics of CRS also depends on the type of costimulatory domain (those with a CD28 costimulatory domain have earlier CRS compared to a 4-1 BB costimulatory domain). There have been different models for CRS prediction based on various cytokines [such as IL-1, IL-6, 1L-10, monocyte chemoattractant protein-1 (MCP-1), macrophage inflammatory protein (MIP)-1α, angiotensin-2, and IFN-γ], measured pre- and post-CAR-T infusion. Among them, most notable is endothelial activation and stress index (EASIX) score [lactate dehydrogenase (LDH; U/L) × creatinine (mg/dL)/platelets (PLTs; 10^9 cells/L)]. It is a marker of endothelial damage and a predictor of survival after acute graft-versus-host disease (GVHD) postallogeneic stem-cell transplant. A modified EASIX score that substitutes C-reactive protein (CRP) (mg/dL) for creatinine better estimates the risk of severe CRS and immune cell associated neurotoxicity syndrome (ICANS) after CAR-T infusion.

How does One Treat Cytokine Release Syndrome, and How does Predictive Scores Help a Physician?

Tocilizumab is a monoclonal antibody against IL-6 receptor and the backbone of CRS treatment. It is recommended for anyone with ≥ Grade 2 CRS. Recently, it has also been recommended by some experts with persistent grade 1 CRS. Steroids are recommended for tocilizumab-refractory CRS. Dexamethasone [10 mg intravenous (IV) Q12 hourly for grade 2 CRS, 10 mg IV Q6 hourly for grade 3 CRS] or methylprednisolone (1 g IV 12 hourly for grade 4 CRS) are recommended for severe CRS. Rarely, in case of no response to steroids, steroid-sparing agents such as anakinra, siltuximab, ruxolitinib, cyclophosphamide, and recently approved anti-IFNγ monoclonal for primary hemophagocytic lymphohistiocytosis (HLH), Emapalumab can be considered. Extensive trials have shown that tocilizumab administration does not seem to affect response durability or survival after CAR-T. On the other hand, there is conflicting data on steroid administration impacting relapse after CAR-T for malignancies. Studies on B-cell malignancies have shown the detrimental effects of steroids, while the same has not been proven for multiple myeloma (MM). This may be due to the lympholytic effect of systemic steroids, which thereby impacts peak levels of CAR-T and its persistence. Predictive scores have helped physicians to administer tocilizumab "pre-emptively," i.e., in patients with persistent grade 1 CRS with a high-risk score, to prevent its progression to higher CRS grades.

Case 2

A 30-year-old male with relapsed diffuse large B-cell lymphoma (DLBCL) after two prior lines of therapy, received CD19 CAR-T (Axi-cel) after fludarabine-cyclophosphamide conditioning. On day 4, he developed grade 3 CRS, for which an injection of tocilizumab was administered. While his fever and hypotension resolved, 3 days later (day +7), he was more somnolent (was sleeping 12–14 hours, instead of usual 7–8 hours) without sedatives. Neurological examination revealed that he was confused but responding to verbal commands. He was oriented to place and person but not to time. He was following commands, able to write simple sentences, name objects, but unable to calculate backward from 100. He was an IT professional, and unable to do simple mathematical calculations was unusual for him. Imaging [magnetic resonance imaging (MRI)] was normal, and the CSF examination revealed no infective cause. He was treated with injection dexamethasone 10 mg IV BD followed by significant improvement within 24 hours. His steroids were tapered by 4 mg every 4th day, and he was discharged on day +24.

The constellation of neurological symptoms that develop after CAR-T is called ICANS. It manifests concomitantly or shortly after clinical manifestations of CRS with symptoms of global cognitive decline (encephalopathy)—somnolence, decreased alertness, and dysphasia which may progress to obtundation. Rarely, it manifests with focal symptoms such as seizures, myoclonus, and motor weakness. Risk factors for ICANS overlap with those of CRS. Seldom, ICANS have been reported after 3 weeks and in the absence of CRS. ICANS happens because CAR-T cells can penetrate the blood-brain barrier (BBB). Moreover, the BBB becomes permeable to many systemic cytokines in severe CRS. An additional risk factor for ICANS is the presence of an underlying clonal hematopoiesis before CAR-T, probably reflecting an underlying "proinflammatory" state. Incidence of severe ICANS (≥grade 3) varies as per product and disease—for large B-cell lymphomas (*Axi-cel* 20–30%, *Tisa-cel* and *Liso-cel* 5–10%), for B-ALL (*Tisa-cel* 9–13%), for mantle cell lymphoma (*Brexu-cel* 30–35%). Increased neurotoxicity in the *axi-cel* and *brexu-cel* studies was likely because of the CD28-derived hinge, transmembrane, and costimulatory domains, which leads to rapid in vivo expansion.

The ICANS is graded by the immune effector cell-associated encephalopathy (ICE) score and the recent ASTCT grading. For children <12 years age, Cornell Assessment of Pediatric Delirium tool is preferred. ICE score involves 5 domains—orientation, naming, following commands, language/writing, and attention (which includes calculation). ASTCT grading involves, in addition to the ICE score, the patient's consciousness, presence of seizures, motor weakness, and presence of cerebral edema. Presence of any feature among the latter three features indicate ≥grade 3 ICANS.

Steroids remain the first line of treatment for ICANS, dexamethasone is recommended for patients with ≥grade 2 ICANS. Intrathecal steroids and anakinra can be used for steroid-refractory ICANS.

A rare neurological event, distinct from ICANS has been recently described. This is a form of delayed neurotoxicity, which is seen in 5% recipients of anti-B cell maturation antigen (BCMA) CAR-T cell therapy for relapsed-refractory MM (RR-MM). Unlike ICANS, it is sporadic, not associated with CRS, happens weeks-months after CAR-T, slowly progressive and steroid unresponsive. These are disease-specific, i.e., for MM. A form of movement disorder manifested by bradykinesia, postural instability, and tremor, occurring 3–4 months post CAR-T infusion, has been described after BCMA-directed CAR-T cell therapies. This is due to expression of BCMA in neurons and microglia in the caudate nucleus, thereby defining this as an "on-target" off-tumor side effect. Similarly, GPRC5D CAR-T cells have been described to lead to cerebellar toxicities (dizziness, gait disturbances). Similar to CRS, risk factors include prior CRS, ICANS, disease burden, high peak (>1,000 cells/μL at any time-point) and persistent blood CAR-T cell levels (>300 cells/μL on day 56). Management relies on its prevention on basis of risk factors—effective bridging therapy to decrease disease burden, early identification, and management of CRS, ICANS, and extended monitoring until 1-year postinfusion. There is anecdotal evidence for use of high dose cyclophosphamide for these toxicities.

Case 3

A 26-year-old boy underwent transplant for Ph+ B-ALL in CR-2, after receiving salvage therapy with hyper CVAD. Posttransplant, he developed cytomegalovirus (CMV) reactivation on day +28 needing ganciclovir for 21 days. On day +90, his bone marrow (BM) examination showed a relapse with 7% B-lymphoid blasts confirmed on flow cytometry. There was 99% CD19 expression on blasts, and he was planned for CD19 CAR-T. Prior to CAR-T, his baseline hemogram was Hb 7 g/dL, total leukocyte count (TLC)—1.1 × 10^9/L, platelet—70 × 10^9/L. Post CAR-T, he developed grade 3 CRS needing tocilizumab. He developed severe cytopenias (grade 3 leukopenia TLC—1 × 10^9/L, and grade 4 thrombocytopenia platelet—15 × 10^9/L), which persisted beyond day +28. He was initiated on injection romiplostim. There was some improvement in his counts by day +75—Hb 9.5 g/dL, TLC 2.4 × 10^9/L, platelet 75 × 10^9/L.

Prolonged cytopenias, especially grade 3–4 lasting for >28 days, have been described in 30–40% CAR-T recipients. The incidence of ≥grade 3 neutropenia and thrombocytopenia for *Ida-cel* and *Cilta-cel* for MM varies between 40 and 60%. The risk of hematotoxicity is a composite of baseline BM reserve (baseline marrow disease burden, lower baseline counts, and prior transplant), inflammatory milieu (higher baseline inflammatory markers) and the inflammation consequent to CAR-T (severe CRS and ICANS, more peak levels of IL-6). Among aforementioned, severe CRS and prior BMT are the most important, and our patient (*Case 3*) had both. Common causes of cytopenias are—lymphodepletion, ongoing CRS (for within 30 days); immune cytopenias, transplant-associated thrombotic microangiopathy (TA-TMA) (for those with prior transplant), large-granular lymphocytosis (LGL) (for cytopenias up to 90 days); and lastly, disease relapse and second malignancy (for cytopenias beyond 90 days). A recent European society for Bone Marrow Transplantation-European Hematology Association (EBMT-EHA) consensus termed this phenomenon of cytopenias post CAR-T as "Immune effector Cell-Associated Hematotoxicity (ICAHT)." They classified ICAHT as early (within 30 days of CAR-T infusion) or late (after day +30). For early ICAHT, neutropenia was graded as absolute neutrophil count (ANC) $\leq 0.5 \times 10^6/\mu L$ for <7 days (Grade 1), 7–13 days (Grade 2), >14 days (Grade 3) and never reached $0.5 \times 10^6/\mu L$ until day 30 (Grade 4).

The chance of hematotoxicity can be predicted before lymphodepletion by the CAR-HEMATOTOX score. It includes the factors of bone marrow reserve (platelet count, ANC, and hemoglobin) and inflammatory markers (CRP, ferritin). Those with a high CAR-HEMATOTOX score (≥2) should undergo a BM examination before CAR-T and be considered for early interventions post-CAR-T. Routine tests for hematotoxicity post-CAR-T include knowing the marrow reserve (reticulocyte count), concomitant medications, vitamin deficiencies (B12, folate), infections (blood cultures, CMV, imaging if required), and ruling out macrophage activation syndrome (serum ferritin, triglycerides). If there is no reversible cause as per the above workup, growth factors (such as G-CSF and thrombopoietin agonists) can be given. Recent data suggests that G-CSF does not impact CAR-T expansion nor worsen the risk of higher-grade CRS/ICANS. If there is no response to growth factors, special tests [Epstein–Barr virus polymerase chain reaction (EBV PCR), Parvovirus PCR, autoimmune workup, and marrow examination for disease relapse] can be considered. Rarely, for cytopenias which are severe, persistent, and refractory to growth factors—autologous stem-cell boosts (if available and cryopreserved before) and allogeneic transplants remain the last options. For patients who receive CAR-T after prior allogeneic BMT and stem-cell boost is contemplated for hematotoxicity, a T-cell depleted CD34 boost is preferred. This is to avoid the immune complications of donor T-cells in a patient who already has modified CAR-T (engineered and transduced) cells in his circulation.

Other toxicities of CAR-T include B-cell aplasia (BCA), infections, and second malignancies. BCA is an "on-target" but "off-tumor" toxicity of CD19 CAR-T. At 1-year post-CD19 CAR-T, approximately 50% patients have persistent BCA. In contrast to rituximab, CD19 CAR-T causes more profound and persistent BCA. BCA has two clinical implications. First, loss of BCA occurs in 60–70% of patients with B-cell lymphomas treated with CD19 CAR-T, at variable time intervals post-CAR-T. Loss of BCA in patients with B-ALL treated with *Tisa-cel* is a harbinger of relapse. A small study showed that initiation of maintenance therapy at loss of BCA in patients with B-ALL can achieve equivalent outcomes to that achieved by a second transplant. This is important because second transplant, although ideal, is not feasible for majority of patients who relapse post CAR-T. Secondly, patients with BCA need long-term intravenous immunoglobulin replacement. While one may think that complete humoral immunity is lost in BCA after CD19 CAR-T, some form is retained due to persistence of long-lived CD19-negative plasma cells. This is not true for patients with MM, as BCMA-directed CART would deplete even the long-lived CD19-negative, BCMA-positive plasma cells, thereby leading to more profound hypogammaglobulinemia. Concerning infections, these patients should be given prophylaxis against pneumocystis carinii-pneumonia (PCP), Varicella-zoster virus, herpes simplex virus (VZV/HSV), and hepatitis-B for 6–12 months postinfusion. Gram-negative and antifungal prophylaxis can be considered in cases of neutropenia for >2 weeks or those on long-term steroids or as per institutional policy.

Similar to transplant, patients with CAR-T are at risk of developing second malignancies. A large retrospective study demonstrated 5-year risk of 15% for second solid tumors and 2% risk for second myeloid neoplasms (SMN). The risk of SMN was reported to be 10% for *cilta-cel*, which compelled the US-FDA to release a black box warning in December 2023. One study showed that preexisting clonal hematopoiesis (CH) increased the risk of second malignancies (19% vs. 4%) after CD19 CAR-T. Similarly, there are anecdotal reports of T-cell malignancies (TCM), after CAR-T. Till December 2023, 22 cases of TCM have been described with five of the six CAR-T products. Interestingly, the CAR transgene was expressed in three of these TCMs. However, it is important to know that >27,000 CAR-T products have been given, and the risk of TCM is exceedingly rare.

LONG-TERM OUTCOMES

The long-term outcomes (LTOs) of CAR-T cell therapy depends on several factors, including the specific indication, the product used, the patient population in the study, disease biology, and the number of prior therapy lines. LTO data have been reported primarily for indications such as relapsed/refractory B-cell lymphoma (RR-BCL) and B-ALL, as CAR-T cell therapy has been available for longer. For LTOs, we have included data from CD19 CAR-T studies, which have reported at least 2-year follow-up. It is important to distinguish whether a study reports intention-to-treat (ITT) analysis or per-protocol analysis, given the significant delays between planning and infusion, which may result in disease progression or death, making some patients ineligible for therapy.

Long-term Outcomes in B-cell Lymphoma Treated with CD19-Targeted Chimeric Antigen Receptor T-cells

SCHOLAR-1 study provided the benchmark for outcomes of patients with primary refractory DLBCL or those with early relapse [<12 months of auto-hematopoietic stem-cell transplant (HSCT)] in the pre-CAR-T era. Among 636 patients, the overall response rates (ORR) to salvage therapy were 25%, with a median survival of <6 months; thereby highlighting the need for more effective therapies.

Table 2 lists studies with 24 months or more follow-up data (24–123 months). These studies report ORRs ranging from 44 to 91%, of which CR rates were

TABLE 2: Long-term outcomes of anti-CD19 CAR-T in LBCL and CLL.

Study (year of publication)	CAR product and trial phase	Cancer types (*n*)	Median follow-up (range)	ORR and CRR	PFS or EFS	DOR in responding patients
Chong et al. (2021)	*Tisa-cel*, single-center case series	DLBCL (24); FL (14)	61 months	ORR: 66%; CRR: 55%	5-year PFS—31% for DLBCL; 5-year PFS for FL—43%	60% remained in response at 5 years
Jacobson et al. (2021)	*Axi-cel*, multicentre phase I/II	DLBCL (77); PMBCL (8); tFL (16)	51 months	ORR: 74%; CRR: 54%	2-year EFS—38%	NR
Cappell et al. (2020)	FMC63-28Z[a], single-centre phase I	DLBCL/PMBCL (28); CLL/SLL (7)	42 months (1–123 months)	ORR: 81%; CRR: 58%	Median EFS: 55 months	76% of patients with a CR remained in response at last follow-up with a DOR ranging from 43 to 113 months
Schuster et al. (2021)	*Tisa-cel*, multicentre phase II	DLBCL, HGBCL or tFL (115)	40 months (38–44 months)	ORR: 53%; CRR: 39%	Median PFS: 2.9 months; median EFS: 2.8 months	Median DOR: Not estimable
Hirayama et al. (2019)	*Liso-cel*, single-centre phase I/II	tFL (13) and FL (8)	38 months for patients with tFL and 24 months for those with FL	ORR: NR for FL and 46% for tFL; CRR: 88% for FL and 46% for tFL	Median PFS: 1.4 months in tFL cohort; NR for FL cohort	All patients with FL with a CR remained in remission at a median follow-up duration of 24 months (range 5–37 months)
Wang et al. (2023)	*Brexu-cel*, multicentre phase II	MCL (68)	36 months (26–56 months)	ORR: 91%; CRR: 68%	Median PFS: 26 months	Median DOR: 47 months in patients with a CR
Frey et al. (2020)	CART-19, single-centre phase II	CLL (38)	32 months (2–75 months)	ORR: 44%; CRR: 28%	Median PFS: 40 months in those with CR	4/9 (44%) of patients with a CR had relapse

(CAR-T: chimeric antigen receptor T-cells; CLL: chronic lymphocytic leukemia; CRR: composite response rate; CR: complete remission; DOR: duration of response; DLBCL: diffuse large B-cell lymphoma; EFS: event-free survival; HGBCL: high grade B-cell lymphoma; LBCL: large B-cell lymphoma; MCL: mantle cell lymphoma; NR: not reached; ORR: overall response rate; OS: overall survival; PMBCL: primary mediastinal B cell lymphoma; PFS: progression free-survival; SLL: small lymphocytic lymphoma; tFL: transformed follicular lymphoma)

between 28 and 68%. A subset of patients continued to show durable responses even at 2 years postinfusion without additional consolidative treatments. Long-term remissions were observed across various lymphoma types, including aggressive B-cell lymphomas, follicular lymphomas, mantle cell lymphoma, and chronic lymphocytic leukemia (CLL), with all currently approved CD19-targeted CAR T-cell products.

Two small single-center studies but with >5-year follow-up data reported that approximately half of the patients achieved a CR, of which 60–70% had a durable response of >4 years. This suggests that it is possible to possibly cure (long-term remission without any further treatment) approximately 30–40% of all patients with relapsed/refractory B-cell lymphomas (RRBCL) who receive CD19 CAR-T, much higher than pre-CAR-T era (<10%).

Long-term Outcomes in B-acute Lymphoblastic Leukemia Treated with CD19-targeted Chimeric Antigen Receptor T-cells

Table 3 includes studies with a median follow-up of >24 months, reporting CR rates between 62 and 86%. Concerning B-ALL, there is a significant difference

TABLE 3: Long-term outcomes of anti-CD19 CAR-T in B-ALL.

Study (year of publication)	CAR design with costimulatory domain, and trial phase	Trial population (*n*)	Median follow-up	CR/CRi	Survival outcomes
Shah et al. (2021)	Mouse scFv, CD28 H/T, CD28 costimulatory domains; single-center phase I	4–30 years (50)	4.8 years	31/50 (62%)	*Median EFS:* 3.1 months [75% patients in CR received allo-HSCT; 7/7 (100%) with MRD-negative CR without allo-HSCT relapsed]
Laetsch et al. (2023) (*Tisa-cel*)	Mouse scFv, CD8α H/T, 4-1BB costimulatory domains; multicenter phase II	3–24 years (79)	39 months	65/79 (82%)	*Median EFS:* 24 months (17% patients in CR received allo-HSCT)
Jacoby et al. (2022)	Mouse scFv, CD28 H/T, CD28 costimulatory domains; single-center phase II	1–36 years (37)	3 years	30/35 (86%)	*Median EFS:* 17 months (83% patients in CR received allo-HSCT)

Continued

Continued

Study (year of publication)	CAR design with costimulatory domain, and trial phase	Trial population (*n*)	Median follow-up	CR/CRi	Survival outcomes
Wayne et al. (2022); (KTE-X19)	Mouse scFv, CD28 H/T, CD28 costimulatory domains; multicenter phase I/II	3–20 years (24)	36 months	16/24 (67%)	*Median RFS:* 5.2 months (88% patients in CR received allo-HSCT)
Hay et al. (2019)	Mouse scFv, CD28 transmembrane, 4-1BB co-stimulatory domains (delivered in a defined $CD4^+$- to-$CD8^+$ cell ratio); CD19 CAR-T cells; single-center phase I/II	20–76 years (53)	31 months	45/53 (85%)	*Median EFS:* 7.6 months (in those achieving MRD-negative CR) (40% patients achieving MRD-negative CR received allo-HSCT)

(allo-HSCT: allogeneic hematopoietic stem cell transplant; B-ALL: B-acute lymphoblastic leukemia; CAR-T: chimeric antigen receptor T-cells; CR/Cri: complete remission/incomplete complete remission; EFS: event-free survival; MRD: minimal residual disease; ScFv: single-chain variable fragment; RFS: relapse-free survival)

for outcomes in pediatric versus adult patients. For adults, CR rates range between 60 and 70%, but median event-free survival (EFS) ranges between 6 and 12 months. On the other hand, for children, CR rates are approximately 80%, with median EFS of 24 months. We have known from the past that transplant is recommended for a standard risk B-ALL in CR-1 for an adult, in contrast to a pediatric patient. This is because of the disease biology of an adult B-ALL, which is more aggressive versus a pediatric B-ALL. The same is reflected in the CAR-T outcomes in the relapsed-refractory setting, too. For the same reason, more physicians have done a consolidative transplant after CAR-T in adults than in pediatric patients. The ELIANA study of *tisa-cel* in children and young adolescents highlighted a 3-year relapse-free survival (RFS) 52% with censoring for HSCT, and 48% without censoring. This suggests a cure may be possible without consolidative HSCT for some pediatric patients treated with *tisa-cel*. However, for adults, the decision to consolidate with allo-HSCT is complex and requires further research to guide treatment decisions.

Since consolidative allo-HSCT is not feasible for all patients, experts have tried to risk stratify patients of CAR-T who are at high-risk of relapse, i.e., patient with EFS of <30%. Factors for risk-stratification are included in **Table 4**. This illustrates the importance of monitoring for BCA and MRD monitoring post-CAR-T for preemptive decisions for consolidative allo-HSCT.

TABLE 4: Preinfusion and postinfusion factors for risk stratification—presence of any one of these factors portends a high risk of relapse post-CAR-T, CAR-T which merits the decision to consolidate with allo-HSCT after CAR-T.	
Preinfusion factors	**Postinfusion variables**
High disease burden prior to CAR-T • >5% blasts preinfusion	*Residual disease by sensitive methods at any time point post-CAR-T* • NGS-MRD positivity at 1 month or 3 months post
Bad disease biology • *KMT2A* rearranged non-CNS extramedullary disease	*Surrogate preemptive marker for CAR-T failure and imminent relapse* • Loss of BCA within 6 months post-CAR-T
Increased risk of CAR-T failure due to less target antigen expression • CD19 dim expression	

(allo-HSCT: allogeneic hematopoietic stem cell transplant; CAR-T: chimeric antigen receptor T-cells; MRD: minimal residual disease; NGS: next-generation sequencing)

Multiple Myeloma—Long-term Outcomes with B-cell Maturation Antigen—Targeted Chimeric Antigen Receptor T-cells

Due to the later development of BCMA-targeted CAR-T, fewer studies have reported LTOs for relapsed/refractory multiple myeloma (RRMM). Progression-free survival (PFS) after *Ida-cel* has been reported to be between 8.8 and 12 months (higher response for higher dose). In contrast to 33% CR rates for Ida-cel, *Cilta-cel* has been reported to have CR rates of 83%. Median PFS with *Cilta-cel* varies between 18 months-not reached (PFS of 55% at 27-month follow-up for not-reached study). Better PFS with *Cilta-cel* than *Ida-cel* could be due to two reasons. Firstly, *Cilta-cel* has two domains against BCMA antigen, in contrast to one in *Ida-cel*. Secondly, *Cilta-cel* was used earlier [1–3 prior lines of therapy (LOT)] as compared to *Ida-cel* (2–4 prior LOT). The survival in MM does not plateau, and relapses continue to happen with longer follow-ups. Nonetheless, median OS for triple-class refractory MM with CAR-T is approximately 36 months, much higher than the pre-CART era (<18 months) **(Table 5)**.

The chance of achieving a long-term remission after CAR-T depends on multiple factors are highlighted in **Table 6**.

CONCLUSION

The CAR-T cell therapy is an efficacious therapy for patients with relapsed-refractory B-cell malignancies and plasma cell neoplasms. Hematologists should be cognizant of its adverse effects, as the principles of management remain the same across all CAR-T products. While CAR-T may serve as one-time final

TABLE 5: Long-term outcomes of patients with RRMM receiving BCMA-targeted CAR-T cells.

Study and year of publication (*n*)	CAR design, name and trial phase	Median follow-up (range)	ORR and ≥ CRR	PFS	DOR
Zhao et al. 2022 (*n* = 74)	Two BCMA-binding domains, CD8α H/T domain, 4-1BB costimulatory domain; LCAR-B38M; multicenter phase I	48 months	ORR: 65/74 (88%); ≥CR: 54/74 (73%)	*Median PFS:* 18 months	*Median DOR:* 23 months
Martin et al. 2023 (*n* = 97)	Two BCMA-binding domains, a CD8α H/T domain, 4-1BB costimulatory domain, *Cilta-cel*; multicenter phase Ib/II	27 months	*ORR*: 95/97 (98%); ≥*sCR:* 80/97 (83%)	27 m PFS: 55% 27 m OS:71%	*Median DOR:* Not estimable (range 23 months to NE)
Mikkilineni et al. 2024 (*n* = 25)	Fully human scFv, heavy chain-only antigen recognition domain, CD8α H/T, 4-1BB costimulatory domain; FHVH33-CD8BBZ	Not mentioned	≥sCR: 52%	*Median PFS:* 78 weeks	*Median DOR:* NR

(BCMA: B-cell maturation antigen; CR: complete response; CRR: composite response rate; DOR: duration of response; H/T: hinge/transmembrane; m: months; NR: not reached; ORR: overall response rate; PFS: progression-free survival; RRMM: relapsed/refractory multiple myeloma; sCR: stringent complete response; ScFv: single-chain variable fragment)

TABLE 6: Factors associated with long-term remissions after CAR-T therapy.

Factors	Characteristics
Depth of response	Patients who achieve deep remissions (MRD negative status) post CAR-T have more likelihood of long-term remission
Type of malignancy	RRBCL vs. B-ALL. For RRBCL—CRs are less, but durable. For B-ALL, CRs are more, but less durable
Tumor burden and location	Patients with lesser disease burden (<5% blasts for B-ALL), nonbulky disease (for lymphomas), and absence of extramedullary disease have best outcomes
Lymphodepletion	Patients who receive fludarabine-cyclophosphamide lymphodepletion have optimal responses. Lymphodepletion depletes the host lymphocytes and its associated cytokines which may possibly reject or mount a response against the engineered CAR-T cells. To simplify, lymphodepletion reduces the presence of endogenous lymphocytes which are "competitors" of infused T-cells
CAR-T cell levels and persistence	• Quantitative PCR assays (like dd-PCR) and multiparametric flow-cytometry can measure CAR-T cell levels • Peak—a peak absolute lymphocyte count (ALC peak >0.67 × $10^9/\mu L$ as per one study) within first 15 days of CAR-T infusion is a surrogate of persistence and activity. Similarly, patients with a high CAR-T cell peak have more durable remission. The peak and expansion are earlier and short-lived with CAR-T cells with CD28ζ costimulatory domain, whereas slower and long-lived with 4-1BBζ. Hence, 4-1BBζ CAR-T may be preferred in patients with high-disease burden • Persistence—studies in RRBCL have shown that CAR-T cells which persist at or beyond 6 months, have lesser likelihood of relapse. The lifespan of CAR-T depends on the costimulatory domain—CD28ζ and 4-1BBζ

(ALC: absolute lymphocyte count; B-ALL: B-acute lymphoblastic leukemia; CAR-T: chimeric antigen receptor T-cells; MRD: minimal residual disease; PCR: polymerase chain reaction; RRBCL: relapsed/refractory B-cell lymphomas)

treatment for patients with RRBCL and pediatric B-ALL, it remains a bridging therapy to allo-HSCT for adults with B-ALL, and provides a long-term remission for patients with myeloma.

Take Home Points

- Cytokine release syndrome is one of the most common toxicities of CAR-T therapy. Noninfectious fever, hypotension, and hypoxia are its cardinal signs.
- Tocilizumab is the drug of choice for CRS, which should be considered once patients develop grade 2 CRS, i.e., requiring low-flow oxygen for hypoxia or fluid-responsive hypotension.
- Steroids are drug of choice for tocilizumab refractory CRS and ≥grade 2 ICANS.
- B-cell aplasia is an "on-target" but "off-tumor" toxicity of CD19 CAR-T, and its "loss" is a surrogate marker for relapse, especially in B-ALL.

- Approximately 30–40% of patients with relapsed-refractory large B-cell lymphomas and approximately 40% of pediatric and adolescent patients with B-ALL get long-term remissions with CD19 CAR-T.
- Patients treated with CD19 CAR-T who are at high risk of relapse (based on preinfusion disease biology and burden; postinfusion factors based on CAR-T expansion and residual disease) merit a consolidative allogeneic HSCT.
- BCMA CAR-T for myeloma has high CR rates and has increased survival of penta-refractory myeloma from <18 to 36 months, the most achieved by any treatment to date in the field of RRMM.

SUGGESTED READINGS

1. Brudno JN, Kochenderfer JN. Current understanding and management of CAR T cell-associated toxicities. Nat Rev Clin Oncol. 2024;21(7):501-21.
2. Perna F, Parekh S, Diorio C, Smith M, Subklewe M, Mehta R, et al. CAR T-cell toxicities: from bedside to bench, how novel toxicities inform laboratory investigations. Blood Adv. 2024;8(16):4348-58.
3. Rejeski K, Subklewe M, Aljurf M, Bachy E, Balduzzi A, Barba P, et al. Immune effector cell-associated hematotoxicity: EHA/EBMT consensus grading and best practice recommendations. Blood. 2023;142(10):865-77.
4. Jain T, Olson TS, Locke FL. How I treat cytopenias after CAR T-cell therapy. Blood. 2023;141(20):2460-9.
5. Myers RM, Shah NN, Pulsipher MA. How I use risk factors for success or failure of CD19 CAR T cells to guide management of children and AYA with B-cell ALL. Blood. 2023;141(11):1251-64.

CHAPTER 6

Noninvasive Prenatal Diagnosis for Sickle Cell Anemia and Thalassemia

Richa Juneja, Reena Das

ABSTRACT

Hemoglobinopathies are inherited in an autosomal recessive pattern and constitute a major healthcare burden in India. If both parents are carriers for sickle or beta thalassemia mutations, there is a 25% risk of having a homozygous baby with clinically significant hemoglobinopathies in each pregnancy. Prenatal diagnosis (PND) is key to the effective prevention of the birth of such babies with symptomatic hemoglobinopathy. Invasive PND requires chorionic villous sampling (CVS) around 10–12 weeks by expert obstetricians and the performance of polymerase chain reaction (PCR) and beta gene sequencing to detect pathogenic mutations in the fetal DNA extracted from the CVS sample. Nonavailability of trained obstetricians to take invasive samples and sophisticated laboratories to perform and report assays is a major hindrance in offering PND services for hemoglobinopathy. More so, some couples refuse to give consent due to the invasive nature of the procedure. Cell-free fetal DNA (cFF DNA) isolated from mothers' plasma at the 10th week of gestation has revolutionized PND of aneuploidies such as Down syndrome. There is a lot of effort from the scientific community across the globe to repeat this success story in the field of monogenic disorders. Testing this cFF DNA from mothers' plasma to predict whether the baby has inherited mutant alleles from both parents is called noninvasive prenatal testing (NIPT). NIPT with high sensitivity can be used as first-line test for mothers at risk of having a child with hemoglobinopathy, and only those testing positive on NIPT can be referred for invasive testing for confirmation. Since the NIPT procedure can be performed a few weeks earlier than CVS, the family can make a well-informed decision regarding the future course of action. The development of robust NIPT for hemoglobinopathy can create a remarkable increase in the reach of PND services for hemoglobinopathies.

INTRODUCTION

Hemoglobinopathies are characterized by a quantitative or qualitative defect in one of the globin chains of the hemoglobin (Hb) molecule. Alpha and beta globin chains with heme form adult hemoglobin (HbA)-constituting >95% of

Hb in adults. Mutations or deletions in alpha and β genes result in either reduced production of globin chain (thalassemia) or production of abnormal hemoglobin (hemoglobinopathy) such as sickle cell disorder (SCD) and HbE. SCD and β-thalassemia is one of the most common genetic diseases worldwide, with high prevalence in sub-Saharan Africa, the Middle East, the Mediterranean regions, and India. Carrier frequencies for sickle hemoglobin (HbS trait) in India can reach up to 40%, with the highest prevalence in central states. The carrier frequency of β-thalassemia (β-thalassemia trait: BTT) varies from 6 to 9.5% in various states. The rate of homozygosity for thalassemia per 1,000 births annually was reported 0.28 in Maharashtra and 0.39 in Gujarat as per one study. Estimates indicate that there would be around 1,00,000 patients with a β thalassemia syndrome and around 1,50,000 cases of sickle cell disease in our country. β thalassemia and SCD require lifelong management and contribute to infant and childhood morbidity and mortality.

The Government of India is determined to eliminate sickle as a public health problem by 2047. It requires community-based screening to identify affected patients and carriers, screening of pregnant women and their partners to identify couples at risk. Offer prenatal testing to couples at risk of having a child with clinically significant hemoglobinopathy and giving the option of termination of pregnancy if fetus is affected on PND.

CONVENTIONAL PRENATAL DIAGNOSIS

Conventional prenatal diagnosis (PND) is well-established for hemoglobinopathies in developed countries and many advanced centers in India. Initial reports of PND for hemoglobinopathies required fetal blood sampling and were done using cumbersome protein analysis or Southern blotting techniques. PND services for monogenic diseases were made feasible by the detection of hemoglobinopathy-causing mutations and deletions with polymerase chain reaction (PCR) modifications or sequencing.

When both partners are detected to have hemoglobinopathy in high-performance liquid chromatography (HPLC), there is a 25% risk of a fetus having a homozygous or compound heterozygous hemoglobinopathy state. Couples at risk of having a child with hemoglobinopathy with severe clinical phenotype such as β-thalassemia major and homozygous HbS are counseled for PND. Mother's and father's blood samples are collected, and disease-causing pathogenic variants in β globin gene are identified in a parental DNA sample. As β thalassemia can be caused by >350 different mutations/genetic changes in β gene, it is important to identify mutations in parents which is subsequently traced in fetal DNA. Fetal DNA is extracted from either a chorionic villus sample (CVS) or amniotic fluid in early pregnancy. CVS is a preferred sample as it provides better quality of fetal DNA, and it can be obtained early in pregnancy (10–12 weeks of gestation). Genetic studies such as amplification refractory mutation system (ARMS), restriction fragment length polymorphism (RFLP), and sequencing are done on extracted fetal DNA to check if the fetus is homozygous or compound heterozygous for parental mutations. In such a situation, an option of medical termination of pregnancy is given to parents after adequate counseling. At the same time, a test for maternal contamination in a fetal sample is conducted by using short tandem repeats (STR) or variable number tandem repeats (VNTR) markers, which are different in both parents, and hence, informative to assess maternal contamination in the CVS sample. Major challenges with existing PND methods are the invasive nature of the test, lack of availability of trained obstetricians to take CVS sample, and complexity of genetic assays. These tests need to be performed by a trained pathologist or geneticist in registered laboratories. Such trained obstetricians who can take out a CVS sample from the placenta at 10–12 weeks are usually not available in the peripheral towns, rural and tribal areas where these diseases are very common. Hence, PND, which is the only hope of effective prevention of hemoglobinopathies, is still not available to many. Researchers across countries are working on finding a solution to this problem to increase the outreach of preventive programs.

NONINVASIVE PRENATAL TESTING

Cell-free fetal DNA (cFF DNA) in maternal plasma is derived from the apoptosis of both maternal cells and placental cytotrophoblast cells. In 1997, the observation was made that fetal DNA can be isolated from maternal plasma and is called cFF DNA, constituting 5–10% of the total and the rest being of maternal origin. Since then, there has been a revolutionary advance in its application for prenatal diagnosis and the development of noninvasive prenatal testing (NIPT) for various diseases. NIPT essentially means testing for disease-causing mutation or genetic event in cFF DNA extracted from maternal plasma to know the risk of disease in the fetus. It is a standard screening method for aneuploidies such as Down syndrome. It is done on next-generation sequencer (NGS) or digital droplet PCR (ddPCR). A number of sequencing reads across various chromosomes are measured and compared to predict aneuploidies. Mothers with positive results on NIPT are only exposed to the risk of invasive CVS/amniotic fluid sampling and confirmatory testing on fetal genetic DNA. This confirmation is needed in view of the possibility of false-positive results on NIPT due to mosaicism in aneuploidy. NIPT has resolved the challenges to increase the outreach of PND for aneuploidies such as Down syndrome and has shown increased acceptance in couples at risk. The rapid development of NIPT for aneuploidies was due to high demand and commercial drive.

Noninvasive prenatal testing has also entered in PND of monogenic disorders. It is used to triage invasive PND testing in sex-linked disorders. For example, in the case of X-linked diseases, real-time PCR is done on cFF DNA to identify the presence of Y chromosome, and invasive PND is offered only when it is a male fetus. Since women are carriers for X-linked diseases, NIPT is used to offer invasive PND only when a male fetus with a risk of being affected with X-linked disorder such as Duchenne muscular dystrophy is to be tested. NIPT is also used to detect autosomal dominant inherited mutations coming from the father. NIPT for maternally inherited dominant mutation and autosomal recessive diseases (such as hemoglobinopathies) is an area of active research. It is very challenging because cell-free DNA has both fetal and maternal, components and the mutation of interest is present in the mother as well.

In conditions such as hemoglobinopathy, it requires detection of inheritance of maternal and paternal alleles in cFF DNA with relative quantification of wild and mutant alleles. It is complex as there is a high level of circulating maternal alleles. There are research papers from various groups on the development of NIPT for hemoglobinopathies using relative mutation dosage (RMD) on a digital droplet PCR platform and relative haplotype dosage (RHDO) using an NGS platform. Both the methods will be discussed in detail in the next section. NIPT has shown accuracy of >90% in screening for hemoglobinopathies in these studies. **Flowchart 1** summarizes the workflow of invasive and non-invasive PND.

There are several advantages of NIPT. It can be offered as early as 8 weeks of pregnancy, reducing apprehension in unaffected pregnancy and giving time for the couple to take further decisions in case of affected pregnancy. It can be done on a venous sample collected by a simple prick. It further reduces the minimal risk of abortion associated with an invasive procedure. These options will boost the acceptance of PND, and hence, the prevention of the birth of affected babies with hemoglobinopathy.

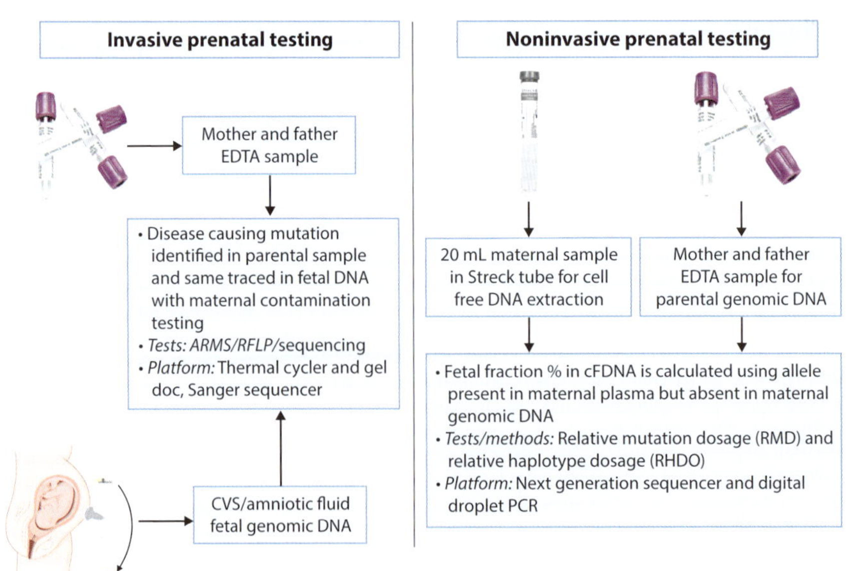

FLOWCHART 1: Comparative workflow of invasive and noninvasive prenatal diagnostic modalities for hemoglobinopathies.

(ARMS: amplification refractory mutation system; CVS: chorionic villus sample; EDTA: ethylenediaminetetraacetic acid; RFLP: restriction fragment length polymorphism)

METHODS OF NONINVASIVE PRENATAL TESTING FOR HEMOGLOBINOPATHY AND CHALLENGES

As discussed earlier, maternal whole blood is collected in special streck collection tubes, and cFFDNA is extracted using either manual methods or a dedicated automated extraction platform for cFFDNA. After quantification of cFDNA, molecular tests are performed. The following molecular approaches have been studied so far for NIPT of various hemoglobinopathies.

Relative Mutation Dosage

Relative proportion of mutant and wild-type allele is determined in cell-free DNA using digital droplet PCR. In a homozygous affected fetus allelic ratio is tilted toward mutant type and vice versa in homozygous wild-type fetus. If both mother and fetus are heterozygous for sickle, then the balance allelic ratio is predicted. In this situation, fetal fraction of cell-free DNA is measured by checking different (polymorphic) allelic markers and checking their relative dosage. It can also be achieved using marker of Y chromosome in case of a male fetus, and in case of a female fetus, other informative polymorphic alleles/indels are used to identify fetal fraction. This technique has been tested in the case of SCD to detect the fetus at risk of homozygous sickle mutation.

Relative Haplotype Dosage Analysis

Since RMD relies on dosage analysis of mutant versus wild alleles only, superior genetic methods were sought for. RHDO analysis has been shown to have an accurate prediction of fetal genotype from cFF DNA. A haplotype is a set of genetic variations inherited together. So, instead of tracking hemoglobinopathy mutation alone, the mutation along with several other adjacent single-nucleotide polymorphisms (SNPs) (haplotypes) are tracked in a fetus. It combines linkage analysis with dosage analysis of alleles.

In this technique, both maternal and paternal haplotypes are detected on blood-derived genomic DNA of parents. Haplotype detection is done by sequencing a large area on chromosome 11. This area includes multiple SNPs adjacent to the mutation site in hemoglobin subunit beta gene (HBB). This is performed using next-generation sequencing platforms. Both amplicon-based and probe capture library preparation strategies are described on different sequencing platforms. Maternal plasma is sequenced for similar SNPs linked to the mutation site. The fetal fraction is calculated in cell-free DNA based on allele reads with SNPs present in maternal plasma but absent in maternal DNA, assumed to be derived from the father, and hence, representing fetal fraction (FF). This is also correlated with paternal haplotyping information. The average of FF at various informative SNPs is taken and multiplied by 2 for final FF calculation. Probability algorithms are applied based on this fetal fraction to arrive at the expected allelic ratio in three possible fetal genotypes, e.g., homozygous for mutation, heterozygous for mutation, or homozygous for wild type. Maternal plasma DNA sequenced on NGS will give information about observed allelic ratios derived from the number of reads with mutation/wild-type reads. The final predicted fetal genotype on NIPT is given by comparing the observed ratios of disease-causing mutant alleles and reference alleles to those expected for the three possible genotypes. A pictorial depiction is in **Flowchart 2**. The major challenges in the RHDO method were limited FF affecting the prediction of fetal genotype in probability algorithm. A recent paper describes that by using bioinformatics tools such as in silico selection, FF in data can be enhanced by selecting short reads of <140 base pairs. They showed it to improve the diagnostic accuracy of NIPT. Specific bioinformatics pipeline and software with algorithms are needed to predict the final fetal genotype.

The following two case scenarios are described to understand NIPT:

- *Scenario 1*: If father and mother are carrying different hemoglobinopathy mutations, the presence of wild-type paternally inherited haplotype will negate significant hemoglobinopathy in a fetus.
- *Scenario 2*: In case of mother and father both are carrying the same mutation, and fetus has inherited mutant haplotype from father. It is very important to

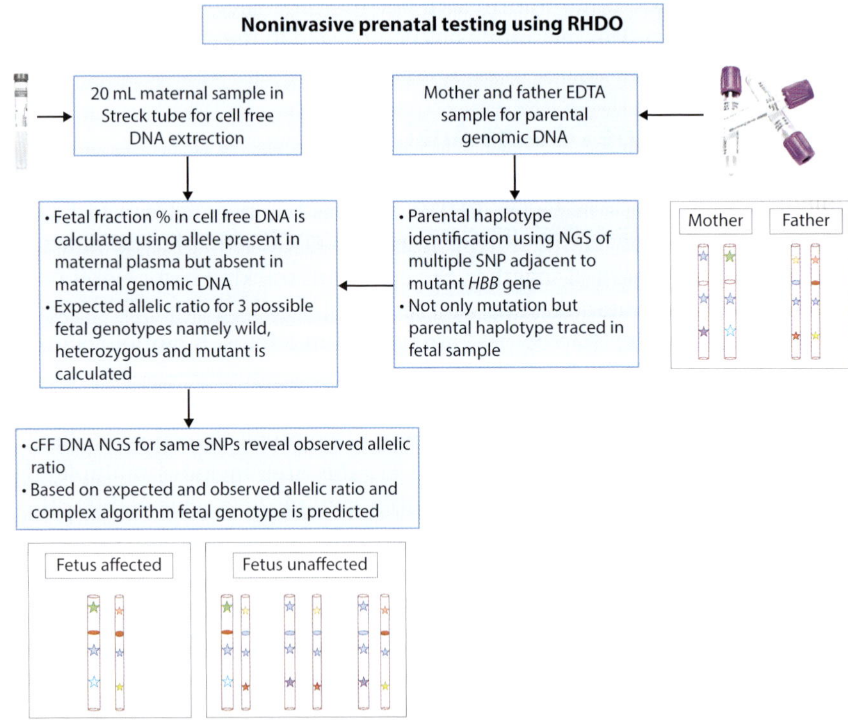

FLOWCHART 2: Diagram explaining noninvasive prenatal testing (NIPT) for autosomal recessive disease using relative haplotype dosage analysis (RHDO). In haplotypes, oval shapes—red (mutant) and blue (wild) indicated β thalassemia-associated alleles. Stars indicate linked single-nucleotide polymorphism (SNPs). Different colored stars indicate informative SNPs used in tracing parental haplotypes in cell-free fetal (cFF) DNA. Fetus is unaffected if father's mutant haplotype is absent in cFF DNA. If it is present along with a maternal mutant haplotype, the fetus is affected.

ensure if fetus has inherited a mutant or wild maternal haplotype. For this SNP, for which father is homozygous and mother is heterozygous will be used for deducing maternally inherited haplotype. Observed and expected allele ratio in cFF DNA will be compared to predict fetal genotype.

CHALLENGES IN ESTABLISHING NONINVASIVE PRENATAL TESTING

Cell-free DNA from maternal plasma has only 5–10% fetal fraction. It depends on several factors such as gestational age, smoking, and preeclampsia. Extraction, estimation of fetal fraction, and maintaining the quality of the same are challenging. Invasive PND testing can be made available with a simple PCR setup, whereas NIPT requires sophisticated and costly sequencing and ddPCR platforms. Trained personnel to perform such cumbersome tests and interpret this complex data are limited. These are certain challenges in the establishment of these NIPT assays. However, with advances in both science and sample shipment logistics, we may be standing on the verge of repeating the success story of NIPT for aneuploidies in the field of hemoglobinopathy.

FUTURE HOPES FOR PREVENTION IN HEMOGLOBINOPATHIES

The cost of prevention is much less than the cost of treatment for hemoglobinopathies. PND of any type adds stress and emotional trauma to a couple at risk. Preimplantation genetic testing (PGT) on embryos and choosing an unaffected embryo for implantation sounds ideal solution for the prevention of hemoglobinopathy. It requires an advanced assisted reproductive technology center and a sophisticated genetic laboratory capable of testing limited genetic material obtained from an embryo for pathogenic mutations with accuracy.

Take Home Points

- Prenatal diagnosis is the only hope to reduce prevalence of genetic diseases like hemoglobinopathies.
- Invasive nature of procedure, nonavailability of trained obstetrician and certified labs is major hindrance in increasing out reach of prenatal diagnosis of these diseases.
- Noninvasive prenatal diagnosis aims to identify the presence of pathogenic parental mutations in cell free fetal DNA from maternal plasma to detect affected fetus.
- Recent studies have shown high sensitivity for NIPT on testing platforms like NGS and ddPCR.
- Robust NIPT can boost the preventive program for hemoglobinopathies.

SUGGESTED READINGS

1. Serjeant GR. Sickle-cell disease. Lancet Lond Engl. 1997;350(9079):725-30.
2. World Health Organization. Guidelines for the control of haemoglobin disorders/edited by Bernadette Modell. [online] Available from https://iris.who.int/handle/10665/66665 [Last accessed May, 2025].
3. Colah R, Mukherjee M, Ghosh K. Sickle cell disease in India. Curr Opin Hematol. 2014;21(3): 215-23.
4. Colah R, Italia K, Gorakshakar A. Burden of thalassemia in India: The road map for control. Pediatr Hematol Oncol J. 2017;2(4):79-84.
5. Mandrile G, Barella S, Giambona A, Gigante A, Grosso M, Perrotta S, et al. First and Second Level Haemoglobinopathies Diagnosis: Best Practices of the Italian Society of Thalassemia and Haemoglobinopathies (SITE). J Clin Med. 2022;11(18):5426.
6. Vrettou C, Kakourou G, Mamas T, Traeger-Synodinos J. Prenatal and preimplantation diagnosis of hemoglobinopathies. Int J Lab Hematol. 2018;40(S1):74-82.
7. Rao E, Chandraker SK, Singh MM, Kumar R. Global distribution of β-thalassemia mutations: An update. Gene. 2024;896:148022.
8. Lo YM, Corbetta N, Chamberlain PF, Rai V, Sargent IL, Redman CW, et al. Presence of fetal DNA in maternal plasma and serum. Lancet Lond Engl. 1997;350(9076):485-7.
9. Ferres MA, Hui L, Bianchi DW. Antenatal noninvasive DNA testing: clinical experience and impact. Am J Perinatol. 2014;31(7):577-82.
10. Jenkins LA, Deans ZC, Lewis C, Allen S. Delivering an accredited non-invasive prenatal diagnosis service for monogenic disorders and recommendations for best practice. Prenat Diagn. 2018;38(1):44-51.
11. Vermeulen C, Geeven G, de Wit E, Verstegen MJAM, Jansen RPM, van Kranenburg M, et al. Sensitive Monogenic Noninvasive Prenatal Diagnosis by Targeted Haplotyping. Am J Hum Genet. 2017;101(3):326-39.
12. Hui WWI, Jiang P, Tong YK, Lee WS, Cheng YKY, New MI, et al. Universal Haplotype-based Noninvasive Prenatal Testing for Single Gene Diseases. Clin Chem. 2017;63(2):513-24.
13. Barrett AN, McDonnell TCR, Chan KCA, Chitty LS. Digital PCR analysis of maternal plasma for noninvasive detection of sickle cell anemia. Clin Chem. 2012;58(6):1026-32.
14. Hudecova I, Chiu RWK. Non-invasive prenatal diagnosis of thalassemias using maternal plasma cell free DNA. Best Pract Res Clin Obstet Gynaecol. 2017;39:63-73.
15. Lam KWG, Jiang P, Liao GJW, Chan KCA, Leung TY, Chiu RWK, et al. Noninvasive prenatal diagnosis of monogenic diseases by targeted massively parallel sequencing of maternal plasma: application to β-thalassemia. Clin Chem. 2012;58(10):1467-75.
16. Tungwiwat W, Fucharoen G, Fucharoen S, Ratanasiri T, Sanchaisuriya K, Sae-Ung N. Application of maternal plasma DNA analysis for noninvasive prenatal diagnosis of Hb E-beta-thalassemia. Transl Res J Lab Clin Med. 2007;150(5):319-25.
17. Xiong L, Barrett AN, Hua R, Tan TZ, Ho SSY, Chan JKY, et al. Non-invasive prenatal diagnostic testing for β-thalassaemia using cell-free fetal DNA and next generation sequencing. Prenat Diagn. 2015;35(3):258-65.
18. Erlich HA, López-Peña C, Carlberg KT, Shih S, Bali G, Yamaguchi KD, et al. Noninvasive Prenatal Test for β-Thalassemia and Sickle Cell Disease Using Probe Capture Enrichment and Next-Generation Sequencing of DNA in Maternal Plasma. J Appl Lab Med. 2022;7(2):515-31.
19. Chen C, Li R, Sun J, Zhu Y, Jiang L, Li J, et al. Noninvasive prenatal testing of α-thalassemia and β-thalassemia through population-based parental haplotyping. Genome Med. 2021;13(1):18.
20. Erlich HA, Ko L, Lee J, Eaton K, Calloway CD, Lal A, et al. Non-invasive prenatal testing of beta-hemoglobinopathies using next generation sequencing, in-silico sequence size selection, and haplotyping. Croat Med J. 2024;65(3):180-9.

CHAPTER 7

Molecular Landscape of Diffuse Large B-cell Lymphoma

Balamurugan Thirunavukkarasu, Sumeet Gujral

ABSTRACT

Diffuse large B-cell lymphoma (DLBCL) is the most common aggressive B-cell non-Hodgkin lymphoma and is molecularly heterogeneous. Gene expression profiling (GEP) classifies DLBCL into germinal-center B-cell-like (GCB), activated B-cell-like (ABC), and unclassifiable types. However, recently, many research groups have grouped DLBCL using various algorithms. They have distinct genetic alterations and prognostic implications. There are overlaps in these research groups indicating that subtypes do exist. It is vital to understand the key pathways such as BCR signaling, PI3K-AKT-mTOR, NF-κB, and antiapoptotic BCL2 signaling, contributing to tumor survival and progression. Advancement in GEP testing has yielded groups such as "Dark-zone signature" and "molecular high-grade" within DLBCL which have poor prognosis. Tailored targeted therapy coupled with immunochemotherapy with improved outcome are available for genetic subtypes of DLBCL.

INTRODUCTION

Diffuse large B-cell lymphoma (DLBCL) is one of the most common aggressive B-cell non-Hodgkin lymphomas. It is a heterogeneous disease at a molecular level. Gene expression profiling (GEP) studies categorize into three groups: (1) Germinal-center B-cell-like (GCB), (2) activated B-cell-like (ABC), and (3) unclassifiable type (UC). 15–20% cases are grouped in UC type if they do not fit into these two categories (Rosenwald et al., 2002). Since GEP is not widely available, many immunohistochemistry algorithms, including he Hans classifier, exist to classify them into their cell of origin, providing prognostic value. However, despite improvement in DLBCL treatment, around 30–40% of cases relapse. This chapter summarizes the various molecular subgroups of DLBCL, not otherwise specified (NOS), and its major signaling pathways and therapeutic implications **(Fig. 1)**.

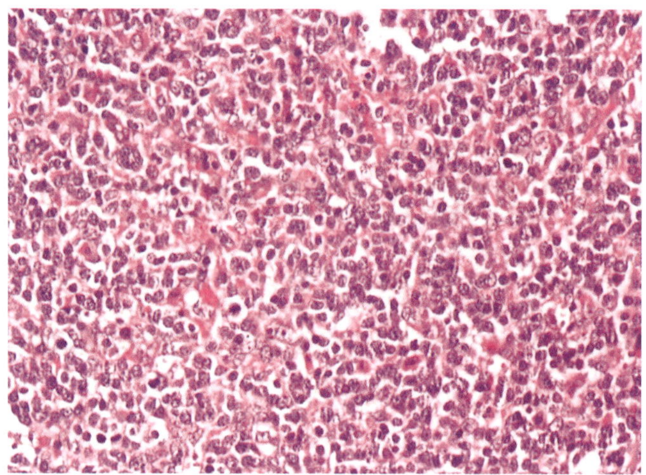

FIG. 1: Morphology of diffuse large B-cell lymphoma, not otherwise specified (NOS) brief.

OVERVIEW OF ALTERATIONS AND CYTOGENETIC CHANGES IN DIFFUSE LARGE B-CELL LYMPHOMA

The genomic alterations in DLBCL, NOS vary with the cell of origin. GCB subtype has histone methylation and acetylation mutations such as *EZH2, EP300, KMT2D,* and genes involving the PIK3 signaling pathway. ABC subtype has frequent mutations in *MYD88, CD79A/B,* and *BCL10* involving the NF-κB pathway and *BLIMP1* mutation. Around 20–30% of cases show *IGH-BCL2* translocation. *BCL6* (3q27) rearrangement is seen in 19–30% cases. *MYC* rearrangement is seen in around 10% of cases carrying adverse prognostic factors and poor outcomes.

MOLECULAR CLASSIFICATION OF DIFFUSE LARGE B-CELL LYMPHOMA

Next-generation sequencing (NGS) of large case numbers of DLBCL has led many author groups to classify DLBCL by novel algorithm/clustering methodologies. *Schmitz et al.* (2018) classified DLBCL into *four subtypes* as MCD (*MYD88*^{L265P} and *CD79B* mutation), BN2 (*BCL6* fusions and *NOTCH2* mutations), N1 (*NOTCH1* mutations), and EZB (based on *EZH2* mutations and *BCL2* translocations) using exome and transcriptome sequencing, DNA copy-number analysis, and targeted amplicon sequencing. There was better outcome in the BN2 and EZB subtypes and inferior survival in the MCD and N1 subtypes.

Wright et al. (2020) with addition of *TP53, TET2, P2RY8, and SGK1* mutations into *six genetic subtypes* that included "MCD (*MYD88* and *CD79B* mutation), BN2 (*BCL6* fusion and *NOTCH2* mutations), N1 (*NOTCH1* mutation), EZB (*EZH2* mutation and *BCL2* translocation), A53 (aneuploid with *TP53* inactivation), ST2 (*SGK1* and *TET2* mutated). In addition, there were composite and unclassifiable groups. A53 carried worse prognosis whereas N1 and MCD were identified mostly in ABC phenotype. ST2 and EZB were seen mostly in GCB cases.

Chapuy et al. (2018) did a comprehensive genetic analysis of 304 cases of DLBCL by whole exome sequencing and identified recurrent mutations, genetic alterations, structural variants, and integrated them into *five major clusters* (C1–C5) and one minor cluster 0 lacking specific driver mutation. Cluster 1 carries somatic variations of *BCL-6,* alterations in NOTCH-2 signaling pathway. There are mutations in *BCL10, TNFAIP3, FAS, B2M,* and CD70. C1 was predominantly classified as ABC subtype. Cluster 2 is characterized by inactivation of *TP53,* loss of *17p, CDKN2A,* and *RB1*. Cluster 3 has somatic variations of *BCL-2,* inactivation mutation and/or copy loss of *PTEN.* Cluster 4 has alterations in histone genes and JAK/STAT pathways. In cluster 5 there is *18q* gain, *MYD88*^{L265P}, and *CD79B* mutation. The majority of the patients in this cluster 5 had systemic DLBCL with testicular involvement indicating extra nodal tropism and similarity to MCD group by Schmitz et al. C1 and C4 had better outcomes while C3 and C5 had unfavorable outcomes. These signatures also predicted prognosis independent of the international prognostic index.

Lacy et al. (2020) identified *five molecular subtypes,* termed *MYD88, BCL2, SOCS1/SGK1, TET2/SGK1,* and *NOTCH2,* along with an unclassified group. Alterations in *BCL2* group have good prognosis while *NOTCH2* had intermediate prognosis and *MYD88* has poor prognosis. The *SOCS1/SGK1* subtype showed biological overlap with primary mediastinal B-cell lymphoma and had best prognosis.

As we can see from the aforementioned discussion, there are overlaps within many groups, indicating that molecular subtypes do exist in DLBCL **(Fig. 2)**.

Method of Testing in Given Studies

It is important to understand the approach, testing methods, and analysis in the aforementioned studies. There can be variability in the sample, study population, sequencing strategy, variant calling, and annotation algorithms leading to differences. For example, Chapuy et al. used whole exome sequencing

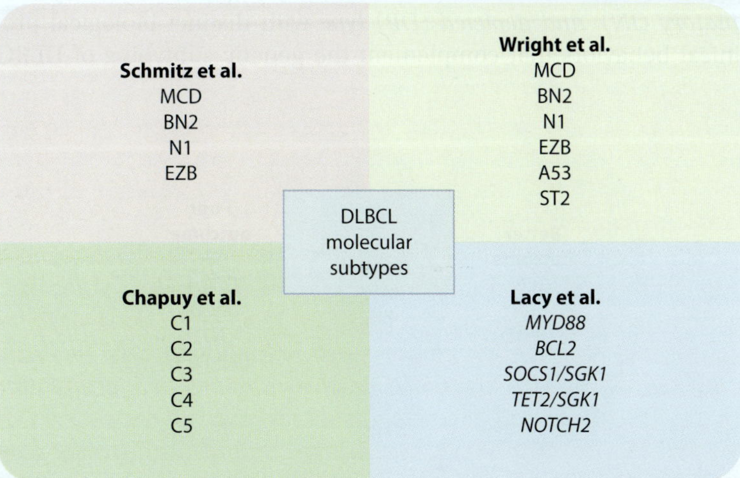

FIG. 2: Molecular subtypes of diffuse large B-cell lymphoma (DLBCL).

Note: For alterations and mutations in the individual group, refer to the paragraph above.

in detecting mutations, mutational signature, chromosomal rearrangement, somatic copy number alterations, and structural variants whereas Lacy et al. used targeted sequencing which lacked *BCL6* fusion data and did not have common copy number analysis and single nucleotide variants with Chapuy et al. leading to discordance in identifying TP53 group in the later. Likewise, LymphGen classifier algorithm cannot predict the classes if the data lacks *BCL2, BCL6* rearrangement data. Thus, to achieve a comprehensive classification, the entire data needs to be available.

ADVANCES ON GENE EXPRESSION-BASED CLASSIFICATION AND INTERPLAY BETWEEN CELL OF ORIGIN AND GENETICS

Recently, the British Columbia group (David Scott et al.) identified GEP double-hit signature in a subset of GCB DLBCLs (lacking *CMYC/BCL2* rearrangement) and Burkitt lymphoma labeling them as *dark-zone signature*. These cases have shorter overall survival, and a shorter diagnosis-treatment interval compared to GCB DLBCL lacking this signature. On a related note, another author has reported "molecular high-grade signature" within DLBCL. These subgroups within DLBCL which may require intense treatment. Within the molecular groups, EZB and ST2 are always GCB-DLBCL while N1 and MCD are ABC type. BN2 group is unclassifiable. Thus, ideally, in all cases of DLBCL, wherever possible, the refined cell of origin (COO) classification needs to be studied in addition to the genetics mentioned earlier **(Fig. 3)**.

MICROENVIRONMENT IN DIFFUSE LARGE B-CELL LYMPHOMA

Transcriptomic analysis of DLBCL has identified four lymphoma microenvironmental (LME) signatures. *Germinal center-like (GC), mesenchymal (MS), inflammatory (IN), and depleted (DP) type* with distinct biological properties and clinical behaviors that complement the genetic subtyping of DLBCL. The

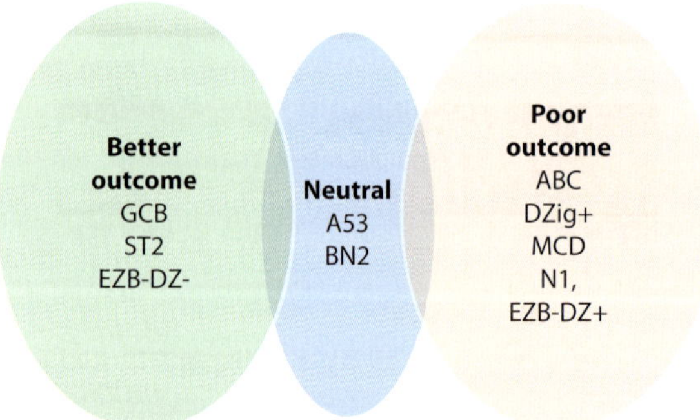

FIG. 3: Outcome of various groups of diffuse large B-cell lymphoma (DLBCL) with R-CHOP (Hilton et al.).

(R-CHOP: cyclophosphamide, doxorubicin, prednisolone and rituximab)

classification was based on the gene expression signature (GES) of the predominant cells found in germinal center, extracellular matrix, and inflammatory cells. The depleted type lacked GES compared to the other types. High grade B-cell lymphoma with *MYC* and *BCL2* rearrangement showed better outcome with GC and MS LMEs compared to IN and DP LMEs. This study highlights the need for personalized treatment and targeted therapy addressing the LME in addition to the genetic subtypes.

Spatial proteomics study in DLBCL has identified three immune microenvironments such as *immune-deficient, dendritic-cell enriched, and macrophage-enriched regions.* In the first group, there is paucity of immune cells with predominance of tumor cells lying distant from blood vessels. In the other group, immune cell-rich areas were found close to blood vessels. Cases with macrophage-enriched regions were identified frequently in DLBCL genetic subgroup with immune evasion. Thus, this variation in the microenvironment leads to variable therapy response to immunotherapy and chimeric antigen receptor T-cell therapy.

■ HIGH GRADE B-CELL LYMPHOMA AND ROLE OF FLUORESCENCE IN SITU HYBRIDIZATION

High grade B cell lymphoma (HGBCL) is an aggressive mature B-cell lymphoma. It is classified as HGBCL with *MYC* and *BCL2* rearrangements (HGBCL-*MYC/BCL2*) and NOS category if it lacks this specific molecular alteration. This category has variable morphology, with DLBCL being the most common. Others include morphology intermediate between DLBCL and Burkitt lymphoma, blastoid resembling lymphoblasts collectively grouped as "Intermediate/blastoid." Lymphoblastic lymphoma, blastoid variant of Mantle cell lymphoma needs to be excluded by relevant immunostaining. For identification of these cases, a sequential strategy of fluorescence in situ hybridization (FISH) testing of *MYC* followed by *BCL2* (and *BCL6*) rearrangement status, and *MYC* translocation partner is advised (refer to **Figs. 4 and 5**). Although there is no current predictive

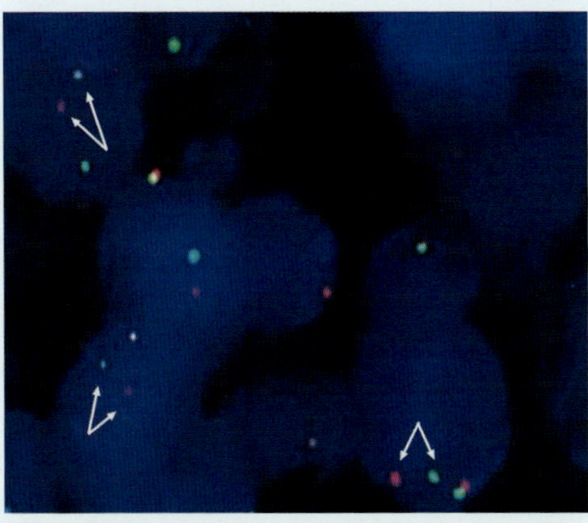

FIG. 4: *MYC* rearrangement using break apart fluorescence in situ hybridization (FISH) (arrows indicating one green and one red split signal).

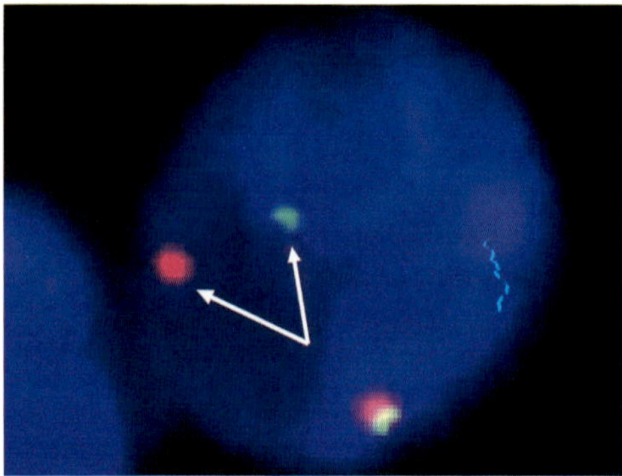

FIG. 5: *BCL2* rearrangement using break apart fluorescence in situ hybridization (FISH) (arrows indicating one green and one red split signal).

immunohistochemical screening tool for identifying these cases, strong MYC expression in > 70% cells is highly predictive. It is important to note that DLBCL/HGBCL with *MYC* and *BCL6* translocations, but lacking *BCL2* translocation, has a distinct presentation, ABC-like gene expression profile, different mutation spectrum it is excluded from this entity and placed in DLBCL, NOS category. In the molecular classification, HGBCL-*MYC/BCL2* belongs to EZB cluster, C3 cluster, or BCL2 cluster while the HGBCL, NOS, in most cases, belong to the unclassified category.

MAJOR SIGNALING PATHWAYS AFFECTED BY GENETIC ALTERATIONS

B-cell receptor (BCR) signaling: The BCR pathway regulates B-cell survival, development, and differentiation. Chronic active or tonic BCR signaling contributes to lymphomagenesis. Loss of function in negative regulators leads to unchecked BCR activation, seen in 38.5% of DLBCL cases. This is more common in *MYD88*-mutated cases with *CD79A/CD79B* activating mutations (56%) compared to MYD88—wildtype cases (36.4%). Such mutations, associated with chronic active BCR signaling, show sensitivity to ibrutinib, a Bruton's tyrosine kinase inhibitor.

PI3K-AKT-mTOR pathway: Altered in 34.3% of DLBCL cases, PI3K indirectly activates the NF-κB pathway and directly promotes target of rapamycin (mTOR) signaling, driving cell proliferation, and tumor progression. Activating mutations in PI3K subunits (e.g., *PIK3CA*) are seen in 6% of ABC DLBCL cases, while PTEN deletions are found in both ABC and GCB subtypes (9–11%).

*BCR-dependent NF-*κB *activation:* In the BN2 subtype, components such as PKCB and *BCL10* of the BCR-dependent NF-κB pathway are altered in 47% of cases.

*NF-*κB *signaling*: Activating mutations in positive regulators (e.g., *TLR2, MYD88*) or inactivation of negative regulators (e.g., *TNIP1, TNFAIP3*) lead to persistent NF-κB activation. In the BN2 subtype, 55% of cases show alterations in negative regulators like *TNFAIP3 or TNIP1*.

Toll-like receptor (TLR2) signaling: TLR2 signaling is mediated by *MYD88* and the IRAK1/4 complex.

MYD88 mutations are common in aggressive DLBCL subtypes.

Antiapoptotic BCL2 family: Mutations in the *BCL2* family, such as the t(14;18) (q32;q21) translocation, occur in 34–44% of GCB DLBCL cases cause constitutive BCL2 activation, promoting tumor survival.

ALTERATIONS IN SPECIFIC SITES

Large B-cell lymphomas of immune-privileged sites occurring in central nervous system, testis, vitreo-retina have frequent mutations in *MYD88* and *CD79B* (MCD)/cluster 5 leading to immune evasion by multiple mechanisms.

Primary mediastinal large B-cell lymphoma—multiple pathways like JAK-STAT, immune evasion, NF-κB are affected. There can be amplification of PD-L1, PD-L2, and mutations in *STAT6, IL4R* have been identified.

Large B-cell lymphoma with IRF4 rearrangement—there is alteration in the *CARD11, CD79B,* and *MYD88* genes involving NF-κB pathway along with loss of 17p13 and gains of chromosome 7.

Primary cutaneous diffuse large B-cell lymphoma, leg type—mutation in *MYD88*, TNFAIP3, and B-cell receptor pathway genes (*CD79A, CD79B, and CARD11*) are identified.

IMPLICATION OF CLASSIFICATION IN TREATMENT DECISION

There are trials (Zhang et al.—GUIDANCE-01 trial) which have combined genetic and microenvironment data with the specific targeted therapy with R-CHOP (cyclophosphamide, doxorubicin, prednisolone and rituximab) demonstrating improvement in response rate and 2-year survival compared to standalone R-CHOP therapy. It has included R-CHOP with ibrutinib for MCD-like and BN2-like group; R-CHOP with lenalidomide for N1-like group; R-CHOP with tucidinostat for EZB-like group; R-CHOP with decitabine for TP53 mutant group and R-CHOP with lenalidomide for NOS group.

Take Home Points

- *Molecular subtypes:* Multiple studies have proven that distinct genetic subtypes exist in DLBCL.
- *Mutations and prognosis*: The refined "cell of origin" testing coupled with genetic subtype testing can provide prognostic value and guide treatment decisions.
- *Mutations and therapy:* Clinical trials incorporating targeted therapies coupled with R-CHOP have given promising results indicating the need for genetic classification driven treatment strategies for DLBCL.

SUGGESTED READINGS

1. Schmitz R, Wright GW, Huang DW, Johnson CA, Phelan JD, Wang JQ, et al. Genetics and pathogenesis of diffuse large B-cell lymphoma. N Engl J Med. 2018;378(15):1396-407.
2. Wright GW, Huang DW, Phelan JD, Coulibaly ZA, Roulland S, Young RM, et al. A probabilistic classification tool for genetic subtypes of diffuse large B-cell lymphoma with therapeutic implications. Cancer Cell. 2020;37(4):551-68.e14.
3. Chapuy B, Stewart C, Dunford AJ, Kim J, Kamburov A, Redd RA, et al. Molecular subtypes of diffuse large B cell lymphoma are associated with distinct pathogenic mechanisms and outcomes. Nat Med. 2018;24(5):679-90.
4. Lacy SE, Barrans SL, Beer PA, Painter D, Smith AG, Roman E, et al. Targeted sequencing in DLBCL, molecular subtypes, and outcomes: a Haematological Malignancy Research Network report. Blood. 2020;135(20):1759-71.
5. Onaindia A, Santiago-Quispe N, Iglesias-Martinez E, Romero-Abrio C. Molecular Update and Evolving Classification of Large B-Cell Lymphoma. Cancers (Basel). 2021;13(13):3352.
6. Hilton LK, Scott DW, Morin RD. Biological heterogeneity in diffuse large B-cell lymphoma. Semin Hematol. 2023;60(5):267-76.
7. Alduaij W, Collinge B, Ben-Neriah S, Jiang A, Hilton LK, Boyle M, et al. Molecular determinants of clinical outcomes in a real-world diffuse large B-cell lymphoma population. Blood. 2023;141(20):2493-507.
8. Zhang MC, Tian S, Fu D, Wang L, Cheng S, Yi HM, et al Genetic subtype-guided immunochemotherapy in diffuse large B cell lymphoma: The randomized GUIDANCE-01 trial. Cancer Cell. 2023;41(10):1705-16.e5

CHAPTER 8

B-ALL Management in the Era of Immunotherapy

Sanjeev Kumar Sharma, Anamika Bakliwal

ABSTRACT

Acute lymphoblastic leukemia (ALL) is considered an aggressive leukemia and is the most common hematological malignancy in pediatric population. The multiagent chemotherapy has significantly improved the survival of children with ALL, though high-risk patients are still at risk of relapse. In adults, B-ALL is a very heterogeneous disease, with increasing age associated with poorer survival. The adults are also treated with pediatric-inspired protocols, though tolerance is a major issue. Treatment of older adults or the elderly is difficult and is associated with a high risk of relapse. Stem cell transplantation (SCT) is reserved for high-risk patients and those with relapsed or refractory disease. The introduction of novel agents has revolutionized the treatment of B-cell ALL. These novel treatment options include inotuzumab, blinatumomab, and chimeric antigen receptor T-cell (CAR-T) cell therapy.

INTRODUCTION

The ALL is a hematological malignancy that results from uncontrolled proliferation of lymphoid precursors. The ALL has an excellent prognosis in children, whereas in adults, the prognosis remains poor. Specific subgroups of ALL such as Philadelphia (Ph+) ALL and Ph-like ALL are being treated with molecularly targeted agents; however, most of them lack a suitable antigen that can be targeted. Many immunotherapeutic agents have been developed for the treatment of relapsed/refractory (R/R) ALL and will improve the survival of these patients.

The chemotherapy for ALL usually consists of four phases—induction, consolidation, and intensification, followed by long-term maintenance. Central nervous system (CNS) prophylaxis is given to prevent relapse in CNS. Allogeneic SCT is reserved for high risk and for relapsed and refractory cases.

The broad expression of CD19 and CD22 on B-cell precursor (BCP)-ALL blasts make them an attractive therapeutic target. In contrast, CD20 is expressed universally on mature B cells and less commonly on B-precursor cells, with 30–50% of BCP-ALL cases having CD20 expression on >20% of blasts. The recent development of targeted therapies, including bi-specific antibodies, antibody-drug conjugates, and CD19 CAR-T cell therapy, has revolutionized B-ALL management. CAR-T therapy is a form of adoptive T-cell immunotherapy, which is based on the infusion of genetically modified T cells that can persist in vivo for a long duration, providing long-term disease control.

Measurable residual disease (MRD) in ALL has become one of the most important tools for remission assessment and treatment strategy. It is defined as the presence of blasts that are not detectable by routine microscopy but may be measured by standardized methods such as flow cytometry, polymerase chain reaction (PCR), and next-generation sequencing (NGS) with a sensitivity of 10^{-4} (i.e., 0.01%) or more. The significance of MRD lies in the fact that if a patient has low but measurable disease after remission induction, then preemptive treatment may prolong overall survival (OS) compared with treatment of overt relapse. MRD persistence indicates resistance to standard chemotherapy and is a significant risk factor for overt relapse. Postinduction MRD persistence may be seen in 30–40% of patients with complete hematologic remission. Based on these findings, MRD eradication has become the goal in patients with B-cell ALL. Nearly all guidelines recommend including MRD assessment in routine clinical practice. The persistence of MRD-positive disease after conventional chemotherapy protocols is a major issue in the management of ALL and results in high relapse rates with continued chemotherapy and even after subsequent SCT.

The time point of MRD assessment is still debatable, with NCCN guidelines suggesting MRD evaluation over the course of sequential phases of therapy (at the end of induction, consolidation, and as a part of surveillance). The European Society for Medical Oncology (ESMO) ALL guidelines recommend MRD monitoring after consolidation to guide the decision of chemotherapy or allo-SCT. The Berlin–Frankfurt–Münster (BFM) ALL 2009 suggests MRD assessment on day 15 of induction chemotherapy in pediatric ALL. With the availability of newer and targeted agents, MRD-positive patients can be converted to MRD-negative, who can then become eligible for allo-SCT. In older patients who are not fit for myeloablative SCT, either reduced intensity conditioning SCT or consolidation or maintenance therapy can be considered.

The treatment of R/R B-ALL patients (Ph+ and Ph–) include:

- *Early relapse or late first relapse*: These patients are initially treated with systemic therapy. If patients achieve second complete remission (CR2) and are MRD-negativity, the options include further chemotherapy or maintenance therapy or allo-SCT. In the case of MRD positivity or if the patient relapses after a prior allo-SCT, the options include chemotherapy, blinatumomab, inotuzumab, CAR-T cell therapy, or second allo-SCT.
- *Multiple relapses*: For patients who have relapsed multiple times, the treatment is challenging and depends upon previous therapies received and the duration of remission by such therapies. Treatment options include chemotherapy, inotuzumab, blinatumomab, CAR-T cell therapy or allo-SCT.

- In R/R Ph+ B-ALL patients [adolescent and young adults (AYA), and adults], after evaluating for ABL1 kinase domain mutation, the treatment includes:
  - Tyrosine kinase inhibitor (TKI) with or without chemotherapy followed by allo-SCT.
  - Blinatumomab with or without TKI followed by allo-SCT.
  - Inotuzumab with or without TKI followed by allo-SCT.
  - CAR-T cell therapy with or without allo-SCT.
- Ph-R/R B-ALL patients can be treated by blinatumomab, inotuzumab, CAR-T cell therapy, or chemotherapy and may be considered for allo-SCT.

CASE 1

A 6-year-old child was diagnosed with a case of B-cell acute lymphoblastic leukemia (B-ALL). He was treated with BFM-2009 protocol and achieved measurable residual disease (MRD)-negative remission and completed further treatment. He, however, relapsed with MRD positivity at the end of treatment. He was planned for salvage chemotherapy followed by allogeneic stem cell transplant (allo-SCT). Which novel agents should be used in salvage chemotherapy?

CASE 2

A 54-year-old male presented with fever and weakness and, on evaluation, was found to have low white cell count and low platelets. His bone marrow examination revealed acute leukemia, and flow cytometry showed B-ALL, with blasts showing positivity for CD19, CD20, and sCD22. His cytogenetics revealed hypodiploidy. He was given rituximab-hyper-CVAD protocol and achieved remission, but had morphological relapse 6 months later. What are the treatment options for him? Should he be considered for blinatumomab, inotuzumab, or rituximab-based therapy followed by allo-SCT or chimeric antigen receptor T-cell (CAR-T) cell therapy?

BLINATUMOMAB

Blinatumomab is a bispecific T-cell engager with an anti-CD19–directed CD3 bi-specific T-cell engager (BiTE) antibody. Patients with measurable residual disease (MRD)-positive chemotherapy-resistant ALL treated with blinatumomab achieved a significant molecular response (MRD negativity) and improved disease-free outcomes among responders compared with nonresponders. Compared to conventional chemotherapy, blinatumomab has a relatively better safety profile, and this is particularly important for older ALL patients where toxicity is a significant limitation for administering chemotherapy. The inclusion of novel targeted agents such as blinatumomab and inotuzumab has allowed the de-escalation of conventional chemotherapy regimens, particularly in older adults, and could improve the poorer long-term survival in this age group. The limitation of blinatumomab is that it is not an optimal choice for patients with relapsed ALL with bulky extramedullary disease and those with central nervous system (CNS) involvement. Blinatumomab administration requires continuous intravenous infusion over 4 weeks. The side effects of blinatumomab include cytokine release syndrome (CRS), pancreatitis, and neurological toxicities.

INOTUZUMAB OZOGAMICIN

Another important target on B cells is CD22, and, like CD19, it plays an important role in B-cell activation and regulation and is present in > 90% of patients with B-ALL. Inotuzumab ozogamicin is a humanized antibody-drug conjugate, consisting of an antibody directed toward cell-surface glycoprotein CD22, and a cytotoxin calicheamicin, derived from micromonospora. The immunoglobulin (Ig)G antibody binds to CD22 on surface of leukemic blasts, resulting in internalization of the antibody-cytotoxin complex into the cell, where calicheamicin intermediate induces breaks in double stranded deoxyribonucleic acid (DNA) and results in apoptosis of sCD22 bearing cells.

Inotuzumab has shown significant activity in relapsed/refractory (R/R) B-cell ALL when used as either a single agent or in combination with chemotherapeutic agents in both adult and pediatric trials. Though single-agent inotuzumab therapy has shown a therapeutic advantage for patients with relapsed/refractory (R/R) ALL, it is not curative, with < 20% of patients achieving long-term survival. Therefore, inotuzumab is combined with chemotherapy and/or blinatumomab with the goal of increasing the depth of response and, thus, the survival outcomes.

In a study, inotuzumab resulted in a rate of complete remission/incomplete complete remission (CR/Cri) of 81% versus 33% after standard salvage chemotherapy. Among those who responded, the rate of MRD negativity was about 78% in the inotuzumab group versus 29% in the control group. Hepatic adverse events were common in the inotuzumab group, with about 11% incidence of sinusoidal obstruction syndrome (SOS) versus 1% in the control group respectively.

Other than hepatic SOS, the toxicities of inotuzumab include marrow suppression and B-cell aplasia, which increases the risk of infection, particularly when used with combination chemotherapy. To overcome the SOS-related toxicity with inotuzumab in stem cell transplant (SCT) patients, it is suggested to avoid dual alkylator conditioning regimens, avoid azole or other known hepatotoxic agents, and use prophylactic ursodiol. Furthermore, if a patient is planned for SCT, it is recommended to administer only up to two cycles of inotuzumab to reduce the risk of hepatic SOS.

CHIMERIC ANTIGEN RECEPTOR T-CELL THERAPY

Chimeric antigen receptor T cell (CAR-T cell) is a form of modified adoptive cell-based immunotherapy that in principle includes transfer of engineered effector T cells to generate immune effector response to kill targeted leukemic cells, therefore offering long-term disease control. CAR-T cell killing of cancer cells is a human leukocyte antigen (HLA)-independent process, unlike native T-cell approach, which recognizes major histocompatibility complex molecules that are often downregulated by cancer cells. The first FDA approved anti-CD19 CAR-T cell product was tisagenlecleucel for B-ALL.

Chimeric Antigen Receptor-T Cell Biology, Manufacturing, and Delivery

T cells are harvested from the patient by leukapheresis. They are then re-engineered ex vivo to acquire monoclonal antibody recognition fragment, specific for the target. After re-engineering and expansion in culture, the cells are shipped to the patient bedside and reinfused. Prior to reinfusion, patients are subjected to lymphodepletion with chemotherapy, such as fludarabine and cyclophosphamide. Once infused, CARs are widely distributed throughout the body, including the CNS, which makes them a promising option for extramedullary relapse. CAR-T cell therapy has obviated the need for SCT in some patients, however, relapses can happen even after CAR-T cell therapy because of antigen escape or downregulation, lack of infused CAR-T cell persistence or T-cell exhaustion.

Adverse Effects of Chimeric Antigen Receptor-T Cell Therapy

Though CAR-T cells infused are autologous, this T-cell therapy is not without side effects. Most of the side effects are self-limited, but severe and life-threatening toxicities can develop with CAR-T cell therapy. The common and potentially severe toxicities include CRS and immune effector cell associated neurotoxicity syndrome (ICANS). CRS manifests as fever and hypotension whereas ICANS is characterized by global encephalopathy, but can also manifest as aphasia, confusion, focal neurological deficits and less often, seizures. Tocilizumab, a humanized anti-interleukin (IL)6 receptor antibody, has been used for the treatment of CRS related toxicity. Other side effects include cytopenias, B-cell aplasia and CAR-T cell associated hemophagocytic lymphohistiocytosis (HLH).

TREATMENT OF POST STEM CELL TRANSPLANT RELAPSED B-CELL ACUTE LYMPHOBLASTIC LEUKEMIA

The B-ALL relapsing after allo-SCT is associated with very poor prognosis. The advents of targeted immunotherapies and CAR-T cell therapy have improved the survival of such patients. It has been seen that patients with relapsed ALL with or without prior allo-SCT respond equally well to blinatumomab, suggesting that blinatumomab maintains its activity independent of previous allo-SCT. Inotuzumab has also been shown to induce remission in such patients. Similarly, studies with CD19 CAR T-cell therapy have shown remarkable response in patients with R/R ALL irrespective of prior allo-SCT. Therefore, both CD19-targeted immunotherapies are valid for relapse after allo-SCT.

HOW TO DECIDE ABOUT THE USE OF NOVEL AGENTS?

Many points need consideration when deciding on which novel agent to use in the management of B-cell ALL. These include the number of prior relapses, disease burden (MRD positivity or frank hematological relapse), sites of disease relapse (medullary or extramedullary), prior therapies including SCT, comorbidities, tolerability to current and previous therapies, toxicities, and remaining therapeutic options. If a patient has received prior immunotherapy or has CD19, CD20, or

CD22-negative blasts, then the treatment will be based on subsequent available options, accordingly. For high disease burden, inotuzumab with chemotherapy is the preferred option, followed by consolidation or maintenance inotuzumab or blinatumumab. If there is only MRD relapse, then the use of blinatumomab may be the primary strategy.

Patients with MRD-positive relapse after intensive reinduction can be treated with blinatumomab along with the continuation of conventional chemotherapy. Blinatumomab consolidation can also be considered as a bridge to SCT. Such patients also have the option of tisagenlecleucel (CAR-T) either as a stand-alone therapy or as a bridge to SCT. Blinatumomab has no benefit in patients with isolated extramedullary disease and therefore lacks efficacy for treatment or prophylaxis of CNS leukemia. Similarly, inotuzumab is also unable to cross the blood-brain barrier and is ineffective for CNS leukemia, though it has some activity against non-CNS extramedullary disease. For such patients, CAR-T therapy is effective as it has significant activity for CNS and other extramedullary diseases and is a preferred treatment approach.

While using subsequent targeted therapies, prior therapies should also be taken into consideration; for example, the use of blinatumomab prior to tisagenlecleucel should be avoided. Both these agents target the same antigen (CD19) and use of blinatumomab may risk the downregulation of CD19 that could impact the efficacy of tisagenlecleucel (CD19 CAR-T). Such patients can be treated with inotuzumab (targeting CD22) as a bridging agent for whom consolidation with tisagenlecleucel is planned since it targets a different antigen. Another important consideration in patients with relapsed disease is the bulk of disease, as inotuzumab is effective in the setting of high disease burden, whereas tisagenlecleucel and blinatumomab work better when used in low disease burden or in MRD settings, which suggests an important role for Inotuzumab in initial debulking.

Cases 1 and 2

The child was treated with one cycle of inotuzumab and then underwent allo-SCT. He developed low-grade SOS which was effectively managed, and the child completely recovered and is well 6 months post-SCT with MRD-negative disease. The second case was treated with inotuzumab-mini-hyper CVD and achieved MDR negativity. He later underwent CD19-CAR-T cell therapy and is in molecular remission 8 months post CAR-T cell therapy.

Take Home Points

- The use of targeted novel immunotherapeutics has led to significant advances in the treatment of R/R B-ALL. The introduction of inotuzumab, blinatumumab, and CAR-T cell therapy has revolutionized the management of relapsed and refractory ALL. In near future these agents will be included in the frontline therapy.
- These immunotherapeutic agents are associated with a unique spectrum of side-effects. The role of stem cell transplantation seems to be reducing.
- Despite the success of immunotherapy, resistance can develop to these novel approaches and mechanisms to mitigate tumor escape are needed.

SUGGESTED READINGS

1. Brown PA, Shah B, Advani A, Aoun P, Boyer MV, Burke PW, et al. Acute lymphoblastic leukemia, version 2.2021, NCCN clinical practice guidelines in oncology. J Natl Compr Canc Netw. 2021;19(9):1079-109.
2. Hoelzer D, Bassan R, Boissel N, Roddie C, Ribera JM, Jerkeman M. ESMO Clinical Practice Guideline interim update on the use of targeted therapy in acute lymphoblastic leukaemia. Ann Oncol. 2024;35(1):15-28.
3. Gökbuget N, Boissel N, Chiaretti S, Dombret H, Doubek M, Fielding A, et al. Management of ALL in adults: 2024 ELN recommendations from a European expert panel. Blood. 2024;143(19):1903-30.
4. Gokbuget N, Dombret H, Bonifacio M, Reichle A, Graux C, Faul C, et al. Blinatumomab for minimal residual disease in adults with B-cell precursor acute lymphoblastic leukemia. Blood. 2018;131(14):1522-31.
5. Kantarjian HM, DeAngelo DJ, Stelljes M, Liedtke M, Stock W, Gökbuget N, et al. Inotuzumab ozogamicin versus standard of care in relapsed or refractory acute lymphoblastic leukemia: Final report and long-term survival follow-up from the randomized, phase 3 INO-VATE study. Cancer. 2019;125(14):2474-87.
6. Kansagra AJ, Frey NV, Bar M, Laetsch TW, Carpenter PA, Savani BN, et al. Clinical utilization of Chimeric Antigen Receptor T-cells (CAR-T) in B-cell acute lymphoblastic leukemia (ALL)-an expert opinion from the European Society for Blood and Marrow Transplantation (EBMT) and the American Society for Blood and Marrow Transplantation (ASBMT). Bone Marrow Transplant. 2019;54(11):1868-80.
7. Hayden PJ, Roddie C, Bader P, Basak GW, Bonig H, Bonini C, et al. Management of adults and children receiving CAR T-cell therapy: 2021 best practice recommendations of the European Society for Blood and Marrow Transplantation (EBMT) and the Joint Accreditation Committee of ISCT and EBMT (JACIE) and the European Haematology Association (EHA). Ann Oncol. 2022;33(3):259-75.
8. Rubinstein JD, O'Brien MM. Inotuzumab ozogamicin in B-cell precursor acute lymphoblastic leukemia: efficacy, toxicity, and practical considerations. Front Immunol. 2023;14:1237738.
9. Sharma SK. What a Clinical Hematologist Should Know about B Cells?. International Blood Research & Reviews. 2022;13(1):8-22.
10. Sharma SK. Stem Cell Transplant for Acute Lymphoblastic Leukemia. In: Basics of Hematopoietic Stem Cell Transplant. Springer; 2023. pp.479-500.

CHAPTER 9

Diagnosis of Ph-like B-ALL: The Ideal Approach in the Indian Setting

Sanjeev Kumar Gupta, Gadha Krishna Leons

ABSTRACT

"*BCR::ABL1*-like acute lymphoblastic leukemia (ALL)" or "Philadelphia-like ALL" (Ph-like ALL) is a genetically heterogeneous group of disorder comprising of entities with a genetic profile similar to *BCR::ABL1* positive B-cell ALL (B-ALL), in absence of positivity for the *BCR::ABL1* fusion. This entity has been identified using the high throughput genomics and gene expression profiling and included as a genetic subtype of B-ALL in the World Health Organization (WHO)-HAEM5 classification of hematolymphoid tumors and the International Consensus Classification. Ph-like ALL cases may not get detected in the initial genetic evaluation of B-ALL for common recurrent translocations and aneuploidies, with karyotyping, fluorescence in-situ hybridization (FISH), reverse transcription polymerase chain reaction (RT-PCR), flow cytometry for DNA ploidy, etc. However, a careful evaluation of the remaining genetically unclassified cases, usually labelled as "B-other ALL", using different techniques such as FISH break-apart probes, RT-PCR for known Ph-like fusions, flow-based cytokine receptor like factor 2 (*CRLF2)/* thymic stromal lymphopoietin receptor *(TSLPR*) overexpression screening, multiplex ligation dependent probe amplification (MLPA) for IKZF1 deletions, targeted RNA sequencing, whole transcriptome sequencing along with the machine learning based genetic classifiers, would be helpful in the detection of most of the B-ALL cases with *BCR::ABL1*-like features.

INTRODUCTION

B-cell acute lymphoblastic leukemia (B-ALL) is a genetically heterogeneous disorder with the wide spectrum of genetic aberrations including recurrent chromosomal translocations like *BCR::ABL1,* aneuploidies, gene copy number alterations and mutations etc. *BCR::ABL1-like ALL or Philadelphia-like ALL (Ph-like ALL)* is a subtype of *BCR::ABL1*-negative B-ALL characterized by DNA alterations resulting in a phenotype similar to that of *BCR::ABL1*-positive B-ALL but lacking the *BCR::ABL1* rearrangement. This entity was simultaneously and independently identified by two groups—Children's Oncology Group (COG)-TARGET-St. Jude consortium and Dutch Childhood Oncology Group in 2009, with overlapping, yet different gene expression signature profiles.

The Ph-like ALL was identified as a clinically important category with aggressive course and was included as a provisional entity in the WHO classification (2016) of B-ALL. Recently, it has been upgraded to a full entity in the WHO-HAEM5 (2022) classification and also included in the International Consensus Classification (ICC) (2022) of B-ALL.

PREVALENCE

The prevalence of Ph-like ALL increases with age and is reported in 10–15% of children, 20% of adolescents, peaks at 25–30% of young adults (21–39 years), 20–25% of adults (>40 years) with B-ALL. Its prevalence is more common in males, Hispanics, and high-risk group patients with higher total leukocyte count (TLC). The frequency reported from India is 9–26% in different studies, depending upon the technique used and the patient profiles.

SUBTYPES OF Ph-LIKE ACUTE LYMPHOBLASTIC LEUKEMIA

Ph-like ALL is genetically heterogeneous and this heterogeneity in the genomic landscape of Ph-like ALL has created a diagnostic challenge for hematopathologists as well as treating physicians. Most of these patients (> 90%) have genomic rearrangements that activate tyrosine kinase or cytokine receptor signaling pathways including that of *ABL1, ABL2, colony stimulating factor 1 receptor (CSF1R), platelet derived growth factor receptor beta (PDGFRB), cytokine receptor like factor 2 (CRLF2), erythropoietin receptor (EPOR), Janus kinase 2 (JAK2), neurotrophic receptor tyrosine kinase 3 (NTRK3),* etc. The recurrent genetic alterations of the kinases and cytokine receptors result in constitutive, ligand independent activation of downstream pathways, resulting in a gene expression profile similar to *BCR::ABL1* B-ALL in the absence of the fusion gene. In the latest ICC classification, *BCR::ABL1*-like B-ALL has been categorized to three distinct subtypes: *ABL1*-class rearranged, Janus kinase/signal transducers and activators of transcription (JAK-STAT) activated, and not otherwise specified (NOS), based on the gene rearrangements present and the pathways activated.

ABL1-class rearranged: Characterized by rearrangements which activate tyrosine kinase pathways. The genes involved in this subgroup are collectively referred to as "ABL-class" and include:

- ABL proto-oncogene 1, nonreceptor tyrosine kinase (*ABL1*),
- ABL proto-oncogene 2, nonreceptor tyrosine kinase (*ABL2*),
- Colony stimulating factor 1 receptor (CSF1R),
- Platelet derived growth factor receptor α and β (*PDGFRA*, *PDGFRB*), etc.

JAK-STAT activated: Characterized by alterations activating the JAK-STAT pathway, and mutations or rearrangements deregulating cytokine receptor expression. JAK-STAT alterations include:

- Rearrangements involving cytokine receptor like factor 2 (*CRLF2*) (e.g., *P2RY8::CRLF2, IGH::CRLF2*),
- Rearrangements involving erythropoietin receptor (*EPOR*) (e.g. *EPOR::IGH*),
- Janus kinase 2 (*JAK2*) mutations (e.g., *JAK2* p.R683G or *JAK1* p.V658F),
- *CRLF2* mutations, etc.

CRLF2 rearrangements are identified in approximately 50% of all Ph-like ALL cases. The *CRLF2* gene, located at Xp22.3/Yp11.3, encodes *CRLF2* (also known as the thymic stromal lymphopoietin receptor, *TSLPR*) which forms a heterodimer with the interleukin-7 receptor α chain (IL7Rα), facilitating the binding of its ligand, TSLP. Deregulation of *CRLF2* occurs through three primary mechanisms: (1) translocation into the immunoglobulin heavy chain enhancer locus (*IGH::CRLF2*), (2) focal interstitial deletion in the pseudoautosomal region upstream of *CRLF2*, leading to *P2RY8::CRLF2* fusion, and (3) less frequent, *CRLF2* point mutations (e.g., F232C).

In pediatric cases, approximately half of *CRLF2*-rearranged patients also carry mutations in *JAK1* or *JAK2*, particularly in the pseudokinase domain at residue R683. These mutations synergize with *CRLF2* overexpression to hyperactivate JAK-STAT signaling, driving cytokine-independent proliferation in hematopoietic cells, as demonstrated in mouse models.

Not otherwise specified: Less common genetic alterations and fusions of FMS-related receptor tyrosine kinase 3 (*FLT3), NTRK3*, etc. may be present.

CONCURRENT GENETIC CHANGES

In addition to the primary driver genetic abnormality, additional secondary genetic events like gene copy number alterations (CNAs) may be present in Ph-like ALL, e.g. *IKZF1* deletions are detectable in 70–80% adults and 40–60% pediatric patients. Other common genes with CNAs include *CDKN2A/B, RB1, ETV6, PAX5*, etc., and can be detected by techniques like multiplex ligation-dependent probe amplification (MLPA).

THERAPEUTIC POTENTIAL

The therapeutic implication of the genetic alterations in Ph-like ALL has generated a lot of interest about this subgroup. Following the identification of Ph-like ALL, higher risk of resistance or relapse must be realized and treatment should be accordingly modified. A highly targetable subgroup within Ph-like ALL consists of patients with ABL1-class gene fusions, which mimic the phenotype of *BCR::ABL1* and thus are susceptible to inhibition by tyrosine kinase inhibitors (TKIs) such as imatinib (an *ABL1* inhibitor) and dasatinib (a dual *ABL1/SRC* inhibitor). Many Ph-like ALL patients are candidates for targeted therapy like TKIs for ABL1-class rearranged cases, *JAK2* inhibitors (ruxolitinib) for JAK-STAT activated cases and other inhibitors depending on the activated pathways. There is evidence of in vitro sensitivity to dasatinib, ruxolitinib, crizotinib, etc., and the clinical trials are also ongoing for targeted inhibitors of kinases.

DIAGNOSIS OF Ph-LIKE ACUTE LYMPHOBLASTIC LEUKEMIA

The diagnosis of Ph-like ALL is challenging because of its genetic heterogeneity, the different types of techniques which can be used for its detection, and lack of a single gold standard test. Thus, diagnosis of Ph-like ALL requires a systematic and integrative approach combining cytogenetic, molecular, and flow cytometry techniques to identify key genetic lesions associated with this subtype. B-ALL cases should be evaluated for Ph-like signature as early as possible. For optimization of genetic workup of a case of B-ALL, a multistep approach is usually employed in the clinical laboratories. It may include a combination of screening tests and more specific methods to detect the aforementioned rearrangements, mutations, and copy number alterations that activate tyrosine kinase, cytokine receptor signaling, JAK-STAT, MAP kinase, or other signaling pathways.

Initial Genetic Workup

The initial genetic assessment is directed toward identifying B-ALL cases with recurrent translocations and aneuploidies for the initial genetic risk stratification. This includes the conventional karyotyping, RT-PCR and/or FISH based detection of *BCR::ABL1, ETV6::RUNX1, TCF3::PBX1, KMT2A::AFF1,* etc.; and the ploidy assessment using conventional karyotyping and/or flow cytometry. The cases with absence of any recurrent translocations or aneuploidies are usually categorized as "B-other" B-ALL. These cases can then be assessed further for *BCR::ABL1*-like features.

Flow Cytometry for CRLF2/TSLPR Expression

The B-other cases or all cases of B-ALL may be screened for *CRLF2* overexpression using flow cytometry (TSLPR antibody) at the initial immunophenotypic assessment **(Fig. 1)**. The cases with *CRLF2* overexpression can further be assessed for specific genomic rearrangements with other partners like *P2RY8, IGH,* etc. using FISH, RT-PCR, or next-generation sequencing (NGS) based testing. Almost half of the cases with *CRLF2* rearrangements may have *JAK2* mutation, particularly R683G, which can be assessed by Sanger sequencing.

Fluorescence In-situ Hybridization Break Apart Probes

In B-other cases with absence of *CRLF2* overexpression, Ph-like screening can be done with FISH break-apart probe strategy. Many Ph-like ALL rearrangements are cytogenetically cryptic, and hence, would be missed on conventional karyotype. The advantage of FISH break-apart probe strategy is that screening of commonly affected genes in Ph-like ALL, e.g., *ABL1, ABL2, PDGFRA, PDGFRB, CRLF2, JAK2,* etc., can be done, especially of genes with multiple fusion partners **(Fig. 2)**. FISH break-apart strategy is widely used for screening in laboratories, particularly where FISH is a routine technique being used for detection of recurrent translocations in B-ALL. Thus, they already have the manpower, necessary infrastructure and expertise for FISH based detection of Ph-like lesions, which may also be the case

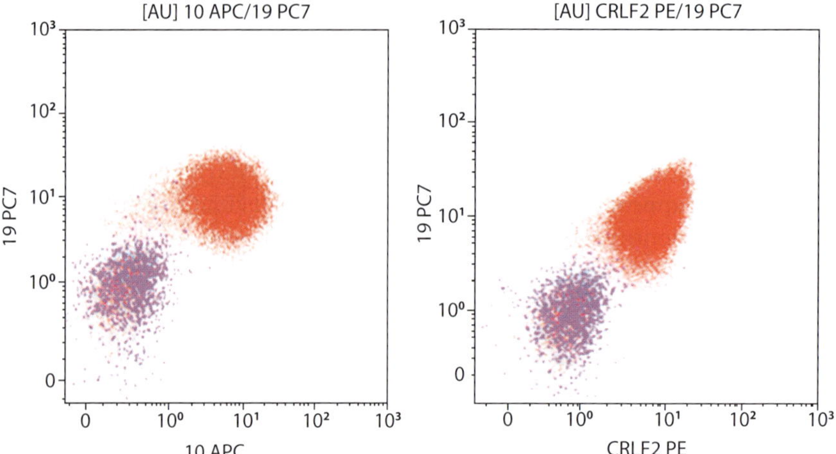

FIG. 1: Flow cytometry for CRLF2/TSLPR showing CRLF2 overexpression in the CD19+ CD10+ blasts (red dots) in a case of B-ALL.

(B-ALL: B-cell acute lymphoblastic leukemia; CRLF2: cytokine receptor like factor 2; TSLPR: thymic stromal lymphopoietin receptor)

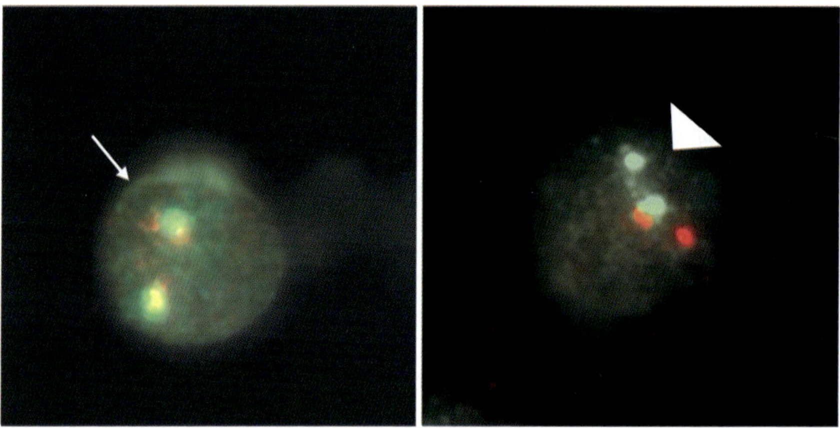

FIG. 2: FISH break apart (BA) probe strategy depicting the normal pattern of 2 fusion (2GR) signals (arrow) of ABL1 BA probe and another cell (arrowhead) showing 1 fusion (1GR) and split of red-green (1G, 1R) signal suggesting ABL1 rearrangement.

(FISH: fluorescence in-situ hybridization)

in many laboratories in India. However, the limitations of this approach are the limited capability to know both the partner genes, the need of multiple sample slides, in addition to being a labor-intensive method.

Reverse Transcription Polymerase Chain Reaction for Known Translocations

An alternative to FISH is to perform multiple sets of multiplex RT-PCRs for known Ph-like fusions. However, the novel breakpoints and novel fusions may be missed. So, the RT-PCR for known Ph-like fusions is not being routinely employed now.

Quantitative Reverse Transcription Polymerase Chain Reaction based TaqMan Low-density Array Screening

Another screening method is the quantitative RT-PCR (qRT-PCR) based TaqMan low-density array (LDA) assay which can rapidly identify the Ph-like ALL as being used by the COG group for screening high-risk B-ALL cases for Ph-like signature. It evaluates the expression levels of 8 selected genes (*JCHAIN, SPATS2L, CA6, NRXN3, MUC4, CRLF2, ADGRF1, BMPR1B*) highly predictive of this subtype and an integrated score is calculated to determine whether the case belongs to Ph-like ALL. However, LDA panel is not available commercially, outside of the clinical trial or institutional setting and difficult to apply across different groups. A similar prediction tool, based on the limited panel qRT-PCR of the 8 selected genes, PHi-RACE, has been devised at PGI, Chandigarh.

IKZF1 Deletions as Marker for Ph-like Acute Lymphoblastic Leukemia

As the frequency of *IKZF1* deletions is higher in Ph-like ALL as compared to the other subtypes of B-ALL, it may act like a surrogate marker to suspect Ph-like ALL. However, all B-ALL cases with *IKZF1* deletions cannot be categorized as Ph-like ALL and need to be investigated for specific Ph-like ALL genomic aberration. MLPA or other techniques like FISH can be useful in the detection of *IKZF1* deletions.

Next-generation Sequencing

The NGS serves as a comprehensive tool to detect:

- *Gene fusions:* Targeted RNA sequencing/whole transcriptome sequencing (WTS)
- *Point mutations:* Whole genome sequencing (WGS)/WTS
- *Gene expression profiles (GEP):* WTS

The recently developed NGS-based assays are highly sensitive in detection of leukemia-associated genetic mutations and fusions. In addition, several commercially-available platforms [e.g., Archer (now IDT) FusionPlex, NanoString Vantage, FoundationOne Heme, and others] can also be used to identify Ph-like ALL-associated alterations. These newer technologies have the potential to identify fusions involving previously-unknown partners.

If the non-NGS based initial tests are noncontributory or one needs to know the partner gene in the FISH break-apart probe positive cases, *targeted RNA sequencing* (e.g., FusionPlex panel) can be done. The limitation of targeted RNA sequencing approach is that it is limited by the number of genes included as well as the coverage of the included genes in the panel and the depth of testing, e.g., Archer FusionPlex panel has 81 lymphoid related genes whereas an in-house developed NARASIMHA panel at ACTREC, Mumbai, has 25 lymphoid related genes, thus having variable capabilities.

The *WTS* would be more reliable to find out the underlying genomic lesions, as the targeted panels would be limited by the gene coverage of the panel. In addition to detecting known and novel fusions, WTS provides comprehensive gene expression signatures which can help detect and define Ph-like ALL. The gene expression data obtained from the transcriptome sequencing can also be analyzed using the machine learning (B-ALL subtype) classifiers such as molecular diagnosis (MD)-ALL or ALLSorts, etc., to improve the ease and accuracy of Ph-like B-ALL diagnosis and subtype prediction. Despite the challenges of bioinformatic data analysis, limited availability, time and cost constraints, the unbiased RNA sequencing (WTS) is the ideal technique for Ph-like ALL and the most comprehensive method for identifying Ph-like ALL fusions, including those not detected by other assays.

The *WGS* can also be employed to detect DNA based translocations, particularly the rare mutations, although some of the detected translocations may not be expressed and may be clinically irrelevant.

Screening Algorithms

The lack of standardized testing for the identification of this prognostically poor and potentially targetable group has necessitated the development of various screening algorithms by different groups and institutions for better treatment stratification. The various approaches used includes comprehensive gene expression profiling or NGS in all newly diagnosed patients or only in selected high-risk patients. While the strategies used to define the Ph-like signature vary, the overall goal of diagnostic testing is accurate identification of the underlying genetic alterations for appropriate targeted therapy.

A tiered approach has been followed by the COG, wherein all newly diagnosed B-ALL patients with National Cancer Institute (NCI) high-risk are screened for the Ph-like GEP with a qRT-PCR-based LDA platform. The LDA card, based on GEP of Ph-like ALL, checks for expression of 8 or 15 genes, and is highly predictive of the Ph-like ALL signature. Subsequently, further tests are performed in those patients who are LDA screen positive. Cases with *CRLF2* overexpression are tested for *P2RY8-CRLF2* fusion and *IGH-CRLF2* rearrangements. *JAK1* and *JAK2* mutation testing is next completed in all patients with confirmed *CRLF2* rearrangements.

In Ph-like cases without *CRLF2* rearrangements, RT-PCR assays are done to detect *ABL* class, *JAK2*, and other known kinase fusions and confirmed by Sanger sequencing. The alternate testing or RNA sequencing is performed on remaining LDA-positive cases and patients with confirmed targetable mutations or fusions are allocated to TKI-containing treatment after induction therapy. This tiered approach optimizes the utilization of available resources especially in the setting of large trials. The limitation, however, is that it involves multiple stages of the workup and is time consuming. Moreover, there is a possibility of novel fusions or other alterations being missed in this targeted approach.

There is no consensus approach to the diagnosis of patients who express a Ph-like signature. These patients are usually adolescents and young adults (AYAs), present with a higher white blood cell (WBC) count and are likely to remain minimal residual disease (MRD)-positive following standard induction regimes. So, the possible population for screening may be AYAs, NCI high-risk, \the Indian Childhood Collaborative Leukemia group (ICiCLe) intermediate-high risk, MRD-positive or relapsed patients, cases with *IKZF1* deletions, *IKZF1* plus profile, MRplus1 (intermediate risk) or MRplus2 (high-risk) profiles based on MLPA, etc. However, selecting an optimal screening method and defining the patient population to be screened are still moving targets. An indicative algorithm is being provided for the stepwise approach and diagnostic approaches for detection and classification of Ph-like ALL **(Flowchart 1)**.

With the rapid advancement in the high throughput techniques, their wider availability, and highly competitive pricing, it is becoming feasible and cost-effective to workup the cases with the high-throughput molecular diagnostic techniques with gene expression profiling rather than the step-wise approaches. The availability of machine learning based B-ALL subtype classifiers like MD-ALL, ALLSorts, etc., have further enabled the usage of gene expression data for B-ALL subtyping. The various underlying genomic lesions in Ph-like ALL and the diagnostic techniques have been summarized **(Fig. 3)**.

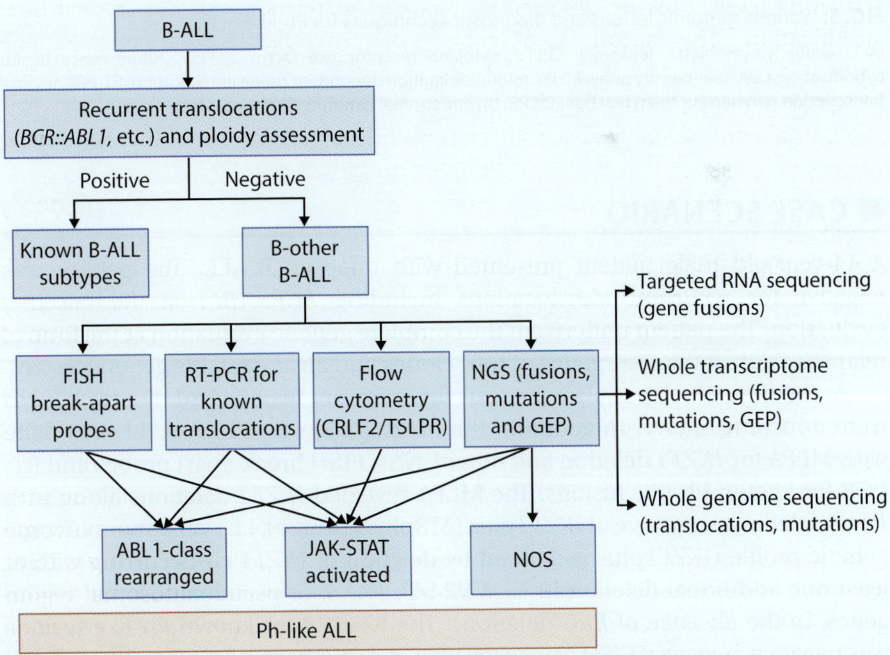

FLOWCHART 1: Algorithm for diagnosis and classification of Ph-like ALL.

(ALL: acute lymphoblastic leukemia; CRLF2: cytokine receptor like factor 2; FISH: fluorescence in-situ hybridization; GEP: gene expression profiles; JAK-STAT: Janus kinase/signal transducers and activators of transcription; NGS: next-generation sequencing; NOS: not otherwise specified; RT-PCR: reverse transcription polymerase chain reaction; TSLPR: thymic stromal lymphopoietin receptor)

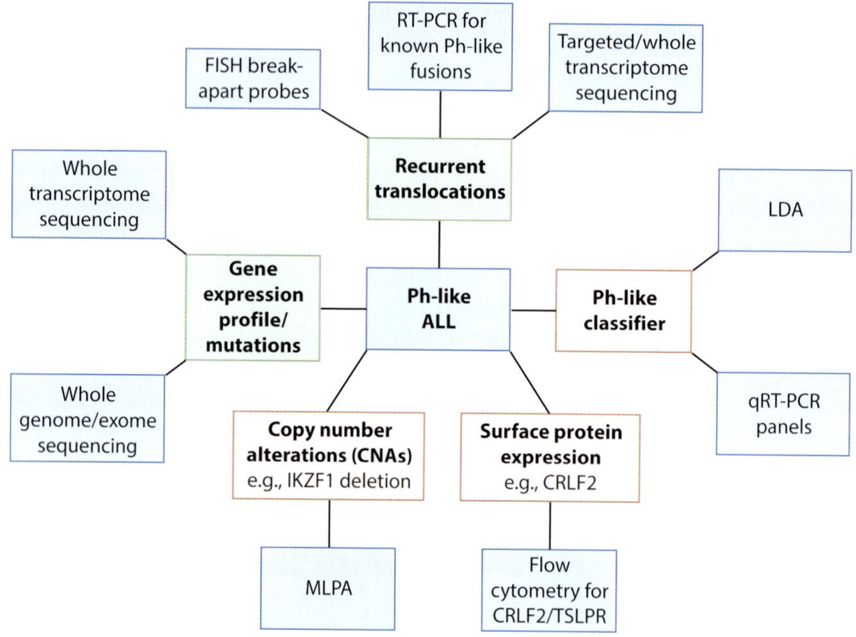

FIG. 3: Various genomic lesions and diagnostic techniques for Ph-like ALL.

(ALL: acute lymphoblastic leukemia; CRLF2: cytokine receptor like factor 2; FISH: fluorescence in-situ hybridization; LDA: low-density array; MLPA: multiplex ligation dependent probe amplification; RT-PCR: reverse transcription polymerase chain reaction; TSLPR: thymic stromal lymphopoietin receptor)

CASE SCENARIO

A 14-year-old male patient presented with relapsed B-ALL. The patient was negative for recurrent translocations including *BCR::ABL1* at the baseline evaluation. The patient underwent the complete genetic evaluation at the time of relapse to detect the resurgence of new clones and any targetable genetic lesion.

At the time of relapse also, the tests for recurrent fusions and ploidy changes were noncontributory. In addition, the investigation for Ph-like ALL was done with MLPA for *IKZF1* deletion and other CNAs, FISH break-apart probes and RT-PCR for known Ph-like fusions. The MLPA revealed *IKZF1* deletions along with *PAX5* deletion suggestive of IKZF1plus (MRplus2 profile), i.e., very poor outcome genetic profile (IKZF1plus is defined by deletion of *IKZF1* co-occurring with at least one additional deletion in *CDKN2A/B, PAX5*, or pseudoautosomal region genes, in the absence of *ERG* deletion). The RT-PCR for known Ph-like fusions was negative, however, FISH was suggestive of *ABL1* rearrangement, although the partner gene could not be known.

In the next step, to know the partner of *ABL1* gene, Archer FusionPlex targeted NGS panel testing was done, which confirmed the fusion of *ABL1* with *SNX2*. Although the *SNX2::ABL1* primers were included in the RT-PCR for known Ph-like fusions performed earlier, it was missed due to novel breakpoint in exon 9 of *SNX2* gene in this case unlike the exon 3 of *SNX2* in previously reported cases. The case was also confirmed with orthogonal testing. The primers were designed based on the breakpoints revealed by targeted NGS and the PCR product was sequenced with Sanger sequencing to visualize the fusion. Later on, the sample was analyzed by whole transcriptome sequencing for additional information and confirmation. It also confirmed the presence of *SNX2::ABL1* fusion. The additional advantage of WTS was that the gene expression data could be analyzed using the machine learning classifier for Ph-like and other new B-ALL subtype detection, such as MD-ALL and ALLCatchR, which predicted the subtype of B-ALL as Ph-like ALL **(Figs. 4A to C)**.

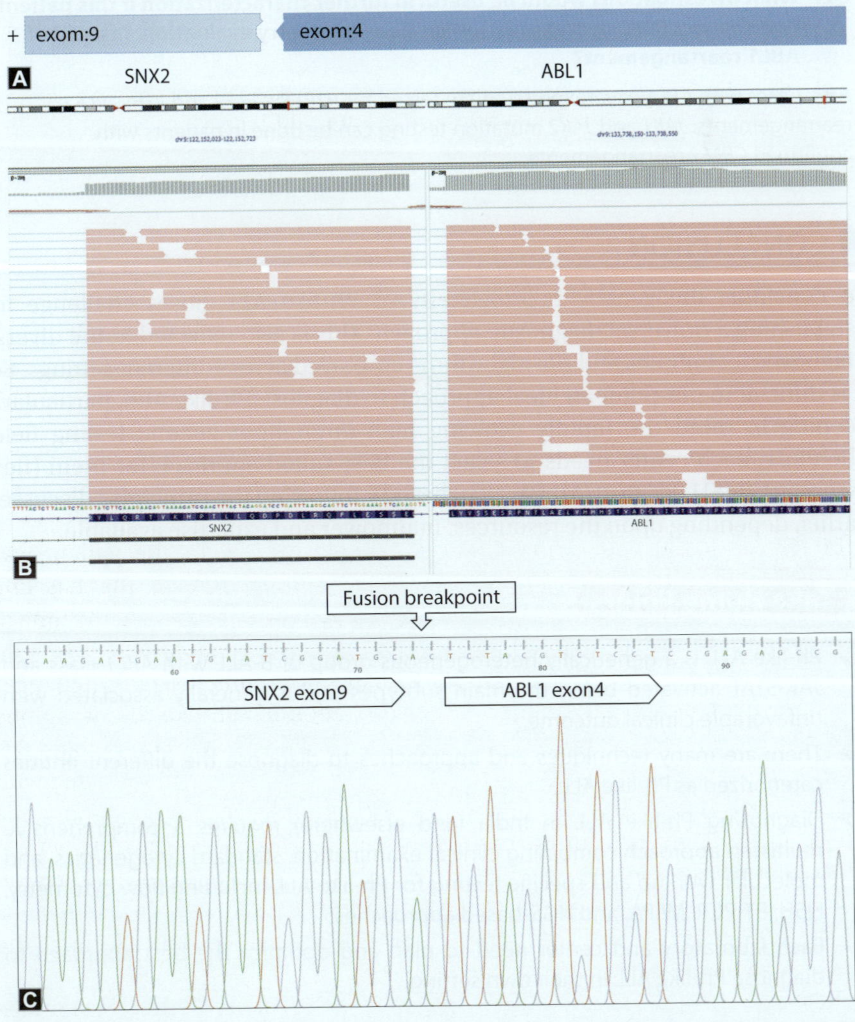

FIGS. 4A TO C: *SNX2::ABL1* fusion in a case with Ph-like ALL detected by: (A) Targeted RNA sequencing (Archer FusionPlex panel); (B) Whole transcriptome sequencing; and confirmed by (C) Sanger sequencing.

(ALL: acute lymphoblastic leukemia)

Case-related Questions

Q1. How the FISH break-apart probes help in diagnosis of Ph-like ALL?

Ans. There are multiple identified fusions categorized as Ph-like fusions. This includes fusions involving genes like *ABL1, ABL2, PDGFRA, PDGFRB,* etc., with multiple other partners. It is not feasible to check all the possible fusion combinations using different set of fusion probes. So, using break-apart FISH probes panel for these commonly involved genes like *ABL1, PDGFRB,* etc., can detect the presence of fusion/ rearrangements involving them. Although laborious, and time consuming, this has proven to be one of the practical approaches of diagnosing Ph-like ALL in Indian settings.

Q2. What investigations would be useful in further characterization if this patient had shown *CRLF2* overexpression on flow cytometry evaluation, instead of ABL1 rearrangement?

Ans. Cases with *CRLF2* overexpression are tested for *P2RY8::CRLF2* and *IGH::CRLF2* rearrangements. *JAK1* and *JAK2* mutation testing can be done in patients with confirmed *CRLF2* rearrangements.

CONCLUSION

To conclude, the genetic heterogeneity of Ph-like ALL poses challenge for establishing a universal diagnostic approach. This is also reflected in the diverse diagnostic techniques and the algorithms employed across different settings. So, it is difficult to pin-point an ideal approach to diagnose Ph-like ALL, particularly keeping in mind the rapidly evolving high-throughput genetic testing field. Therefore, each center needs to select the best-suited approach for them (flow cytometry/FISH/RT-PCR/MLPA/NGS based), following the principles discussed earlier, depending upon the resources, manpower and expertise available.

Take Home Points

- Ph-like ALL is a genetically heterogeneous group of B-ALL with *ABL1*-class and JAK-STAT activated being the main subtypes and is generally associated with unfavorable clinical outcome.
- There are many techniques and approaches to diagnose the different entities categorized as Ph-like ALL.
- Diagnosing Ph-like ALL in India (and elsewhere) requires a comprehensive multistep approach combining clinical examination, standard cytogenetics, and molecular workup and specific testing for Ph-like ALL including flow cytometry, FISH, RT-PCR, MLPA, and NGS-based approaches.
- Each laboratory and center need to plan and optimize the best approach to diagnose Ph-like ALL in their own setting.

SUGGESTED READINGS

1. Mullighan CG, Su X, Zhang J, Radtke I, Phillips LA, Miller CB, et al. Deletion of IKZF1 and prognosis in acute lymphoblastic leukemia. N Engl J Med. 2009;360(5):470-80.
2. Den Boer ML, van Slegtenhorst M, De Menezes RX, Cheok MH, Buijs-Gladdines JG, Peters ST, et al. A subtype of childhood acute lymphoblastic leukaemia with poor treatment outcome: a genome-wide classification study. Lancet Oncol. 2009;10(2):125-34.
3. Pui CH, Roberts KG, Yang JJ, Mullighan CG. Philadelphia chromosome-like acute lymphoblastic leukemia. Clin Lymphoma Myeloma Leuk. 2017;17(8):464-70.
4. Roberts KG, Li Y, Payne-Turner D, Harvey RC, Yang YL, Pei D, et al. Targetable kinase-activating lesions in Ph-like acute lymphoblastic leukemia. N Engl J Med. 2014;371(11):1005-15.
5. Reshmi SC, Harvey RC, Roberts KG, Stonerock E, Smith A, Jenkins H, et al. Targetable kinase gene fusions in high risk B-ALL: a study from the Children's Oncology Group. Blood. 2017;129(25):3352-61.
6. Jain N, Roberts KG, Jabbour E, Patel K, Eterovic AK, Chen K, et al. Ph-like acute lymphoblastic leukemia: a high-risk subtype in adults. Blood. 2017;129(5):572-81.
7. Gupta SK, Bakhshi S, Kamal VK, Sharma P, Pushpam D, Sahoo RK, et al. Proposal and clinical application of molecular genetic risk scoring system, "MRplus", for BCR-ABL1 negative pediatric B-cell acute lymphoblastic leukemia-report from a single centre. Leuk Res. 2021;111:106683.
8. Leons GK, Sharma P, Gupta SK, Gupta R, Rani L, Gajendra S, Roy A, et al. Detection of a novel SNX2 gene breakpoint in the SNX2::ABL1 fusion transcript in Ph-like B-cell acute lymphoblastic leukemia. Pediatr Blood Cancer. 2023;70(10):e30546.
9. Gupta SK, Leons GK. Genetics of B-Cell Acute Lymphoblastic Leukemia (B-ALL): Recent Updates and Indian Perspective. Indian J Hematol Blood Transfus. 2025.

CHAPTER 10

Point-of-Care Testing in Coagulation

Vandana Puri, Jasmita Dass

ABSTRACT

Point-of-care testing (POCT) devices in coagulation provide rapid, bedside evaluation of hemostatic function, measuring parameters such as prothrombin time (PT), activated partial thromboplastin time (aPTT), international normalized ratio (INR), activated clotting time (ACT), and comprehensive viscoelastic tests like thromboelastography (TEG) or ROTEM. These devices are invaluable in critical care, trauma, cardiac surgery, and anticoagulation clinics, where immediate results guide urgent interventions, transfusion decisions, or anticoagulant dosing. POCT minimizes delays by eliminating sample transport and lab processing, reduces blood volume requirements—beneficial for pediatric or ICU patients—and enables decentralized testing, including at-home monitoring for patients on long-term anticoagulation therapy. This enhances patient compliance, improves safety, and may lower overall healthcare costs by preventing complications and enabling early intervention.

INTRODUCTION

Point-of-care (POC) testing is defined as testing performed at or near the patient's bedside with the aim that results will possibly change the patient's therapy/affect patient care. POC testing is sometimes performed by patients themselves or by staff not primarily trained for laboratory testing. The tests in general have a higher reagent cost per test than laboratory assays but offer advantages in certain situations such as managing anticoagulant therapy with warfarin, perioperative heparin management in cardiac surgeries, patient blood management in situations like trauma, obstetric care, liver transplant surgeries, etc., managing antiplatelet therapy, etc., as the measurement durations (25–45 minutes) are shorter as compared to conventional coagulation tests (CCTs) (40–60 minutes). There are lesser chances of sample degradation as no transport or minimal transport time is required. There is also a potential for round-the-clock patient monitoring if required.

PHASES OF COAGULATION

The process of coagulation in vivo begins after endothelial injury that exposes von Willebrand factor antigen (vWF) which binds to platelets by the glycoprotein (Gp)Ib-IX-V receptor causing platelet activation. This is referred to as primary hemostasis. Simultaneously, the tissue factor exposure activates the extrinsic pathway of coagulation and forming small amounts of thrombin by extrinsic tenase complex and is referred as the initiation phase of coagulation. The small amount of thrombin produced activates the factor IX and VIII leading to formation of the intrinsic tenase complex leading to a much higher formation of thrombin as by this time the extrinsic tenase complex is already inhibited by tissue factor pathway inhibitor. This is the amplification phase. The last phase is propagation which results in the formation of a stable fibrin clot. Platelets play an important role as the intrinsic and extrinsic tenase complex and prothrombinase complex are formed on their surface.

CONVENTIONAL TESTS OF COAGULATION AND THEIR DRAWBACKS

Traditionally CCTs—prothrombin time (PT) with international normalized ratio (INR) which measure extrinsic and common pathway, activated partial thromboplastin time (APTT) that measures intrinsic and common pathway, thrombin time (TT), fibrinogen are used as an initial screen. However, these CCTs suffer from some drawbacks and do not measure the entire process of hemostasis. These drawbacks are listed in the following text:

- Cannot predict which patients will bleed.
- Not proportional to the severity of the bleed.
- Does not take into account other components of coagulation system such as the platelets and cellular components.
- Does not take into account fibrinolytic pathway and the effect of factor XIII.
- Do not yield to monitoring of newer anticoagulants.
- False negative for mild factor deficiencies.
- Does not explain why hemophiliacs bleed despite normal extrinsic pathway.
- Patients with similar PT and APTT results may have significantly different bleeding profiles.

Some of these drawbacks are taken care of by viscoelastic testing such as thromboelastography (TEG) and rotational thromboelastometry (ROTEM) where the contribution of fibrinogen, platelets, and fibrinolytic pathway can be assessed within an hour of sample collection.

Point-of-care Tests in Coagulation

Point-of-care devices and their functions are listed in **Flowchart 1**.

POC market in coagulation is expanding at a rapid pace and is expected to grow from $1.53 billion in 2021 to $2.44 billion in 2028 at a compound annual growth rate (CAGR) of 6.9% with the largest market share occupied by anticoagulant monitoring devices followed by platelet function monitoring.

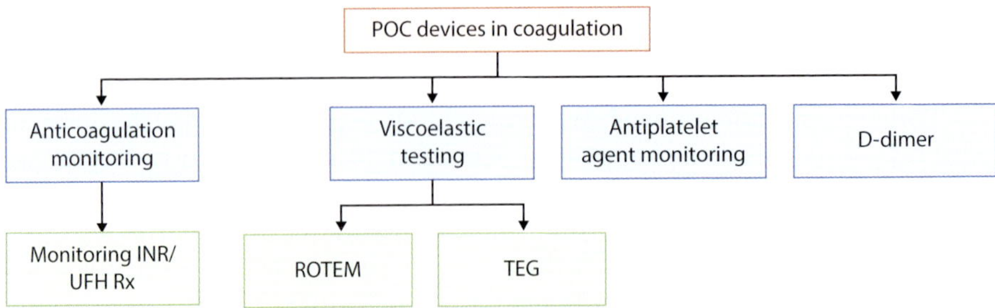

FLOWCHART 1: Point-of-care (POC) testing devices that can be used for platelet and coagulation testing.

(INR: international normalized ratio; ROTEM: rotational thromboelastometry; TEG: thromboelastography; UFH: unfractionated heparin)

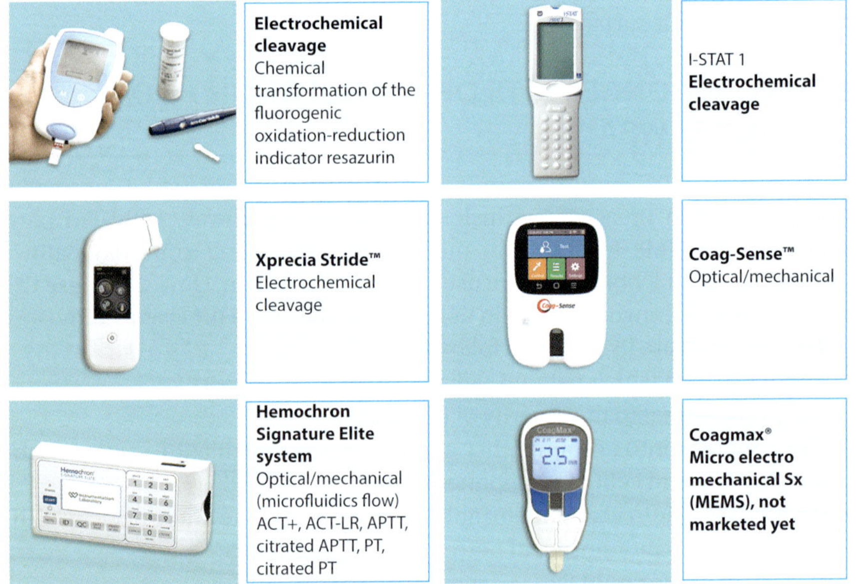

FIG. 1: Point-of-care (POC) devices for international normalized ratio (INR) monitoring.

(PT: prothrombin time; APTT: activated partial thromboplastin time)

We will look at the utility and details of these devices by looking at four case scenarios.

Case 1

A 41-year-old doctor, posted at primary healthcare center (PHC) is diagnosed with right lower limb deep venous thrombosis (DVT). He was started on warfarin, INR stabilized at 2.6. He is having problems in getting frequent INR done.

Vitamin K antagonists (VKA) including warfarin have a narrow therapeutic window and therefore require frequent monitoring of INR. Traditionally, this is done by the citrated samples tested in the laboratory. There are multiple POC devices that can monitor INR. These devices and their principle are shown in **Figure 1**.

The POC INR devices are approved for monitoring of VKA therapy. These offer significant advantages for outpatient monitoring as the need to travel to give samples can be obviated. These devices are also useful in the thrombosis clinic to take quick decisions to manage VKA therapy for patients. The use of POC INR devices for at-home management are recommended for patients who can self-adjust their VKA therapy. A meta-analysis has shown that the use of POC INR led to a significant rise of 6.14% in the time in INR in therapeutic range compared to laboratory PT/INR measurements.

These devices typically require 10–30 µL of blood mostly the capillary blood collected by fingerprick. This is applied to a test strip which is inserted in the INR device. Testing is performed on the whole blood (WB) rather than plasma as in the CCT with testing optimized to function across a hematocrit range of 25–55%. Of these systems, the ones based on optical/mechanical clot detection require WB samples while electrochemical devices do not necessarily require WB samples. Calibration is performed and International Sensitivity Index (ISI) for these devices is assigned by the manufacturers. Calibration data and mean normal PT (MNPT) is encoded in the test strips or in a batch-specific code chip. The POC INR devices have a coefficient of variation (CV) of 3–5%. Quality control (QC) on these systems involve the electronic QC by testing the optical/electronic system within the device. Some of the manufacturers also have liquid QC (LQC) material and are recommended for all POC instruments at the start of a new batch of strips, when results are in doubt or every 6 months. LQC is sometimes waived for at-home testing. Devices used for anticoagulation use should be enrolled in external quality assurance program with the caveat that the samples sent as a part of external quality assessment (EQA) is a citrated sample while most of these devices test WB, and hence, measure precision rather than accuracy. The devices usually overestimate INR at a value of ≥3.5 while at low INR values, they have a tendency to underestimate. POC INR devices are not approved for anticoagulation monitoring for lupus anticoagulant (LA) positive patients. A detail of these devices with ISI and QC are given in **Table 1**.

The patient bought a CoaguChek XS and comfortably could monitor INR on fortnightly basis.

Case 2

A 68-year-old male with triple vessel disease, due for coronary artery bypass grafting (CABG). Monitoring of unfractionated heparin (UFH) is required during surgery.

Activated clotting time (ACT) was first described by Hattersley in 1966 and is used for monitoring UFH therapy in patients on cardiopulmonary bypass (CPB), on extracorporeal membrane oxygenation (ECMO), undergoing percutaneous transluminal coronary angioplasty, on hemofiltration or hemodialysis. ACT is a one-stage WB clotting coagulation test for intrinsic pathway using celite/kaolin/particulate glass as activators with platelets as the source of phospholipids. CPB is performed with systemic anticoagulation to prevent both thrombosis and consumptive coagulopathy. Dependent on the circuits, an ACT of 300–600 seconds is targeted with a dose of UFH of 300–400 IU/kg with boluses thereafter.

TABLE 1: Point-of-care (POC) devices with thromboplastin and quality control (QC) details.

POC devices with thromboplastin					
Instrument, manufacturer	**Sample**	**Thrombo-plastin, ISI, heparinase**	**Clot detection method**	**Calibration method**	**QC**
CoaguChek XS, Roche	Capillary/ venous whole blood (WB) noncitrated	Recombinant human; 1.0; Yes	Electrochemical cleavage (amperometric)	Code chip	On board QC, strip integrity check; LQC NA
CoaguChek Pro II, Roche	Capillary/ venous WB noncitrated	Recombinant human; 1.0; Yes	Electrochemical cleavage (amperometric)	Code chip	On board QC, strip integrity check; liquid QC (LQC) available
Coag-Sense, CoagSense Inc	Capillary WB/ recalcified plasma	Rabbit brain; 1.0; No	Optical/ mechanical	Barcode on cuvette, automatic	Additional QC strips
Hemochron Signature Elite, Werfen	Capillary/ venous WB citrated/ noncitrated	Rabbit brain; 1.0; No	Optical/ mechanical/ microfluidics flow	Barcode on cuvette, automatic	Electronic QC and LQC available
I-STAT, Abott	WB noncitrated	Human recombinant; 1.05; Yes	Electrochemical cleavage	On board software	Electronic QC and LQC

ACT is done 60 minutes before starting CPB and then every 30–60 minutes after heparinization. At such doses of UFH, PT and APTT are unmeasurable and therefore ACT is used for UFH monitoring. For uncoated circuits, an ACT value of >480 seconds is the target. For patients who have a contraindication to heparin, bivalirudin can be used with a target ACT of 2.5 times the baseline value. ACT is also used to check for completeness of protamine reversal after CPB is concluded. The reference range for unheparinized blood is 70–180 seconds with a linearity of the test for approximately 8.0 U/mL heparin. There are multiple factors that influence ACT including antithrombin deficiency, factor or fibrinogen deficiency, thrombocytopenia, anemia, hemodilution, hypothermia, and LA. ACT is sensitive to deficiencies in FVIII (<25% of normal), IX, X, XI, XII deficiency, in patients receiving oral anticoagulants or with liver disease. The ACT is insensitive to deficiencies of factor VII and factor XIII. ACT is also prolonged by direct thrombin inhibitors and lesser prolongation is seen with anti-Xa drugs.

Direct thrombin inhibitors will prolong the ACT. The direct Xa inhibitors (apixaban, edoxaban, and rivaroxaban) have a lesser effect on the ACT although this is dependent upon the precise drug being used. Various devices that monitor ACT are listed in **Table 2**.

The ACT-low range is typically used for monitoring of ECMO, percutaneous coronary intervention (PCI), and hemodialysis as these use a lower concentration of UFH (0.5–3.0 U/mL). It is recommended that LQC is done for ACT devices daily along with electronic QC.

Modifications of ACT include Xa-ACT, MAX-ACT, and plasma ACT. Xa-ACT uses bovine Xa instead of the contact activator and was designed to monitor low molecular weight heparin (LMWH) therapy. MAX-ACT uses a combination of kaolin, celite, and glass to maximally activate factor XII making the test more sensitive to heparin and less affected by hypothermia and hemodilution.

The patient was put on CPB after checking the baseline ACT and could achieve an ACT of 500 seconds at 30 minutes post the first UFH bolus. His ACT continued to be >480 seconds throughout the procedure and after protamine reversal, fell to 100 seconds. His surgery was uneventful and he made a complete recovery.

Case 3

A 40-year-female presents with acute abdomen and fever. He has received 2L NS and colloid, noradrenaline and meropenem and was on mechanical ventilation.

TABLE 2: Point-of-care (POC) devices for activated clotting time (ACT).

POC devices for ACT					
Instrument, manufacturer	**Sample**	**ACT activator**	**Clot detection method**	**Analytical imprecision**	**Other assays available**
Hemochron Signature Elite, Werfen	Capillary/ venous whole blood (WB) citrated/ noncitrated	ACT+ uses a mixture of silica, kaolin and phospholipids; ACT-LR uses a celite activator	Optical/ mechanical/ microfluidics flow	≤10%	ACT+, ACT low range, POC INR, POC aPTT
I-STAT, Abott	WB noncitrated	Kaolin, celite	Electrochemical cleavage (amperometry)	<6%	ACT, POC INR
Actalyke Mini II and Actalyke XL, Helena Laboratories	Venous WB, noncitrated	Celite, kaolin, glass particulate	Magnet rotation	0.1% mean difference of duplicates	ACT, MAX-ACT, ACT-low range, heparinase
ACT plus, Medtronic cardiac surgery	Venous WB, native and citrated	Kaolin	Plunger motion	~15% duplicate values showed >12% difference	ACT, heparin dose response,
HMS plus, Medtronic cardiac surgery	Venous WB, noncitrated	Kaolin	Plunger motion		Heparin protamine titration

(ACT-LR: low range activated clotting time; APTT: activated partial thromboplastin time; INR: international normalized ratio)

He was posted for exploratory laparotomy. Her CBC is hemoglobin (Hb): 8.2 g/dL, platelets: 80,000/μL, INR: 1.4.

To predict the risk of bleeding in this patient, viscoelastic testing can be used. The common viscoelastic tests are TEG and ROTEM which are global tests of hemostasis. TEG was first described by Hartert in 1948. Pentapharm GmbH (Munich, Germany) marketed a modified instrumentation using the terminology ROTEM. Both TEG and ROTEM provide continuous information from initial fibrin formation to clot retraction and fibrinolysis to assess clot formation, strength, and dissolution by measuring the effect of a continuously applied rotational force on WB that is transmitted to an electromechanical transduction system (TEG) or optical detection system (ROTEM). **Figure 2** shows the principle of TEG and ROTEM.

The tracings produced by these look similar and have fairly similar parameters. These are shown in **Figure 3**.

TEG and ROTEM can be performed on WB postrecalcification called native-TEG and nonactivated thromboelastometry (NATEM) respectively or can be performed using different agonists as shown in **Table 3**.

MA/MCF measure the contribution of platelets and fibrinogen, R time or CT are dependent on the clotting factors and fibrinolysis is measured by the CL30/Ly30 and CL60/Ly60. Various parameters and their measurement are shown in **Table 4**.

The ROTEM images from Case 3 and the management done are shown in **Figure 4**. The EXTEM and INTEM both show a reduced maximum clot firmness (MCF) while FIBTEM was normal indicating that fibrinogen was not the cause of reduced MCF. Despite a platelet count of 80,000/μL, the patient was at a risk of increased bleeding and the same was managed by giving pooled platelets to the patient following which ROTEM normalized.

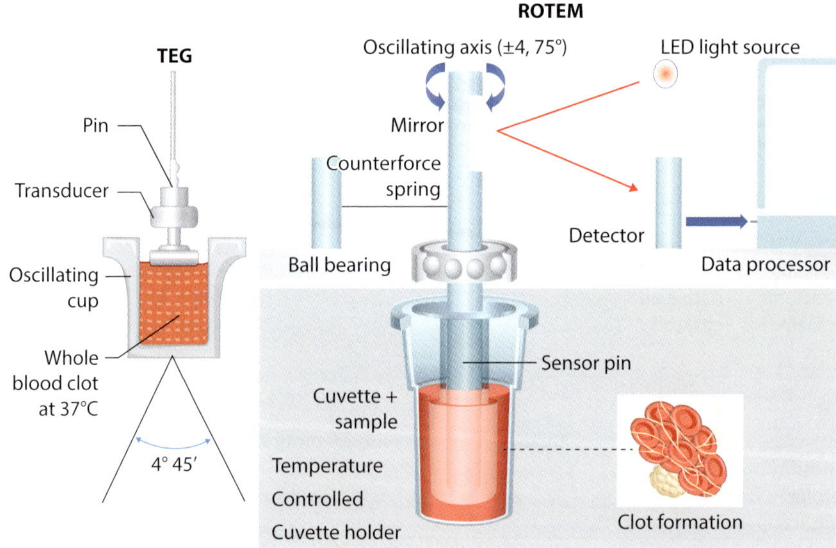

FIG. 2: Principles of thromboelastography (TEG) and rotational thromboelastometry (ROTEM).

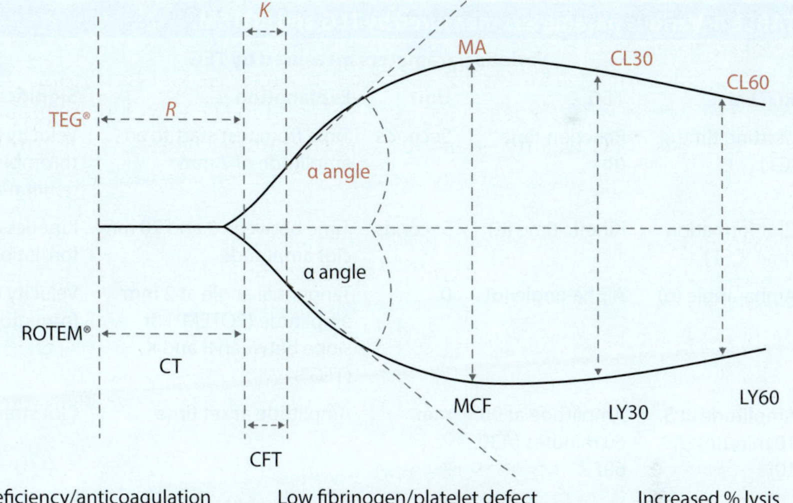

FIG. 3: Thromboelastography (TEG) and rotational thromboelastometry (ROTEM).
(CT: clotting time; CFT: clot formation time; MCF: maximum clot firmness)

TABLE 3: Pathways assessed by various agonists using TEG and ROTEM.

Pathways assessed by various agonists		
	TEG	**ROTEM**
Intrinsic pathway	Kaolin-TEG	INTEM—ellagic acid activator
Extrinsic pathway	-	EXTEM—tissue factor activator
Both extrinsic and intrinsic pathway	Rapid TEG—TF and kaolin	-
Heparin	Heparinase TEG—kaolin + heparinase	HEPTEM—kaolin + heparinase
Fibrinogen	Functional fibrinogen TEG—TF + abciximab	FIBTEM—TF + cytochalasin D
Fibrinolysis inhibition	-	APTEM—TF + aprotinin/tranexamic acid
Recalcification alone	Native TEG	NATEM

(APTEM: anti-plasminogen-activated-tissue-factor; EXTEM: extrinsic thromboelastometry; HEPTEM: heparinase thromboelastography; NATEM: nonactivated thromboelastometry; ROTEM: rotational thromboelastometry; TEG: thromboelastography; TF: tissue factor)

There are various algorithms to guide patient management based on TEG/ROTEM results for trauma, obstetric emergencies, cardiac surgery, etc. Also, their usage in many settings has led to reduction in the overall units transfused and optimization of blood product usage.

The ROTEM sigma and TEG-6s are cartridge-based systems that will require minimal pipetting and are available in the market. A soon-to-be launched system is the Quantra which will be a purely automated system with no manual pipetting based on ultrasound to detect clot. The measurements will be clotting time, clot stiffness, and platelet and fibrinogen contributions to clot stiffness.

TABLE 4: Various parameters measured by TEG and ROTEM.

Various parameters measured by TEG				
ROTEM	**TEG**	**Unit**	**Explanation**	**Significance**
Clotting time (CT)	Reaction time (R)	Seconds	Time from test start to an amplitude of 2 mm	Velocity of thrombin generation
Clot formation time (CFT)	Kinetic time (K)	Seconds	Time between 2 and 20 mm clot amplitude	Kinetics of clot formation
Alpha-angle (α)	Alpha-angle (α)	0	Tangential angle at 2 mm amplitude (ROTEM®) or slope between R and K (TEG®)	Velocity of clot formation
Amplitude at 5, 10 minutes (A5, 10)	Amplitude at 30, 60 minutes (A30, 60)	mm	Amplitude at set time	Clot strength
Maximum clot firmness (MCF)	Maximum amplitude (MA)	mm	Greatest width achieved	Maximal cloth strength
Lysis index at 30, 60 m (L130, 60)	Clot lysis at 30, 60 m (CL30, 60)	%	Residual clot firmness at set time, as % of MCF/MA	Clot stability and fibrinolysis

(TEG: thromboelastography; ROTEM: rotational thromboelastometry)

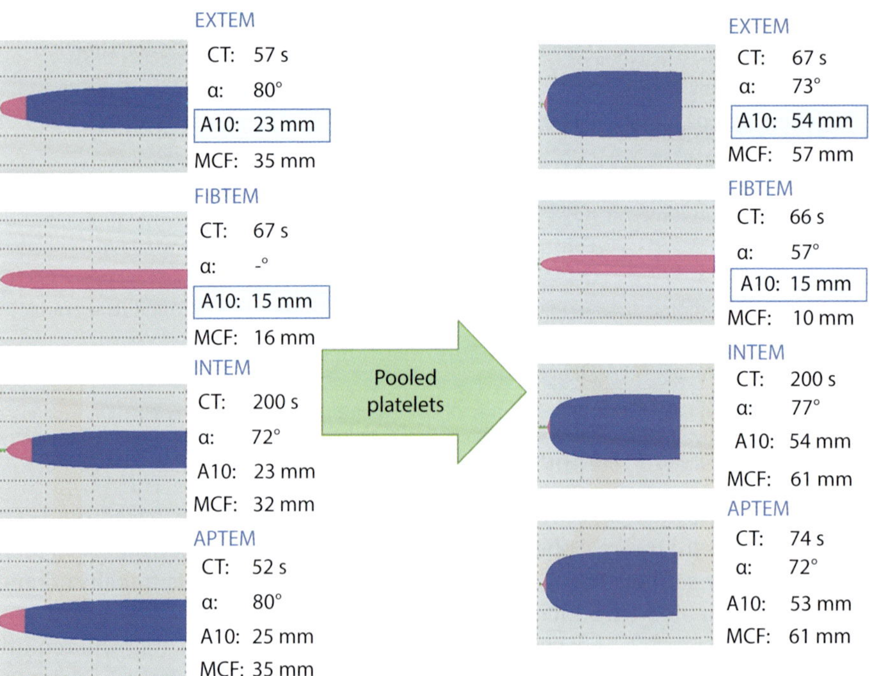

FIG. 4: Baseline rotational thromboelastometry (ROTEM) traces from case 3 and the effect after transfusion of pooled platelets.

(APTEM: anti-plasminogen-activated-tissue-factor; CT: clotting time; FIBTEM: fibrinogen-based ROTEM test; EXTEM: extrinsic thromboelastometry; MCF: maximum clot firmness)

Case 4

A 62-year-male presented with pain in right leg. He had history of deep vein thrombosis (DVT) 2 years back. On examination, swelling of right leg is seen. Clinically, he is suspected to have recurrent DVT. Can any POC test be used to predict recurrence?

D-dimer along with a low pretest probability score is the parameter that has a high negative predictive for DVT in the outpatient setting. In this scenario, referrals for D-dimer testing to central laboratories take time and delay the diagnosis. There are multiple POC devices that can measure D-dimer and can aid in diagnosis especially at the primary care or emergency setting. Some of the POC devices for D-dimer are listed in **Table 5**.

TABLE 5: Point-of-care (POC) devices for D-dimer.

Test	Quantitative				Qualitative
	Pathfast D-dimer	***Vidas D-dimer test***	***Cardiac D-dimer***	***Triage D-dimer***	***Clearview simplify D-dimer***
Sample volume	100 μL citrated plasma	200 μL of citrated plasma	150 μL whole blood anticoagulated with Li-heparin	250 μL of EDTA whole blood	35 μL of capillary whole blood
Methodology	Chemiluminescent enzyme immunoassay with two D-dimer monoclonal antibodies, one labeled with alkaline phosphatase and the other coated with magnetic particles	Two-step enzyme immunoassay sandwich method with fluorescent detection. It uses an alkaline phosphatase–labeled anti-FbDP monoclonal antibody (P2C5A10)	Dual monoclonal antibody sandwich comprising a poly-(streptavidin)-biotin capture system with a gold particle label	Single-marker fluorescence sandwich immunoassay uses the 3B6 D-dimer antibody	Immunochromatography, and the test uses two D-dimer–specific murine monoclonal antibodies, one of which (DD3B6/224) is conjugated to colloidal gold particles
Results	The analyzer displays a quantitative result within a range of 5–5000 μg/L FEU, with a cutoff value of 570 μg/L FEU	The Vidas analyzer displays a quantitative result within a range of 45–10,000 μg/L FEU, with a cutoff value of 500 μg/L FEU	The cardiac D-dimer displays a quantitative result within a range of 100–4,000 μg/L FEU, with a cutoff value of 500 μg/L FEU	The Triage Meter Plus displays a quantitative result within a range of 56 –2,800 μg/L FEU (or 100 –5,000 μg/L D-DU), with a cutoff value of 196 μg/L FEU (or 350 μg/L D-DU)	A visible pink-purple colored line is formed at the test zone (T) when D-dimer concentrations exceed 80 μg/L (positive test result). Test results are valid if a pink-purple line is present at the control zone (PC)

(EDTA: ethylenediaminetetraacetic acid; FEU: fibrinogen equivalent units; FbDP: fibrin degradation products)

Case 5

A 62-year-male, case of ischemic stroke was started on clopidogrel 75 mg + aspirin. He suffered one more stroke while on therapy. The neurologist wants to assess if antiplatelet therapy is working or not.

The gold standard technique to measure platelet function is light transmission aggregometry (LTA). However, it requires patient preparation, fasting state, operator skill-intensive, is laborious, and requires a large volume of blood. Some POC devices that are used to assess platelet function are described in **Table 6**.

TABLE 6: Point-of-care (POC) devices of platelet function monitoring.

System	PFA-100 (Siemens Healthcare)	VerifyNow assay (Werfen)	Multiplate analyzer (Roche Diagnostics)	TEG platelet mapping (Hemonetics corp.)	ROTEM platelets system (Werfen)
Methodology	WB is drawn through a small capillary tube and an aperture coated with collagen and other agonists under high shear. The reading stops when platelet adhesion and aggregation obstruct blood flow through the aperture (closure time). Three cartridges are available (collagen/ADP, collagen/epinephrine and collagen/prostaglandin E1), which enable detection of the effects of aspirin or P2Y12 receptor inhibitor	Turbidometry-based optical detection system that assesses the antiplatelet response of aspirin and P2Y12 receptor inhibitors in whole blood. Agonist-stimulated platelets bind to fibrinogen-coated polystyrene beads, leading to aggregation and changes in light transmission in citrated whole blood after addition of different activators, including lyophilized ADP and prostaglandin E1. The result is shown as platelet reaction units (PRU) calculated from changes in light transmission	WB using electrical impedance aggregometry. Hirudin-anticoagulated blood is mixed with saline in a disposable test cuvette containing two independent highly conductive metallic wires. Specific platelet activators (e.g., AA, ADP + PGE1, or TRAP) are added to induce platelet aggregation. Electrical impedance between the wires increases, which is monitored for 6-minutes. Results are averaged to a calculated area under the curve and are expressed as aggregation units	Evaluation of platelet function through direct activation of AA and ADP receptors, with analysis of the resulting formation of TEG curves. Comparison of these curves with the standard kaolin activated TEG assay allows for the quantification of platelet aggregation and inhibition at both AA and ADP receptors	Impedance aggregometry to assess platelet function in citrated whole blood. ADP-TEM for Clopidogrel, ARA-TEM for Cox inhibitors, TRAP-TEM for GpIIb/IIIa inhibitors

(AA: arachidonic acid; ADP: adenosine diphosphate; PGE1: prostaglandin E1; TEG: thromboelastography)

Of these devices, VerifyNow is a cartridge-based system that lends itself to platelet function monitoring in a very simplified manner.

Verify, Now was used for our case 5. Platelet reaction unit (PRU) was 240 in the P2Y12 cartridge and indicated inadequate inhibition of platelet function. The antiplatelet therapy was modified to aspirin 100 mg and clopidogrel dose was increased to 150 mg. Reassessment revealed a PRU of 145 and the patient did not suffer any subsequent events on the revised doses.

CONCLUSION

POC tests in coagulation are an expanding market. The biggest share is the monitoring of vitamin K antagonist therapy with many devices such as CoagChek XS and Pro, Xpercia Stride, etc. These devices are of use for patients who can monitor and self-adjust their therapy. In addition, they are also used in the anticoagulation clinics to reduce turn-around time. The second large market is to monitor UFH therapy and for that ACT is used with a target value of >480 seconds for nonheparin bound circuits and is also used for protamine reversal. The third segment is viscoelastic testing with use of ROTEM and TEG which study all the phases of coagulation and also the contribution of platelets and fibrinolytic pathway. They have led to an optimization of patient blood management during many operative procedures. D-dimer testing at primary care settings can also be done using multiple POC devices. The last segment is for assessing antiplatelet therapy for which VerifyNow, MultiPlate, etc., are available and can be used to tailor therapy in patients started on antiplatelet therapy.

Future directions: The POC devices are going to expand with additions in the automated equipment such as Quantra, higher uptake of TEG-6s, ROTEM Sigma, INR monitoring devices, as well as antiplatelet therapy adjustment.

Take Home Points

- POC testing in coagulation is expanding.
- POC tests have a higher cost per test but can be performed with less skilled individuals and some tests even by patients themselves.
- VKA monitoring by INR estimation is the largest component of POC market.
- ACT-UFH monitoring for cardiac surgeries.
- Viscoelastic testing—TEG/ROTEM/(Quantra).
- Antiplatelet monitoring by VerifyNow, MultiPlate. Platelet function modules on TEG and ROTEM are also available.
- D-dimer estimations at primary care centers—Vidas®, Pathfast™, Cardiac®, and Triage®, LumiraDx, AQT90 Flex, etc.

SUGGESTED READINGS

1. Wool GD. Benefits and Pitfalls of point-of-care coagulation testing for anticoagulation management. Am J Clin Pathol. 2019;151(1):1-17.
2. Ferreira CN, Sousa M de O, Dusse LMS, Carvalho MG. Revista Brasileira de Hematologia E Hemoterapia. 2010;32:416-21.
3. Fortune Business Insights. (2028). Point of care coagulation testing devices market growth. [online] Available from https://www.fortunebusinessinsights.com/industry-reports/point-of-care-coagulation-testing-devices-market-101235 [Last accessed May, 2025].
4. CADTH optimal use reports. Guidance on the use of point-of-care testing of international normalized ratio for patients on oral anticoagulant therapy. Ottawa (ON): Canadian Agency for Drugs and Technologies in Health; 2014.
5. CADTH optimal use reports. Point-of-care testing of international normalized ratio for patients on oral anticoagulant therapy: systematic review and economic analysis. Ottawa (ON): Canadian Agency for Drugs and Technologies in Health; 2014.
6. Hattersley PG. Activated coagulation time of whole blood. JAMA. 1966;196(5):436-40.
7. Wahba A, Milojevic M, Boer C, De Somer FMJJ, Gudbjartsson T, van den Goor J, et al. 2019 EACTS/EACTA/EBCP guidelines on cardiopulmonary bypass in adult cardiac surgery. Eur J Cardiothorac Surg. 2020;57(2):210-51.
8. Sahli SD, Rössler J, Tscholl DW, Studt JD, Spahn DR, Kaserer A. Point-of-care diagnostics in coagulation management. Sensors. 2020;20(15):4254.

CHAPTER 11

MicroRNAs in Hematology

Ruchi Gupta, Manish Kumar Singh, Ghazala Sabereen

ABSTRACT

MicroRNAs (miRNAs) have emerged as pivotal post-transcriptional regulator in various biological processes. In hematology, they have the capability of delicately balancing various hematopoietic pathways like self-renewal of hematopoietic precursors, lineage commitment, and apoptosis within the entire spectrum of hematopoietic hierarchy. Many miRNAs such as miR-142, miR-144, miR-150, miR-155, and miR-223 are highly hematopoiesis-specific and fine-tune each step from stem cell quiescence to terminal differentiation. A dysregulation of the miRNAs can thus perturb differentiation, and their imbalance are likely to contribute toward the development of hematological malignancies. There are numerous studies in individual disease states which have attempted to uncover the role of miRNAs in different hematological diseases; this chapter aims to briefly discuss the complex biogenesis of miRNAs, and their responsibility in normal hematopoiesis and in various benign and malignant hematological disorders.

INTRODUCTION

The role of genetic and epigenetic modifiers in normal and malignant hematopoiesis has long been established and is still unraveling. The epigenetic alterations do not directly hamper the genetic sequences but disturb the physiological balance between gene activation and gene repression, resulting in an aberrant gene expression. Epigenetic alterations are mediated through DNA modifications, histone modifications, chromatin remodeling, and noncoding RNAs (ncRNAs). MicroRNAs (miRNAs) are among the most extensively researched ncRNAs, and there is mounting evidence to highlight the role of miRNAs in fine-tuning normal hematopoiesis and regulating oncogenes and tumor suppressors in hematological malignancies. miRNAs regulate more than 1,500 encoding genes in the human genome. Numerous studies have revealed that miRNAs have a remarkable ability to move between various subcellular compartments, body fluids and microvesicles. This mobility plays a crucial role in regulating various cellular processes; they can act as signaling molecules, facilitating communication between cells and mediating cell-cell interactions. In this review, a brief overview of the genesis of miRNAs, their role in normal hematopoiesis and in some of the hematological disorders is provided.

BIOGENESIS OF MicroRNAs

The miRNAs are non-coding small RNAs, with an average length of 22 nucleotides. They were originally discovered in *Caenorhabditis elegans*. The genes transcribing miRNA occur singly or in clusters, and are located majorly in the intronic regions of the protein encoding. They may also be found in intergenic regions of the genome. When miRNAs are located in the intronic region, the host genes may regulate their expression. The biogenesis of miRNA is a complex process and involves multiple steps; originating in the nucleus in the precursor form and then further processing in the cytoplasm to form the mature miRNA in the cytoplasm. The key steps involved in the generation of miRNA is briefly depicted in **Figure 1**. In the nucleus the miRNA is double stranded, and is transported to the cytoplasm through exportin. In the cytoplasm, one strand is retained (guide strand) based on

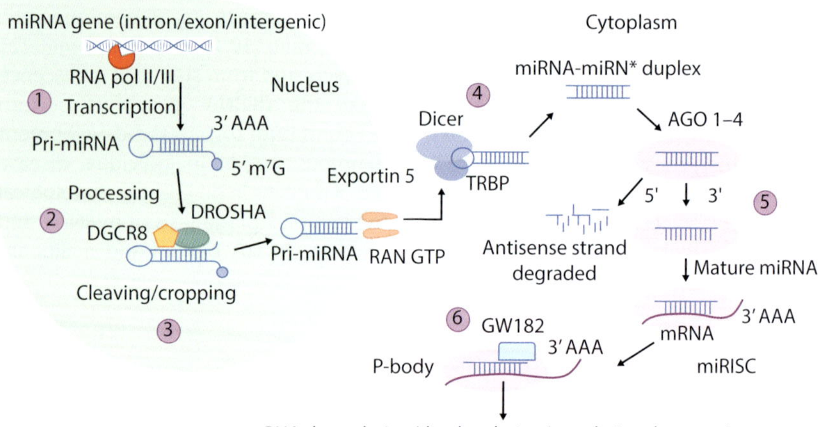

FIG. 1: Summary of miRNA biogenesis pathway. Biogenesis of miRNAs consists of the stepwise processing of pri-miRNAs in the nucleus and the cytoplasm. Briefly, 1, 2 depict the formation of primary miRNAs (pri-miRNA), which is a distinct hairpin-like structure that is recognized and cleaved by the "microprocessor", a heterodimer complex formed by DROSHA and DGCR8. The microprocessor cleavage site is defined by multiple structural and sequence motifs. The resulting product is exported into the cytoplasm via Exportin-5, for a second cleavage event by DICER. The resulting duplex is loaded into one of the AGO paralogs for strand selection and assembly of mature RISC complexes. Recognition chambers inside AGO facilitate the recognition of target RNAs, and the subset of nucleotides involved in these facilitated pairings is known as the seed sequences (sky blue color) and the complementary pairing regions. The miRISC molecules and repressed mRNAs accumulate in specific areas of cytoplasm, such as P bodies, GW bodies, and stress granules, where the presence of deadenylating enzymes and AGO proteins in these areas leads to the decay of mRNA.

the thermodynamic stability and accessible 5' end, while the other one is degraded (passenger strand). The guide strand is critical for the recognition of mRNA target in the RNA induced silencing complex (RISC). The 2nd to the 8th nucleotide from the 5' end of the guide strand is called the "seed region" and is critical for the recognition of target RNAs. The interaction of the mRNA with miRNA requires a perfect, or a near-perfect sequence complementarity to this seed region. The suppression of gene expression occurs either through the complementarity with the seed region, leading subsequently to mRNA degradation or translational repression

MicroRNAs IN HEMATOPOIESIS

Hematopoiesis is a well-ordered step-wise lineage restriction, originating from a very small population of self-renewing stem cells. The multipotent progenitors (MPP) differentiate either into lymphoid-restricted common lymphoid progenitors or form myeloid and erythroid/megakaryocytic (MEK) specific common progenitors. All the stages of hematopoiesis are tightly regulated by an intricate network of dedicated transcription factors and miRNAs. Petrov et al. studied 27 different hematopoietic subsets from all parts of the hematopoietic hierarchy in adult mice and defined a comprehensive profile of 288 miRNA in different cell lineages. Differential expression of miRNAs was appreciated in the progenitor populations as compared to the differentiated cell types. The miRNAs overexpressed in the stem cells, included, miR-125b, miR-196a, miR-196b, let-7d, miR-148b, miR-130a, and miR-351, while many miRNAs like miR-484, miR-200c, miR-331, miR-320, miR-210, miR-324–5p, miR-212, and miR-690, are downregulated in progenitors, but expressed across differentiated cells. Interestingly, although a distinct profile of miRNAs has been observed in different cell lineages, only five miRNAs have been reported to be highly specific for hematopoietic cells; miR-142, miR-144, miR-150, miR-155, and miR-223.

Moreover, their analysis revealed that there were no lineage specific miRNAs in the 27 populations studied, rather a bi- and sometimes trimodal expression patterns was observed in different stages of maturation of the cells. A diagrammatic representation of some of the differentially expressed miRNAs at each step of hematopoietic hierarchy is provided in **Figure 2**.

MicroRNAs IN HEMATOLOGICAL DISORDERS

MicroRNAs are extensively involved in all cellular processes, and hence covering the role of miRNAs in all aspects of hematological disorders would be difficult in this review; hence, the authors have focused on some of the routinely encountered, benign, and malignant hematological states, as detailed here.

MicroRNAs and Anemia

MicroRNA remains stable and is thus able to interact and modulate transporters, enzymes, and receptors in distant cells/organs. Several studies have demonstrated that various miRNAs, viz. miR-15a, miR-24, miR-150, and miR-223,

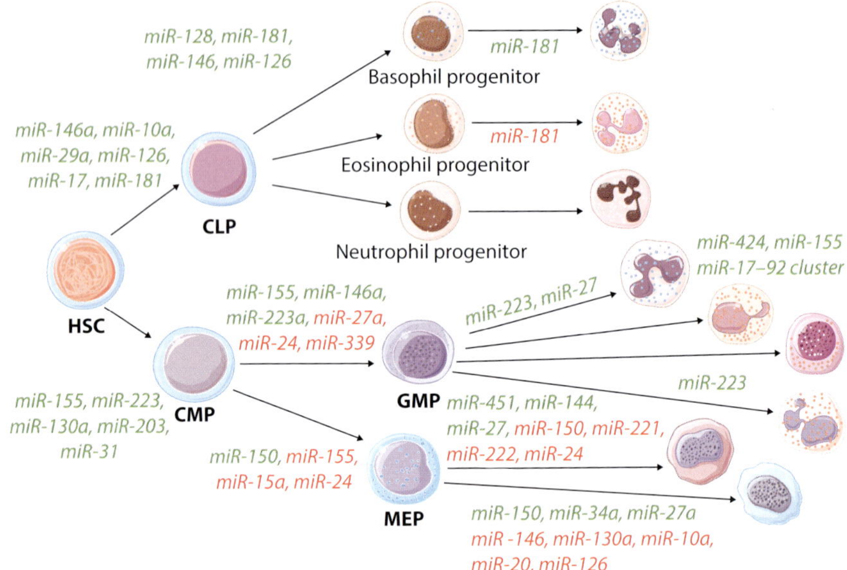

FIG. 2: Hematopoietic hierarchy with key regulatory microRNAs (miRNAs). The miRNAs in green color are upregulated, while the red color depicts the downregulated miRNAs.

(CLP: common lymphoid progenitor; CMP: common myeloid progenitor; GMP: granulocyte/macrophage progenitor; HSC: hematopoietic stem cells; MEP: megakaryocyte/erythroid progenitor; MPP: multipotent progenitors; Pro-B: B lymphocyte progenitor; Pro-NK: NK-cell progenitor; Pro-T: T-cell progenitor)

influence anemia by regulating erythropoiesis. These miRNAs have been found to deregulate erythropoiesis in several diseases such as iron deficiency anemia (IDA), thalassemia, sickle cell disease, leukemia, and other cancers. miR-15a suppresses erythropoiesis by inhibiting c-Myb, and it also ameliorates the severity of thalassemia and sickle cell disease by increasing HbF levels. miR-24 impairs heme biosynthesis through ALK4 regulation, while miR-150 and miR-223 modulate critical hematopoietic pathways affecting cell differentiation and apoptosis. miR-146a, miR-125b, and miR-122 were significantly upregulated with lower hepcidin expression in adolescents with iron deficiency and IDA, when compared with iron overloaded individuals. The downregulation of these miRNAs was found to be associated with higher hepcidin levels. These miRNA-protein interactions suggest that targeted therapies such as protein-based miRNA modulators could optimize erythropoiesis.

MicroRNAs and Acquired Aplastic Anemia

A perturbed T-cell homeostasis and immune-mediated hematopoietic stem cell (HSC) destruction are known to be the key pathogenetic mechanism of acquired aplastic anemia (aAA). Inhibitory cytokines such as interferon-gamma (IFN-γ) and TNF-α play a significant role in suppressing human HSC. aAA simulates an autoimmune like state, where there is immune mediated destruction of the hematopoietic stem cells leads to marrow failure and pancytopenia. The immune deregulation includes a Th1 polarization and Th17/Treg cell imbalance. Inhibitory cytokines like IFN-γ and TNF-α play a significant role in suppressing human hematopoietic stem cells (HSCs). miRNAs are closely intertwined with T cell differentiation and can modulate their cytokine-related functional outputs. miR-17 and miR-19b, are the key players controlling Th1 responses, supporting IFN-γ production while miR-155 and miR-17 lead to downregulation of SHIP-1 and PTEN, respectively, which leads to T cell expansion. Some of the miRNAs known to be deregulated in the activated T cells in aAA are miR-126, miR-155, miR-146b-5p, miR-150, and miR-1. The miR-150 is upregulated in activated T cells and has been shown to serve as a biomarker for AA and help monitor its progression. It also supports the survival of effector CD8+ T cells and reduces their differentiation into memory cells by attenuating IL-2 signaling. Downregulation of miR-16, and upregulation of both of its targets, NF-κB and MYC, has been reported in aAA patients, thereby facilitating a proinflammatory milieu.

MicroRNAs and Immune Thrombocytopenia

miRNA-150 regulates megakaryocyte differentiation and maturation by targeting MYB, a transcription factor that inhibits megakaryopoiesis. As in other autoimmune disorders such as systemic lupus erythematosus, and rheumatoid arthritis, miRNAs have a critical role in immune thrombocytopenia (ITP), by deregulating the immune response. miRNAs such as miR-155, miR-146, mir-142, and miR-181 have been shown to be deregulated in ITP. miR-146a acts such as a "break" and is a regulator of T-cell activation; it is downregulated in ITP, leading to excessive immune activation and destruction of platelets. Results of genome-wide expression analysis of mRNA and microRNA in the T cells of patients with ITP showed that there were 1,915 genes and 22 miRNAs differentially expressed in ITP when compared to controls. *miR-142-3p, miR-21,* and *miR-146a* can serve as biomarkers for diagnosing and monitoring thrombocytopenia, and levels of miR-199a-5p and miR-221-3p are helpful in predicting the response of patients to thrombopoietin receptor agonists.

MicroRNAs in Acute Leukemias

Acute lymphoblastic leukemias reflect lymphoid maturation arrest in distinct stages resulting in specific immunophenotypic and miRNA signatures. Recently Turk et al. reviewed the literature on miRNA in leukemias (ALL, AML, CML, and CLL), and miR-155-5p, miR-181a-5p, miR-125b-5p, and miR-19a-3p, reportedly had the highest number of miRNA-target interactions (MTIs). The target genes with the highest number of MTIs were TP53, BCL2, KIT, ATM, RUNX1, and ABL1. Interestingly, amongst the other miRNAs, they observed that 82 miRNAs were differentially expressed in only one type of leukemia while 55 miRNAs were associated with two or more subtypes. Some of the miRNAs which are deregulated in B-ALL, T-ALL, and AML and the ones with prognostic and therapeutic relevance are shown in **Figure 3**.

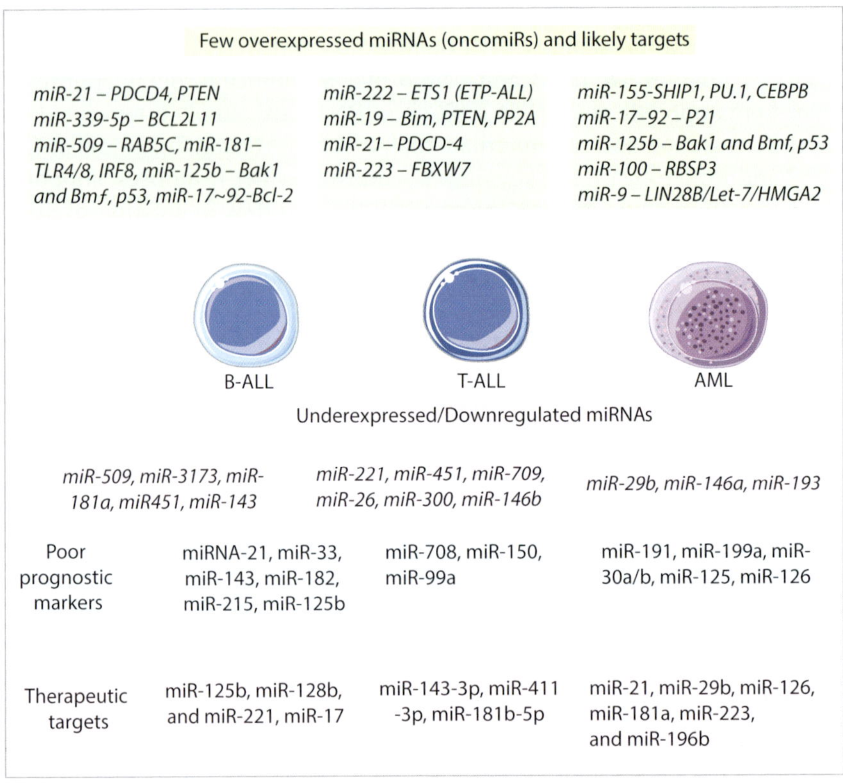

FIG. 3: MicroRNAs in acute leukemia.

MicroRNAs in B-cell Non-Hodgkin Lymphoma

MicroRNAs are actively involved in the B-cell ontogeny and finely regulate the genesis of lymphocyte subsets, and thus their dysregulation in lymphoid neoplasms is evident. They are critical players involved in the pathogenesis, diagnosis, and prognosis of these malignancies. Studies have been carried out to delineate individual miRNA expression and ascertain miRNA signatures for specific stages of cell differentiation. The levels of miRNA-155, miRNA-200c, miRNA-130a, miRNA-125b, and miRNA-21 were found to be significantly upregulated, whereas miRNA29c, miRNA451, and miRNA145 were downregulated in B-NHL patients when compared with healthy controls. Some of the salient miRNAs involved in the genesis or prognosis of some of the B-NHL are documented here.

- *Chronic lymphocytic leukemia (CLL)*: Interestingly, the first genetic alteration of a miRNA locus, and was reported in CLL, which was the deletion of miR-15a/16-1. It has been identified in approximately 70% of CLL patients. The deletion of the 13q14 region in CLL, corroborates with loss of miRNA-15 and miRNA-16. Prognostically, down-regulation of miR-29 has been noted with an aggressive form of the disease. A downregulation of miR34a has been seen in CLL patients with del17p or TP53 mutation; thereby making it an important biomarker of poor treatment response. The therapeutic potential of some miRNAs has also been explored in CLL like miR-181a. It plays an important role in the regulation of apoptosis. It has been considered a potential candidate for the management of CLL cases which over-express TCL-1 in preclinical studies. Similarly, a synthetic locked nucleic acid (LNA anti-miR) of miR-155 inhibitor, cobomarsen (MRG-106) has been tested in a phase I clinical trial in many lymphomas including CLL

- *Diffuse large B-cell lymphoma*: Some of the highly expressed miRNAs in DLBCL are miRNA-17-92, miRNA-222, miR-15a/16-1 clusters, and let-7f. Forced overexpression of miRNA-155 leads to the suppression of the growth inhibition of BMP2/4 and TGF-β1 via SMAD5 inhibition leading to the development of DLBCL. Like CLL, miRNA-15a/miRNA-16-1 are decreased which otherwise target BCL2; thereby reducing apoptosis of lymphoma cells. The upregulation of miRNA-17-92 in GCB-DLBCL correlates with increased MYC expression, and aggressiveness of lymphomas by affecting apoptosis. Fassina et al. reported significant overexpression of miRNA-17-92 cluster, miRNA-150, and miRNA-210 in GCB-DLBCL and allowed correct subtyping of DLBCLs and correctly identified 97% of GCB-DLBCL cases. miR-34a, miR-181a and miR-222, while miR-142, miR-146-5p, and miR-223 were notable for treatment-free survival in patients with DLBCL.
- *Follicular lymphoma (FL)*: Overexpressed miRNAs distinct to FL are miRNA-20a/b and miRNA-194 and they target cell proliferation inhibitors such as CDKN1A and SOCS2, respectively.
- *Mantle cell lymphoma (MCL)*: miRNAs such as miRNA-124a, miRNA-155, miRNA-328, miRNA-326, miRNA-302c, miRNA-345, miRNA-373, and miRNA-210 were identified as upregulated in patients with MCL, while the miRNA-29 family (miRNA-29a, -29b, and -29c) is downregulated. The upregulated miRNA inhibits CDK6 expression as well as phosphorylation of RB1. As in CLL, miR-16-1 regulates the expression of cyclin D1 in MCL. Due to truncated cyclin D1 mRNA, there is a deletion of miR-16-1 binding sites within the cyclin D1 mRNA 3′-UTR, resulting in increased total cyclin D1 mRNA and protein expression. Prognostically, miRNA-142-3p/5p, miRNA-150, and miRNA-15a/b were found to be associated with short overall survival of patients with MCL.
- *Nodal marginal zone lymphoma (NMZL)*: NMZL has been shown to overexpress miRNA-221, miRNA-223, and let-7f, in contrast to FL, which shows upregulation of miRNA-494. The germinal center-related genes LMO2 and CD10 are the potential targets of miRNA-223 and miRNA-221 and thus may be considered as marginal zone miRNA signature.

MicroRNAs in Multiple Myeloma

miRNAs can influence the pathogenesis and progression of MM. Global miRNA expression profiles were evaluated by Pichiorri et al. in four normal plasma cell samples, five MGUS patients and, 10 MM patients. A differential miRNA expression of miR-21, miR-32, and miR-17–92 cluster, miR-106b~25 cluster, miR-181a/b was noted in MM and MGUS, in comparison to normal PCs . In plasma cell leukemia, overexpression of 4 miRNAs (miR-106b, miR-497, miR-181b, and miR-181a*) was reported by Lionetti et al. and these patients exhibited a poor treatment response to lenalidomide and low-dose dexamethasone. In comparison to responders. The downregulation of miR-15a/16, and IL-6 induced miR-21 expression via STAT3-dependent pathways in MM cells, favors cell proliferation and decreasing apoptosis in MM. The miRNA expressions are also in tune with the chromosomal abnormalities. For example, gain of chromosome 1q correlates with the overexpression of miRNAs located at 1q which include: miR-1231, miR-205, miR-215, and miR-488. Similarly, MM patients with t(14; 16) show a higher expression of miR-1 and miR-133a, and a downregulation of miR-135b and miR-146a is seen in MM with t(4; 14). miRNAs can influence p53-dependent tumor suppressor activities as well; like miR-125b and miR-504 are direct negative regulators of p53, while miR-125a-5p acts as an oncomiR. Furthermore, MM cells exhibiting drug resistance, show upregulation of the miR-21, miR-125a, b miR-221/222, and miR-451, while aberrant expression of miR-137 sensitizes the cells to bortezomib, thereby becoming potential therapeutic targets.

MicroRNAs in Myeloproliferative Neoplasms

It is well established that the mutations in tyrosine kinase and other related genes lead to constitutively active proteins, which leads to myeloproliferative. While the generation of the BCR-ABL1 oncogene, encoding the chimeric BCR-ABL1 protein with constitutive kinase activity is the driving force for CML, the key driver mutations in polycythemia vera (PV), essential thrombocythemia (ET), primary myelofibrosis (PMF), and chronic neutrophilic leukemia, include *JAK2, CALR, MPL,* and *CSF3R,* which result in constitutive activation of the Janus kinase/signal transducer and activator of transcription (JAK-STAT) pathway. The role of miRNAs in MPN is divided into two broad categories as described here:

1. *MiRNAs in CML*: Many miRNAs reported to be de-regulated in CML, some of which include, miR-155, miR-152-3p, miR-362-5p, miR-140, miR-409, miR-50, miR-320a, miR-92a-1-5p, which are directly or indirectly involved in disease pathogenesis. Some of these are depicted in **Figure 4**. These miRNAs

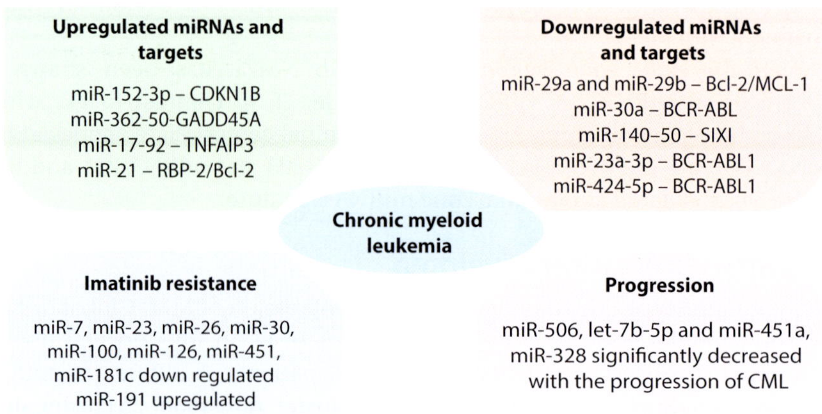

FIG. 4: MircoRNAs alteration in chronic myeloid leukemia (CML).

are involved in various pathways involving cell proliferation, apoptosis, cell cycle regulation and, differentiation. The therapeutic importance of miRNAs has also been documented in various studies and the expression of miR-17, miR-18a, and miR-20a was significantly higher in the imatinib (IM) resistant patients when compared to IM-responsive patients, and miR-21 and miR-451 have been appear to be good biomarkers to predict optimal TKI responders.

2. *miRNAs in BCR-ABL1 negative MPNs*: Overexpression of miR29a and miR125b in mouse hematopoietic stem/progenitor cells results in biased myeloid expansion and the development of a myeloproliferative disorder that progresses to AML. It is interesting to note that JAK2 positivity is seen in all three conditions, viz, ET, PV, and MF >95% PV patients and in 50–60% of ET and PMF patients. However, it is interesting to note that the same mutation could result in three different phenotypes. This may be explained by the regulation mediated by the disease-specific miRNA. Their deregulations may contribute to the specific phenotypes of PV, ET, and PMF and can be used to differentiate the three disorders. Studies in mouse models have shown that a myeloproliferative disorder phenotype may be developed by sustained expression of a single miRNA, miR-125b or miR-155, or knock-out of miR-146a. miR-125b inhibits apoptosis leading to an expansion of HSC, by probable regulation of the TP53 pathway genes. Tombak A et al. observed discriminatory expression of miR-221 and miR-223 particularly in ET and PMF groups ($p < 0.05$) , while miR-451, miR-144, and miR-145 have been reported to be higher in PV samples.

A summary of the commonly observed deregulated miRNAs in a few hematological disorders is provided in **Table 1**.

TABLE 1: Summary of the miRNAs and their targets in some of the hematological diseases.

Diseases	miRNA	Regulatory functions
B-acute lymphoblastic leukemia	miR-125b	miR-125b can target apoptosis regulators like Bak1 and Puma and cyclin C
	miR-99a	miRNA-99a regulates the FKBP51 and IGF-1R/mTOR signaling pathways, which suppress proliferation and promote apoptosis
	miR-100	Overexpression of miRNA-99a and miR-100 is associated with a poor prognosis and resistance to vincristine and daunorubicin
	Let-7e	Let-7e miRNAs act as tumor suppressors and are involved in the pathogenesis of various hematological malignancies, including leukemia. Let-7e miRNA profiles can be used to classify ALL subtypes and recognize ALL patients

Continued

Continued

Diseases	miRNA	Regulatory functions
B-acute lympho-blastic leukemia	miR-181b	It is also a potential therapeutic target for the treatment of leukemia patients. miRNA-181b-5p regulates cell proliferation by targeting SSX2IP, also enriched in vesicles/exosomes of circulating leukemic cells, hence can be used as a prognosis biomarker for childhood ALL
T-acute lyampho-blastic leukemia	miR-146b-5p	Overexpression of miR-146b-5p delays T-ALL progression. Therefore, miR-146b-5p is a functional tumor suppressor miRNA in T-ALL
	miR-223	Upregulation of miR-223 leads to decreased FBXW7 expression, which can increase MYC, MYB, NOTCH1, and cyclin E levels
	miR-19	miR-19, the cluster component with the highest expression in T-ALL, enhances lymphocyte survival and cooperates to promote leukemogenesis in a mouse model of T-ALL
	miR-146a	microRNA-146a promotes the growth of leukemic cells by downregulating CNFR and activating JAK2/STAT3 signaling
	miR-150	Downregulation of miRNA-150 in T-ALL correlates with a higher relapse rate, indicating its prominent role in T-ALL pathogenesis
	miR-155	miRNA-155 is overexpressed in patients with T-ALL and may contribute to the initiation and progression of the disease. Downregulation correlates with poor prognosis; BCL2 is a potential target for this miRNA
Acute myeloid leukemia	miR-17~92 cluster,	Overexpression of miR-17, 20-a, and miR-106-a suppresses AML-1 protein expression, which leads to decreased monocyte differentiation and maturation, and enhanced blast proliferation
	miR-9 and 9* (miR-9/9*)	Overexpression of miR-9 acts as an oncomiR and promotes proliferation and cell survival in MLL-rearranged AMLs. In t(8;21) positive AMLs, it facilitates monocytic differentiation and has a tumor suppressor function.
	miR-326	miR-326 may act as a tumor suppressor gene, regulating cell growth, apoptosis, migration, and invasion. miR-326 mimics are able to artificially inhibit tumor growth and metastasis
	miR-194	miR-194-5p expression declines in AML, and restoration of miR-194-5p retards proliferation and triggers cell apoptosis
	miR-301b	miR-301b induces proliferation and suppresses apoptosis in AML cells by modulating the FOXF2/Wnt/β-catenin axis
	miR-324	miR-324-5p is upregulated in AML and is a therapeutic target in AML
	miR-328	Downregulation of miR-328 in AML patients is associated with a poor prognosis, including shorter RFS and worse OS

Continued

Continued

Diseases	miRNA	Regulatory functions
Myelodysplastic syndrome (MDS)	miR-205-5p	miR-205-5p can act as an oncogene in MDS by suppressing PTEN
	miR-320a	High levels of miR-320 in MDS may be associated with a poor prognosis
	miR-125a	miR-125a plays a crucial role in MDS by regulating the expression of genes that control cell proliferation and differentiation. Overexpression of miR-125a in CD34+ cells of MDS patients can arrest erythroid differentiation and modulate the NF-κB activation pathway
	miR-378-3p	miR-378-3p is underexpressed in most cases of MDS, which is associated with hypermethylation of its promoter
	miR-29b	Downregulation of miRNA-29b promotes the transformation of MDS into AML
	miRNA-126	MicroRNA-126 (miR-126) plays a crucial role in maintaining MDS stem and progenitor cells. A study found that targeting miR-126 can increase cell cycling, enhance apoptosis, partially reverse pancytopenia, and block leukemic transformation
B-NHL	miR-155	miR-155 is oncogenic, and transgenic mice that express miR-155 in B cells develop lymphoma. In CLL, high levels of miR-155 are associated with increased cell division, apoptosis inhibition, and more aggressive disease
	miR-17-92	This cluster promotes cell survival, proliferation, and angiogenesis. Conditional knockout of miR-17/92 in Myc-driven lymphomas increases apoptosis and reduces tumorigenicity and tumor progression, making it an attractive therapeutic target
	miR-15a and miR-16-1	miRNA-15a is part of the miR-15/16 cluster, which suppresses tumorigenicity, promotes apoptosis, and inhibits cell proliferation. miRNA 15a targets oncogenes such as BCL2, MCL1, CCND1, and WNT3A. In CLL, miR-15a and miR-16-1 expression levels are inversely correlated with BCL2 expression
	miR-181	miRNA-181a in CLL acts as a tumor suppressor gene. miR-181a, along with miR-221 and miR-223, has the greatest diagnostic potential for CLL
	miR-19	miR-19a is an oncogenic miRNA that promotes c-MYC-induced lymphomagenesis by repressing apoptosis by the activation of PTEN. miR-19a alters cellular sensitivity to chemotherapy drugs, such as cisplatin, 5-FC, and adriamycin
	miR-224	miR-224 expression may play a significant role in the development and progression of DLBCL. Low expression is associated with a poor clinical outcome in DLBCL patients treated with R-CHOP

Continued

Continued

Diseases	miRNA	Regulatory functions
B-NHL	miR-34a	Decreased expression levels of miRNA-34a are associated with prognosis in lymphomas such as diffuse large B-cell lymphoma (DLBCL). It can induce apoptosis in B-cell lymphoma by reducing the expression of B-cell lymphoma 2 (BCL2) and sirtuin-1
	miR-150	Overexpression of miR-150 can lead to reduced mature B-cell levels, increased apoptosis, and severe defects in B-cell development. miR-150 may be a novel therapeutic target for B-NHLs
	miR-146	Low levels of miR-146b-5p and miR-320d in DLBCL patients are associated with poor clinical outcomes, such as reduced overall and progression-free survival

(AML: acute myeloid leukemia; CNFR: complement network factor receptor; miRNA: microRNA; MLL: mixed lineage leukemia; mTOR: mechanistic target of rapamycin; OS: overall survival; RFS: relapse-free survival; T-ALL: T-cell acute lymphoblastic leukemia)

TECHNIQUES FOR THE DETECTION OF MicroRNAs

The widely deployed methods for miRNA detection include Northern blotting, microarrays, and quantitative real-time polymerase chain reaction (qRT-PCR). These methods have been used for high-throughput miRNA analysis with reliable outputs and high sensitivity. With the advent of technology, next-generation sequencing (NGS), high-performance liquid chromatography, coupled with long and short probes to detect multiple miRNAs, single-molecule sequencing, have been explored for miRNA detection. Similarly, point-of-care testing such as lateral flow assays has also been explored for miRNA detection but has a long way to go in terms of improving sensitivity. Moreover, numerous innovative biochemical detection methods and miRNA sensing methods, which may be fluorescence-based, electrochemical, or Raman-scattering readouts, have been reported recently to improve sensitive multiplex detection.

Take Home Points

- MicroRNAs are small regulatory molecules, which can fine-tune numerous biological functions and are extensively intertwined with normal hematopoiesis.
- The deregulated miRNAs provide a valuable insight to the disease mechanism, and highlight that there is extensive genetic and epigenetic interplay in the genesis of a hematological malignancy, and miRNAs play a role in cell proliferation or reducing apoptosis.
- Upregulation of oncogenic miRNAs and downregulation of tumor suppressor miRNAs are associated with the genesis of many hematological malignancies, particularly leukemia.

- Unfortunately, the miRNAs are not disease specific, and they have a complex spatiotemporal relationship. Consequently, the type of miRNA and its expression vary among different diseases, and this is possibly due to the heterogeneity of the sample tested (peripheral blood, bone marrow, plasma, and extracellular vesicles) and the techniques used for ascertaining their levels.
- Summarily, miRNAs can serve as biomarkers in the diagnosis and prognostication of hematological diseases. Since many of these miRNAs have oncogenic or tumor-suppressive functions, miRNAs have been the focus of research as therapeutic targets.

SUGGESTED READINGS

1. Zhao A, Zhou H, Yang J, Li M, Niu T. Epigenetic regulation in hematopoiesis and its implications in the targeted therapy of hematologic malignancies. Sig Transduct Target Ther. 2023;8:71.
2. O'Brien J, Hayder H, Zayed Y, Peng C. Overview of MicroRNA Biogenesis, Mechanisms of Actions, and Circulation. Front Endocrinol (Lausanne). 2018;9:402.
3. Nassiri SM, Ahmadi Afshar N, Almasi P. Insight into microRNAs' involvement in hematopoiesis: current standing point of findings. Stem Cell Res Ther. 2023;14:282.
4. Petriv OI, Kuchenbauer F, Delaney AD, Lecault V, White A, Kent D, et al. Comprehensive microRNA expression profiling of the hematopoietic hierarchy. Proc Natl Acad Sci USA. 2010;107(35):15443-8.
5. Davis M, Clarke S. Influence of microRNA on the maintenance of human iron metabolism. Nutrients. 2013;5(7):2611-28.
6. Garavelli S, De Rosa V, de Candia P. The Multifaceted Interface Between Cytokines and microRNAs: An Ancient Mechanism to Regulate the Good and the Bad of Inflammation. Front Immunol. 2018;9:3012.
7. Sabreen G, Rahman K, Gupta R, Chaturvedi CP, Srivastava J, Chandra D, et al. Role of miRNAs in T-cell activation and Th17/Treg-cell imbalance in acquired aplastic anemia. Int J Lab Hematol. 2024;46(3):515-22.
8. Lu S, Yadav AK, Qiao X. Identification of potential miRNA-mRNA interaction network in bone marrow T cells of acquired aplastic anemia. Hematology. 2020;25(1):168-75.
9. Jafarzadeh A, Marzban H, Nemati M, Jafarzadeh S, Mahjoubin-Tehran M, Hamblin MR, et al. Dysregulated expression of miRNAs in immune thrombocytopenia. Epigenomics. 2021;13(16):1315-25.
10. Zhao Y, Cui S, Wang Y, Xu R. The Extensive Regulation of MicroRNA in Immune Thrombocytopenia. Clin Appl Thromb Hemost. 2022;28:10760296221093595.
11. Turk A, Calin GA, Kunej T. MicroRNAs in Leukemias: A Clinically Annotated Compendium. Int J Mol Sci. 2022;23(7):3469.
12. Tapeh BEG, Alivand MR, Solali S. The role of microRNAs in acute lymphoblastic leukemia: From biology to applications. Cell Biochem Funct. 2020;38(4):334-46.
13. Autore F, Ramassone A, Stirparo L, Pagotto S, Fresa A, Innocenti I, et al. Role of microRNAs in Chronic Lymphocytic Leukemia. Int J Mol Sci. 2023;24(15):12471.
14. Getaneh Z, Asrie F, Melku M. MicroRNA profiles in B-cell non-Hodgkin lymphoma. EJIFCC. 2019;30(2):195-214.
15. Witten L, Slack FJ. miR-155 as a novel clinical target for hematological malignancies. Carcinogenesis. 2020;41(1):2-7.
16. Handa H, Murakami Y, Ishihara R, Kimura-Masuda K, Masuda Y. The Role and Function of microRNA in the Pathogenesis of Multiple Myeloma. Cancers (Basel). 2019;11(11):1738.

17. Pichiorri F, Suh SS, Ladetto M, Kuehl M, Palumbo T, Drandi D, et al. MicroRNAs regulate critical genes associated with multiple myeloma pathogenesis. Proc Natl Acad Sci USA. 2008;105(35):12885-90.
18. Lionetti M, Musto P, Di Martino MT, Fabris S, Agnelli L, Todoerti K, et al. Biological and clinical relevance of miRNA expression signatures in primary plasma cell leukemia. Clin Cancer Res. 2013;19(12):3130-42.
19. Jang MA, Choi CW. Recent insights regarding the molecular basis of myeloproliferative neoplasms. Korean J Intern Med. 2020;35(1):1-11.
20. Navabi A, Akbari B, Abdalsamadi M, Naseri S. The role of microRNAs in the development, progression, and drug resistance of chronic myeloid leukemia and their potential clinical significance. Life Sci. 2022;296:120437.
21. Zhan H, Cardozo C, Raza A. MicroRNAs in myeloproliferative neoplasms. Br J Haematol. 2013;161(4):471-83.
22. Li XJ, Luo XQ, Han BW, Duan FT, Wei PP, Chen YQ. MicroRNA-100/99a, deregulated in acute lymphoblastic leukemia, suppresses proliferation and promotes apoptosis by regulating the FKBP51 and IGF1R/mTOR signaling pathways. Br J Cancer. 2013;109(8):2189-98.
23. Yan W, Song L, Wang H, Yang W, Hu L, Yang Y. Extracellular vesicles carrying miRNA-181b-5p affect the malignant progression of acute lymphoblastic leukemia. J Transl Med. 2021;19:511.
24. Pomari E, Lovisa F, Carraro E, Primerano S, D'Amore ESG, Bonvini P, et al. Clinical impact of miR-223 expression in pediatric T-Cell lymphoblastic lymphoma. Oncotarget. 2017;8(64): 107886-98.
25. Wang L, Zhang H, Lei D. microRNA-146a Promotes Growth of Acute Leukemia Cells by Downregulating Ciliary Neurotrophic Factor Receptor and Activating JAK2/STAT3 Signaling. Yonsei Med J. 2019;60(10):924-34.
26. Mendiola-Soto DK, Bárcenas-López DA, Pérez-Amado CJ, Cruz-Miranda GM, Mejía-Aranguré JM, Ramírez-Bello J, et al. MiRNAs in Hematopoiesis and Acute Lymphoblastic Leukemia. Int J Mol Sci. 2023;24(6):5436.
27. Mogilyansky E, Rigoutsos I. The miR-17/92 cluster: a comprehensive update on its genomics, genetics, functions, and increasingly important and numerous roles in health and disease. Cell Death Differ. 2013;20:1603-14.
28. Chen P, Price C, Li Z, Li Y, Cao D, Wiley A, et al. miR-9 is an essential oncogenic microRNA specifically overexpressed in mixed lineage leukemia-rearranged leukemia. Proc Natl Acad Sci USA. 2013;110(28):11511-6.
29. Lu Y, Zhong L, Luo X, Liu C, Dan W, Chu X, et al. MiRNA-301b-3p induces proliferation and inhibits apoptosis in AML cells by targeting FOXF2 and regulating Wnt/β-catenin axis. Mol Cell Probes. 2022;63:101805.
30. Eryaskina YA, Titov SE, Kovynev IB, Fedorova SS, Pospelova TI, Zhimulev IF. MicroRNAs in the Myelodysplastic Syndrome. Acta Naturae. 2021;13(2):4-15.
31. Fang J, Varney M, Starczynowski DT. Implication of microRNAs in the pathogenesis of MDS. Curr Pharm Des. 2012;18(22):3170-9.
32. Wang H, Sun J, Zhang B, Zhao D, Tong H, Wu H, et al. Targeting miR-126 disrupts maintenance of myelodysplastic syndrome stem and progenitor cells. Clin Transl Med. 2021;11(10):e610.
33. Jet T, Gines G, Rondelez Y, Taly V. Advances in multiplexed techniques for the detection and quantification of microRNAs. Chem Soc Rev. 2021;50(6):4141-61.

CHAPTER 12

How to Assess Measurable Residual Disease in Acute Myeloid Leukemia

Narasimhapriyan Kannan, Tanishq Khatavkar, Nikhil Patkar

ABSTRACT

Measurable residual disease (MRD) refers to detection of disease below the morphologic threshold (<5% blasts in bone marrow) for remission. Currently, the main techniques used to detect MRD in acute myeloid leukemia (AML) are: (1) Multiparametric flow cytometry MRD (MFC)-MRD along with leukemic stem cell MRD (LSC)-MRD. (2) Molecular MRD that includes polymerase chain reaction (PCR), droplet digital PCR (dd-PCR), and next-generation sequencing (NGS). With current techniques, the sensitivity of MRD detection reaches up to 10^{-5}. Various studies have highlighted that MRD positivity is an independent predictive factor of inferior outcome in AML. Also, MRD positivity detected by a combination of methods (MFC and NGS) accentuates its prognostic significance. Therefore, detection of AML-MRD has been incorporated into clinical decision making. AML-MRD assessment is still challenging due to applicability of different methods used for detection, determining time-point of assessment, standardization of the technique used, comparability of the methods of detection, its utility in patients treated with less intensive therapy, etc. In this chapter, we will discuss how to assess MRD by the aforementioned techniques and its clinical impact.

INTRODUCTION

Acute myeloid leukemia (AML) is a biologically heterogeneous disease with heterogeneous outcomes. Therefore, risk stratification of the patients is necessary to prognosticate them. Earlier, the risk stratification of AML was solely based on cytogenetics which considered t(8;21), t(15;17), and inv(16) as favorable risk group and presence of complex karyotype, -5, del(5q), -7, and 3q abnormalities as adverse risk group. The cases not encompassed in favorable and adverse groups along with trisomies 8, 21, 22, and 11q abnormalities, etc., were considered intermediate risk. However, with discovery of recurrent gene mutations observed in AML, techniques such as polymerase chain reaction (PCR), Sanger sequencing as well as next-generation sequencing (NGS) were required to detect these mutations. The massive parallel sequencing attribute of NGS helps in simultaneous detection of multiple mutations in a short time. Also, the detection of gene mutations is essential for risk stratification such as mutations in *NPM1* (without *FLT3*-ITD), *CEBPA* are considered as favorable risk AMLs and presence of AML-myelodysplasia related (AML-MR) mutations such as *ASXL1, BCOR, EZH2,* etc., and AML with *TP53* mutations are considered as adverse risk AMLs. The European Leukemia Net (ELN) 2022 stratifies adult AML patients into favorable, intermediate, and adverse risk for patients receiving intensive chemotherapy by incorporating the cytogenetic and molecular subgroups discussed earlier with few modifications. The therapy of AML is changing vastly with development of targeted therapies such as midostaurin for *FLT3* mutations, *IDH1/2* inhibitors such as ivosidenib and enasidenib, etc., and less intensive therapies such as azacytidine and venetoclax combination for patients unfit for conventional 3+7 induction. NGS plays a vital role in risk stratification of patients receiving less intensive therapy too, as the 2024 ELN recommendation stratifies patients with *NPM1/IDH1/2/ DDX41* as favorable risk and *TP53* mutation as adverse risk group and patients with *RAS* pathway and *FLT3* mutations are considered intermediate risk.

Earlier the response assessment for therapy was based on morphologic assessment of blast percentage and peripheral blood counts, with patients having < 5% blasts in bone marrow and platelet count of 100,000/μL and absolute neutrophil count (ANC) of 1,000/μL being considered in complete morphologic remission (CR). However, a majority of patients achieving CR eventually relapse. Therefore, it is essential to identify those patients who might relapse. One such parameter to predict the outcome is measurable residual disease (MRD). MRD refers to detection of residual disease below the cutoff for morphologic remission (< 5% blasts) and its assessment helps in (1) Quantitative measurement for evaluation of deeper remission status; (2) Disease surveillance, prediction of relapse and starting pre-emptive therapy; (3) Disease monitoring post-transplant; (4) As a surrogate endpoint for drug trials. In a systematic review and meta-analysis of 81 articles comprising 11,151 AML patients, it was found that MRD-positive patients have an inferior disease-free survival (DFS) 25% versus 64% and overall survival (OS) 34% versus 68% compared to MRD-negative patients. Additionally, end of induction MRD status had prognostic significance even in patients who did not achieve morphologic remission (> 5% blasts), suggesting that detection of abnormal myeloid blasts determines the outcome since morphologic evaluation may also include normal/regenerating myeloid blasts.

ACUTE MYELOID LEUKEMIA-MEASURABLE RESIDUAL DISEASE ASSESSMENT

Currently, AML-MRD is assessed by:

- Multiparametric flow cytometry (MFC-MRD) assessment
- Leukemic stem cell MRD (LSC-MRD) assessment
- Assessment of MRD using quantitative polymerase chain reaction (qPCR)
- Assessment of MRD using NGS

A summary of comparison between the methods is described in **Table 1**.

TABLE 1: Summary comparing different methods of AML-MRD assessment.

Method	MFC-MRD	qPCR	NGS-MRD
Applicability	> 90%	40–60%	> 90%
Sensitivity	10^{-3}–10^{-4}	10^{-4}–10^{-5}	10^{-3}–10^{-4}
Turnaround time	1–2 days	3–5 days	10–14 days
Cost	Relatively costlier	Cheap	Relatively costlier
Merits	• Widely available across various labs • Applicable in over 90% patients of AML • Dead/degenerated cells can be excluded from the assay • Shorter turnaround time (1–2 days) • Additional clones can be detected that may be missed with targeted molecular MRD/PCR • With high events acquired, the sensitivity may reach 10^{-5}	• Higher sensitivity • More objective assay compared to MFC-MRD • Can be performed in peripheral blood as well as bone marrow	• Applicability in > 90% cases • Useful in cases with heterogeneous expression of FCM markers • Accentuates the prognostic significance of MRD positivity in MFC-MRD-positive cases • Peripheral blood samples can also be used in follow-up
Demerits	• Needs expertise in sample processing and analysis • Bone marrow sampling is required • Immunophenotypic shifts are common and hence results may be false negative • Compared to B or T ALL MRD, the maturation pattern is not defined by stages, therefore identifying abnormal blasts may be difficult	• Applicability only in ~40–60% of AML, limited to *NPM1* mutation, *RUNX1::RUNX1T1* and *CBFB::MYH11* currently • Missense mutations and small insertions/deletions are difficult to quantify reliably at high sensitivity due to false positivity • Mutational profile of diagnostic sample is required • Development of new clone during the course of the disease may be missed	• Limited availability of centers performing the assay • Processing steps are comparatively complex • False negativity in cases with targeted therapy when performed by single gene assays

(AML: acute myeloid leukemia; MFC: multiparametric flow cytometry; MRD: measurable residual disease; NGS: next-generation sequencing; qPCR: quantitative polymerase chain reaction)

Multiparametric Flow Cytometry—Measurable Residual Disease

Principle: It relies on identification of abnormal myeloid blasts from the regenerating/normal myeloid blasts by abnormal antigen expression **(Figs. 1A to D)**. The abnormal antigen expression refers to:

- Overexpression of markers (or) (e.g., CD34, HLA-DR, CD117 overexpression)
- Underexpression of markers (or) (e.g., CD38, CD13, CD33 underexpression)
- Cross-lineage expression of markers (or) (e.g., CD19, CD7, CD56 expression)
- Asynchronous expression of markers (aberrant coexpression of markers expressed in mature cells on immature cells, e.g., CD15, CD11b expression)

There are two main approaches in detecting these abnormal blasts:

1. *Leukemia associated aberrant immunophenotype (LAIP) based approach:* The aberrant expression of antigens present during the diagnostic time-point are tracked during the MRD (follow-up) time-points. Presence of two or more LAIP markers on blasts are considered abnormal (e.g., CD56, CD7 expression on myeloid blasts during diagnostic time-point can be tracked during MRD time-point).

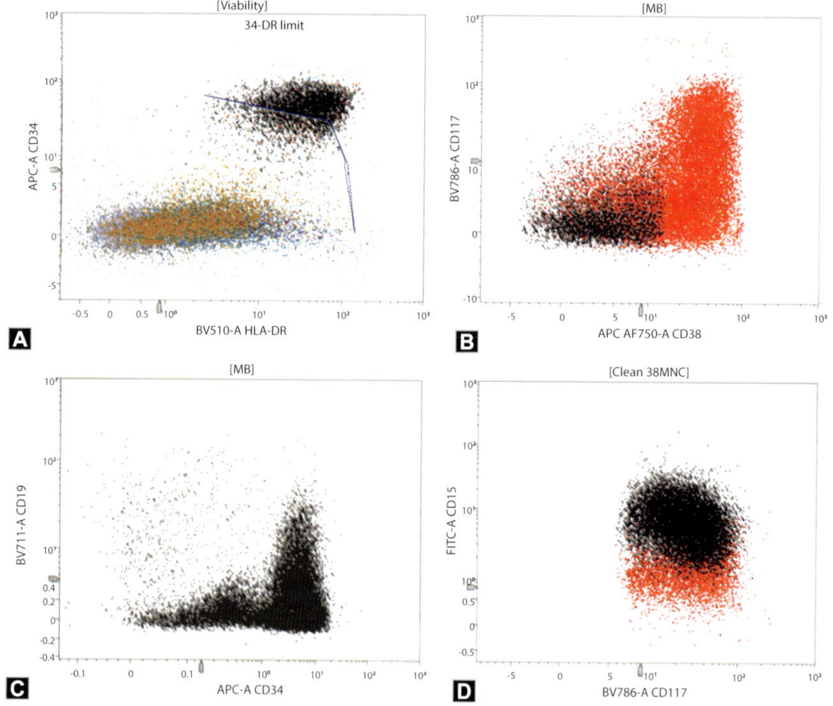

FIGS. 1A TO D: Abnormal myeloid blasts (black population) showing (A) Overexpression of CD34 and HLA-DR, (B) Underexpression of CD117 and CD38, (C) Cross-lineage expression of CD19, and (D) Asynchronous expression of CD15 on blasts.

2. *Different from normal (DFN):* The aberrant expression of antigens is detected based on difference from normal maturation pattern of control samples **(Fig. 2)** (e.g., when the immunophenotype of diagnostic time-point is not available, the abnormal blasts at MRD time-points are detected by bright CD34 and HLA-DR compared to templates created using control samples). **Figures 3A to C** shows normal antigen expression pattern of maturing myeloid cells, monocytes, and erythroids.

As per 2021 ELN recommendation for AML-MRD detection, a combination of both approaches is recommended. The gating strategy for AML-MRD is described in **Figures 4A to Q**.

Sample preparation and prerequisites: The ELN 2021 update on MRD in AML suggested that the first pull sample needs to be submitted for MRD analysis and the sample has to be processed within 3 days of storage at ideal conditions [although it is preferable to process it as early as possible since ethylenediaminetetraacetic acid (EDTA) anticoagulant can affect antigen expression of certain myeloid antigens with prolonged storage]. Sample preparation can be done by either (1) bulk lysis (preferred method), or (2) stain/lyse/wash or no wash techniques. A minimum of 500,000 events and at least 100 viable events in the blast window is recommended. However, to improve the sensitivity, as many events as possible need to be acquired. For LSC-MRD, a minimum of 4 million events are recommended.

Panel design: The panel used by ELN members consisted of 8–10 colors for AML-MRD. The markers used for AML-MRD should comprise a backbone of markers

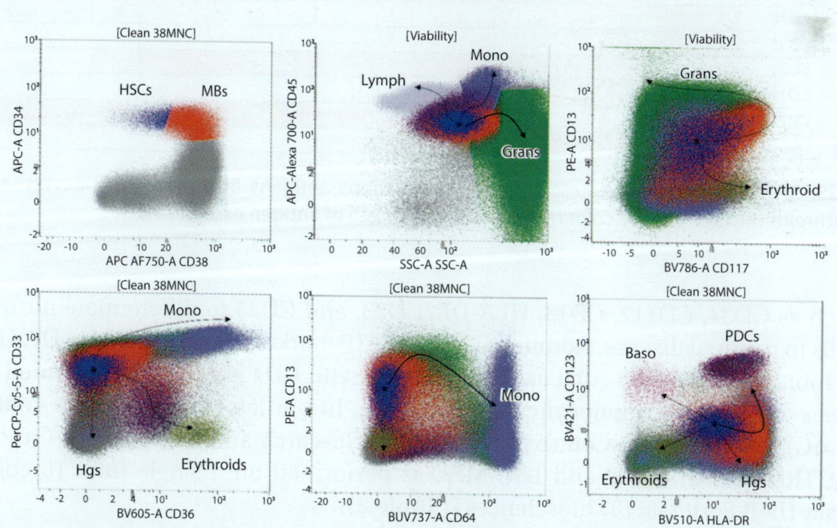

FIG. 2: Normal maturation pattern of various hematopoietic cells.

(HSCs: hematopoietic stem cells; MBs: myeloblasts; Mono: monocytes; Lymph: lymphocytes; Grans: granulocytes; Hgs: hematogones; PDCs: plasmacytoid dendritic cells; Baso: basophils)

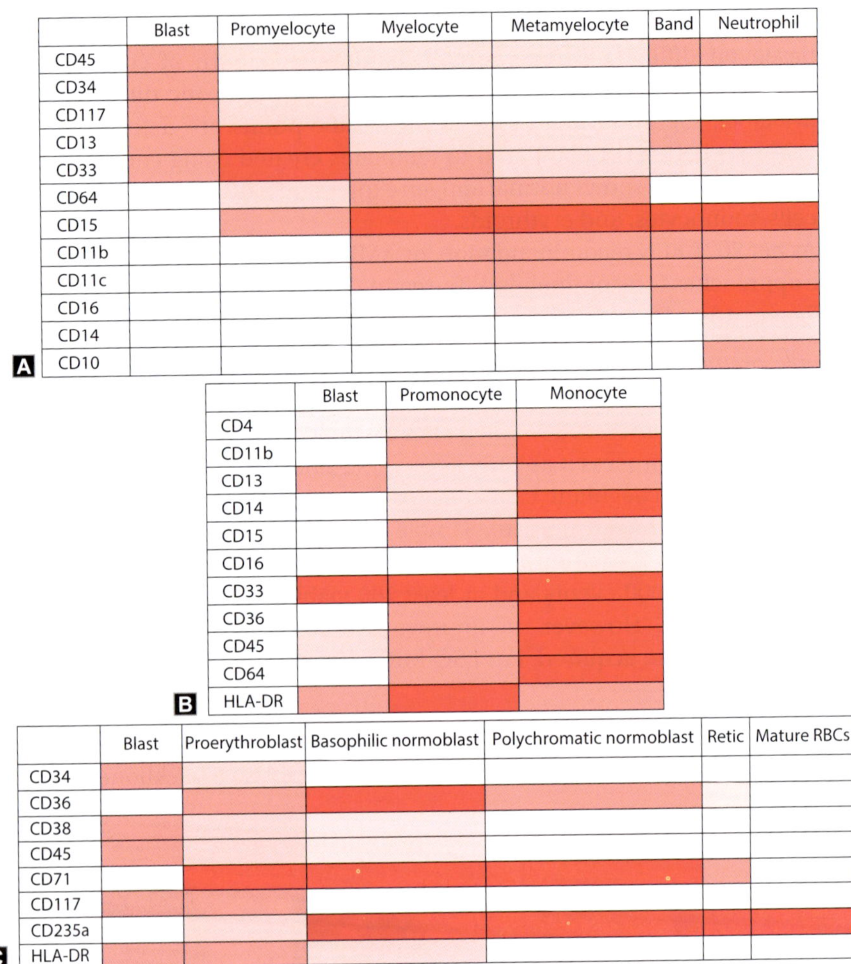

FIGS. 3A TO C: Normal expression pattern of various antigens in myeloid, monocytes, and erythroids (Intensity of the color represents the strength of antigen expression).

such as CD34, CD117, CD13, HLA-DR/CD33, and CD45 to differentiate normal cells to residual disease. Additional useful LAIP markers include CD56, CD7. Use of monocytic markers such as CD64, CD11b, and CD4 is also recommended in cases of AML with monocytic differentiation. In our lab [Tata memorial centre (TMC), the Advanced Centre for Treatment, Research and Education in Cancer (ACTREC)] AML-MRD and LSC-MRD is performed on a single tube 16 color assay (LSR Fortessa, BD biosciences) **(Table 2)**.

Limit of blank (LOB), limit of detection (LOD), and limit of quantification (LOQ): These assays must be established individually for the panel used in the laboratory. A minimal cluster of 20 and 50 events could represent reproducible LOD and LOQ, respectively.

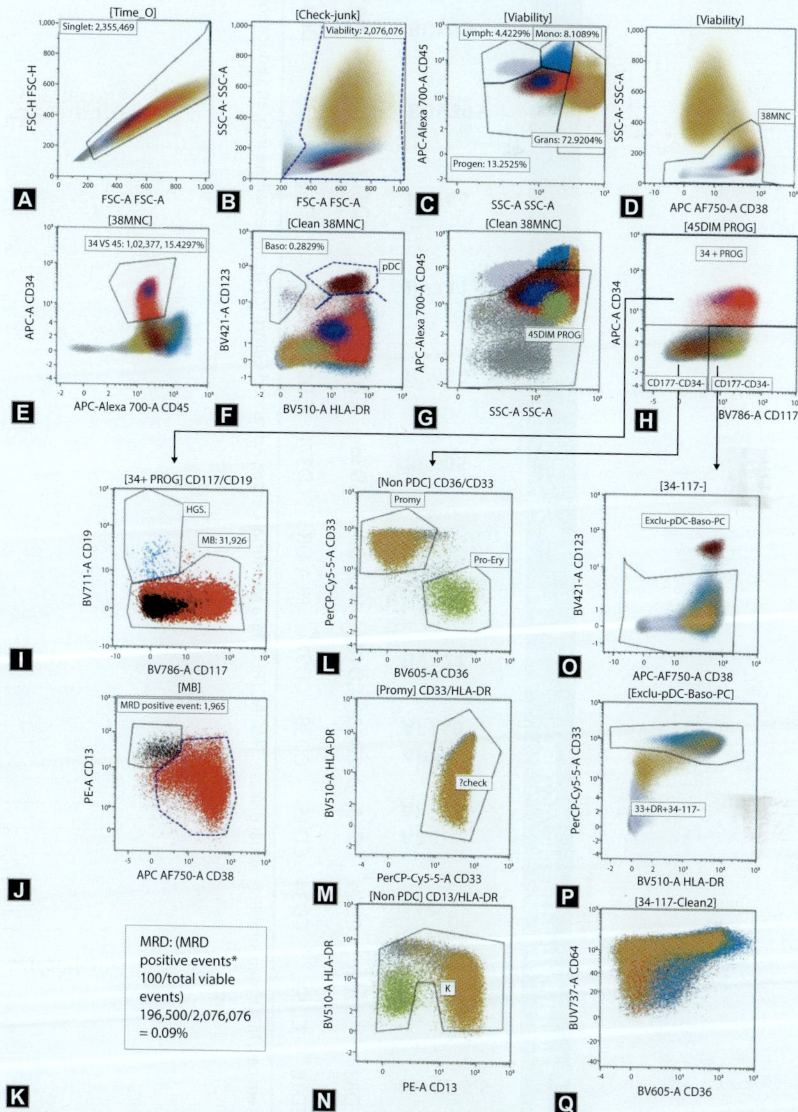

FIGS. 4A TO Q: Gating strategy for AML-MRD: (A) After gating the singlets, (B) the debris are removed using FSC-A versus SSC-A. (C) The major populations are gated in CD45 versus SSC scatter plot. (D) The granulocytes are removed using mononuclear cell gate in CD38 versus SSC plot. (E and F) CD34+ population, basophils, and plasmacytoid dendritic cells are visualized as they fall in CD45dim window. (G) The CD45bright lymphocytes and monocytes are removed from the mononuclear cells using a CD45dim progenitor gate. (H) The events in the CD45dim progenitor gate are separated into three populations based on CD34 and CD117 expression, (1) CD34+, (2) CD34-CD117+, and (3) CD34-CD117- populations. (I) The CD34+ stage 1 hematogones are excluded using CD19 versus CD117 plot. (J) Abnormal myeloid blasts (MRD) are detected expressing bright CD13, dim CD38, and negative CD117 (black population). Similarly, in CD34- cases, the CD34-CD117+ and CD34- CD117- populations are further analyzed using LAIP/DFN approach for various markers (Figs. L to N and O to Q, respectively). (K) Finally, the MRD is quantified.

(AML: acute myeloid leukemia; MRD: measurable residual disease; DFN: different from normal; LAIP: leukemia associated aberrant immunophenotype)

TABLE 2: AML-MRD and LSC-MRD panel currently used in TMC, ACTREC.

	FITC	PE	ECD	PerCP 5.5	PC7	APC	APC AF_700	APC AF750	BV421	BV510	BV605	BV650	BV711	BV786	BUV395	BUV737
AML-MRD	CD15	CD13	CD7	CD33	CD203c	CD34	CD45	CD38	CD123	HLA-DR	CD36	CD14	CD19	CD117	CD56	CD64
LSC-MRD	CD96	CD13	CD7	CD18	CD52	CD34	CD45	CD38	CD97	HLA-DR	CD371	CD54	CD33	CD117	CD71	CD64

(AML: acute myeloid leukemia; LSC: leukemic stem cell; MRD: measurable residual disease; TMC ACTREC: Tata Memorial Centre, Advanced Centre for Treatment, Research, and Education in Cancer)

Control samples: The panel of markers needs to be analyzed on a minimum of 10 samples (preferably age-matched) and this has to be performed again if there is a change in the methodology.

Leukemic Stem Cell—Measurable Residual Disease

Detection of residual LSC is still at an experimental stage, however it is recommended in patients enrolled in clinical studies. LSCs are identified by aberrant expression of markers such as CD45RA, CD52, CD54, CD96, CD97, CD366, and CD371 on CD34+ CD38- CD45 dim population. LSC-MRD has higher sensitivity and less false negativity for prognosis over MFC-MRD.

Various studies have shown the prognostic significance of AML-MRD by MFC, few of them are discussed in **Table 3**.

Molecular Measurable Residual Disease Assessment

The MRD assessment by molecular techniques consists of PCR [qPCR, digital droplet (ddPCR)] and error-corrected NGS using unique molecular identifiers (UMI). The principle of molecular MRD assessment is tracking the molecular alterations (mutations/fusions) which were found during diagnosis. As per ELN 2021 guidelines, the sensitivity of molecular techniques should reach a minimum of 10^{-3} or lower. The types of molecular alterations assessed for MRD are as follows:

- *Single nucleotide variations:* Mutations usually seen in genes such as *TP53, KRAS, NRAS,* myelodysplasia-related genes (*U2AF1, SRSF2, SF3B1*), etc.

TABLE 3: Summary of different studies on AML-MRD by immunophenotyping.

Study	Summary	FCM approach and MRD cutoff for positivity	MRD status on outcome
Boddu, 2018	194 adult AMLs, MRD assessed at morphologic response	DFN approach with cluster of > 20 events considered positive	Correlated with CIR
Patkar, 2019	451 adult AMLs, post-induction, post-consolidation MRD assessment	DFN + LAIP approach, any MRD events were taken positive	Post-induction MRD correlated with OS and RFS
Brodersen, 2020	1,022 pediatric AMLs, MRD assessed after 1st induction	DFN approach, with events > 0.5 decades (log10 U) considered positive	Correlated with OS, RR, DFS, TRM
Lowenberg, 2021	780 adult AMLs, MRD assessed after 2nd cycle	LAIP approach, with 0.1% or more events considered positive	Correlated with RFS
Maiti, 2021	97 adult AMLs, treated with venetoclax + decitabine. MRD assessed after 1, 2, 4 months	DFN approach, with 0.1% or more events considered positive	Correlated with CR, RFS, EFS, OS

(AML: acute myeloid leukemia; CIR: cumulative incidence of relapse; CR: complete remission; MRD: measurable residual disease; DFN: different from normal; DFS: disease free survival; EFS: event free survival; LAIP: leukemia associated aberrant immunophenotype; MRD: measurable residual disease; OS: overall survival; RFS: relapse free survival; RR: relapse risk; TRM: treatment related mortality)

- *Insertions/deletions (Delins):* Mutations usually seen in genes such as *NPM1, FLT3-ITD, CEBPA*, etc.
- *Gene fusions:* Fusions such as *RUNX1::RUNX1T1, CBFB::MYH11, PML::RARA, KMT2A* rearrangements, etc.
- *Overexpression:* Genes such as *WT1, BAALC, ERG*, etc.

Preanalytical considerations: EDTA samples from peripheral blood and bone marrow can be used for MRD assessment, although the sensitivity in peripheral blood is 1 log lower than bone marrow. If bone marrow is used, then only 5 mL of first pull sample is preferred to avoid hemodilution. If a peripheral blood sample is used then a minimum of 10 mL sample depending on white blood cell (WBC) count is preferred.

Measurable Residual Disease Analysis by Quantitative Polymerase Chain Reaction

Patients with recurrent genetic abnormalities such as *NPM1* mutation as well as *RUNX1::RUNX1T1, PML::RARA,* and *CBFB::MYH11* fusions are currently monitored by PCR. Hence, the applicability of the assay is limited to ~40–60% cases. In addition, gene expression (*WT1, EVI1*) can also be evaluated by qPCR.

The starting material is ribonucleic acid (RNA) for detection of fusions and gene expression analysis. Whereas, either deoxyribonucleic acid (DNA)/RNA can be used for detection of gene mutations such as (*NPM1, FLT3, IDH*, etc.)

While assessing MRD by qPCR, the test has to be done in triplicate. In addition to the target gene, a housekeeping gene (*ABL1*) also needs to be amplified. In our lab, a minimum of 100,000 copies of *ABL1* is considered optimal for reporting. The copy numbers of the gene/transcript of interest are then normalized to *ABL1* copies and is reported as the MRD. Results are taken as positive when at least two of the triplicates are amplified within a cycle threshold of 40, with a cycling threshold of 0.1. The sensitivity of qPCR reaches 10^{-4}–10^{-5}. The limitations of MRD assessment by real-time quantitative polymerase chain reaction (RQ-PCR) is that it requires separate assays for each mutation, e.g., *NPM1* mutations and *FLT3* internal tandem duplication (ITDs) can have numerous permutations and it is practically impossible to develop and validate separate assays for each.

Gene expression analysis: As per ELN 2021 recommendations, assessment of *WT1* expression is not recommended as a MRD marker due to its low specificity. However, if there are no other MRD markers (including MFC-MRD) *WT1* expression can be assessed using a validated *WT1* MRD assay preferably in peripheral blood. In a recent study, overexpression of *WT1* at MRD time-point was associated with shorter OS and relapse-free survival (RFS).

Digital Droplet Polymerase Chain Reaction

The ddPCR is used for the absolute quantification of target nucleic acids. For a high-quality run, the number of total copies should be > 32,000, the total droplet count should be > 15,000, and empty droplets should be > 100. The advantages of this technique over qPCR are: (1) Absolute quantification and hence does not require calibration curves, (2) Can be multiplexed, (3) Lower impact of PCR inhibitors. The disadvantages include subsampling errors and partitioning errors. The optimal cutoff for positivity is yet to be established, however a variant allele frequency (VAF) of 0.2 or more is provisionally taken as positive. Similar to the PCR assays, the main limitation here again is that every mutation still requires a different primer and probe and multiplexing beyond 3–4 targets is not feasible.

Next-generation Sequencing—Measurable Residual Disease

The NGS-MRD analysis in AML relies on tracking the mutations/gene fusions detected during diagnosis at MRD time-points. NGS-MRD is particularly useful for AML, because somatic alterations are seen in > 90% patients of AML at diagnosis. Detection of MRD by NGS is based on two approaches. (1) Single gene assays. (2) Panel-based assays.

Single Gene Assays

In our laboratory, single gene assays are used to detect *NPM1* mutation and *FLT3*-ITDs. It is an amplicon-based assay which involves PCR by adding adapter linked primers for exon 12 of *NPM1* and exon 14 of *FLT3* followed by sequencing. The main advantages of this assay are (a) More than half the patients of AML with normal karyotype can be monitored, (b) High sensitivity (up to 0.002%), and (c) Detects all types of *NPM1* and *FLT3*-ITDs involving exon 12 and 14 respectively. The limitation is that rare mutations involving other exons cannot be monitored.

Panel-based Assays

In panel-based assays, multiple genes are assessed for mutations simultaneously. In our lab (TMC, ACTREC), the NGS-MRD is done using a panel-based approach comprising whole/specific exons of 26 genes (*ASXL2, FLT3, IDH2, KRAS, PTPN11 CSF3R, JAK2, NRAS, RAD21, IDH1, KIT, PHF6, RUNX1, NPM1, TP53, U2AF1, WT1, SF3B1, BCOR, CALR, CEBPA, EZH2, GATA2, SRSF2, STAG2,* and *ZRSR2*). The region of interest is enriched during library preparation by various techniques discussed in the following text.

Molecular inversion probes (MIPs) based assays: MIPs are single stranded oligonucleotides with complementary domains for the gene of interest which are flanked by UMIs and linked by a backbone sequence common to all probes. Once it hybridizes to the gene of interest, the sequence is copied by polymerase and ligated to form a circle. This is followed by PCR amplification of the capture events and sequencing.

Archer based assays: This is a nested PCR based technique in which molecular adapters that consist UMI, indices as well as universal primer binding site are added to the fragmented DNA and gene specific primers consisting indices are added. This helps in identification of novel fusion partner.

Capture-based assays: Following DNA fragmentation, end-repair and A-tailing, adapter ligation (with presence of UMIs) is done followed by low cycle PCR amplification. The hybridization and capture are done using biotin labeled probes targeting the gene of interest.

The main challenge in assessing MRD is to differentiate the actual mutations from the errors that occur during PCR (~1% error) and sequencing (~0.1% error). This is especially true for substitution mutations and is overcome by "error corrected NGS" using UMIs and computational methods [for insertion mutations (e.g., *NPM1, FLT3*) and deletion mutations, error correction may not be required since PCR/sequencing errors are minimal-absent for insertion/deletions].

UMIs: The DNA/cDNA molecules are barcoded with unique sequences (usually 6–12 nucleotides) during library preparation, prior to PCR. The individual molecules are grouped into read families based on the UMI during sequencing. PCR/sequencing errors are distinguished from the actual variants once the consensus reads are taken from the read family **(Figs. 5A and B)**. The UMIs can be incorporated in a single strand or both the strands (duplex sequencing). Duplex sequencing improves the sensitivity and specificity at the cost of coverage, hence are currently limited to research settings.

Computational methods of error correction: Includes removal of (1) base with high error rates (Q score < 30), (2) reads with low mapping scores, (3) additional methods include performing NGS on control samples to identify baseline error rates in each position of the target, and (4) use of algorithms for specific genes (e.g., *FLT3*).

Both targeted as well as panel-based approaches are considered for MRD analysis. If a panel-based approach is used and the presence of variants which

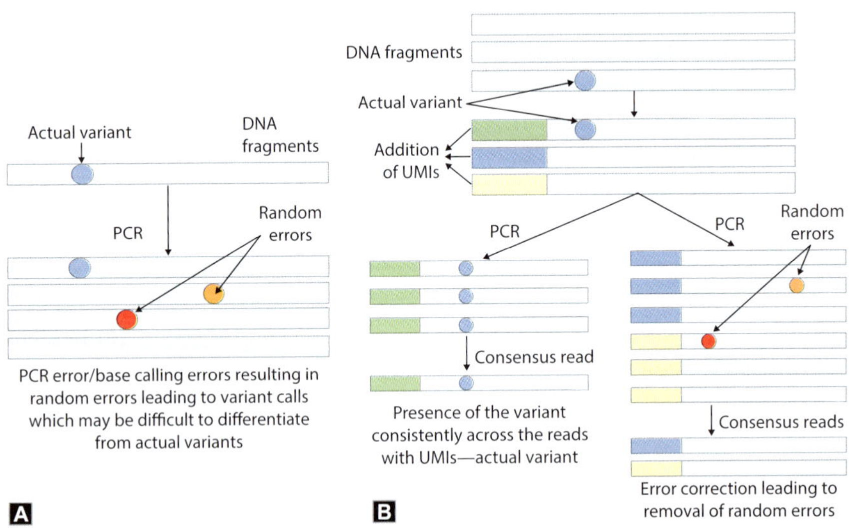

FIGS. 5A AND B: (A) NGS-MRD without addition of UMIs leading to difficulty in interpretation of actual variant, (B) compared with MRD with addition of UMIs that differentiates actual variant from random errors.

(DNA: deoxyribonucleic acid; MRD: measurable residual disease; NGS: next-generation sequencing; PCR: polymerase chain reaction; UMIs: unique molecular identifiers)

were not found in the diagnostic sample is detected, it should be reported only when it can be confidently reported above the background noise. The depth of coverage should be well enough (>20,000) to differentiate the actual variant from background noise.

LOD: LOD for NGS is ~2–5% VAF which improves to 0.1–0.5% VAF when UMIs are used for error correction.

Panel design: The NGS panel in MRD should be designed in such a way that it covers the common genes which are mutated in AML (e.g., *NPM1*, *RAS* pathway mutations, etc.), along with genes which have prognostic significance, e.g., *TP53*. Care should be taken to avoid common mutations seen in age-related clonal hematopoiesis (e.g., *DNMT3A*, *TET2*, and *ASXL1*) and germline variants should not be assessed. Also, with targeted therapies (e.g., Midostaurin) detection of *FLT3*-ITDs alone could lead to false negativity, hence it should be evaluated along with the comutations/to be checked by other methods such as MFC-MRD.

As per ELN 2021 recommendations, for error-corrected sequencing approach ≥10,000 read families and >10 mutant reads are minimum requirements and a read family should contain at least three reads. For nonerror-corrected sequencing approaches the minimum recommendation is to have ≥60,000 reads and >60 mutant reads.

Using background error correction, MRD positivity is taken as VAF more than the mean background error + 3*SD (standard deviation) of the background error.

TIME-POINTS OF ASSESSMENT

As per ELN 2022 recommendations, AML-MRD is assessed after two cycles of intensive chemotherapy followed by the end of consolidation. For acute promyelocytic leukemia (APL), qPCR for *PML::RARA* is done at the end of consolidation.

For AML with NPM1 mutation: The qPCR assay should be performed in peripheral blood samples at the end of two cycles of intensive therapy. Patients who have persistent transcript levels have increased risk of relapse at 3 years. In addition, ELN 2022 recommendation suggests *NPM1* qPCR in bone marrow at the end of therapy. This is followed by serial monitoring by qPCR in peripheral blood every 4–6 weeks/in bone marrow for every 3 months for next 2 years. Presence of low level MRD positivity (< 2% but more than the detection limit) at end of consolidation has low risk of relapse.

COMBINATION OF METHODS FOR DETECTION

The presence of MRD by any one method (MFC/molecular MRD) carries an inferior outcome than patients who are MRD negative by both methods. However, the risk of relapse is comparatively lesser than patients who test positive by both methods.

UTILITY OF MEASURABLE RESIDUAL DISEASE

As per ELN 2022, in clinical practice, the presence or absence of MRD positivity can allow either reclassification into favorable or intermediate risk, especially in *NPM1* mutated AML. Nonadverse risk patients who are MRD positive after two cycles of intensive therapy and adverse risk AML patients are candidates for allogeneic stem cell transplant, whereas nonadverse risk patients with MRD negativity after two cycles of intensive therapy may be considered for autologous transplant, although not widely preferred. Patients with *NPM1* MRD positivity after two cycles of intensive therapy may benefit from early transplant. The same applies to end-of-treatment MRD positivity, wherein the options include—immediate transplantation/intensive chemotherapy/less intensive therapy to eradicate MRD followed by transplant. For patients of AML with *NPM1* mutation receiving less intensive therapy, the patients who achieved MRD negativity had longer OS compared to MRD-positive patients. This is also verified by a recent study in which, patients who achieved MRD negativity after four cycles had superior OS compared to MRD-positive patients.

Take Home Points

- The MRD positivity confers inferior outcome. In addition, the detection of MRD by a combination of methods accentuates its impact.
- The MFC-MRD assessment depends on the detection of aberrant immunophenotype on abnormal myeloid blasts from normal/regenerating myeloid blasts.
- The MRD by qPCR is currently limited to core binding factor fusion AML, AML with *NPM1* mutation, and APL with *PML::RARA* fusion.
- The NGS-MRD is based on tracking the mutations found at diagnostic time points using unique molecular identifiers and error correction.

SUGGESTED READINGS

1. Heuser M, Freeman SD, Ossenkoppele GJ, Buccisano F, Hourigan CS, Ngai LL, et al. 2021 Update on MRD in acute myeloid leukemia: a consensus document from the European LeukemiaNet MRD Working Party. Blood. 2021;138(26):2753-67.
2. Döhner H, Wei AH, Appelbaum FR, Craddock C, DiNardo CD, Dombret H, et al. Diagnosis and management of AML in adults: 2022 recommendations from an international expert panel on behalf of the ELN. Blood. 2022;140(12):1345-77.
3. Patkar N, Kakirde C, Shaikh AF, Salve R, Bhanshe P, Chatterjee G, et al. Clinical impact of panel-based error-corrected next generation sequencing versus flow cytometry to detect measurable residual disease (MRD) in acute myeloid leukemia (AML). Leukemia. 2021;35(5):1392-404.
4. Jongen-Lavrencic M, Grob T, Hanekamp D, Kavelaars FG, Al Hinai A, Zeilemaker A, et al. Molecular minimal residual disease in acute myeloid leukemia. N Engl J Med. 2018;378(13):1189-99.
5. Zeijlemaker W, Grob T, Meijer R, Hanekamp D, Kelder A, Carbaat-Ham JC, et al. CD34+CD38-leukemic stem cell frequency to predict outcome in acute myeloid leukemia. Leukemia. 2019;33(5):1102-12.

CHAPTER 13

Relevance of Screening of Myeloid/ Lymphoid Neoplasms for Germline Predisposition

Ganesh Kumar V

ABSTRACT

Hematologic malignancies, including acute leukemias, myeloproliferative neoplasms (MPNs), and myelodysplastic syndromes (MDS), are often driven by somatic mutations, yet increasing evidence points to inherited genetic predispositions. Germline mutations in genes such as *RUNX1*, *CEBPA*, *GATA2*, and *TP53* are associated with familial cancer risk. Similarly, lymphoid neoplasms such as B-cell acute lymphoblastic leukemia (B-ALL), chronic lymphocytic leukemia (CLL), non-Hodgkin lymphoma (NHL), and Hodgkin lymphoma (HL) are linked to genetic variants in PAX5, SH2B3, IKAROS, and POT1. Advances in precision genomics emphasize the value of identifying these mutations for personalized treatment, genetic counseling, and family risk assessment. These insights guide clinical management, improving outcomes through tailored therapies and innovations in gene-editing technologies.

INTRODUCTION

Hematologic malignancies, including acute leukemias, mature lymphoid neoplasms, myeloproliferative neoplasms (MPNs), and myelodysplastic syndromes (MDS), are typically associated with somatic mutations. While these diseases are mainly acquired through genetic mutations during a patient's lifetime, growing evidence suggests that a subset may also be linked to inherited genetic predispositions. Germline mutations or variants refer to DNA alterations passed through generations and are increasingly recognized as playing a role in various cancers, including hematologic malignancies. Traditionally, research and clinical focus have been on somatic mutations and environmental factors, but the importance of identifying germline predispositions has gained recognition. Advances in precision genomics have underscored the growing recognition of hereditary or germline predisposition to hematopoietic neoplasms. This shift has major implications for both the individual patient and their family, who may face an increased risk of developing similar or other cancers. The identification of a germline variant also opens the possibility of malignancies beyond hematopoietic tissue. Screening for germline mutations in myeloid and lymphoid neoplasms is an emerging area in clinical practice, with the potential to influence disease management, prevention strategies, and genetic counseling. This chapter explores the significance of screening for germline predispositions in myeloid/lymphoid neoplasms, focusing on its impact on diagnosis, treatment, genetic counseling, and family risk assessment. It also examines the types of germline mutations associated with these cancers and current screening strategies.

The initial identification of familial platelet disorder with a tendency to myeloid malignancies (FPD/MM) linked to pathogenic (P) or likely pathogenic (LP) germline *RUNX1* variants occurred in 1999. The significance and increasing recognition of these syndromes are emphasized by their first inclusion in the WHO classification of hematopoietic tumors in 2016, "Myeloid Neoplasms with Germline Predisposition" chapter. Familial clustering was initially observed in chronic lymphocytic leukemia (CLL) and acute myeloid leukemia (AML). This led to the identification of germline variants such as *RUNX1, CEBPA, GATA2, ANKRD26, DDX41,* and *ETV6*, which are now linked to an increased risk of developing myeloid neoplasms. Additionally, germline predispositions extend to lymphoid and plasma cell neoplasms, with recent findings associating germline variants in genes such as *IKZF1, SH2B3, PAX5* [familial acute lymphoblastic leukemia (ALL)], and KDM1A/LSD1 [familial multiple myeloma (MM)] and *DIS3* genes with these cancers. Inherited bone marrow failure (BMF) syndromes, such as *GATA2* haploinsufficiency syndrome, short telomere syndromes, Shwachman-Diamond syndrome, Diamond-Blackfan anemia (DBA), SCN, and familial thrombocytopenias, are also associated with an elevated risk of myeloid neoplasms. Inherited immune deficiency syndromes, including ataxia-telangiectasia, Bloom syndrome, Wiskott-Aldrich syndrome, and Bruton agammaglobulinemia, are linked to a higher likelihood of lymphoid neoplasms. Early detection of germline predisposition syndromes (GPS) is crucial for proper donor selection, tailoring conditioning regimens for allogeneic hematopoietic stem-cell transplantation, and developing personalized, genomics-based treatment strategies.

GERMLINE PREDISPOSITION TO MYELOID MALIGNANCIES

In myeloid disorders with germline predisposition, cytopenias often manifest early but can also appear intermittently or later in life. Risk of progression to MDS/AML is influenced by factors such as clonal evolution, bone marrow dysplasia, and genetic mutations, particularly TP53 and RUNX1. Specific genetic changes such as monosomy 7 or CSF3R variants are markers for leukemia transformation. Hematopoietic stem cell transplantation (HSCT) is often required due to severe BMF, though timing is crucial. In some cases, early HSCT may influence leukemia risk, especially when multi-hit TP53 mutations or other somatic alterations are present. High malignant penetrance syndromes include CEBPA, GATA2, SAMD9/SAMD9L, and TP53, while variable malignant penetrance syndromes are represented by ANKRD26, DDX41, ETV6, RUNX1, and various BMF syndromes.

Classification of Myeloid Neoplasms with Germline Predisposition by WHO 2022

- *Myeloid neoplasms with germline predisposition without a pre-existing platelet disorder or organ dysfunction:*
  - Germline CEBPA P/LP variant (CEBPA-associated familial AML)
  - Germline DDX41 P/LP variant
  - Germline TP53 P/LP variant (Li–Fraumeni syndrome)
- *Myeloid neoplasms with germline predisposition and preexisting platelet disorder:*
  - Germline RUNX1 P/LP variant [familial platelet disorder with associated myeloid malignancy (FPDMM)]
  - Germline ANKRD26 P/LP variant (thrombocytopenia 2)
  - Germline ETV6 P/LP variant (thrombocytopenia 5)
- *Myeloid neoplasms with germline predisposition and potential organ dysfunction:*
  - Germline GATA2 P/LP variant (GATA2-deficiency)
  - Bone marrow failure syndromes
  - Severe congenital neutropenia (SCN)
  - Shwachman–Diamond syndrome (SDS)
  - Fanconi anemia (FA)
  - Telomere biology disorders RASopathies [neurofibromatosis type 1, CBL syndrome, Noonan syndrome or Noonan syndrome-like disorders, Down syndrome, germline SAMD9 P/LP variant (MIRAGE syndrome)], germline SAMD9L P/LP variant (SAMD9L-related ataxia pancytopenia syndrome), Bi-allelic germline BLM P/LP variant (Bloom syndrome)
- *Additional cancer predisposition syndromes that have been associated with myeloid neoplasms: CHEK2, MPL, RECQL4, BRCA1, BRCA2, MLH1, MSH2, MSH6, PMS2, NBN, and WAS*
- *Emerging disorders:* Germline variants in *CSF3R, ERCC6L2, JAK2, MBD4, MECOM/EVI1, NPM1, RBBP6, SRP72, TET2,* and *GATA-1*

Germline mutations in TP53, RUNX1, GATA2, CEBPA, DKC1, and TERT are associated with various hematologic malignancies. TP53 mutations are linked to a wide range of cancers, including myeloid malignancies, and are a hallmark of Li–Fraumeni syndrome. GATA2 mutations increase susceptibility to MDS, AML, and lymphoid malignancies, while mutations in CEBPA are associated with familial AML. DKC1 and TERT mutations, which affect telomerase, increase the risk of MDS, AML, and other cancers. Initial linkage studies in families with AML and familial platelet disorders identified a clustering at the chromosome 21q22.1-22.2 loci, leading to the discovery of germline RUNX1 haploinsufficiency, also known as RUNX1-familial predisposition syndrome. Additional findings include autosomal dominant variants in the 5' untranslated region of the *ANKRD26* gene, which is associated with an elevated risk of MDS and AML. Germline missense pathogenic variants in the *ETV6* gene have also been linked to an increased susceptibility to a range of hematologic malignancies, including MM, pre-B cell ALL, MDS, chronic myelomonocytic leukemia (CMML), and biphenotypic acute leukemia. Emberger syndrome, associated with *GATA2* gene alterations, manifests as lymphedema and MDS/AML due to disruptions in a transcription factor essential for vascular development and hematopoietic stem-cell differentiation. Related conditions such as MonoMAC syndrome, which results in deficiencies in dendritic cells, monocytes, B cells, and NK cells, are also caused by GATA2 variants, collectively referred to as "GATA2 haploinsufficiency syndrome." This syndrome is marked by phenotypic variability and a heightened risk of MDS/AML. Inherited defects in the nucleotide excision repair pathway, such as XPC germline variants in xeroderma pigmentosum, are also linked to an increased risk of Tp53/complex karyotype MDS/AML. Additionally, MIRAGE syndrome, identified in 2016, is caused by germline-activating SAMD9 variants and is characterized by myelodysplasia, infection, growth restriction, and other systemic abnormalities. Germline variants in RUNX1, ETV6, and ANKRD26 predispose individuals to myeloid malignancies (MDS/AML) and platelet disorders, with these genes exhibiting autosomal dominant inheritance. Carriers of RUNX1 or ETV6 mutations experience mild to moderate lifelong thrombocytopenia, while ANKRD26 mutations lead to severe thrombocytopenia with complete penetrance. Platelet function is generally normal in size but may show defects in aggregation, particularly in RUNX1 carriers. Malignant penetrance varies: RUNX1 carriers have a 50% risk of developing hematologic malignancies, with MDS/AML most common, while ETV6 mutations have a 30% lifetime malignancy risk, primarily resulting in B-cell ALL. ANKRD26 mutations confer the lowest risk (8%) of myeloid malignancies. The mechanisms behind leukemia development in these conditions are not fully understood. RUNX1 mutations often lead to haploinsufficiency, and somatic mutations in genes such as *BCOR* are common in MDS/AML cases, though they do not correlate with malignancy risk. In contrast, somatic mutations in ETV6 and ANKRD26 carriers are less well understood, though some patients develop clonal hematopoiesis or additional mutations in genes such as *ASXL1* and *KRAS*. The delay in malignant onset suggests that additional somatic mutations are required for leukemogenesis.

Variants with Germline Predisposition to Myeloid Neoplasms

CEBPA encodes a transcription factor involved in myeloid development, and germline mutations in CEBPA are linked to AML predisposition. In 7–15% of biallelic CEBPA-mutated AML cases, one mutation is inherited, usually affecting the N-terminal, while the other is acquired at the 3′ end. Germline 5′-end mutations have 90% penetrance and typically present in young adulthood, with a favorable prognosis but frequent recurrence, often due to new leukemic clones. Germline 3′-end mutations have lower penetrance (46%) and a quicker recurrence rate (median 9 months), but still a favorable outlook, especially with indel bZIP variants. Co-occurring mutations such as GATA2 are common in these cases.

GATA2 encodes a transcription factor crucial for hematopoiesis, and germline mutations cause GATA2 deficiency syndrome, predisposing individuals to myeloid malignancies, immunodeficiency, and lymphedema. The syndrome, often de novo, presents with variable symptoms, including hematologic issues and infections, and myeloid neoplasms such as MDS and AML affect 75% of carriers, typically starting around age 20. GATA2 deficiency is common in pediatric MDS, especially with monosomy 7. Germline mutations are typically loss-of-function, often in the ZF2 domain, while somatic mutations in AML usually affect the ZF1 domain. MDS/AML in these patients often involve karyotypic abnormalities such as monosomy 7 and mutations in MDS/AML driver genes (e.g., *STAG2* and *RUNX1*). Bone marrow findings range from normal to MDS/AML, with different mutations linked to disease progression.

SAMD9 and *SAMD9L* are genes on chromosome 7 involved in hematopoietic cell function. Germline variants in SAMD9 cause MIRAGE syndrome (early-onset MDS, infections, growth restriction, and adrenal hypoplasia), while SAMD9L variants cause ataxia-pancytopenia syndrome (cerebellar dysfunction and pancytopenia). Both syndromes are strongly linked to young-onset MDS with monosomy 7, with nearly complete penetrance for SAMD9 variants and 70% for SAMD9L variants. These variants typically involve gain-of-function mutations in the C-terminus. Germline SAMD9/9L variants account for 8–17% of childhood MDS, with a median diagnosis age of 9.6 years. Clonal evolution often leads to loss of the mutated chromosome 7, complicating detection. MDS progression is associated with additional mutations in driver genes such as *SETBP1* and *ASXL1*. While pediatric patients with SAMD9/9L variants have favorable HSCT outcomes (85% 5-year survival), those with severe multiorgan involvement have a poorer prognosis. Rare cases of spontaneous remission occur through somatic revertant mosaicism.

TP53 is a critical tumor suppressor gene that plays essential roles in DNA repair, cell cycle regulation, apoptosis, senescence, and differentiation. Germline mutations in TP53 lead to Li-Fraumeni syndrome (LFS), a hereditary cancer predisposition condition with a high lifetime cancer risk (≥70% for men, ≥90% for women). The most common cancers in LFS include adrenocortical carcinomas, breast cancer, CNS tumors, soft tissue sarcomas, and osteosarcomas, though patients are also at an elevated risk for other malignancies such as ALL, MDS, and AML (which account for 2–4% of cases). LFS patients are especially vulnerable to second cancers due to chemotherapy and radiation, with about 45% developing a second malignancy. TP53 mutations are found in around 6% of therapy-related AML (t-AML) cases, and LFS patients with t-AML often exhibit a complex karyotype and loss of the wild-type TP53 allele.

Germline DDX41 variants, located on chromosome 5, predispose individuals to MDS and AML, typically presenting at ages 66–68, similar to sporadic cases. These variants are found in 2–6% of adult MDS/AML patients and have a 50% penetrance for developing myeloid malignancies, with a higher progression rate in men. MDS/AML linked to DDX41 often presents with hypocellular bone marrow and a normal karyotype. Prognoses tend to be more favorable compared to sporadic cases. In addition to MDS/AML, DDX41 variants are also associated with aplastic anemia, MPNs, lymphoid malignancies, and solid tumors, though the causal link is unclear. Common DDX41 variants include missense, frameshift, and splice-site mutations, with specific variants common in certain regions, such as North America, the UK, and Japan. Malignant transformation often involves somatic mutations in DDX41 on the trans allele, found in 55–70% of cases. Acquired variants such as c.1574G > A (p.Arg525His) are frequent across populations. Other somatic mutations, including ASXL1, DNMT3A, and TP53, are also observed, with CUX1 mutations notably over-represented in DDX41-mutated cases. The acquisition of somatic mutations occurs early in malignancy development. A study by Peng Li et al. examined hematologic malignancies in individuals carrying germline DDX41 variants, using data from 9,821 patients across six institutions. Germline DDX41 mutations are the most common predisposition to adult AML/MDS, often presenting in elderly individuals without a family history. These cases exhibit a distinct disease course with favorable outcomes, independent of somatic mutations or other risk factors. Among the 82 germline DDX41 variants identified, 39 were classified as causal variants, associated with concurrent somatic DDX41 mutations in 79% of cases, reduced somatic mutation burdens, and rare canonical mutations such as NPM1 or FLT3. DDX41 mutations also predispose individuals to MPNs, B-cell lymphomas, and other neoplasms.

Several BMF syndromes predispose individuals to MDS and AML. These syndromes are often caused by defective DNA repair (e.g., Fanconi anemia), ribosome biogenesis issues (e.g., Shwachman–Diamond syndrome), or telomeropathies. Symptoms typically include cytopenias and other phenotypic features such as exocrine pancreatic insufficiency or radial ray abnormalities. The risk of MDS/AML varies depending on the underlying condition. For instance, ADH5/ALDH2 deficiency has an 80% risk of MDS/AML, while conditions such as Fanconi anemia and Shwachman–Diamond syndrome have a moderate risk of 10–30%, and Diamond–Blackfan anemia has a lower risk (<10%).

Yang et al. explored the genetic landscape of 391 adult AML patients, focusing on somatic mutations and germline variants. The cohort had a mean age of 59 years at diagnosis, with 59% of patients aged 60 or older. Of the 321 patients with cytogenetic reports, 44% had a normal karyotype. The most common somatic mutations identified were FLT3, NPM1, FLT3-ITD, DNMT3A, and IDH2. Germline analysis revealed that 13.6% of patients carried pathogenic or likely pathogenic variants (P/LP), with 64.45% harboring variants of uncertain significance. These pathogenic variants were found in 34 genes, including known hematologic malignancy predisposition genes such as *DDX41*, *FANCM*, and *BRIP1*. Germline mutations in DNA damage response genes, including *CHEK2*, were also identified, with a significant correlation between pathogenic variants and adverse or intermediate-risk AML. RUNX1 mutations predispose individuals to familial platelet disorder with a propensity to develop myeloid neoplasms (FPD-MPN). A study by Yu et al. analyzed 27 families with research genomic data and detected 26 different germline RUNX1 variants. Among 51 patients without hematologic malignancy, somatic mutations were found in at least one clonal hematopoiesis of indeterminate potential (CHIP) or an AML driver gene. *BCOR* was the most frequently mutated gene, and sequential sequencing data from 19 patients demonstrated dynamic changes in somatic mutations over time, with stable clones being more frequent in older patients. This study emphasizes the importance of monitoring somatic mutations in patients with familial platelet disorder with propensity to develop myeloid neoplasms (FPD-MPN). Familial predisposition to MPNs is linked to genetic factors such as JAK2 polymorphisms and germline duplications on chromosome 14q32, enhancing the development of MPNs. Nonsyndromic familial myeloid predisposition syndromes, such as those linked to CEBPA and DDX41, are associated with MDS/AML. Inherited bone marrow failure syndromes (IBMFS), including Fanconi anemia, short telomere syndrome, and GATA2 haploinsufficiency syndrome, also increase the risk of MDS/AML. These syndromes have specific genetic variants influencing prognosis, and conditions such as SCN and thrombocytopenia can evolve into AML.

Relevance of Coexisting Somatic Mutations

Coexistence of recurrent somatic mutations is common in GPS. CEBPA-associated familial AML is characterized by an alteration in the second CEBPA allele; DDX41 mutations, in the second DDX41 allele (DDX41 p.R525H); and TP53 mutations are often accompanied by a complex karyotype and alteration in the second TP53 allele. In Familial platelet disorder with associated myeloid malignancy, alteration in the second RUNX1 allele is common, as well as mutations in GATA2, CBL, DNMT3A, KRAS, FLT3, and monosomy 7. In GATA2 haploinsufficiency syndromes, mutations in RUNX1, SETBP1, IKZF1, and CRLF2, along with monosomy 7 and trisomy 8 are common. SCN is associated with monosomy 7, RUNX1 mutations, and CSF3R mutations. Shwachman–Diamond syndrome often presents with TP53 mutations and monosomy 7 or del7q. While TP53 mutations in Shwachman–Diamond syndrome are not diagnostic of MDS nor do they predict impending malignant transformation, they can persist at low VAF for many years without progression. Common cytogenetic abnormalities that are not associated with a high risk of progression to MDS/AML include 20q deletion and isochromosome 7q. Fanconi anemia is associated with gain of 3q, deletion 7q, monosomy 7, complex karyotypes, and RUNX1 mutations. Casitas B-lineage lymphoma (CBL) syndrome often features acquired uniparental disomy of the mutated allele, except in occasional cases with splice-site mutations. Neurofibromatosis type 1 is characterized by a loss-of-function alteration of the second allele. SAMD9-related and SAMD9L-related syndromes involve monosomy 7 and loss of (partial) chromosome 7 carrying the SAMD9L variant.

■ GERMLINE PREDISPOSITION TO LYMPHOID NEOPLASMS

Clinical studies have shown that first-degree relatives of patients with CLL, non-Hodgkin lymphoma (NHL), and Hodgkin lymphoma (HL) have significantly higher rates of developing the same lymphoid malignancy. Genome-wide association studies have identified genetic susceptibilities, but familial predisposition is attributed to select genes. For example, inherited pathogenic variants in PAX5, SH2B3, and IKAROS are linked to familial B-ALL, while the *POT1* gene is associated with familial CLL. Specific inherited immune deficiency syndromes, such as ataxia telangiectasia (ATM), Bloom syndrome (BLM), Wiskott–Aldrich syndrome (WAS), and others, increase the risk of B- and T-cell lymphomas. Cartilage hair hypoplasia, linked to telomere dysfunction and immunodeficiency, also predisposes to lymphoid neoplasms. These disorders often involve DNA damage susceptibility and impaired immune surveillance, which contribute to an increased risk of cancer. Familial clusters of monoclonal gammopathy of undetermined significance, MM, and Waldenstrom macroglobulinemia have been observed in population studies. In 2018, KDM1A/LSD1 was identified as the first autosomal dominant gene linked to an increased predisposition to MM. It encodes a tumor-suppressor protein that acts as an epigenetic repressor by demethylating histone H3 on lysine 4 and regulating hematopoietic stem cell renewal. Additionally, recent exome sequencing has identified variants in the *DIS3* gene in two families with MM.

Recent studies are increasingly identifying the role of germline predisposition in B-ALL, including SNPs in genes such as *IKZF1*, *ARID5B*, and *GATA3*, which provide insights into leukemia biology and drug responsiveness. RAD21 germline variants can predispose to childhood lymphoblastic leukemia. A noncoding germline variant in GATA3 has been linked to Philadelphia chromosome-like ALL (Ph-like ALL), driving disease susceptibility through enhancer activation and chromatin reorganization. This variant upregulates GATA3 transcription, which directly regulates the CRLF2 oncogene and potentiates JAK-STAT signaling in leukemogenesis. A germline ETV6 deletion, identified through whole-genome sequencing (WGS), was found to segregate in a family with thrombocytopenia, B-progenitor ALL, and diffuse large B-cell lymphoma. This deletion causes exon skipping and protein truncation, highlighting the role of structural variants in familial leukemia and the importance of structural variant analysis in identifying genetic predispositions. Pathogenic or likely pathogenic germline variants in genes associated with ALL or other cancers are reported in 8% of adult and 11% of pediatric ALL patients, highlighting the significance of hereditary predisposition in ALL leukemogenesis. ETV6 mutations predispose to leukemia by aberrant cellular localization, decreased transcriptional repression, and disrupted megakaryocyte maturation. Autosomal dominant germline PAX5 variants reduce PAX5's transcriptional activity, highlighting its role in a new syndrome of susceptibility to pre-B cell neoplasia and expanding the understanding of PAX5's involvement in B-ALL pathogenesis.

Systemic Cancer Predisposition Syndromes

In addition to specific genomic variants linked to myeloid, lymphoid, or plasma cell neoplasms, established cancer predisposition syndromes such as Li-Fraumeni, Lynch, and Down syndrome also increase the risk of hematopoietic neoplasms. Li-Fraumeni syndrome, caused by germline variants in the *TP53* gene, is associated with early-onset cancers, including soft tissue and osteosarcomas, as well as leukemia. Lynch syndrome, resulting from defects in mismatch repair genes (*MSH1*, *MLH1*, *MSH6*), has been linked to leukemia (AML and CLL), MM, and NHL, particularly with MSH2 defects. Down syndrome, characterized by trisomy 21 and truncating variants in the *GATA1* gene, predisposes individuals to leukemia, including acute megakaryocytic leukemia and B-cell ALL. An oncogenic gain-of-function variant in the *CSF2RB* gene has been shown to drive leukemic transformation in patients with Down syndrome, cooperating with acquired mutations in cohesion complex and epigenetic regulators.

Clinical Importance of Germline Predisposition Syndromes Identification

Precision genomics has not only improved the speed and accuracy of diagnosing hereditary predisposition syndromes (HPS)/GPS but also plays a critical role in therapy, particularly in the management of BMF and malignancy. In patients with germline predisposition to hematological malignancies, allogeneic hematopoietic cell transplantation (HCT) remains an integral part of treatment, but it requires careful donor selection. Excluding pathogenic germline variants in sibling or haploidentical donors is crucial to avoid posttransplant donor-derived malignancies. Patients with germline predisposition to hematological malignancies are more sensitive to chemotherapy and radiation therapy, increasing the risks of transplant-related morbidity and mortality, particularly in conditions involving chromosomal breakage and short telomere syndromes. These patients are at an elevated risk (~10–20%) for graft failure due to bone marrow dysfunction, immune dysregulation, and use of a less intensive conditioning regimen. Genomic evaluation is essential in customizing treatment plans for these patients to optimize outcomes and reduce complications.

Furthermore, recognizing GPS can guide screening for family members. Incomplete penetrance and somatic reversion can result in relatives carrying gene variants without exhibiting symptoms. Genetic counseling and testing are recommended for these individuals, even if no immediate interventions are available. Specific therapies, such as danazol for short telomere syndromes and azithromycin for GATA2 haploinsufficiency, can also be crucial for managing symptoms and preventing complications.

Management and surveillance for individuals with P/LP germline variants linked to myeloid malignancies (MDS/AML) are based largely on expert opinion due to the lack of rigorous evidence-based guidelines. For those with variants in genes associated with platelet dysfunction (such as RUNX1, ETV6, or ANKRD26), platelet aggregation studies are recommended, especially if there is a history of easy bruising or bleeding. Antifibrinolytic agents or desmopressin may be used for patients with mild bleeding or undergoing high-risk procedures. Regular CBC monitoring is suggested, with tests every 3–4 months for individuals with RUNX1 variants and every 6–12 months for ETV6 or ANKRD26 variants. Bone marrow biopsy, including cytogenetic and molecular profiling, should be conducted if any abnormalities persist. For individuals with P/LP germline RUNX1 variants, the development of somatic RUNX1 variants indicates a higher risk of MDS/AML and warrants early HSCT work-up. In contrast, preemptive HSCT is not recommended for these variants due to incomplete penetrance. For DDX41 variant carriers, screening for MDS/AML should start around age 40, or 10 years younger than the earliest family case. Bone marrow biopsies and molecular testing are recommended if persistent cytopenias or other abnormalities develop. HSCT is considered upon MDS/AML onset, and the use of posttransplant cyclophosphamide is advised to reduce severe graft-versus-host disease (GVHD). In BMF syndromes, monitoring CBC every 6 months is recommended, with HSCT considered when severe BMF, MDS/AML, or related complications arise. Tailored conditioning regimens are recommended, particularly to avoid the risk of secondary solid tumors, as seen in conditions such as Fanconi anemia.

Approach to Diagnosis

A systematic approach is employed to identify GPS in patients, especially those with unexplained cytopenias or hematopoietic neoplasms. Clinical indicators prompting screening include younger age at the onset of cytopenias or hematopoietic malignancy (typically under 40 years), unexplained macrocytosis, elevated fetal hemoglobin levels, a personal or family history of hematopoietic neoplasms or cancers linked to hereditary syndromes, and syndromic features such as HPV-driven warts and lymphedema for GATA2 haploinsufficiency, or reticulocytopenia for DBA. When these clinical signs are observed, patients are referred to genetics clinics or specialized hematologists/oncologists for further evaluation. This process includes a comprehensive history and physical examination, genetic counseling, and informed consent for precision genomics testing. The evaluation may also involve bone marrow assessments (if clinically indicated), specific clinical tests such as flow cytometry-fluorescence in situ hybridization (FISH) for telomere length, chromosomal breakage assays for Fanconi anemia, and custom-designed genetic testing panels. If a pathogenic variant is found, confirmation is sought through germline testing in affected and unaffected family members or by analyzing germline tissues such as skin fibroblasts, hair follicles, nail clippings, or buccal swabs. Each tissue type has advantages and limitations—for instance, nail clippings may yield lower DNA, and T-cells may not be ideal for all HPS cases. Skin fibroblasts are preferred due to their reliability. In cases of variants of uncertain significance (VUS), a bioinformatics team evaluates the variant using in-silico tools, sequence conservation, and various databases to predict its potential impact. The case is reviewed by a team of expert clinicians, geneticists, and bioinformaticians. Final confirmation of the variant is carried out through functional validation in the laboratory. If no results are obtained from targeted panel testing, whole-exome sequencing is performed for further exploration of potential genetic causes.

FUTURE DIRECTIONS

Genomic characterization of GPS has significantly advanced our understanding of the biological mechanisms behind these unique disorders. By studying the clonal evolution and neoplastic transformation in patients with GPS, researchers are uncovering new insights into how these conditions progress. Key areas of focus include how genetically deficient cells manage to survive and proliferate, leading to clonal selection. Understanding these mechanisms could reveal specific vulnerabilities that could be targeted by novel drug development strategies. Additionally, the emergence of gene-editing technologies provides a promising therapeutic avenue. By directly manipulating the genetic material of affected cells, it may be possible to correct defects and alter the course of these hereditary syndromes, offering potential new treatments for patients with hematopoietic neoplasms associated with germline predisposition.

CONCLUSION

Early recognition of germline predisposition to hematopoietic neoplasms is essential for timely diagnosis and personalized treatment. A stepwise genomics approach allows for accurate diagnoses and helps avoid inappropriate treatments. Future research will focus on expanding the feasibility of specialized precision medicine clinics, developing innovative methods for variant validation, improving transplant conditioning strategies, and creating novel therapies to prevent clonal evolution and reverse genetic discrepancies in GPS. These advances aim to enhance patient care, optimize treatment decisions, and ultimately improve outcomes for individuals with hereditary blood cancers.

Take Home Points

- Germline mutations contribute significantly to the development of hematologic malignancies, including leukemias, MPNs, and lymphoid neoplasms, alongside somatic mutations.
- Key genetic variants in genes such as *RUNX1*, *CEBPA*, *PAX5*, and *TP53* are linked to familial predispositions, underscoring the importance of genetic screening for early detection.
- Precision genomics plays a crucial role in diagnosing germline predispositions, guiding personalized treatment plans, and influencing disease management strategies.
- Genetic counseling and family risk assessment are essential for individuals with inherited mutations, ensuring informed decisions regarding treatment and screening.

SUGGESTED READINGS

1. Klco JM, Mullighan CG. Advances in germline predisposition to acute leukemias and myeloid neoplasms. Nat Rev Cancer. 2021;21(2):122-37.
2. Hayashi Y, Harada Y, Huang G, Harada H. Myeloid neoplasms with germ line RUNX1 mutation. Int J Hematol. 2017;106(2):183-8.
3. Swerdlow SH, Campo E, Harris NL, Jaffe ES, Pileri SA, Stein H, et al. WHO Classification of Tumours of Haematopoietic and Lymphoid Tissues. [online] Available from https://publications.iarc.fr/Book-And-Report-Series/Who-Classification-Of-Tumours/WHO-Classification-Of-Tumours-Of-Haematopoietic-And-Lymphoid-Tissues-2017 [Last accessed May, 2025].
4. Hansen MC, Nyvold CG, Roug AS, Kjeldsen E, Villesen P, Nederby L, et al. Nature and nurture: a case of transcending haematological pre-malignancies in a pair of monozygotic twins adding possible clues on the pathogenesis of B-cell proliferations. Br J Haematol. 2015;169(3):391-400.
5. Rio-Machin A, Vulliamy T, Hug N, Walne A, Tawana K, Cardoso S, et al. The complex genetic landscape of familial MDS and AML reveals pathogenic germline variants. Nat Commun. 2020;11(1):1044.

6. Mangaonkar AA, Patnaik MM. Hereditary Predisposition to Hematopoietic Neoplasms: When Bloodline Matters for Blood Cancers. Mayo Clin Proc. 2020;95(7):1482-98.
7. Cuccuini W, Collonge-Rame MA, Auger N, Douet-Guilbert N, Coster L, Lafage-Pochitaloff M. Cytogenetics in the management of bone marrow failure syndromes: Guidelines from the Groupe Francophone de Cytogénétique Hématologique (GFCH). Curr Res Transl Med. 2023;71(4):103423.
8. Feurstein S. Emerging bone marrow failure syndromes—new pieces to an unsolved puzzle. Front Oncol. 2023;13:1128533.
9. Przychodzen B, Makishima H, Sekeres MA, Balasubramanian SK, Thota S, Patel BJ, et al. Fanconi Anemia germline variants as susceptibility factors in aplastic anemia, MDS and AML. Oncotarget. 2018;9(2):2050-7.
10. Trottier AM, Feurstein S, Godley LA. Germline predisposition to myeloid neoplasms: Characteristics and management of high versus variable penetrance disorders. Best Pract Res Clin Haematol. 2024;37(1):101537.
11. Board WC of TE. Haematolymphoid Tumours. [online] Available from https://publications.iarc.fr/Book-And-Report-Series/Who-Classification-Of-Tumours/Haematolymphoid-Tumours-2024 [Last accessed May, 2025].
12. Kubota Y, Zawit M, Durrani J, Shen W, Bahaj W, Kewan T, et al. Significance of hereditary gene alterations for the pathogenesis of adult bone marrow failure versus myeloid neoplasia. Leukemia. 2022;36(12):2827-34.
13. Martin ES, Ferrer A, Mangaonkar AA, Khan SP, Kohorst MA, Joshi AY, et al. Spectrum of hematological malignancies, clonal evolution and outcomes in 144 Mayo Clinic patients with germline predisposition syndromes. Am J Hematol. 2021;96(11):1450-60.
14. Brown AL, Hiwase DK. What's germane in the germline? Finding clinically relevant germline variants in myeloid neoplasms from tumor only screening. Leuk Res. 2020;96:106431.
15. Yoshida K. Myeloid neoplasms with germline predisposition. Rinsho Ketsueki. 2023;64(9):949-54.
16. Arai H, Matsui H, Chi S, Utsu Y, Masuda S, Aotsuka N, et al. Germline Variants and Characteristic Features of Hereditary Hematological Malignancy Syndrome. Int J Mol Sci. 2024;25(1):652.
17. Sullivan MJ, Palmer EL, Botero JP. ANKRD26-Related Thrombocytopenia and Predisposition to Myeloid Neoplasms. Curr Hematol Malig Rep. 2022;17(5):105-12.
18. Chin HL, Lam JCM, Christopher D, Michelle PL, Junrong BY. Challenges associated with the identification of germline variants on myeloid malignancy genomic profiling-a Singaporean experience. Front Oncol. 2023;13:1182639.
19. Kongkiatkamon S, Niparuck P, Rattanathammethee T, Kobbuaklee S, Suksusut A, Wudhikarn K, et al. Prevalence and clinical outcomes of germline variants among patients with myeloid neoplasms. J Clin Pathol. 2025;78(4):259-65.
20. Carraway HE, LaFramboise T. Myeloid neoplasms with germline predisposition: Practical considerations and complications in the search for new susceptibility loci. Best Pract Res Clin Haematol. 2020;33(3):101191.
21. Yang F, Long N, Anekpuritanang T, Bottomly D, Savage JC, Lee T, et al. Identification and prioritization of myeloid malignancy germline variants in a large cohort of adult patients with AML. Blood. 2022;139(8):1208-21.
22. Harrigan AM, Trottier AM. Hereditary acute myeloid leukemia associated with C-terminal CEBPA germline variants. Fam Cancer. 2023;22(3):331-9.
23. Homan CC, Venugopal P, Arts P, Shahrin NH, Feurstein S, Rawlings L, et al. GATA2 deficiency syndrome: A decade of discovery. Hum Mutat. 2021;42(11):1399-421.
24. Yoshida M, Tanase-Nakao K, Shima H, Shirai R, Yoshida K, Osumi T, et al. Prevalence of germline GATA2 and SAMD9/9L variants in paediatric haematological disorders with monosomy 7. Br J Haematol. 2020;191(5):835-43.
25. Link DC, Schuettpelz LG, Shen D, Wang J, Walter MJ, Kulkarni S, et al. Identification of a novel TP53 cancer susceptibility mutation through whole-genome sequencing of a patient with therapy-related AML. JAMA. 2011;305(15):1568-76.

26. Taylor J, Xiao W, Abdel-Wahab O. Diagnosis and classification of hematologic malignancies on the basis of genetics. Blood. 2017;130(4):410-23.
27. Wan Z, Han B. Clinical features of DDX41 mutation-related diseases: a systematic review with individual patient data. Ther Adv Hematol. 2021;12:20406207211032433.
28. Dirse V, Norvilas R, Gineikiene E, Matuzevičienė R, Griskevicius L, Preiksaitiene E. ETV6 and NOTCH1 germline variants in adult acute leukemia. Leuk Lymphoma. 2018;59(4):1022-4.
29. Makishima H, Saiki R, Nannya Y, Korotev S, Gurnari C, Takeda J, et al. Germ line DDX41 mutations define a unique subtype of myeloid neoplasms. Blood. 2023;141(5):534-49.
30. Liu C, Ballerini P, Nguyen G, Mincheva Z, Copin B, Bouslama B, et al. Germline RUNX1 variants in paediatric patients in a French specialised centre. E J Haem. 2023;4(1):145-52.
31. Poggi M, Canault M, Favier M, Turro E, Saultier P, Ghalloussi D, et al. Germline variants in ETV6 underlie reduced platelet formation, platelet dysfunction and increased levels of circulating CD34+ progenitors. Haematologica. 2017;102(2):282-94.
32. Bannon SA, Routbort MJ, Montalban-Bravo G, Mehta RS, Jelloul FZ, Takahashi K, et al. Next-Generation Sequencing of DDX41 in Myeloid Neoplasms Leads to Increased Detection of Germline Alterations. Front Oncol. 2020;10:582213.
33. Ernst MPT, Kavelaars FG, Löwenberg B, Valk PJM, Raaijmakers MHGP. RUNX1 germline variants in RUNX1-mutant AML: how frequent? Blood. 2021;137(10):1428-31.
34. Li P, Brown S, Williams M, White T, Xie W, Cui W, et al. The genetic landscape of germline DDX41 variants predisposing to myeloid neoplasms. Blood. 2022;140(7):716-55.
35. Matsui H, Hirata M. Evaluation of the pathogenic potential of germline DDX41 variants in hematopoietic neoplasms using the ACMG/AMP guidelines. Int J Hematol. 2024;119(5): 552-63.
36. Kim K, Ong F, Sasaki K. Current Understanding of DDX41 Mutations in Myeloid Neoplasms. Cancers. 2023;15(2):344.
37. Bataller A, Loghavi S, Gerstein Y, Bazinet A, Sasaki K, Chien KS, et al. Characteristics and clinical outcomes of patients with myeloid malignancies and DDX41 variants. Am J Hematol. 2023;98(11):1780-90.
38. Qu S, Li B, Qin T, Xu Z, Pan L, Hu N, et al. Molecular and clinical features of myeloid neoplasms with somatic DDX41 mutations. Br J Haematol. 2021;192(6):1006-10.
39. Thompson C, Ariagno S, Kohorst MA. Pediatric Germline Predisposition to Myeloid Neoplasms. Curr Hematol Malig Rep. 2022;17(6):266-74.
40. Steinberg-Shemer O, Orenstein N, Krasnov T, Noy-Lotan S, Marcoux N, Dgany O, et al. Congenital thrombocytopenia associated with a heterozygous variant in the MEIS1 gene encoding a transcription factor essential for megakaryopoiesis. Platelets. 2022;33(4):645-8.
41. Veitia RA, Innan H. Pathogenic "germline" variants associated with myeloproliferative disorders in apparently normal individuals: Inherited or acquired genetic alterations? Clin Genet. 2022;101(3):371-4.
42. Bellanné-Chantelot C, Rabadan Moraes G, Schmaltz-Panneau B, Marty C, Vainchenker W, Plo I. Germline genetic factors in the pathogenesis of myeloproliferative neoplasms. Blood Rev. 2020;42:100710.
43. Tapper W, Jones AV, Kralovics R, Harutyunyan AS, Zoi K, Leung W, et al. Genetic variation at MECOM, TERT, JAK2 and HBS1L-MYB predisposes to myeloproliferative neoplasms. Nat Commun. 2015;6:6691.
44. Rumi E, Cazzola M. Advances in understanding the pathogenesis of familial myeloproliferative neoplasms. Br J Haematol. 2017;178(5):689-98.
45. Lu C, Xie M, Wendl MC, Wang J, McLellan MD, Leiserson MDM, et al. Patterns and functional implications of rare germline variants across 12 cancer types. Nat Commun. 2015;6:10086.
46. Alsultan A, Essa M, Aljefri A, Ayas M, Alharbi M, Alkhayat N, et al. Frequency of pathogenic/ likely pathogenic germline variants in cancer-related genes among children with acute leukemia in Saudi Arabia. Pediatr Blood Cancer. 2020;67(7):e28340.
47. Fukuhara S, Oshikawa-Kumade Y, Kogure Y, Shingaki S, Kariyazono H, Kikukawa Y, et al. Feasibility and clinical utility of comprehensive genomic profiling of hematological malignancies. Cancer Sci. 2022;113(8):2763-77.

48. Di Fede E, Massa V, Augello B, Squeo G, Scarano E, Perri AM, et al. Expanding the phenotype associated to KMT2A variants: overlapping clinical signs between Wiedemann-Steiner and Rubinstein-Taybi syndromes. Eur J Hum Genet. 2021;29(1):88-98.
49. Trottier AM, Godley LA. Inherited predisposition to haematopoietic malignancies: overcoming barriers and exploring opportunities. Br J Haematol. 2021;194(4):663-76.
50. Nishii R, Baskin-Doerfler R, Yang W, Oak N, Zhao X, Yang W, et al. Molecular basis of ETV6-mediated predisposition to childhood acute lymphoblastic leukemia. Blood. 2021;137(3):364-73.
51. Hofer KD, Bühler MM, Roncador M, Rechsteiner M, Maggio EM, Tchinda J, et al. Mutational patterns in therapy-related acute lymphoblastic leukemia subgroups: one step closer to unveiling the genetic odyssey. Leuk Lymphoma. 2024;65(6):808-15.
52. Schedel A, Friedrich UA, Morcos MNF, Wagener R, Mehtonen J, Watrin T, et al. Recurrent Germline Variant in RAD21 Predisposes Children to Lymphoblastic Leukemia or Lymphoma. Int J Mol Sci. 2022;23(9):5174.
53. Shah S, Schrader KA, Waanders E, Timms AE, Vijai J, Miething C, et al. A recurrent germline PAX5 mutation confers susceptibility to pre-B cell acute lymphoblastic leukemia. Nat Genet. 2013;45(10):1226-31.
54. Douglas SPM, Lahtinen AK, Koski JR, Leimi L, Keränen MAI, Koskenvuo M, et al. Enrichment of cancer-predisposing germline variants in adult and pediatric patients with acute lymphoblastic leukemia. Sci Rep. 2022;12(1):10670.
55. Porter CC, Di Paola J, Pencheva B. ETV6 Thrombocytopenia and Predisposition to Leukemia. In: Adam MP, Feldman J, Mirzaa GM, Pagon RA, Wallace SE, Amemiya A (Eds). GeneReviews®. Seattle (WA): University of Washington, Seattle; 1993.
56. Rampersaud E, Ziegler DS, Iacobucci I, Payne-Turner D, Churchman ML, Schrader KA, et al. Germline deletion of ETV6 in familial acute lymphoblastic leukemia. Blood Adv. 2019;3(7):1039-46.
57. Noetzli L, Lo RW, Lee-Sherick AB, Callaghan M, Noris P, Savoia A, et al. Germline mutations in ETV6 are associated with thrombocytopenia, red cell macrocytosis and predisposition to lymphoblastic leukemia. Nat Genet. 2015;47(5):535-8.
58. Duployez N, Jamrog LA, Fregona V, Hamelle C, Fenwarth L, Lejeune S, et al. Germline PAX5 mutation predisposes to familial B-cell precursor acute lymphoblastic leukemia. Blood. 2021;137(10):1424-8.
59. Yang H, Zhang H, Luan Y, Liu T, Yang W, Roberts KG, et al. Noncoding genetic variation in GATA3 increases acute lymphoblastic leukemia risk through local and global changes in chromatin conformation. Nat Genet. 2022;54(2):170-9.
60. Bloom M, Maciaszek JL, Clark ME, Pui CH, Nichols KE. Recent advances in genetic predisposition to pediatric acute lymphoblastic leukemia. Expert Rev Hematol. 2020;13(1):55-70.

CHAPTER 14

Recent Advances in the Diagnosis and Treatment of Hodgkin Lymphoma

Mukul Aggarwal, Rakhee Kar, Kaniyappan Nambiar

ABSTRACT

Classic Hodgkin lymphoma (CHL) is characterized by key genetic alterations, particularly in the nuclear factor κB (NF-κB), Janus kinase-signal transducers and activators of transcription (JAK/STAT), and phosphatidylinositol 3-kinase (PI3K)/AKT pathways, contributing to cancer development and immune evasion. Atypical cells in CHL require careful differentiation from similar disorders. There are rare instances where CHL coexists with other lymphomas, known as composite lymphoma. Additionally, transformations between CHL and other lymphomas can occur infrequently, particularly from B-cell non-Hodgkin lymphoma. New markers, such as STAT6, Fascin, and GATA3, help distinguish CHL from other lymphomas.

Additionally, circulating tumor DNA is an effective tool for monitoring treatment response and residual disease, with decreasing levels indicating a positive response to therapy. Nodular lymphocyte-predominant Hodgkin lymphoma (NLPHL) is now considered closely related to T-cell/histiocyte-rich large B-cell lymphoma. It may be renamed nodular lymphocyte-predominant B-cell lymphoma. NLPHL arises from germinal center B cells and is influenced by specific bacterial antigens.

The patient usually presents with cervical or mediastinal lymphadenopathy with or without internal lymphadenopathy. They are investigated with lymph node biopsy and commonly positron emission tomography–computed tomography (PET-CT) for staging and diagnosis. The treatment is chemotherapy-based or chemoradiotherapy based and associated with good prognosis in most of the patients. Targeted therapy with brentuximab and checkpoint inhibitors is revolutionizing the management of advanced Hodgkin lymphoma and relapsed refractory patients.

INTRODUCTION

The classification of Hodgkin lymphoma (HL) includes two primary types: (1) classic Hodgkin lymphoma (CHL) and (2) nodular lymphocyte-predominant Hodgkin lymphoma (NLPHL). This article explores recent advancements in the pathogenesis, diagnostic approaches, and management of HL.

PATHOLOGICAL FEATURES OF HODGKIN LYMPHOMA

The standard characteristics of HL are summarized in **Table 1**. The first four types [nodular sclerosis (NS), lymphocyte rich, mixed cellularity, and lymphocyte depleted] belong to CHL.

Pathogenesis of Classic Hodgkin Lymphoma

Cell of Origin

The Hodgkin and Reed–Sternberg (HRS) cells are believed to originate from germinal center (GC) B cells due to the presence of somatic hypermutations in immunoglobulin variable genes. The HRS cells likely arise from preapoptotic GC B cells with harmful mutations that would typically undergo apoptosis. However, they evade this process through similar transforming events occurring in the normal GC CD30+ B cells. The normal CD30+ B cells in the GC are distinguished populations in the light zone that evade apoptosis by activating the nuclear factor κB (NF-κB) and Janus kinase-signal transducers and activators of transcription (JAK/STAT) signaling pathways. In contrast to the HRS cells, these cells maintain a fully preserved B-cell program.

TABLE 1: Pathological characteristics of Hodgkin lymphoma.

Type	Morphology	Background	EBV	Immunophenotype
Nodular sclerosis	• HRS cells, including Lacunar cells • Cellular nodules are surrounded by partial or complete collagen band	T cells, eosinophils, macrophages, plasma cells	Usually	CD30+, CD15+, MUM1+, CD45–, CD20–/+, CD3–, PAX5 weak+
Lymphocyte rich	• HRS cells + mononuclear cells • Nodular or diffuse architecture	• Background of small lymphocytes (B and T) • B cells are most prominent in LRCHL. Other cells are rare	+	
Mixed cellularity	HRS cells + mononuclear cells	T cells, neutrophils, eosinophils, macrophages, plasma cells	++	
Lymphocyte depleted	HRS cells + pleomorphic variant	A paucity of reactive lymphocytes	++	
Nodular lymphocyte predominant Hodgkin lymphoma	• Popcorn cells • Nodular architecture (rarely diffuse architecture)	B cells and follicular dendritic cells (rarely T cells predominant)	–	CD20+, OCT2+, BOB1+, PAX5+, BCL6+, CD30–, CD15–, and MUM1–

(EBS: Epstein–Barr virus; HRS: Hodgkin and Reed–Sternberg; LRCHL: lymphocyte-rich classical Hodgkin lymphoma)

Morphogenesis and Giant Cell Formation

Giant multinucleated HRS cells are formed from dividing mononuclear Hodgkin cells that undergo incomplete cytokinesis. This phenomenon in HL arises due to sustained microtubule connections between daughter cells, ultimately resulting in their refusion. Endomitosis is another minor way of giant multinucleated HRS cell formation, where all mitosis stages occur within the nuclear membrane without spindle formation.

Cyclin A, mainly active in the S phase and found in the nucleus, may influence CHL morphogenesis. Abnormal cytoplasmic levels can lead to multinucleation, and downregulating this pathway may cause apoptosis in HL cells, resulting in mummified cells.

Role of Epstein–Barr Virus

The Epstein–Barr virus (EBV) in CHL typically displays a latency type II pattern, exhibiting Epstein–Barr virus nuclear antigen 1 (EBNA1), latent membrane protein 1 (LMP1), and latent membrane protein 2A (LMP2A) expression. **Table 2** summarizes the primary function and role of latent genes and microRNA (miRNA). Research indicates that EBV-positive CHL exhibits a lower mutation burden and fewer chromosomal abnormalities than EBV-negative CHL. This phenomenon can be ascribed to the survival signals conferred by viral proteins, particularly LMP1 and LMP2A.

Genetic Alterations

The CHL exhibits various driver mutations, which are summarized in **Table 3**, along with the affected pathways. Besides the pathways in the table, the NOTCH1 signaling pathway may show constitutive activation in HRS cells.

TABLE 2: Primary function and role of Epstein–Barr virus (EBV) latent genes and miRNA.

EBV latent genes and miRNA	Function	Major role in CHL
EBNA1	• Key viral replication factor • Responsible for tethering viral genomes to the chromosomes of the host cell	• Ensures viral genomes are retained during cell division • Act as a transcription factor • Inhibits TGFβ signaling
LMP1	• The cytoplasmic domain mimics a signaling motif of CD40 • Enhance cyclin A expression	Activation of NF-κB and other signaling pathways
LMP2A	The cytoplasmic domain mimics signaling modules of the B-cell receptor (BCR) components	Act as a survival signal for BCR-negative GC B cells
EBV-encoded miRNA	Regulation of viral and modulation of host gene expression	• Suppress lytic cycle and BCR signaling • Role in immune evasion

(EBNA1: Epstein–Barr virus nuclear antigen 1; LMP1: latent membrane protein 1; LMP2A: latent membrane protein 2A; NF-κB: nuclear factor κB; TGFβ: transforming growth factor)

TABLE 3: Significant pathways affected with frequent mutations identified in classical Hodgkin lymphoma (CHL).

Pathways	Genes with recurrent mutations
NF-κB pathway	*NFKBIA, NFKBIE, TNFAIP3, TRAF3, CYLD, REL, MAP3K14*, and *BCL3*
JAK/STAT pathway	*SOCS1, PTPN1, CSF2RB, JAK2,* and *STAT6*
PI3K/AKT pathway	*GNA13* and *ITPKB*

(NF-κB: nuclear factor κB; JAK/STAT: Janus kinase-signal transducers and activators of transcription; PI3K/AKT: phosphatidylinositol 3-kinase)

An additional set of recurring genetic alterations in HRS cells significantly impacts immune evasion strategies, aiding their escape from immune surveillance. The commonly impacted genes include *B2M, MHC2TA, PDL1, and PDL2*. Recent evidence indicates that aberrant expression of receptor tyrosine kinases and dysregulation of activator protein 1 (AP-1) transcription factors also play a significant role in the pathogenesis of CHL.

The HRS cells also exhibit a significant prevalence of aneuploidy and hypertetraploidy, characterized by recurrent chromosomal gains (e.g., 2p, 9p, 17q, 19q, 20q) as well as losses (e.g., 6q, 13q).

MORPHOLOGY

The morphology of atypical cells utilized for diagnosing HL may be observed in four clinical scenarios: (1) CHL, (2) composite CHL, (3) reactive lymphoid hyperplasia, and (4) lymphoproliferative disorders not classified as CHL.

Hodgkin Reed–Sternberg-like Cells and Composite Classic Hodgkin Lymphoma

The large, atypical cells resembling HRS cells are referred to as HRS-like cells in cases of reactive lymphoid hyperplasia and lymphoproliferative disorders not classified as CHL. A comprehensive list of these entities is presented in **Table 4**.

Exceedingly rare instances have been documented in which CHL coexists with non-Hodgkin lymphoma or NLPHL as a composite lymphoma. These cases may present either synchronously or as a result of transformation between the two lymphoma types. Composite CHL has been documented in the literature in conjunction with various other types of lymphoma, namely follicular lymphoma, marginal zone lymphoma, diffuse large B-cell lymphoma, mantle cell lymphoma, NLPHL, and T-cell lymphomas.

Transformations from and to Classic Hodgkin Lymphoma

The transition from low-grade B-cell non-Hodgkin lymphoma to CHL occurs more commonly than the progression of CHL into other lymphoma types. Chronic lymphocytic leukemia, follicular lymphoma, marginal zone lymphoma, and mantle cell lymphoma can show transformation to CHL **(Figs. 1A to I)**.

TABLE 4: Entities with HRS-like cells.	
B-cell-derived lymphoproliferative disorders	Diffuse large B cell lymphoma NOS
	EBV-positive diffuse large B-cell lymphoma
	T cell/histiocyte-rich large B-cell lymphoma
	ALK+ large B-cell lymphoma
	Primary mediastinal large B-cell lymphoma
	Mediastinal gray-zone lymphoma
	Lymphomatoid granulomatosis
	Primary effusion lymphoma
	Mantle cell lymphoma
	Follicular lymphoma
	Marginal zone lymphoma
	Chronic lymphocytic leukemia/small lymphocytic lymphoma
	Polymorphic lymphoproliferative disorders arising in immune deficiency/dysregulation and EBV-positive mucocutaneous ulcer
	Primary cutaneous marginal zone lymphoma and primary cutaneous follicle center lymphoma
T-cell-derived lymphoproliferative disorders	Anaplastic large cell lymphomas
	Nodal T follicular helper cell lymphomas
	Peripheral T-cell lymphoma NOS
Reactive hyperplasia	Infectious mononucleosis

(EBV: Epstein–Barr virus; HRS: Hodgkin Reed–Sternberg; NOS: not otherwise specified)

The CHL infrequently transforms into diffuse large B-cell lymphoma (DLBCL), with < 1% of cases presenting such an occurrence. The development of DLBCL appears to be de novo in nature rather than arising clonally from preexisting cells in patients with a history of CHL. Gene expression profiling has revealed the presence of both GC type and unclassifiable subtypes in these DLBCL cases.

Morphological Prognostic Indicators

Morphological variants in CHL subtypes also have important prognostic implications. The syncytial variant of NS CHL and the reticular variant of Lymphocyte-depleted (LD) CHL are linked to a poorer prognosis. The NS CHL exhibits heterogeneous morphology and clinical behavior. Several morphological grading systems have been developed to identify tumors with adverse behavior tumors. The British National Lymphoma Investigation grading system classifies CHL into grade 1 and grade 2 based on the presence of pleomorphic HRS cells, with or without lymphocyte depletion or increased fibrotic components. Another grading system classifies NS CHL as high risk based on the presence of any of the following criteria: eosinophilia (>5% of all cells or clusters in at least five high-power fields), lymphocyte depletion (<33% of all cells), and atypia (>25% of HRS cells being bizarre and anaplastic) **(Figs. 2A to I)**.

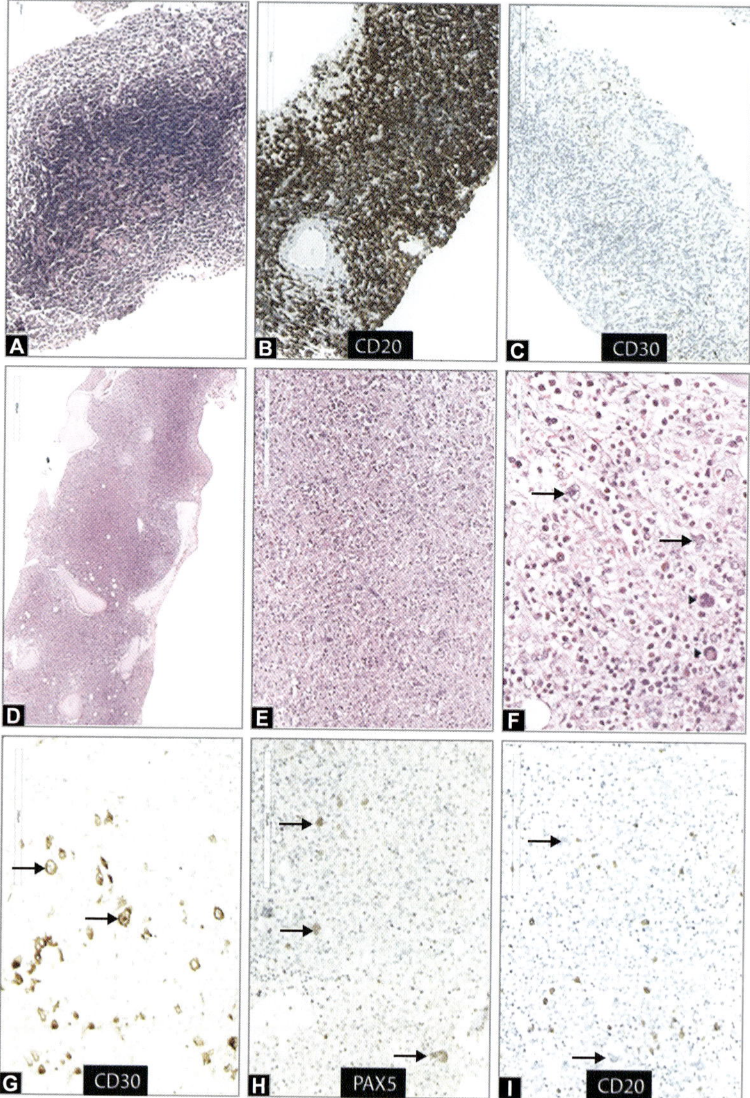

FIGS. 1A TO I: The transformation of splenic marginal zone lymphoma to classic Hodgkin lymphoma is illustrated from panels A to I. (A) Initially, the presentation was splenic marginal zone lymphoma, with biopsy revealing small lymphoma cells that replaced the white pulp and infiltrated the red pulp. (B) These cells were found to express CD20, (C) while CD30 was negative throughout the biopsy. (D) During follow-up, bone marrow analysis demonstrated diffuse infiltration by classic Hodgkin lymphoma. (E) Many scattered large cells were observed against a background of histiocytes, small lymphocytes, and eosinophils. (F) The Hodgkin and Reed–Sternberg cells displayed abundant cytoplasm, enlarged nuclei, vesicular chromatin, and prominent nucleoli (as indicated by the arrows). Additionally, mummified cells (arrowheads) with hyperchromatic chromatin and loss of cellular details were also noted. (G) Immunohistochemical stains revealed that the neoplastic cells (indicated by the arrows) were positive for CD30 and (H) showed weak positivity for PAX5, (I) while they were negative for CD20. There was no evidence of marginal zone lymphoma.

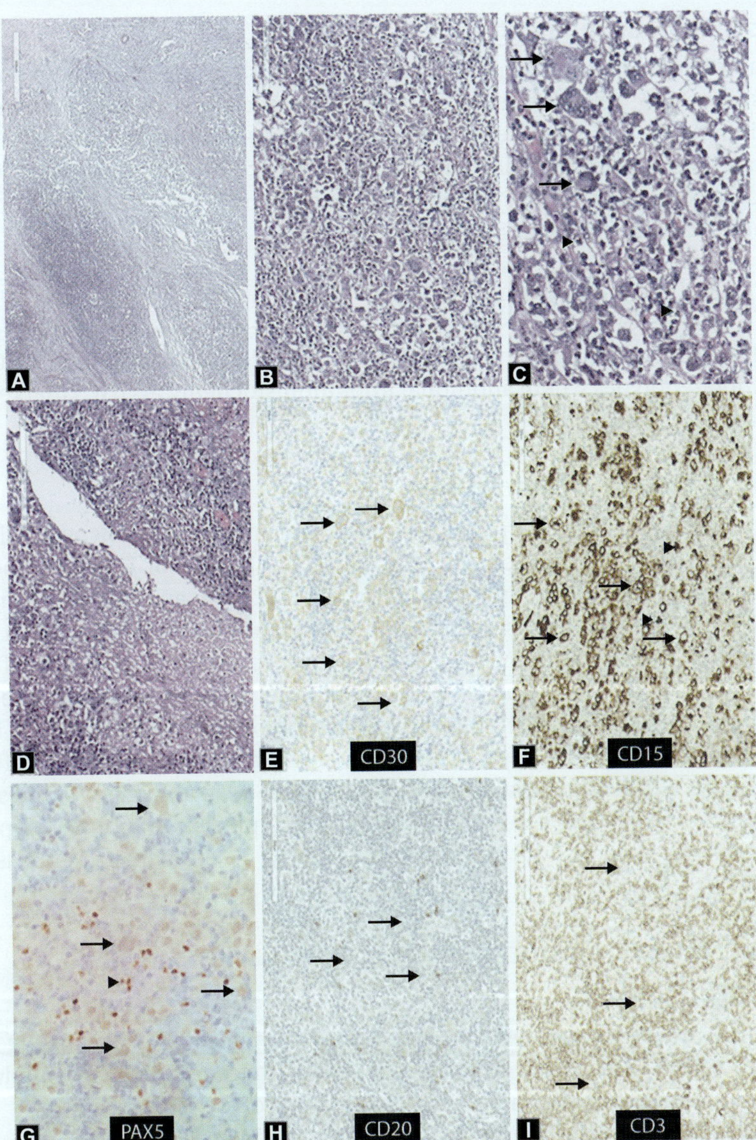

FIGS. 2A TO I: High-grade classic Hodgkin lymphoma, nodular sclerosis subtype. (A) The lymph node biopsy demonstrates an effaced architecture characterized by extensive collagenous bands that compartmentalize the node into multiple distinct nodules. (B) Large, atypical cells are predominant, accounting for >25% of the cellular composition, (C) displaying pleomorphic and bizarre features as indicated by arrows. The background contains numerous neutrophils (arrowhead), lymphocytes, and histiocytes, (D) with foci of necrosis also observed. Immunohistochemical staining highlights the neoplastic cells (arrows), which are positive for CD30 (E) and CD15 (F), showing weak positivity for PAX5 (G). In contrast, they are negative for CD20 (H) and CD3 (I).

Tumor Microenvironment

The tumor microenvironment (TME) and HRS cells share a symbiotic relationship. Senescent HRS cells induce a senescence-associated secretory phenotype, contributing to the characteristic microenvironment observed in CHL, which facilitates tumor progression. The TME in CHL comprises various cell types, including T cells, B cells, plasma cells, eosinophils, neutrophils, histiocytes, stromal cells, and fibroblasts.

IMMUNOHISTOCHEMISTRY

The classic immunophenotype is described in **Table 1**. Rare cases show atypical immunophenotypes where additional immunohistochemical (IHC) markers can aid diagnosis.

Atypical Immunophenotype

A limited subset of CHL may present with atypical immunophenotypes, including CD20 expression, diminished CD30 expression, absence of PAX5, or aberrant T-cell marker expression. In instances where CD20 or another B-cell marker exhibits uniform and intense expression, the identification of CHL from other stromal-rich B-cell lymphomas necessitates the loss of additional B-cell differentiation markers. Positivity for B-cell markers other than PAX5 is more frequent in lymphocyte-rich (LR) CHL than in other subtypes. The diagnosis of a PAX5-negative CHL should be approached with considerable caution, and differentiation from a T-cell lymphoma may require gene rearrangement studies. In a minor subset of NS CHL exhibiting an otherwise typical immunophenotype, the HRS cells may demonstrate atypical expression of T-cell markers, such as CD4 and CD2.

Useful Newer Immunohistochemical Markers in Special Situations

In routine practice, weak PAX5 may be the sole indicator for diagnosing CHL, whereas CD30 and CD15 may be expressed in morphological mimickers. In certain situations, the interpretation of PAX5 can be uncertain, and other positive markers may be beneficial. The list is provided in **Table 5**.

TABLE 5: Newer immunohistochemical (IHC) markers for diagnosis of CHL.

IHC markers	The pattern of expression in CHL
STAT6^{YE361}	Nucleocytoplasmic/nuclear expression
GATA3	Nuclear expression
Fascin	Cytoplasmic expression
MDC/CCL22, CD83*	Cytoplasmic and Golgi zone expression
STAT3*	Nucleocytoplasmic expression
TUBB2B*	Cytoplasmic expression

*At least two positive markers favor classical Hodgkin lymphoma (CHL) over anaplastic lymphoma kinase (ALK)-negative anaplastic large cell lymphoma (ALCL).

Liquid Biopsy

Circulating tumor DNA (ctDNA) is a valuable tool for biomarker-driven therapies, enhancing the monitoring of minimal residual disease and identifying treatment resistance. Although CHL tumors have a low proportion of tumor cells, they release a significant amount of ctDNA. Notably, a reduction in ctDNA levels after the initial treatment strongly indicates a response to therapy and predicts disease course. STAT6 mutation in ctDNA has been utilized to assess residual disease in CHL. The clinical utility of ctDNA in CHL remains in its nascent stages and is expected to progress over time.

DIFFERENTIAL DIAGNOSIS

A list of differential diagnosis and their distinguishing features to differentiate from CHL is given in **Table 6**.

TABLE 6: List of differential diagnoses and distinguishing characteristics from classical Hodgkin lymphoma (CHL).

Differential diagnoses	Features that favor the listed entity over CHL
EBV + Diffuse large B cell lymphoma	• *Positive:* CD45; OCT2, BOB1, PAX5, CD79a (strong B-cell immunophenotype) • EBV latency type III, if present
Mediastinal gray zone lymphoma	• Neoplastic cells with more centroblastic cytology and loss of typical CHL architecture and inflammatory background • Strong B-cell immunophenotype, exhibiting strong expression of at least 2 B-cell markers
Primary mediastinal large B-cell lymphoma	• *Positive:* MAL, P63, CD23, CD45, CD20, OCT2, BOB1, PAX5, CD79a (strong B-cell immunophenotype) • CD30—heterogeneous and weak expression • *Negative:* EBER-ISH
Nodular lymphocyte predominant Hodgkin lymphoma	• *Positive:* J chain, MEF2B; CD20, OCT2, BOB1, PAX5, CD79a (strong B-cell immunophenotype) • *Negative:* EBER-ISH, CD30, MUM1, GATA3, Fascin, STAT6
Polymorphic lymphoproliferative disorders arising in immune deficiency/dysregulation	EBER is positive in the full morphological spectrum from small and medium-sized B cells to immunoblasts and mature plasma cells
Anaplastic large cell lymphoma, ALK-negative	• *Negative:* PAX5, EBER-ISH • *Positive:* CD45, pan T cell antigens, and cytotoxic markers (granzyme, perforin, and TIA1)
Peripheral T-cell lymphoma NOS with HRS-like cells	Loss of T-cell antigens, presence of *TCR* gene rearrangement/monoclonal T cells
T-cell lymphomas of follicular helper origin	Expression of two or more T follicular helper cell markers (CD10, BCL6, PD1, CXCL13, CXCR5, ICOS, SAP)

(ALK: anaplastic lymphoma kinase; EBV: Epstein–Barr virus; EBER: Epstein–Barr encoding region; HRS: Hodgkin Reed–Sternberg; NOS: not otherwise specified)

Nodular Lymphocyte-predominant Hodgkin Lymphoma

Traditionally, NLPHL has been categorized alongside CHL due to the morphological similarities observed between the neoplastic cells of both conditions and the predominance of these neoplastic cells relative to the non-neoplastic immune cells present. New terminology has been proposed for NLPHL, renaming it nodular lymphocyte-predominant B-cell lymphoma as they show a close relationship with T-cell/histiocyte-rich large B-cell lymphoma (THRLBCL).

Nodular lymphocyte-predominant Hodgkin lymphoma also arises from GC B cells; however, it shows an intact B-cell program, in contrast to CHL. Recent studies suggest a potential role for bacterial antigens, specifically *Moraxella catarrhalis* and *Rothia mucilaginosa*, in NLPHL pathogenesis. Pathways such as NFκB and JAK/STAT that are altered in CHL may also be activated in NLPHL; however, the specific genes impacted differ. Recurrent mutations have been identified in genes including *PAX5, PIM1, RHOH (TTF), MYC, JUNB, DUSP2, SGK1, SOCS1,* and *CREBBP*. A grading system has been introduced in NLPHL that consists of two grades. Grade 1 encompasses Fan patterns A, B, and C, while grade 2 comprises Fan patterns D, E, and F.

The NLPHL cases with a high risk of transforming into aggressive B-cell non-Hodgkin lymphoma, like THRLBCL or DLBCL, require more intensive clinical follow-up. The following factors are associated with this increased risk of transformation:

- Older age
- Negative immunoglobulin D (IgD)
- High B-cell clonality along with increased intraclonal diversification
- Absence of the characteristic immunoglobulin heavy chain (IgH) rearrangement (long CDR3) typically seen in most NLPHL patients.

Progressive transformation of germinal center (PTGC) is closely associated with NLPHL, as many patients with PTGC may progress to or present synchronously with NLPHL. When pattern 5 of PTGC, which resembles a small primary follicle, is observed, it is imperative to comprehensively examine the entire specimen for the potential coexistence of NLPHL. This pattern is notably more prevalent in cases that exhibit synchronous involvement of both conditions, as opposed to instances involving PTGC alone.

The classic immunophenotype associated with LP cells is summarized in **Table 1**, while additional markers utilized to distinguish them from LR CHL are detailed in **Table 6**. Notably, the accompanying non-neoplastic B cells display weak staining for OCT-2; however, the expression is stronger in LP cells. PD-1 positive T follicular helper cells form tight rosettes around the LP cells.

MANAGEMENT OF HODGKIN LYMPHOMA

Approach to Patient

Most patients of HL present with palpable nontender lymphadenopathy typically in the neck, supraclavicular area, and axilla. About half of them have enlarged mediastinal nodes at diagnosis. Subdiaphragmatic nodes, though uncommon, can be seen in elderly males or advanced stage/late diagnosis. Often, HL is diagnosed during the evaluation of "PUO" (Pyrexia of unknown origin). "Pel-Ebstein" fever can be seen rarely which manifests as persistent fever for weeks interspersed with intervals of afebrile period.

The evaluation of CHL patients is summarized in **Flowchart 1**. After a detailed history, a physical examination should be done to palpate for involved lymph nodes and other extramedullary sites, assess for comorbidities, and proceed by biopsy of the involved tissue. In a proven case on lymph node (LN) biopsy, staging with PET may suffice without bone marrow by biopsy. But in cases with B symptoms, without peripheral LN, bone marrow may be involved, and biopsy often gives the primary diagnosis.

STAGING

Staging for CHL is anatomically based as the disease tends to spread from one node group to another in a contiguous manner. **Table 7** depicts the Lugano classification for staging.

- Hilar nodes should be "lateralized" and when involved on both sides, constitute stage II disease.
- To define the number of anatomic regions, all nodal disease within the mediastinum is a single lymph node region, and hilar involvement constitutes an additional site of involvement.
- The number of anatomic regions should be indicated by a subscript (e.g., II-3).
- All cases are subclassified to indicate the absence (A) or presence (B) of the B symptoms.
- The designation "E" refers to extranodal contiguous extension (i.e., proximal or contiguous extranodal disease) that can be encompassed within an irradiation field appropriate for nodal disease of the same anatomic extent. The more extensive extranodal disease is designated stage IV.
- *Bulky disease:* A single nodal mass, in contrast to multiple smaller nodes, of 10 cm or more than or equal to one-third of the transthoracic diameter at any level of thoracic vertebrae as determined by CT; record the longest measurement by CT scan. The term "X" (used in the Ann Arbor staging system) is no longer necessary.
- The subscript "RS" is used to designate the stage at the time of relapse.

Patients are stratified based as early or advanced disease as shown in **Box 1**.

Depending on the uptake of the involved sites on the PET-CT, Deauville scoring is given as described in **Table 8**, at the time of diagnosis, suspected relapse, and treatment response assessment.

TREATMENT

A majority of patients with HL are cured with treatment by chemotherapy alone or in combination with radiation. Common regimens and agents used for therapy are:

- ABVD—Adriamycin, bleomycin, vinblastine, dacarbazine
- Involved-site radiation therapy (ISRT)

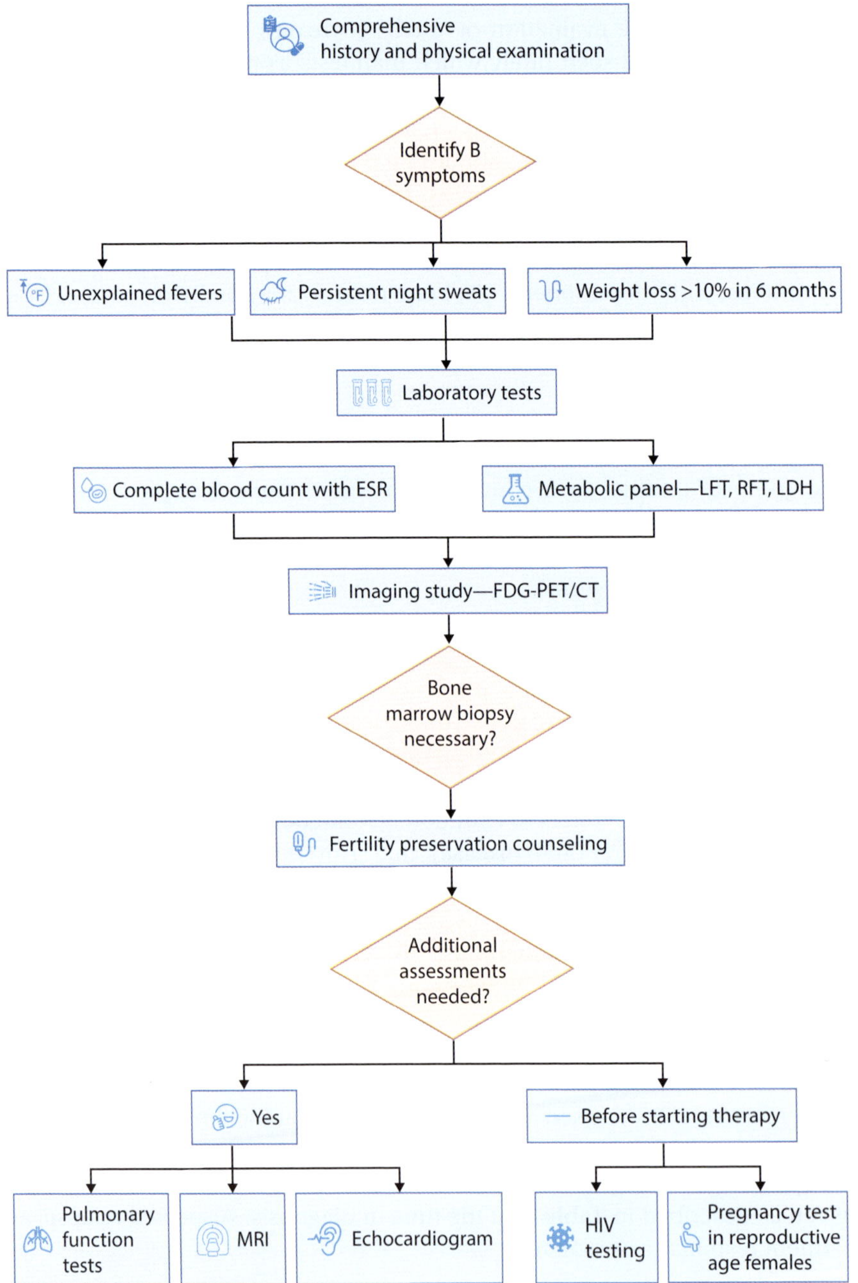

FLOWCHART 1: Initial diagnostic evaluation of a patient with Hodgkin lymphoma (HL).

(ESR: erythrocyte sedimentation rate; FDG: fluoro-2-deoxy-D-glucose; HIV: human immunodeficiency virus; LDH: lactate dehydrogenase; LFT: liver function test; MRI: magnetic resonance imaging; PET/CT: positron emission tomography–computed tomography; RFT: renal function test)

TABLE 7: Lugano classification for staging of lymphomas (derived from Ann Arbor staging with Cotswolds modifications).

Stage	Definition
I	Involvement of a single lymph node region (e.g., cervical, axillary, inguinal, mediastinal) or lymphoid structure such as the spleen, thymus, or Waldeyer's ring
II	Involvement of two or more lymph node regions or lymph node structures on the same side of the diaphragm
III	Involvement of lymph node regions or lymphoid structures on both sides of the diaphragm: • *Stage III-1:* Involvement of spleen or splenic hilar, celiac, or portal nodes • *Stage III-2:* Involvement of paraaortic, iliac, inguinal, or mesenteric nodes
IV	Diffuse or disseminated involvement of one or more extranodal organs or tissue beyond that designated "E," with or without associated lymph node involvement

BOX 1: Classification of patients as early-stage and advanced-stage Hodgkin lymphoma (HL).

- Early-stage disease (stage I or II), a better prognosis
- Depending on the classification system, it is "unfovarable" in the presence any of the following:
  - B symptoms
  - Existence of bulky mediastinal disease as indicated by chest skiagram
  - Lymphadenopathy greater than 10 cm
  - Erythrocyte sedimentation rate (ESR) exceeding 30/50 mm
  - Involvement of extralymphatic regions
  - Involvement of >2 or 3 nodal sites
- Advanced-stage disease (stage III or IV), a worse prognosis
- Hasenclever index or international prognostic score (IPS) is used for prognosis, where 1 point ascribed to (higher score = worse prognosis):
  - Male sex
  - Age ≥ 45 years
  - Serum albumin < 4 g/dL
  - Hemoglobin < 10.5 g/dL
  - Stage IV disease
  - Leukocytosis ≥ 15,000/cumm
  - Lymphocytopenia, i.e., <8% of white blood cell (WBC) on differential or absolute lymphocyte count < 600/cumm

TABLE 8: Deauville scoring system.

Score	PET/CT	Remark
Negative	1	No uptake
	2	Uptake ≤ mediastinum
	3	Uptake > mediastinum but ≤ liver
	4	Uptake moderately higher than liver and visually above adjacent background activity
Positive	5	Uptake markedly higher than liver and/or new lesions

- Brentuximab vedotin (BV)—monoclonal antibody brentuximab (targets CD30 on the cell surface) linked with antimitotic agent monomethyl auristatin E.
- Check point inhibitors (CPI)—Nivolumab (Nivo) and Pembrolizumab (Pemb)—monoclonal antibodies against PD-1 receptor that blocks interaction with PD-L1 and PD-L 2, thereby releasing PD-1 mediated antitumor inhibition of T cells.

Early-stage Disease Favorable Disease

The treatment protocol for stage IA/IIA favorable CHL conventionally is to administer two cycles of ABVD chemotherapy. Following this, the response is assessed with an interim fluoro-2-deoxy-D-glucose (FDG)-Positron emission tomography/computed tomography (PET/CT) scan, categorized by the Deauville scoring system, and managed as shown in **Flowchart 2**.

Early-stage Disease Unfavorable Disease

The initial treatment is:

- Two cycles of ABVD followed by two more cycles with 30 Gy ISRT or four more cycles of AVD among Deauville 1–3 after interim PET/CT.
- BrECADD (BV, etoposide, cyclophosphamide, doxorubicin, dacarbazine, dexamethasone)—granulocyte-colony stimulating factor (GCSF) for two cycles with ISRT.
- Nivo-AVD for four cycles with ISRT.
- BV-AVD-GCSF with ISRT for four cycles.

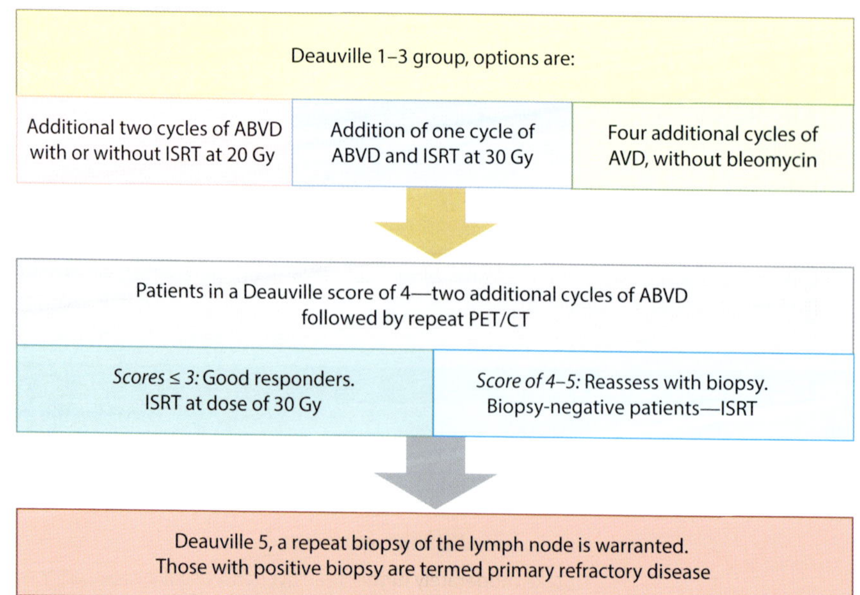

FLOWCHART 2: The management of early-stage favorable disease.

(ABVD: adriamycin, bleomycin, vinblastine, dacarbazine; ISRT: involved-site radiation therapy)

For those with Deauville 4–5, an additional two cycles of ABVD or BrECADD are to be given before restaging with PET/CT. Favorable responders (Deauville 1–4) can be further consolidated with ISRT.

Deauville 5 is reassessed with a repeat biopsy. If positive on biopsy, managed as primary refractory.

Advanced-stage Disease

Patients with advanced-stage disease do not benefit from the addition of radiation therapy and should be treated with chemotherapy alone as depicted in **Flowchart 3**.

It is important to schedule interim PET just before the next cycle and end of treatment PET CT after 6 weeks, as chemotherapy or radiation-induced changes can confound the results and interpretation.

Refractory/Relapsed Disease

Patients who relapse or are refractory to primary therapy require alternative salvage chemotherapy to document chemosensitivity and achieve maximum reduction of tumor mass. Poor prognostic factors are depicted in **Figure 3**.

Treatment for primary refractory or early relapse within 3 months of therapy are summarized in **Box 2**.

For patients who achieve PET complete/partial response, autologous stem cell transplantation can cure over half of patients. Common conditioning regimens are BEAM, LEAM, CBV based for lymphoma transplants.

BV has also been used as maintenance postautologous stem cell transplantation (ASCT), for up to 16 cycles. These can be used as salvage to allogenic transplants in chemo-refractory diseases.

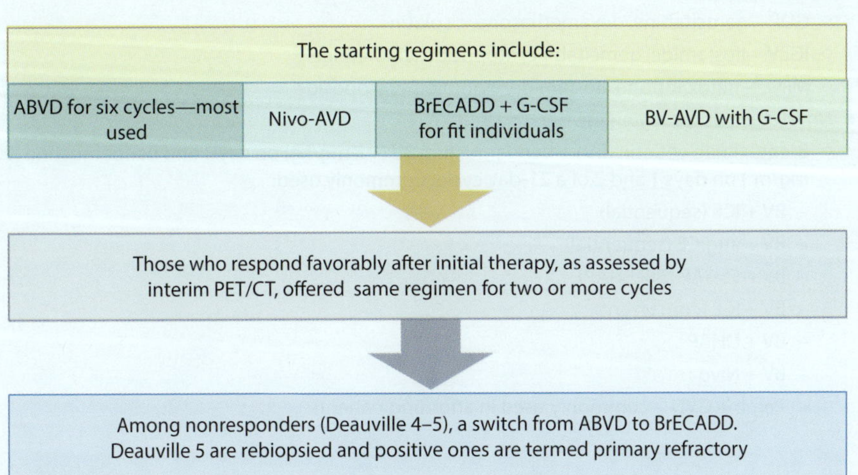

FLOWCHART 3: The management of advanced-stage disease.

(ABVD: adriamycin, bleomycin, vinblastine, dacarbazine; BrECADD: brentuximab vedotin, etoposide, cyclophosphamide, doxorubicin, dacarbazine, dexamethasone; G-CSF: granulocyte-colony stimulating factor; PET/CT: positron emission tomography–computed tomography)

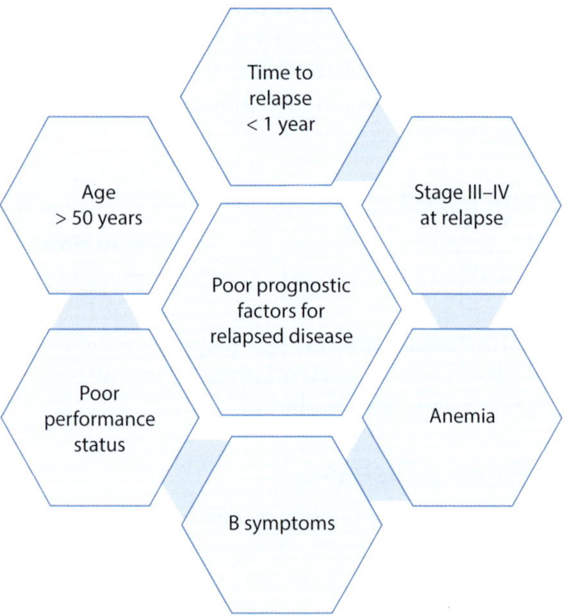

FIG. 3: Poor prognostic factors in relapsed disease.

BOX 2: Treatment options for relapsed/refractory disease.

- *Salvage chemotherapy regimens*:
  - ICE—ifosfamide, carboplatin, etoposide
  - DHAP—dexamethasone, ara-C, cisplatin
  - GVD—gemcitabine, vinorelbine, doxorubicin (liposomal doxorubicin)
  - GDP—gemcitabine, dexamethasone, cisplatin
  - IGEV—ifosfamide, gemcitabine, etoposide, vinorelbine
  - MINE—mitoxantrone, ifosfamide, vinorelbine, etoposide
- *Novel agent based regimens*:
  - Brentuximab vedotin (BV) + bendamustine BV (1.8 mg/kg) on day 1 and bendamustine (90 mg/m^2) on days 1 and 2 of a 21-day cycle. Commonly used:
    - BV + ICE (sequential)
    - BV + augICE (sequential)
    - BV + ESHAP (BRESHAP)
    - BV + ICE (concurrent)
    - BV + DHAP
    - BV + Nivo
    - Pemb + GVD—commonly used in affording patients

Therapeutic options are limited in patients resistant to newer agents like BV and CPI. Chimeric antigen receptor T-cells directed against CD30 have shown promising results in early clinical trials. Antibody-drug conjugates against CD25 are also being studied in relapsed refractory patients.

FOLLOW-UP AFTER COMPLETION OF TREATMENT AND MONITORING FOR LATE EFFECTS

All patients after remission are followed up closely for at least five years after treatment to detect any recurrence and long-term side effects of therapy. Physician visit is scheduled:

- Every 3 months for the first 2 years (when relapse risk is higher),
- Every 6 months until year 3,
- Annually thereafter.
- Imaging should only be performed if there is significant clinical concern for relapse and if deemed necessary. Surveillance FDG-PET/CT should not be routinely performed.

Due to excellent response to therapy, long-term complications like second malignancies and cardiac injury are a concern. Long term follow-up is summarized in **Box 3**.

MANAGEMENT DURING PREGNANCY

The CHL accounts for 6% of all cancers in pregnancy. Clinical features and prognostic factors are similar. Management requires a multidisciplinary approach including high-risk obstetrics care. Complete radiologic staging of CHL is not required and may include a chest X-ray with an abdominal shield and an abdominal ultrasound (US) or magnetic resonance imaging (MRI) without gadolinium. Treatment approaches are summarized in **Flowchart 4**.

Breastfeeding should be avoided in patients receiving chemotherapy in the postpartum period.

BOX 3: Long-term complications following therapy.

- *Secondary leukemia*:
  - After chemotherapy regimens that contain alkylating agents plus radiation therapy
  - Risk is higher after BEACOPP-like regimens, multiple treatments after relapse, age > 60 years, prior transplant, etc.
- Cervical radiation accelerates carotid atherosclerosis as well as thyroid disorders
- *Infertility*:
  - Regimens containing alkylating agents may induce permanent infertility
  - Younger women are more likely to recover fertility
  - Rare with ABVD
- *Cardiac*: Long-term cardiac toxicity-myopathy, heart failure, etc., after anthracycline-containing regimen and chest radiation

(ABVD: adriamycin, bleomycin, vinblastine, dacarbazine; BEACOPP: bleomycin, etoposide, doxorubicin, cyclophosphamide, vincristine, procarbazine, and prednisone)

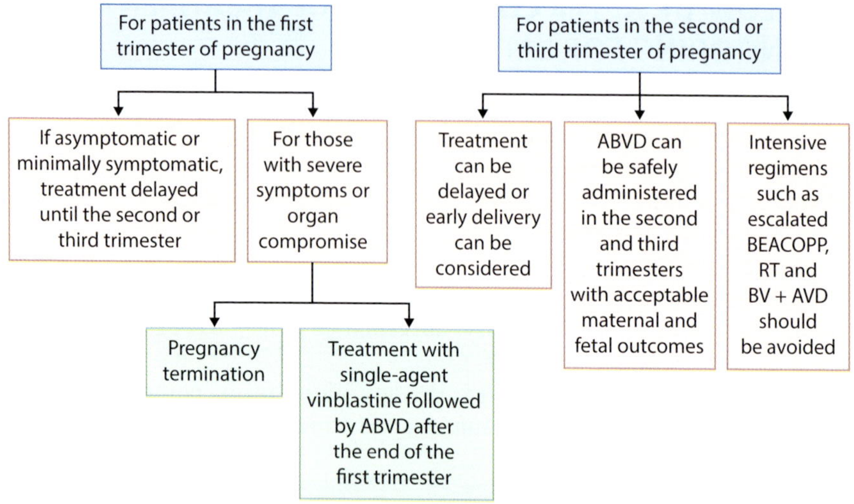

FLOWCHART 4: Management options in pregnancy.

(ABVD: adriamycin, bleomycin, vinblastine, dacarbazine; BEACOPP: bleomycin, etoposide, doxorubicin, cyclophosphamide, vincristine, procarbazine, and prednisone)

HODGKIN'S LYMPHOMA IN HUMAN IMMUNODEFICIENCY VIRUS PATIENTS

Human immunodeficiency virus (HIV)-positive patients and CHL have the following characteristics:

- 10-fold higher risk of developing HL.
- Almost all cases are EBV-positive.
- Most common subtype is mixed cellularity.
- Typically present with advanced stages and B symptoms, leading to poorer prognosis.

Treatment regimens are like those for non-HIV patients, utilizing BEACOPP (bleomycin, etoposide, doxorubicin, cyclophosphamide, vincristine, procarbazine, and prednisone), or ABVD chemotherapy. The complete response rates for these patients stand at 82%, with a 5-year overall survival rate of 76%, and an event-free survival rate of 71%.

NODULAR LYMPHOCYTE-PREDOMINANT HODGKIN LYMPHOMA

The NLPHL represents <5% of cases of HL and has several characteristics that suggest its relationship to NHL. NLPHL tends to have a chronic, relapsing course, and sometimes transforms to diffuse large B-cell lymphoma. Most patients have stage I or II disease (75%). "B" symptoms are uncommon. Management is summarized in **Box 4**.

BOX 4: Management options for nodular lymphocyte-predominant Hodgkin lymphoma (NLPHL).

- *Early stage disease at diagnosis*:
  - Treated with radiotherapy
  - Observed
  - This is associated with a 15-year nonrelapse survival rate of 82%
- *Advanced stage NLPHL*:
  - No treatment of asymptomatic disease
  - If symptoms and signs of organ function impairment, ABVD or CHOP can be considered, in addition to rituximab

(ABVD: adriamycin, bleomycin, vinblastine, dacarbazine; CHOP: cyclophosphamide, doxorubicin, vincristine, prednisone)

Take Home Points

- The HRS cells likely arise from preapoptotic GC B cells with harmful mutations.
- The genetic alteration and EBV virus in CHL aid antiapoptotic mechanisms.
- The EBV virus in CHL typically displays a type II latency pattern.
- Anaplastic cells, an increased proportion of HRS cells, a decreased proportion of lymphocytes, and tissue eosinophilia appear to be adverse prognostic indicators in NS CHL.
- Pathological assessment will be crucial in introducing advanced therapeutic options, such as EBV-specific T-cell therapy and CD30-specific chimeric antigen receptor (CAR-T) therapy.
- NLPHL is closely related to THRLBCL.
- Hodgkin lymphoma is a highly curable hematologic malignancy.
- Accurate diagnosis and careful staging of the disease are paramount.
- Identification of poor prognostic features and response to therapy are crucial for risk-adapted therapy to increase the likelihood of cure and minimize toxicity potentially.
- Nonchemotherapy-based approaches including combinations with BV and CPI are rapidly changing treatment algorithms.
- In relapsed disease, salvage therapy with ASCT helps cure at least 50% of patients.

Case-based Questions

1. A 45-year-old male presents with an enlarged lymph node in the cervical region, which was biopsied. Histopathological examination reveals a predominantly diffuse infiltrate of large neoplastic cells, some resembling lymphocyte-predominant (LP)-like cells with background small lymphocytes. In addition, a few focal nodular areas are identified within the biopsy. IHC staining shows positive markers for B-cells both in the large cells and in the nodules, and T-cells are seen in the background in the diffuse areas.

The patient has a history of HL but has not had any prior treatment for the current lymphadenopathy.

Q. What is the most likely diagnosis based on the histological findings?

Ans: NLPHL Grade 2.

Explanation: The presence of focal B cell-rich nodular areas in the biopsy, despite the overall diffuse pattern, is characteristic of NLPHL. The diffuse infiltrate of LP-like cells (Grade 2 areas) along with the nodular (Grade 1) areas distinguish it from THRLBCL. Without these nodular areas, the diagnosis would lean toward de novo THRLBCL. Therefore, the case should be classified as Grade 2 NLPHL (Pattern E) based on the nodular structure present.

2. A 56-year-old male presents with a history of rapidly enlarging cervical lymphadenopathy, fever, night sweats, and weight loss. Imaging reveals multiple enlarged lymph nodes. Histological examination of a lymph node core biopsy shows large, atypical cells admixed with few small lymphocytes. IHC staining of large, atypical cells reveals the following:

- *CD30:* Strongly positive
- *CD20:* Variably positive (expression noted in < 50% of atypical cells)
- *CD79A:* Positive
- *OCT2:* Positive
- *EBER-ISH:* Positive in 90% of the atypical cells
- *EBNA2 (EBV latency type III marker):* Positive

Q. Which of the following is the most likely diagnosis?

A. Classical HL
B. Nodular lymphocyte-predominant Hodgkin lymphoma
C. EBV + Diffuse large B-cell lymphoma
D. T-cell/histiocyte-rich large B-cell lymphoma

Ans: (C) EBV + Diffuse large B-cell lymphoma

Explanation:

- *CD30 expression:* CD30 is strongly positive in this case, which is a hallmark feature of both CHL and EBV + DLBCL. However, in the context of other markers, this suggests a DLBCL rather than CHL.
- *CD20 expression:* The weak expression of CD20 (<50%) is consistent with EBV + DLBCL, which may show downregulation of B-cell markers.
- *Retained expression of CD79A and OCT2:* These B-cell markers are typically retained in EBV + DLBCL and lost in CHL, further supporting this diagnosis.
- *EBNA2 positive:* EBV latency type III with EBNA2 expression is seen in about 10% of EBV + DLBCL cases. EBNA2 positivity excludes CHL.

Thus, with predominant cells positive for EBER-ISH, the most likely diagnosis is EBV + DLBCL.

SUGGESTED READINGS

1. O'Malley DP, Dogan A, Fedoriw Y, Medeiros LJ, Ok CY, Salama ME. American Registry of Pathology Expert Opinions: Immunohistochemical evaluation of classic Hodgkin lymphoma. Ann Diagn Pathol. 2019;39:105-10.
2. Brune MM, Juskevicius D, Haslbauer J, Dirnhofer S, Tzankov A. Genomic Landscape of Hodgkin Lymphoma. Cancers (Basel). 2021;13(4):682.
3. Satou A, Takahara T, Nakamura S. An Update on the Pathology and Molecular Features of Hodgkin Lymphoma. Cancers (Basel). 2022;14(11):2647.
4. Maco M, Kupcova K, Herman V, Ondeckova I, Kozak T, Mocikova H, et al. Circulating tumor DNA in Hodgkin lymphoma. Ann Hematol. 2022;101(11):2393-403.
5. Tousseyn TA, King RL, Fend F, Feldman AL, Brousset P, Jaffe ES. Evolution in the definition and diagnosis of the Hodgkin lymphomas and related entities. Virchows Arch. 2023;482(1):207-26.
6. Simonin M, Jardin F, Leblanc T, Latour S, Landman Parker J. An update on molecular features and therapeutic perspectives of pediatric classical Hodgkin Lymphoma. What the clinician needs to know? Eur J Med Genet. 2023;66(1):104672.
7. Küppers R. Advances in Hodgkin lymphoma research. Trends Mol Med. 2025;31(4):326-43.
8. Ding Y, Jaffe ES. Histopathologic features and differential diagnosis in challenging cases of nodular lymphocyte predominant B-cell lymphoma/nodular lymphocyte predominant Hodgkin lymphoma. J Clin Transl Pathol. 2024;4(2):61-9.
9. Hoppe RT, Advani RH, Ai WZ, Ambinder RF, Armand P, Bello CM, et al. Hodgkin Lymphoma, Version 2.2020, NCCN Clinical Practice Guidelines in Oncology. J Natl Compr Canc Netw. 2020;18(6):755-81.
10. Bonadonna G. Historical review of Hodgkin's disease. Br J Haematol. 2000;110(3):504-11.
11. Swerdlow SH, Campo E, Pileri SA, Harris NL, Stein H, Siebert R, et al. The 2016 revision of the World Health Organization classification of lymphoid neoplasms. Blood. 2016;127(20): 2375-90.
12. Ng AK. Current survivorship recommendations for patients with Hodgkin lymphoma: focus on late effects. Blood. 2014;124(23):3373-9.
13. Bachanova V, Connors JM. Hodgkin lymphoma in pregnancy. Curr Hematol Malig Rep. 2013;8(3):211-7.
14. Hasenclever D, Diehl V. A prognostic score for advanced Hodgkin's disease. International prognostic factors project on advanced Hodgkin's disease. N Engl J Med. 1998;339(21): 1506-14.
15. Barrington SF, Mikhaeel NG, Kostakoglu L, Meignan M, Hutchings M, Müeller SP, et al. Role of imaging in the staging and response assessment of lymphoma: consensus of the International Conference on Malignant Lymphomas Imaging Working Group. J Clin Oncol. 2016;34(21):2562.
16. Lister TA, Crowther D, Sutcliffe SB, Glatstein E, Canellos GP, Young RC, et al. Report of a committee convened to discuss the evaluation and staging of patients with Hodgkin's disease: Cotswolds meeting. J Clin Oncol. 1989;7(11):1630-6.
17. Chen R, Zinzani PL, Lee HJ, Armand P, Johnson NA, Brice P, et al. Pembrolizumab in relapsed or refractory Hodgkin lymphoma: 2-year follow-up of KEYNOTE-087. Blood. 2019;134(14): 1144-53.
18. Gillessen S, Plütschow A, Fuchs M, Markova J, Greil R, Topp MS, et al. Intensified treatment of patients with early stage, unfavourable Hodgkin lymphoma: Long-term follow-up of a randomised, international phase 3 trial of the German Hodgkin Study Group (GHSG HD14). Lancet Haematol. 2021;8(4):e278.
19. Moskowitz CH, Walewski J, Nademanee A, Masszi T, Agura E, Holowiecki J, et al. Five-year PFS from the AETHERA trial of brentuximab vedotin for Hodgkin lymphoma at high risk of progression or relapse. Blood. 2018;132(25):2639-42.
20. Rashidi A, Ebadi M, Cashen AF. Allogeneic hematopoietic stem cell transplantation in Hodgkin lymphoma: A systemic review and meta-analysis. Bone Marrow Transplant. 2016;51(4):521-8.

21. Straus DJ, Jung SH, Pitcher B, Kostakoglu L, Grecula JC, Hsi ED, et al. CALGB 50604: Risk-adapted treatment of non-bulky early-stage Hodgkin lymphoma based on interim PET. Blood. 2018;132(10):1013-21.
22. Straus DJ, Długosz-Danecka M, Connors JM, Alekseev S, Illés Á, Picardi M, et al. Brentuximab vedotin with chemotherapy for stage III or IV classical Hodgkin lymphoma (ECHELON-1): 5-year update of an international, open-label, randomised, phase 3 trial. Lancet Haematol. 2021;8:e410-e421.

CHAPTER 15

Updates in the Diagnosis of the Antiphospholipid Syndrome

Ankur Ahuja, Dinesh Chandra, Himil Parikh

ABSTRACT

Antiphospholipid syndrome (APS) is a systemic autoimmune disorder characterized by vascular thrombotic events, as well as pregnancy-related complications. The presence of antiphospholipid antibodies (APA), including lupus anticoagulant (LA), anticardiolipin (aCL), and anti-β2 glycoprotein I (aβ2GPI), play a crucial role in its diagnosis. The *revised Sapporo criteria (2006)* remain the standard classification system, requiring the presence of at least one clinical and one laboratory criterion confirmed twice at least *12 weeks apart*. The *2023* American College of Rheumatology/European League Against Rheumatism *(ACR/EULAR) classification* introduces a scoring-based system incorporating additional features, including the incorporation of thrombocytopenia as an entry criterion followed by additional scores based on different clinical and laboratory findings, increasing the specificity of APS diagnosis.

Laboratory testing for APS must be carefully managed, especially in *anticoagulated patients, as warfarin, heparins, and direct oral anticoagulants (DOACs)* can interfere with LA detection, leading to false positives or negatives. Standard testing includes *dilute Russell's Viper Venom Time (dRVVT) and activated partial thromboplastin time (APTT)*, with mixing studies recommended to differentiate LA positivity from factor deficiencies. Additionally, *noncriterion antibodies* such as *antiphosphatidylserine/prothrombin (aPS/PT)* may help refine risk stratification, particularly in *triple-positive* patients with persistent antiphospholipid positivity.

The *lupus cofactor phenomenon*, in which the inhibitory effect of LA is enhanced in the presence of β2GPI or prothrombin, highlights the complexity of LA testing and the necessity of *three-step testing (screening, mixing, and confirmation)*. Proper preanalytical sample handling, storage, and *timing of testing in relation to anticoagulation status* are crucial for accuracy. Finally, a *comprehensive approach to APS diagnosis* involves correlating laboratory results with clinical presentation, considering thrombotic history, pregnancy complications, and systemic autoimmune conditions to establish a high-risk aPL profile.

INTRODUCTION

Lupus anticoagulant (LA), when present in plasma, is due to the in vitro phenomenon caused by the autoantibodies, which interferes with phospholipid-dependent coagulation, resulting in prolonging of the clotting times, especially activated partial thromboplastin time (APTT). It is a paradoxical situation because, though the LA presence prolongs the clotting tests in vitro, it is accompanying by hypercoagulability and thrombosis in vivo.

Antiphospholipid syndrome (APS), which is a systemic autoimmune disease, is characterized by thrombosis in arterial, venous, and micro-vessels. In obstetrics, it leads to morbidity in pregnancy. The insistent presence of antiphospholipid antibodies (APA) leading to nonthrombotic manifestations was not mentioned in the literature much prior. The classification of the APS is currently based upon the Sapporo criteria, which were published in 1991 and further revised in 2006.

The revised Sapporo criteria for APS included the clinical features (thrombosis or pregnancy morbidity) and the laboratory tests [for lupus anticoagulant (LAC), immunoglobulin (Ig)G/IgM anticardiolipin antibodies (aCL), and/or IgG/IgM anti-β2-glycoprotein I antibodies (anti-β2GPI)] with repetition of the tests at least twice in a span of least 12 weeks apart. This criteria is mentioned in **Box 1**.

BOX 1: Revised Sapporo classification criteria for the antiphospholipid syndrome (APS).

Clinical criteria:
- *Vascular thrombosis:* One or more clinical episodes of arterial, venous, or small vessel thrombosis, in any tissue or organ
- *Pregnancy morbidity*:
  - One or more unexplained deaths of a morphologically normal fetus at or beyond the 10th week of gestation, with normal fetal morphology documented by ultrasound or by direct examination of the fetus, or
  - One or more premature births of a morphologically normal neonate before the 34th week of gestation because of:
    - Eclampsia or severe preeclampsia, or
    - Recognized features of placental insufficiency
  - Three or more unexplained consecutive spontaneous abortions before the 10th week of gestation, with maternal anatomic or hormonal abnormalities and paternal and maternal chromosomal causes excluded

Laboratory criteria:
- Lupus anticoagulant (LA) present in plasma, on two or more occasions at least 12 weeks apart, detected according to the guidelines of the International Society on Thrombosis and Haemostasis (ISTH)
- Anticardiolipin (aCL) antibody of immunoglobulin (Ig)G and/or IgM isotype in serum or plasma, present in medium or high titer (i.e., > 40 GPL or MPL, or > 99th percentile), on two or more occasions, at least 12 weeks apart, measured by a standardized ELISA
- Anti-β2 glycoprotein-I antibody of IgG and/or IgM isotype in serum or plasma (in titer > 99th percentile), present on two or more occasions, at least 12 weeks apart, measured by a standardized ELISA

Antiphospholipid syndrome (APS) is present if at least one of the clinical criteria and one of the laboratory criteria that follow are met

(ELISA: enzyme linked immunosorbent assay; GPL: G phospholipid; MPL: M phospholipid)

INDICATIONS FOR TESTING FOR ANTIPHOSPHOLIPID ANTIBODIES IN PATIENTS PRESENTING WITH THROMBOSIS OR OBSTETRIC COMPLICATIONS

- Unprovoked/minor provoked venous thromboembolism (VTE), involvement of unusual sites by VTE without any evident risk factors [cerebral venous sinus thrombosis, splanchnic vein thrombosis (including portal vein, mesenteric vein, and splenic vein thrombosis, and the Budd–Chiari syndrome)].
- Arterial thrombosis in young (<50 years of age) without any evident risk factors.
- Thrombosis/pregnancy-related complications in patients having autoimmune disorders or systemic lupus erythematosus (SLE).
- Inexplicable thrombosis at microvascular sites.
- Presence of livedoid vasculopathy/livedo reticularis.
- Prolonged PT/APTT with unexplained causes
- Thrombosis developing recurrently unexplained even on therapeutic anticoagulation.
- Thrombocytopenia
- Recurrent severe preeclampsia/stillbirths/miscarriages or evidence of placental insufficiency < 34 weeks of onset.
- Unexplained cardiac valve abnormalities.

LABORATORY DIAGNOSIS OF ANTIPHOSPHOLIPID SYNDROME

Preanalytics

- *Problem*: LA is done frequently during anticoagulation in routine practice, resulting in false negative/positive results.
  - *Solution*: LA testing should be deferred until anticoagulation is discontinued.
- *Problem*: Both unfractionated heparin (UFH) and low molecular weight heparin (LMWH) interfere with LA clotting assays at supratherapeutic anti-Xa levels (high chances of false positivity).
  - *Solution*:
    - *Adopting three-step procedure*: False-positive LA can be abolished.
    - *Testing with heparin neutralizer* contained dilute Russell's viper venom time (dRVVT) reagents and LA-specific APTT reagents.
    - *Timing of the sample*: Sample from the patient should be taken:
      - ◊ Not before 12 hours after the administration of the last dose of LMWH.
      - ◊ As near as possible to the next dosage of LMWH.
- *Problem*: False negativity/positivity with vitamin K antagonists (VKAs).
  - *Solution*:
    - Use of Ecarin clotting time (ECT) and Taipan snake venom time (TSVT) in such cases.
    - In 2009 guidelines, dilution of the patient sample with normal pooled plasma (NPP) was suggested, however, many studies do not recommend it.

- *Problem*: False positives APTT and dRVVT based tests with the direct oral anticoagulants (DOACs) even if they are in low concentrations.
  - *Solution*:
    - Plasma can be pretreated with adsorbents such as activated charcoal products which are available commercially also to eliminate the effect of DOACs.

The LA tests can be done after 48 hours of the last dosage of DOACs and are more prolonged in patients with renal impairment. Testing algorithm of APS for patients on anticoagulants is mentioned further in the **Table 1**.

Testing in Acute Phase or during Pregnancy

- *Problems*:
  - As we are aware that physiologically FVIII is increased in the acute phase or pregnancy, hence APTT assays may become shortened, possibly leading to false negativity.
  - Besides, C-reactive protein gets elevated in the acute phase/pregnancy, which may prolong APTT, thus leading to false positives or negatives.

TABLE 1: Suggested APA testing algorithm for patients on anticoagulants.

Anticoagulant	Laboratory assays	Laboratory notes	Clinical notes
Patient not anticoagulated, or anticoagulation status not known	• PT, APTT, TT, fibrinogen • DRVVT • LAR-APTT • aCL/aβ2GPI	• If DRVVT is raised, one should check for the presence of Xa-inhibitors by executing an anti-Xa assay • If TT is raised, one should check for liver coagulopathy, any IIa-inhibitors or the presence of paraprotein	LA testing (if have been performed during an acute phase of thrombotic event) should be interpreted with caution
VKA	PT, APTT, TT, fibrinogen DRVVT, LAR-APTT aCL/ aβ2GPI	• DRVVT and LAR-APTT in neat plasma can be testified if INR < 1.5 • TSVT/ET can be done if INR ≥ 1.5 • ACP is ineffective	• LA testing ideally to be performed 1–2 weeks after discontinuation of the VKA, along with contemplation bridging of LMWH • False negatives are conceivable if we perform only mixing studies
LWMH	• PT, APTT, fibrinogen • Heparin-specific anti-Xa assay • DRVVT, LAR-APTT aCL/ aβ2GPI	• DRVVT and/or LAR-APTT can only be performed if heparin level below level acceptable in the assay • TSVT/ET cannot be used • ACP ineffective	• LA testing to be performed after 12 h of the last dose of LMWH was given along with as near as possible to the next dose of LMWH • LA testing if have been performed during an acute phase of thrombotic event should be interpreted with caution

Continued

Continued

Anticoagulant	Laboratory assays	Laboratory notes	Clinical notes
UFH	• PT, APTT, fibrinogen • Heparin-specific anti-Xa assay • DRVVT, LAR-APTT • aCL/aβ2GPI	• DRVVT/ LAR-APTT shall be performed only if heparin levels are below acceptable levels in the assay and TT is normal • TSVT/ET cannot be used. • ACP ineffective	LA testing if have been performed during an acute phase of thrombotic event should be interpreted with caution
Direct FXa-inhibitors	• PT, APTT, Clauss fibrinogen • Drug-specific anti-Xa assay • DRVVT, LAR-APTT • aCL/aβ2GPI	• DRVVT shall be performed only if drug-specific anti-Xa assay is below lower limit of quantification (LLoQ) • TSVT/ET can be done if drug-specific anti-Xa assay is above LLoQ • ACP effective	DOAC shall be stopped temporarily for > 48 hours after the last dose, which was prolonged in with renal impairment
Dabigatran	• PT, APTT, TT, fibrinogen • Dabigatran assay • DRVVT, LAR-APTT • aCL/aβ2GPI	• DRVVT and LAR-APTT shall be done only if dabigatran assay and TT are below LLoQ • TSVT/ET cannot be used • ACP effective	
• Argatroban • Bivalirudin	• PT, APTT, TT, fibrinogen • Drug-specific anti-IIa assay • DRVVT, LAR-APTT • aCL/aβ2GPI	• DRVVT and LAR-APTT shall be performed only if drug-specific anti-IIa assay is below LLoQ • TSVT/ET cannot be used • ACP partially effective	LA testing if have been performed during an acute phase of thrombotic event should be interpreted with caution
• Fondaparinux • Danaparoid	• PT, APTT, fibrinogen • Drug-specific anti-Xa assay • DRVVT, LAR-APTT • aCL/aβ2GPI	• TSVT/ET cannot be used • ACP ineffective	Ideally, LA testing is to be performed as near as possible to the next dose, with monitoring of the drug-specific anti-Xa activity levels
• Direct FXIa-inhibitors • Direct FXIIa-inhibitors	• PT, APTT, TT, fibrinogen • DRVVT • aCL/aβ2GPI	• Effects on LAR-APTT/ TSVT/ET are not known • Effectiveness of ACP not known	No data yet available

(aCL/aβ2GPI: solid-phase assays for anticardiolipin and anti-β2GPI antibodies; ACP: activated charcoal product effective; APTT: activated partial thromboplastin time; DRVVT: dilute Russell's viper venom time; ET: ecarin time; FXa: factor Xa; FXIa: factor XIa; FXIIa: factor XIIa; LAR-APTT: lupus anticoagulant responsive; LLoQ: lower limit of quantification; LMWH: low molecular weight heparin; PT: prothrombin time; TSVT: taipan snake venom time; TT: thrombin time; UFH: unfractionated heparin; VKA: vitamin K antagonist; LLqQ: lower limit of quantitation)

Source: Adapted from BSH 2024 guidelines.

- *Solution*: Repetition of LA after 6 weeks of postdelivery and ideally it has to be done after 3 months.

Sample Preparation

- *Collection*:
    - Samples for LA assays to be collected into 0.105–0.109 M (3.2%) trisodium citrate (Light blue topped vacutainer).
    - *Order of collection:* 2nd just after blood culture.
- *Processing*:
    - Double centrifugation at 2,000 g for 15 minutes to attain the platelet count (Plt) of $<10 \times 10^9$/L. After the first centrifugation, plasma is to be separated before performing the second centrifugation step.
    - Ideally, finish processing within 4 hours of sample collection.
- *Storage*:
    - Frozen plasma for LA assays is to be stored in a polypropylene tube.
    - Frozen plasma should be stored below –70°C and can be used for up to 6 months.
    - Plasma or serum to be stored below –30°C for up to 6 months.
    - Frozen samples must be thawed in a temperature-controlled water bath at 37°C avoiding freeze/thawing cycles.
- *Preanalytical issue*: Hemolysis may get APTT shortened leading to false-negative LA results.

Routine Coagulation Screening Tests in Diagnosis of Lupus Anticoagulant

- *Initial steps*:
    - PT and lupus-unresponsive APTT to be performed to assess sample integrity and to reduce superfluous investigation of prolonged clotting times.
    - Thrombin time (TT) to be done to screen for the presence of direct thrombin inhibitors and heparin.
    - Fibrinogen assay as an indicator of an acute phase response.

Assays Available for Lupus Anticoagulant Testing

- Commonly performed LA assays are dRVVT, silica clotting time (SCT), hexagonal phase phospholipid neutralization (STACLOT-LA), Kaolin clotting time (KCT), dilute prothrombin time (dPT), platelet neutralization procedure (PNP), tissue thromboplastin inhibition (TTI), and less commonly used assays, the Taipan Venom Time (TVT), and Textarin:Ecarin ratio.
- Interaction of these LAC assays in the coagulation cascade can be seen in **Figure 1**.

As shown in **Figure 2A**, if LA is present, it will interfere with the prothrombinase complex binding to the phospholipid surface of platelets and prolong the clotting time. **Figure 2B** shows that in presence of excess phospholipids, even if LA is present, it will neutralize the antibody, facilitating binding of the prothrombinase complex onto the platelet phospholipid surface and normalizing the clotting time.

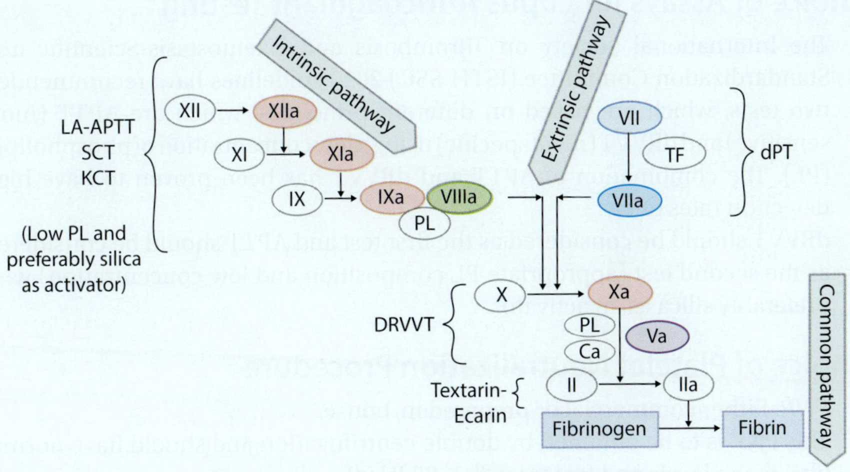

FIG. 1: Interaction of specific LAC assays within the coagulation cascade.

(dPT: dilute prothrombin time; dRVVT: dilute Russell viper venom time; KCT: Kaolin clotting time; PL: phospholipid; SCT: silica clotting time)

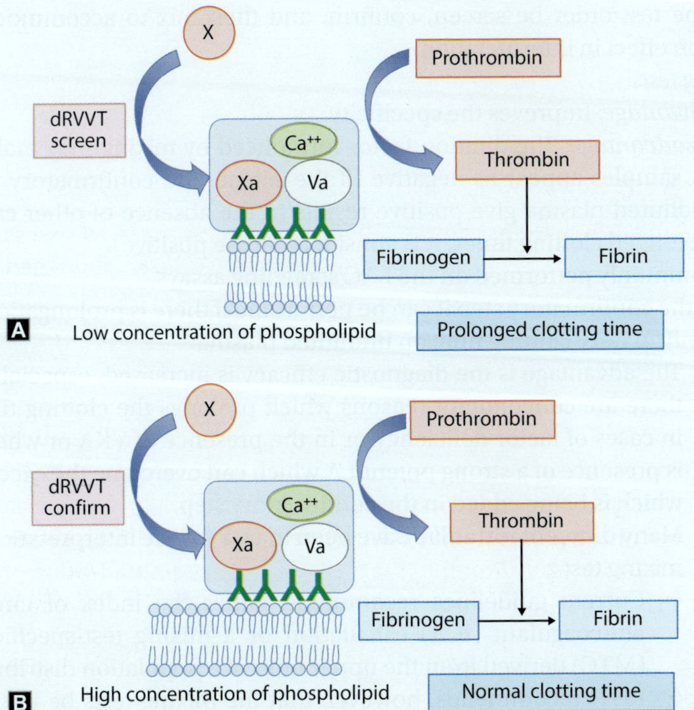

FIGS. 2A AND B: (A) dRVVT screening assay contains a low amount of phospholipid. (B) dRVVT confirm assay requires a reagent containing an increased phospholipid concentration.

(dRVVT: dilute Russell viper venom time)

Choice of Assays for Lupus Anticoagulant Testing

- The International Society on Thrombosis and Haemostasis-Scientific and Standardization Committee (ISTH-SSC) 2020 guidelines have recommended two tests, which are based on different principles, which are APTT (most sensitive) and dRVVT (most specific) using a low concentration of phospholipid (PL). The combination of APTT and dRVVT has been proven to have high detection rates of LA.
- dRVVT should be considered as the first test and APTT should be considered as the second test (appropriate PL composition and low concentration) with preferably silica as an activator.

Choice of Platelet Neutralization Procedure

- *PNP:* Either commercial or prepared in-house.
- This PNP is to be obtained by double centrifugation and should have normal fibrinogen levels and factor levels > 80 IU/dL.

Three Step Procedure

- As per the ISTH and the British Society of Haematology (BSH) guidelines, all three steps (screening, mixing, and confirmation) are vital. However, the Clinical and Laboratory Standards Institute (CLSI) guidelines recommend that the test order be screen, confirm, and then mix to accommodate the dilution effect in interpretation.
- *Mixing tests*:
    - *Advantage*: Improves the specificity.
    - *Disadvantage*: The dilution factor introduced by mixing may make weak LA samples appear as negative (if the screen and confirmatory tests on undiluted plasma give positive results in the absence of other causes of prolonged clotting times, it is considered to be positive).
    - Commonly performed on the LAC screening assays.
    - In the confirmatory step it can be performed if there is prolongation of the confirmatory clotting time on undiluted plasma.
        - The advantage is the diagnostic efficacy is increased, especially when there are concomitant reasons which prolongs the clotting time e.g., in cases of factor deficiency or in the presence of VKA or when there is presence of a strong potent LA which can overcome the excess of PL which is being added in the confirmatory step.
        - Many different formulae have been in task for the interpretation of the mixing tests:
            - ◊ Current guidelines recommend either the index of circulating anticoagulant (ICA) calculation or a mixing test-specific cutoff (MTC) derived from the upper limit of a population distribution.
            - ◊ ISTH recommends, however, that the mixing tests be interpreted with a mixing test-specific cutoff expressed as a normalized ratio, as this improves sensitivity.
            - ◊ Results of the mixing test results suggest LA when the normalized clotting time is greater than the local cutoff value.

Lupus Cofactor Phenomenon

- Sometimes in the screening tests of the LA, moderate prolonged coagulation times is noted. Still, when mixed with the normal pooled plasma, they exhibit coagulation times that are paradoxically longer than those of the index plasma alone. This paradoxical effect infers that in such scenarios the LA would be needing the existence of a cofactor to express its full anticoagulant activity.
- The LA is directed against the complex of proteins (prothrombin or β2GPI) having negatively charged phospholipids. Thus, the "lupus cofactor" could be β2GPI or prothrombin.
- The manifestation of the "lupus cofactor phenomenon" suggests that if we perform only screening and confirmatory procedures by skipping the mixing tests like we do in the integrated tests, it will be unsuitable.

Normalization of Results

- Normalized ratio is—clotting time of the patient/clotting time of the PNP.
- The patient's and the PNP's clotting time must be measured in the same run so that we can reduce the analytical variations related to the reagent, instrument, and operator.
- The mean of a reference interval which is determined per lot of reagents used in the denominator of the formula as per the CLSI guidelines is less applied.

Cutoff Values

The ISTH-SSC 2020 guidelines recommend for the screening and mixing procedures.

- Use of the 99th percentile to determine the cutoff value.
- At least 120 donors.
- For the confirmation procedure mean percentage of correction is being used.
- Can we use the manufacturer's cutoff values?—Yes, as an alternative, after verification, it is possible, especially if it is in agreement with guidelines and by suitable statistical models after using an adequately large donor population.
- Can cutoff values be transferred across the labs?—No, because there are varied variables from the sample collection system to the varied sample tubes, to the different demographics, to the variation in PNP, and batches of reagents.
- Screening/mixing tests are considered positive if the normalized clotting time is more than the established cutoff.
- *Confirmatory test*:
  - Needs to be executed if the screening test advocates LA presence, regardless of the mixing results.
  - Confirmatory test is executed on a mix of 1:1 PP and PNP if the confirmatory clotting time is prolonged.
  - Results are expressed as ratio of patient-to-PNP run in parallel with the test plasma for all procedures (screening, mixing, and confirm).
- For paired tests, the LA ratio (screen/confirm) is expressed as a normalized ratio of both the screen and the confirm times.

Report of Results

- The final report of LA is reported as positive or negative.
- Borderline or uncertain LA reports should not be used. In such scenarios, the report should read "suggest retesting after 1 week or more."
- Local cutoff values must be reported alongside the analytical results for the screening/mixing and confirmatory steps.
- Results should be explained clearly.
- LA results should always be corelated with the results of aCL and aβ2GPI for assessing the risk profile.
- APA results should always be interpreted in a clinical context with the knowledge of history, personal history, symptoms, signs, and ongoing treatment.
- The report must incorporate all of the aforementioned clinical aspects besides the patient's anticoagulation status.
- In case of use of DOAC adsorbents, it needs to be mentioned in a report.

Solid-phase Tests for Antiphospholipid Antibodies

- Screening for APS should incorporate IgG and IgM aCL and aβ2GPI assays.
- These assays are performed by enzyme-linked immunosorbent assays (ELISA) preferably on fully automated platforms.

Noncriteria Antiphospholipid Antibodies

- Antiphosphatidylserine/prothrombin antibodies (anti-PS/PT) are the options available.
- They foresee the risk of recurrence in patients with previous thrombosis.
- They are frequently found in triple-positive patients.
- The independent diagnostic utility of them, however in thrombotic and obstetric APS is ambiguous.

Confirmation of Persistent Lupus Anticoagulant Positivity

- Why it is necessary to repeat to confirm persistent positivity?
    - It will exclude the transient LA which are being induced by infection/ drugs.
- How much duration is advised to repeat the tests?
    - The guidelines advise that the positive results be repeated after 12 weeks of the last performed confirmation tests.
- How does repeated positive confirmation test will help?
    - It will further render the test more reliable and assurance of a test result even if there are possibilities of poor standardization and interference factors which may affect the test result.

WHAT ARE THE RECENT ADDED UPDATES AND THEIR REQUIREMENT?

Till recently, we were following the Sapporo criteria which were published in 1991 and were revised in 2006 for the diagnosis of APS, but in due course of time there has been expansion of knowledge in the pathophysiology, clinical features including some nonthrombotic clinical contexts, involvement of additional systemic diseases and risk stratification. In addition, the Sapporo criteria did not integrate the evidence-based definitions which created the confusion and heterogeneity. In view of aforementioned reasons hence there was a dire need of another classification which fills up the lacunae of the previous classification providing more stringent criteria for patient enrolment into clinical trials.

Of late, in 2023, American College of Rheumatology (ACR) and European League Against Rheumatism (EULAR) have developed a newer classification system for the APS **(Box 2 and Flowchart 1)**. In this classification many parameters have been incorporated so that the sensitivity and specificity of APS diagnosis are improved especially in patients with additional clinical parameters like thrombocytopenia, SLE, microvascular manifestations, and cardiac valvular disease.

If any clinical criteria or APA test is evident of APS and that test(s) is positive within 3 months of the clinical symptoms/signs then the scoring needs to be done as per **Box 2 and Table 2** and APS is classified when the total scores of each of both clinical and lab domains are more than at least 3 (Research purpose only right now).

ISOLATED POSITIVITY (SINGLE POSITIVITY) OF THE LUPUS ANTICOAGULANT AND ANTI-B2-GLYCOPROTEIN I ANTIBODY

Scenario 1—isolated (single) positivity of lupus anticoagulant without any anti-β2GPI, aCL, anti-PS/PT.

Potency of isolated LA positivity is mild and therefore the thrombotic risk is low, though in comparison to general population the risk is still high. However, some studies show comparable results of thrombotic tendency.

- In contrast, elderly population is more affected.
- Among all APA, LA has the highest thrombotic risk.
- In the single LA-positivity with the negativity for anti-β2GPI and anti-PS/PT antibodies, it has been observed that the antibody is directed against the unknown plasma proteins.
- Samples having isolated LA positivity exhibits weaker activity than the LA in triple-positive samples.

BOX 2: 2023 ACR/EULAR antiphospholipid syndrome (APS) classification clinical criteria).

Clinical criteria:

Domian 1—Macrovascular (venous thromboembolism) (score)

Domain 2—Macrovascular (arterial thrombosis) (score)

- Unexplained without risk factor—Carries a score of 4
- Unexplained with risk factor—Carries a score of 2

Domain 3—Microvascular (score)

- Suspected etiology—Carries a score of 2
  - Livedo racemosa (physical examination): Nonuniform, irreversible, broken, and asymetric persistent discoloration are the ones only which are scored
  - Livedoid vasculopathy lesions (by physical examination)
  - Antiphospholipid antibody nephropathy (physical exam or lab test)
  - Pulmonary hemorrhage (by clinical symptoms and imaging)
- Established etiology—Carries a score of 5
  - Livedoid vasculopathy confirmed by pathology
  - Histopathology (HPE) confirmed microthrombosis/endothelial cell proliferation
  - Histopathology confirmed aPL nephropathy
  - Cytopathology/HPE confirmed pulmonary hemorrhage
  - Imaging/HPE confirmed otherwise unexplained myocardial disease
  - Imaging/HPE confirmed otherwise unexplained adrenal hemorrhage or microthrombosis

Domain 4—Obstetrics (score)

- Prefetal death/early fetal death—Carries a score of 1
- Fetal death in absence of preeclampsia with severe featured or placental insufficiency—Carries a score of 1
- Preeclampsia with severe featured or placental insufficiency with severe features—Carries a score of 3
- Preeclampsia with severe featured and placental insufficiency with severe features—Carries a score of 4

Domain 5—Cardiac valve (score)

- Unexplained valve thickening—Carries a score of 2
- Unexplained valve vegetation—Carries a score of 4

Domain 6—Hematology (score)

- Unexplained thrombocytopenia—Carries a score of 2

Laboratory criteria

Domain 7—aPL test by the coagulation based functional assay (score)

Lupus anticoagulant (LA) assay

- 3-step (screening – mixing study – confirmation) with two screening test systems
- Positive if at least 1 test systems yields a positive result following all three steps
- Positive LA at a single time—Carries a score of 1
- Positive persistent LA at a two times—Carries a score of 5

Domain 8 — aPl test by solid phase based assay only ELISA methodology (score)

Anticardiolipin antibody (aCl) and/or anti–β2-glycoprotein I antibody (anti-β2 GPI)

- Moderate (positive 40–79 units)—Carries a score of 1
- Moderate positive IgG (40–79 units)—Carries a score of 4
- High positive IgG aCL or anti-β2 GPI (>80 units)—Carries a score of 5
- High positive IgG aCL and anti-β2 GPI (>80 units)—Carries a score of 7

(ACR: American College of Rheumatology; EULAR: European League Against Rheumatism)

Source: Adapted from Devreese KMJ, de Groot PG, de Laat B, Erkan D, Favaloro EJ, Mackie I, et al. Guidance from the scientific and standardization committee for lupus anticoagulant/antiphospholipid antibodies of the International Society on Thrombosis and Haemostasis: update of the guidelines for lupus anticoagulant detection and interpretation. J Thromb Haemost. 2020;18(11):2828-39.

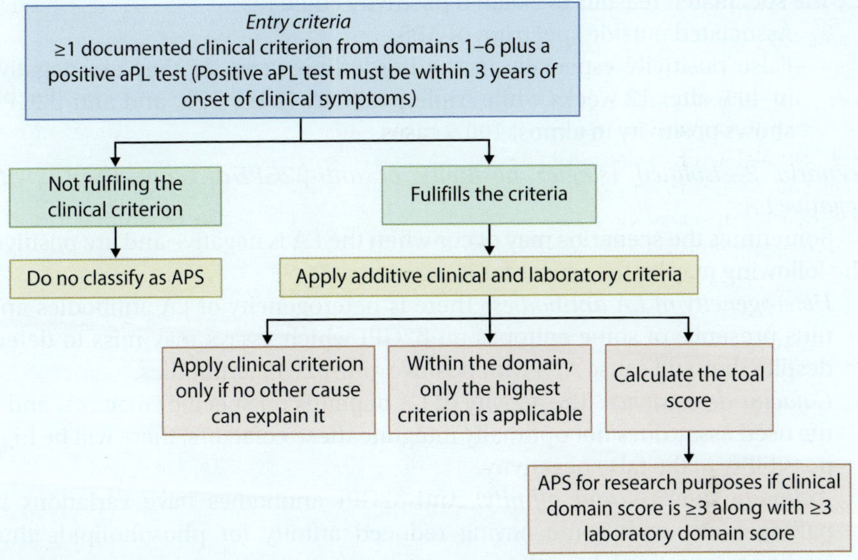

FLOWCHART 1: 2023 ACR/EULAR APS classification criteria.

(ACR: American College of Rheumatology; APS: antiphospholipid syndrome; EULAR: European League Against Rheumatism)

TABLE 2: Lupus anticoagulant testing-example showing calculation of LAC test.

	Diluted Russel Viper Venom Test (dRVVT)		**Silica clotting time (SCT)**	
	Clotting time (second)	**Ratios**	**Clotting time (second)**	**Ratios**
Pt plasma (screen)	69.2 s	Screen ratio = 1.82	161 s	Screen ratio = 3.67
PNP (screen)	37.9 s (3S D cutoff—49.53 s)		43.8 s (3 SD cutoff—64 s)	
Mix Pt plasma (screen)	62.1 s	Mix ratio = 1.63	85 s	Mix ratio = 1.94
PNP (screen)	37.9 s (3 SD cutoff—49.53 s)		43.8 s (3SD cutoff—64 s)	
Pt plasma (confirm)	39.5 s	Confirm ratio = 1.14	42 s	Confirm ratio = 1.11
PNP (confirm)	34.5 s (3 SD cutoff—38.05 s)		37.6 s (3 SD cutoff—57 s)	
	Normalized ratio = 1.59		Normalized ratio = 3.30	
Result: Lupus anticoagulant positive *Advice:* Repeat testing after 12 weeks				

- The speculated reasons of isolated positivity could be:
  - Associated outside spectrum of APS.
  - False positivity especially in the borderline cases, as they are negative in 40% after 12 weeks while triple positivity (LAC, aCL, and anti-β2GPI) shows positivity in almost 100% cases.

Scenario 2—isolated (single) positivity of anti-β2GPI/aCL/anti-PS/PT with negative LA.

Sometimes the scenarios may occur when the LA is negative and are positive. The following may be the causes for it.

- *Heterogeneity of LA antibodies:* There is heterogeneity of LA antibodies and thus presence of some epitopes on β2GPI which assays may miss to detect despite they still cause APS with positive anti-β2GPI antibodies.
- *Cofactor dependence:* The activity of LA depends on specific cofactors, and if the used assay does not optimally integrate these cofactors, there will be high possibility of the false negativity.
- *Antibody subclass and affinity:* Anti-β2GPI antibodies have variations in pathogenicity with some having reduced affinity for phospholipids thus leading to negative LA results.
- *Technical factors:* The preanalytical and analytical factors such as the sample collection, storage, and the performance of assay can influence the test results.
- *Presence of interfering factors:* Some medications, illnesses can interfere with the LA assays, thus leading to a false negativity.

Case

A 29-year-old male diagnosed presented with unprovoked left leg deep vein thrombosis. He was referred for the workup for antiphospholipid antibody testing. There was no family history of thrombosis and not receiving any anticoagulant therapy.

Laboratory Investigations

- PT—12 second (10–13 second)
- APTT—69 second (27–26.7 second)
- TT—17.2 second (16–21 second)
- Fibrinogen—258 mg/dL (200–400 mg/dL)
- IgM and IgG anti-β2 glycoprotein 1 antibody—moderately positive (40–79 units) which carries the score of 4.
- IgM and IgG anti-cardiolipin antibody—negative <40 units.

Lupus Anticoagulant Testing **(Table 2)**

- $\text{Screen ratio} = \dfrac{\text{Screen CT of patient's plasma}}{\text{Screen CT of PNP}}$
- $\text{Mix ratio} = \dfrac{\text{Mix CT of patient's plasma}}{\text{Mix CT of PNP}}$
- $\text{Confirm ratio} = \dfrac{\text{Confirm CT of patient's plasma}}{\text{Confirm CT of PNP}}$
- $\text{Normalized ratio} = \dfrac{\text{Screen ratio}}{\text{Confirm ratio}}$

Diagnosis: Possible antiphospholipid syndrome (double positive for LA and anti-β2 glycoprotein 1 antibody).

The positive tests should be repeated after 12 weeks for confirmation.

Take Home Points

- APS is a paradoxical hypercoagulable state, despite causing prolonged clotting times in vitro.
- Revised Sapporo criteria (2006) and 2023 ACR/EULAR classification provide structured diagnostic frameworks for APS classification.
- APS may be diagnosed even if the above classification criteria are not met.
- Persistent APA positivity (12 weeks apart) is essential for APS confirmation.
- dRVVT and APTT are primary LA screening tests; mixing studies improve specificity.
- Anticoagulation affects LA testing; specific protocols are needed for warfarin, heparins, and DOACs.
- Noncriteria antibodies (aPS/PT) are emerging as potential markers for risk assessment.
- Lupus cofactor phenomenon suggests that LA effects are enhanced by β2GPI or prothrombin.
- APS testing should always be interpreted in a clinical context, considering patient history and systemic conditions.
- Newer classification criteria incorporate additional systemic features, improving diagnostic sensitivity and specificity.
- Proper sample collection, storage, and processing are critical for accurate APS testing.

SUGGESTED READINGS

1. Yao K, Zhang L, Zhou H, Tang N, Li D. Plasma antiphospholipid antibodies effects on activated partial thromboplastin time assays. Am J Med Sci. 2017;354:22-26.
2. Wilson WA, Gharavi AE, Koike T, Lockshin MD, Branch DW, Piette JC, et al. International consensus statement on preliminary classification criteria for definite antiphospholipid syndrome: report of an international workshop. Arthritis Rheum. 1999;42(7):1309-11.
3. Miyakis S, Lockshin MD, Atsumi T, Branch DW, Brey RL, Cervera R, et al. International consensus statement on an update of the classification criteria for definite antiphospholipid syndrome. J Thromb Haemost. 2006;4(2):295-306.
4. Arachchillage DRJ, Laffan M. What is the appropriate anticoagulation strategy for thrombotic antiphospholipid syndrome? Br J Haematol. 2020;189(2):216-27.
5. Devreese KM. Antiphospholipid antibody testing and standardisation. Int J Lab Hematol. 2014;36(3):352-63.
6. De Kesel PM, Devreese KMJ. The effect of unfractionated heparin, enoxaparin and danaparoid on lupus anticoagulant testing. Can activated carbon eliminate false positive results? Res Pract Thromb Haemost. 2019;4(1):161-8.
7. Favaloro EJ, Mohammed S, Curnow J, Pasalic L. Laboratory testing for lupus anticoagulant (LA) in patients taking direct oral anticoagulants (DOACs): potential for false positives and false negatives. Pathology. 2019;51(3):292-300.
8. Arachchillage DJ, Platton S, Hickey K, Chu J, Pickering M, Sommerville P, et al. Guidelines on the investigation and management of antiphospholipid syndrome. Br J Haematol. 2024;205(3):855-80.

9. Schouwers SM, Delanghe JR, Devreese KM. Lupus anticoagulant (LAC) testing in patients with inflammatory status: does C-reactive protein interfere with LAC test results? Thromb Res. 2010;125(1):102-4.
10. Kristoffersen AH, Hammer IJ, Vannes S, Åsberg A, Aakre KM. Impact of different preanalytical conditions on results of lupus anticoagulant tests. Int J Lab Hematol. 2019;41(6):745-53.
11. Kitchen S, Adcock DM, Dauer R, Kristoffersen AH, Lippi G, Mackie I, et al. International Council for Standardization in Haematology (ICSH) recommendations for processing of blood samples for coagulation testing. Int J Lab Hematol. 2021;43(6):1272-83.
12. Ahuja A, Tyagi S, Pati HP, Saxena R, Somasundaram V, Manivannan P, et al. Utility of Lupus Anticoagulant Assays (APTT-LA, KCT, DPT and DRVVT) in Detection of Antiphospholipid Syndrome (APS) in High Risk Pregnancy Cases. Indian J Hematol Blood Transfus. 2019;35(3):478-84.
13. Tripodi A. To mix or not to mix in lupus anticoagulant testing? That is the question. Semin Thromb Hemost. 2012;38(4):385-9.
14. Loeliger A. Prothrombin as cofactor of circulating anticoagulant in systemic lupus crythematosus. Thromb Diath Haemorrh. 1959;3:237-56.
15. Devreese KMJ, de Groot PG, de Laat B, Erkan D, Favaloro EJ, Mackie I, et al. Guidance from the scientific and standardization committee for lupus anticoagulant/antiphospholipid antibodies of the International Society on Thrombosis and Haemostasis: update of the guidelines for lupus anticoagulant detection and interpretation. J Thromb Haemost. 2020;18(11):2828-39.
16. Barbhaiya M, Zuily S, Naden R, Hendry A, Manneville F, Amigo MC, et al.; ACR/EULAR APS Classification Criteria Collaborators. 2023 ACR/EULAR antiphospholipid syndrome classification criteria. Ann Rheum Dis. 2023;82(10):1258-70.
17. Yin D, de Groot PG, Ninivaggi M, Devreese KMJ, de Laat B. Clinical Relevance of Isolated LAC Positivity in Thrombotic APS Patients. Thromb Haemost. 2021;121(09):1220-7.
18. Yin D, de Laat B. Commentary on: circulating plasmablasts contribute to antiphospholipid antibody production, associated with type I interferon upregulation. J Thromb Haemost. 2019;17(7):1030-2.

CHAPTER 16

Heparin-induced Thrombocytopenia and Vaccine-induced Thrombocytopenia

Narender Kumar, Jasmina Ahluwalia

ABSTRACT

Heparin-induced thrombocytopenia (HIT) and vaccine-induced thrombosis and thrombocytopenia (VITT) are rare, immune-mediated, and prothrombotic conditions involving platelet activation. HIT arises from pathogenic anti-platelet factor 4 (PF4)-heparin antibodies, typically occurring 5–14 days after heparin exposure. It is classified into type I (nonimmune, mild, and transient) and type II (immune-mediated, with high thrombotic risk). HIT pathogenesis involves PF4-heparin complex formation, immune response activation, and platelet activation via FcγRIIa, with contributions from monocytes, neutrophils, and endothelial cells. Genetic polymorphisms may influence susceptibility to HIT and thrombosis. Clinical diagnosis of HIT utilizes the 4Ts or HIT expert probability (HEP) scoring systems, with laboratory testing required for intermediate/high scores. HIT diagnostics include immunoassays [enzyme-linked immunosorbent assay (ELISA), latex, chemiluminescence, etc.] for anti-PF4 antibodies and functional assays (serotonin release and platelet aggregation/activation assays). VITT, a rare adverse event post-coronavirus disease 2019 (COVID-19) vaccination, results from pathogenic anti-PF4 antibodies independent of heparin, often causing thrombosis in atypical sites like cerebral venous sinuses. VITT diagnosis requires ELISA and PF4-enhanced functional assays due to its unique pathophysiology.

INTRODUCTION

Heparin-induced thrombocytopenia (HIT) is a highly prothrombotic, immune-mediated condition characterized by platelet activation. It is triggered by the formation of pathogenic antibodies targeting the complex between heparin and platelet factor 4 (PF4). HIT can be classified into two distinct types: Type I is heparin-associated thrombocytopenia, and type II is the classical HIT. Type I HIT is a nonimmune phenomenon triggered by the direct interaction of heparin with circulating platelets, leading to their clumping or sequestration. This form is relatively common, affecting approximately 10–30% of patients treated with heparin. It usually develops within 48–72 hours of starting heparin therapy and results in mild, transient thrombocytopenia. Importantly, type I HIT is self-limiting, with platelet counts returning to normal within 4 days after discontinuing heparin, and is not linked with thrombotic risk. Type II or classical HIT, on the other hand is immune-mediated. It is significantly less common, with an incidence of 0.1–7%, depending on factors such as the type of heparin, treatment length, and the patient population. This form is associated with a heightened risk of thrombotic events, occurring in 25–50% of affected individuals. The risk of type II HIT is approximately 10 times greater with unfractionated heparin (UFH) than low molecular weight heparin (LMWH). Typically, it manifests 5–14 days following the heparin administration and requires prompt recognition and management due to its potential complications.

In addition to classical HIT, several other conditions are linked to anti-PF4 antibodies. In these conditions, anti-PF4 antibodies are formed against platelets without heparin involvement. These disorders can be broadly categorized as follows:

- *Autoimmune HIT (aHIT):* In this condition both heparin-dependent and heparin-independent anti-PF4 antibodies can be seen. Subtypes of aHIT include delayed-onset HIT (thrombocytopenia develops or deteriorates after heparin discontinuation), persistent HIT (lasting more than a week postheparin cessation), heparin flush HIT, and maximum cases associated with fondaparinux. In aHIT, immunoglobulin (IgG) anti-PF4 antibodies can activate platelets even in absence of heparin.
- *Spontaneous HIT:* This variant arises in the absence of heparin and is often triggered by factors such as knee replacement surgery or infections. It is primarily driven by platelet-activating antibodies that are produced without heparin.
- *Vaccine-induced thrombosis and thrombocytopenia:* This condition involves highly pathogenic anti-PF4 antibodies that causes platelet activation in the absence of heparin and typically occurs following immunization for coronavirus disease 2019 (COVID-19). This is an extremely rare adverse event linked to various vaccines like adenovirus-based vaccines, mRNA vaccines, and whole inactivated virus vaccines. VITT typically occurs 5–30 days after getting vaccine and is defined by thrombocytopenia, high D-dimer, and the manifestation of thrombosis in unusual sites.

PATHOGENESIS OF HEPARIN-INDUCED THROMBOCYTOPENIA

The HIT arises from a complex interplay between PF4, heparin, and anti-PF4-heparin antibodies.

Interaction between PF4, Heparin, and Platelets

The PF4, a chemokine released by activated platelet α granules, is a tetramer composed of two identical homodimers. This structural arrangement allows two HIT (or VITT) antibodies to bind to one PF4 molecule. PF4, characterized by a strong positively charged equatorial band, is nonimmunogenic in its native state. However, conformational changes expose a neoepitope, forming the HIT antigen.

Heparin, a negatively charged glycosaminoglycan, binds to the positively charged amino acids on PF4. This interaction neutralizes PF4's charge and promotes the formation of antigens at the "north" and "south" poles of the molecule. Heparin-independent antigens, on the other hand, form at the equatorial sites. The PF4-heparin interaction facilitates the clustering of PF4 molecules, exposing hidden epitopes for that anti-PF4-heparin antibodies. These interactions lead to the development of ultra-large complexes (ULCs), which consist of at least 16 PF4 molecules bound to heparin chains **(Flowchart 1A)**. These ULCs are electrostatically developed on the surface of platelets and are more prominent with UFH compared to LMWH. Fondaparinux, which lacks sufficient saccharide chains, does not form ULCs, explaining its lower HIT risk.

Immune Response and Anti-PF4-heparin Antibody Production

The immune response in HIT may have evolved to recognize negative charges on bacterial surfaces, particularly gram-negative bacteria. Heparin exposure triggers ULCs formation, which activates the complement system, leading to C3 and C4 deposition on the ULCs. This enables the complexes to attach to complement receptor 2 on B cells, promoting their activation and the transport of antigens to lymphoid follicles. This process culminates in the production of anti-PF4-heparin antibodies, predominantly IgG, within 4–14 days of heparin exposure. While IgM and IgA antibodies can also form, their clinical significance is less clear.

The maturation of B cells into plasma cells is a time-dependent process, necessary for the secretion of large quantities of IgG antibodies. These antibodies bind to the ULCs, triggering platelet activation via the FcγRIIa receptor. This interaction induces platelet degranulation, aggregation, and a self-amplifying loop that increase PF4 availability for further complex formation **(Flowchart 1B)**. Activated platelets generate procoagulant microparticles, enhancing thrombin production and contributing to a hypercoagulable state.

Impact of Monocytes, Neutrophils, and Endothelial Cells

In addition to platelets, other cell types play critical roles in the thrombotic complications of HIT:

- *Monocytes:* PF4 exhibits a higher binding affinity for monocytes compared to platelets, attributed to differences in the glycosaminoglycan composition of their glycocalyx. This enhances the binding of HIT antibodies. Antibody-antigen complexes on monocytes surface result in interleukin-8 secretion and tissue factor expression. Tissue factor-expressing microparticles from monocytes contribute to thrombin generation and enhance the procoagulant state.
- *Neutrophils:* Neutrophils are activated through the interaction of platelet P-selectin and FcγRIIa with anti-PF4-heparin antibodies. This activation

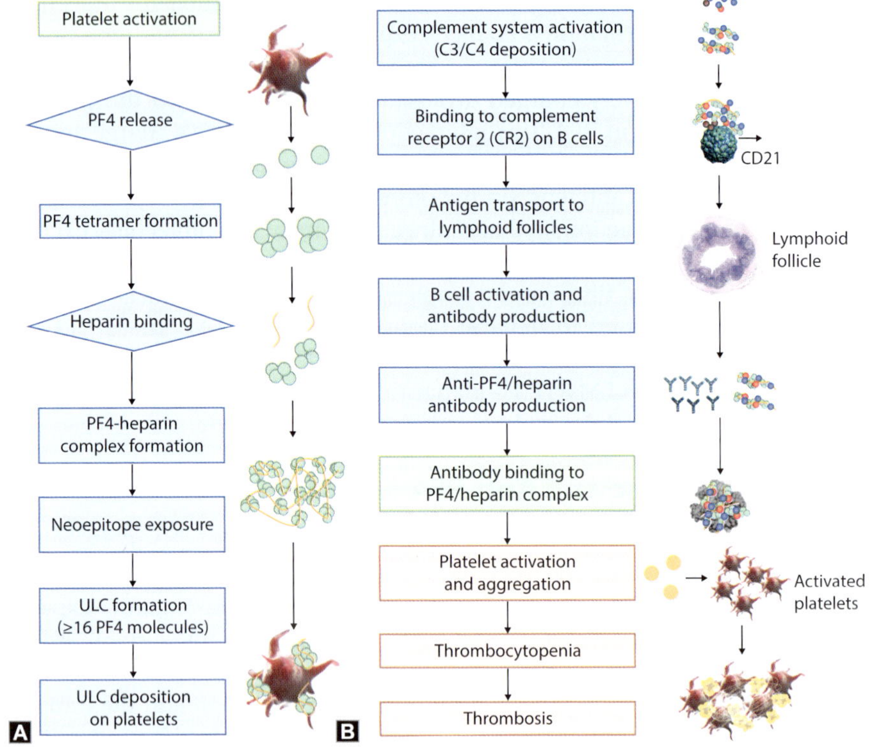

FLOWCHARTS 1A AND B: Pathophysiology of heparin-induced thrombocytopenia. (A) The interaction between PF4, heparin, and platelet. (B) Immune response and anti-PF4-heparin antibody production.

(PF4: platelet factor 4; ULC: ultra-large complexes)

triggers the formation of neutrophil extracellular traps (NETs), which bind PF4 and enhance immune complex formation. The NETs provide a procoagulant surface that directly promotes thrombin generation. NETs are integral to the hypercoagulability seen in HIT.

- *Endothelial cells:* Anti-PF4-heparin antibodies bind to PF4 on endothelial cells possibly via the fragment antigen-binding region of antibodies. This binding is preferentially targeted to microvascular endothelial cells. This interaction, often stimulated by tumor necrosis factor-α released during platelet activation, leads to endothelial injury. Injured endothelial cells express tissue factors, adhesion molecules, and alter their glycocalyx, promoting thrombosis. Additionally, endothelial cells release thrombomodulin, potentially reducing local anticoagulant activity and favoring clot formation.

Genetic Influences in Heparin-induced Thrombocytopenia Pathogenesis

The presence of anti-PF4-heparin antibodies does not always result in the development of HIT, nor do all HIT patients experience thrombotic complications.

Genetic polymorphisms may influence these variable responses. Polymorphisms in Fc receptor genes, such as FcγRIIIA 158V and FcγRIIA 131R have been linked to increased susceptibility to HIT and thrombosis in HIT, respectively. Future research may uncover additional genetic factors contributing to individual variability in HIT responses, providing insights into patient-specific risks and therapeutic strategies.

PATHOGENESIS OF VACCINE-INDUCED THROMBOSIS AND THROMBOCYTOPENIA

The VITT is thought to result from the formation of PF4-dependent antigens, triggered by interactions between PF4 and viral proteins such as hexons. Notably, VITT occurs approximately three times more frequently with ChAdOx1 nCoV-19 compared to Ad26.COV2.S vaccine. The prevailing theories regarding VITT antibody development suggest that immunogenic PF4/polyanionic complexes form upon vaccine administration. These complexes can circulate systemically, activating monocytes and neutrophils through FcγIIa receptor-dependent pathways. This activation may promote the differentiation of B cells into plasma cells, leading to the production of anti-PF4 antibodies. Additionally, vaccine excipients, including extracellular nucleic acids and proteins derived from human cell lines used in adenovirus propagation, might contribute to neoepitope formation and the generation of anti-PF4 antibodies.

In addition to neoepitope formation, vaccine excipients might promote proinflammatory responses and localized thrombosis. For example, studies indicate that components of the ChAdOx1-S vaccine, including adenosine triphosphatase (ATPase) activity potentially associated with heat shock proteins and chaperones, may facilitate limited ADP production and activation of platelet at the site of vaccination. Additionally, ethylenediaminetetraacetic acid (EDTA), an excipient in the ChAdOx1-S vaccine, was found to induce vascular hyperpermeability. EDTA by chelating calcium ions (Ca^{2+}) can alter E-cadherin, a key element of endothelial cell connections, compromising their integrity. This disruption increases vascular permeability in animal models such as mice and zebrafish and is thought to have similar effects in humans, allowing vaccine ingredients to invade the circulation and potentially contribute to inflammation.

CLINICAL PRESENTATION OF HEPARIN-INDUCED THROMBOCYTOPENIA AND VACCINE-INDUCED THROMBOSIS AND THROMBOCYTOPENIA

Both HIT and VITT are highly prothrombotic disorders associated with significant mortality if not managed promptly. Clinical symptoms typically emerge after 5 days from the initiating event. Thrombosis rapidly becomes widespread, involving arterial, venous, and microvascular circulations, often affecting multiple vascular beds simultaneously.

Heparin-induced Thrombocytopenia: Clinical Evaluation and Scoring Systems

In patients receiving heparin, HIT should be suspected by clinical assessment, particularly if there is a significant drop in platelet count. The probability of HIT can be assessed by the "4Ts" scoring criteria, which considers four key clinical features: thrombocytopenia, timing of platelet count decline, presence of thrombosis or other sequelae, and alternative causes for thrombocytopenia **(Table 1)**. Thrombosis in HIT is influenced by the patient's clinical profile. Venous thrombosis is more frequent in postoperative patients, whereas approximately 30% of cardiovascular surgery patients develop arterial thrombosis.

The platelet count should be measured prior to starting heparin therapy. Since most HIT cases develop 5–14 days after heparin initiation, platelet count should be monitored within this timeframe. For a score of ≤ 3, laboratory testing is typically unnecessary unless specific intensive care unit (ICU) circumstances warrant it. The instant discontinuation of heparin should be done if the score is ≥4 and a therapeutic-dose alternative anticoagulant should be initiated while awaiting laboratory confirmation.

Another scoring method, the HIT expert probability (HEP) score, was introduced in 2010. While both the HEP and 4Ts scoring systems have similar sensitivity and specificity, the HEP score is more effective in ICU patients with multiple alternative causes of thrombocytopenia. Either system can be used in clinical practice.

Vaccine-induced Thrombosis and Thrombocytopenia: Clinical Characteristics

VITT typically develops 5–30 days after vaccination. It is characterized by thrombocytopenia, high D-dimer results, anti-PF4 antibodies that stimulate platelets,

TABLE 1: The pretest probability scoring system for heparin-induced thrombocytopenia.

Score	Thrombocytopenia	Timing of platelet count fall	Thrombosis or other sequelae	Other cause for thrombocytopenia
0	<30% decrease or platelet nadir ≤10 × 10^9/L	Thrombocytopenia develops ≤ 4 days	None	Definite other cause is present
1	30–50% decrease or platelet nadir 10–19 × 10^9/L	After day 10	Progressive/recurrent thrombosis; erythematous lesions; suspected thrombosis not yet proven	Possible other cause is evident
2	>50% decrease or platelet nadir ≥20 × 10^9/L	Clear onset between days 5 and 10	New thrombosis; skin necrosis; acute systemic reaction postheparin bolus	No other cause for platelet count falls evident

Note: Pretest probability scores: High (6–8), Intermediate (4–5), Low (0–3).

and thrombosis at unusual sites, such as cerebral venous sinuses (CVT) and splanchnic veins. Unlike HIT, VITT primarily affects healthy vaccine recipients, with symptoms becoming evident only when thrombosis develops. The degree of platelet count reduction is crucial for both conditions. HIT is associated with a ≥ 30% drop, while VITT often involves a ≥ 50% decline. At presentation, platelet counts may still be within the normal range. Thrombosis in VITT is notable for its predilection for CVT, a rare thrombotic site. While CVT is observed in HIT, it occurs in fewer than 2% of cases.

LABORATORY DIAGNOSIS OF HEPARIN-INDUCED THROMBOCYTOPENIA

The accurate and prompt diagnosis of HIT in the laboratory is critical for informing clinical management and minimizing thrombotic complications. Laboratory testing becomes essential for cases with intermediate or high 4T scores. Typically, diagnostic evaluation involves a combination of immunoassays assays for screening and functional assays for confirmation. These tests include immunoassays that identify anti-PF4-heparin antibodies and functional assays that assess platelet activation. **Table 2** outlines the diagnostic tests available for HIT.

Qualitative immunoassays, which detect anti-PF4-heparin antibodies, are extensively used due to their high sensitivity and rapid turnaround time (usually within 1 hour). However, these tests are not suitable as standalone screening tools because they do not quantify antibody levels. Automated quantitative immunoassays, such as latex immunoassay and chemiluminescence immunoassay (CLIA), offer faster results with less hands-on time. The latex immunoassay, which is performed using widely available analyzers, has better sensitivity and specificity than manual rapid assays. The CLIA is particularly advantageous due to its high sensitivity and specificity, making it the preferred choice in the absence of functional assays. ELISA is another widely used immunoassay with excellent sensitivity. A negative result from a high-sensitivity ELISA effectively rules out HIT. Strong optical density signals in ELISA are often indicative of a positive functional assay result. However, the test's labor-intensive nature, high cost, and long turnaround time (4–24 hours) can pose challenges, especially in resource-limited settings.

Functional assays, which measure platelet activation or aggregation, require donor platelets that are pretested for responsiveness to patient serum containing anti-PF4-heparin antibodies. These assays detect platelet activation in the presence of patient plasma and specific heparin concentrations, with confirmation achieved through inhibition of activation using excess heparin. The complex nature of these tests limits their use to specialized centers. Flow cytometry-based assays, a more recent addition to HIT diagnostics, rely on detecting platelet activation markers such as Annexin V and P-selectin. While these tests demonstrate good sensitivity and specificity, their restricted accessibility is due to the need for specialized instruments and standardized protocols. The serotonin-release assay (SRA), long considered the gold standard

TABLE 2: Diagnostic tests for screening and diagnosis of HIT, along with the associated technology and turnaround time.

Test category	Technique	Turnaround time	Comments
Qualitative immunoassay (rapid tests)	Lateral flow immunoassay	<1 hour	Requires fresh samples for best results
	Gel immunoassay	<1 hour	Limited availability
	Immunofiltration assay	<1 hour	Limited availability
Quantitative immunoassay (automated)	Latex immunoassay	<1 hour	Commonly available, efficient, and standardized
	Chemiluminescent immunoassay	<1 hour	Recommended in the absence of functional assays
Quantitative immunoassay (manual)	ELISA	4–24 hours	High sensitivity, but labor-intensive
Functional assays (platelet activation based)	Heparin-induced platelet activation	2–3 hours	Requires pretested PF4-reactive donor platelets
	Light transmission aggregometry	2–3 hours	Requires pretested PF4-reactive donor platelets
	Multiple electrode aggregometry	2–3 hours	Whole blood assay, limited availability
	Flow cytometry	2–3 hours	Recently introduced, promising test but needs standardization
	Serotonin-release assay	4–24 hours	Original gold standard, but radioisotope use limits availability

(ELISA: enzyme-linked immunosorbent assay)

for functional HIT testing, boasts high sensitivity and specificity. However, its reliance on radioactive isotopes and live platelets makes it labor-intensive and impractical for widespread use. Efforts are underway to develop alternative methods, such as high-performance liquid chromatography, ELISA, and flow cytometry, to circumvent the need for radioactive materials.

When combined with 4T score, rapid screening tests may effectively exclude many HIT cases, especially in peripheral centers with limited resources. Automated assays such as latex-based immunoassays and CLIAs provide rapid, reliable results, and are ideal for primary diagnostic workflows. Functional assays, though highly accurate, are reserved for confirmation in expert centers.

For diagnosing VITT, immunoassays beyond ELISA have limited utility. While rapid assays like CLIA are sensitive for HIT, they lack specificity for VITT. Functional assays modified for VITT, such as PF4-enhanced platelet activation assays and PF4-enhanced SRAs, offer greater sensitivity and are better suited for this condition.

Take Home Points

Heparin-induced Thrombocytopenia

- The HIT is a prothrombotic, immune-mediated disorder caused by antibodies against the complex of PF4 and heparin.
- The interaction between PF4, heparin, and anti-PF4-heparin antibodies leads to activation of platelets, thrombin generation, and a hypercoagulable state. Monocytes, neutrophils, and endothelial cells amplify the thrombosis process.
- Use of the "4Ts" or HEP scores to assess pretest probability. Scores ≥ 4 warrant laboratory testing and discontinuation of heparin.
- The screening by immunoassays and confirmation by functional assays are needed for the diagnosis.

Vaccine-induced Thrombosis and Thrombocytopenia

- VITT is associated with COVID-19 vaccines and involves anti-PF4 antibodies with heparin-independent mechanism for platelet activation.
- It primarily affects healthy individuals 5–30 days postvaccination, leading to thrombocytopenia, elevated D-dimer levels, and thrombosis at atypical sites.
- Formation of PF4-dependent antigens triggered by vaccine components or excipients, leads to robust anti-PF4 antibody production and a hypercoagulable state.
- In addition to ELISA, functional assays modified for VITT, such as PF4-enhanced platelet activation or SRAs, provide higher specificity.

SUGGESTED READINGS

1. Salter BS, Weiner MM, Trinh MA, Heller J, Evans AS, Adams DH, et al. Heparin-induced thrombocytopenia. J Am Coll Cardiol. 2016;67(21):2519-32.
2. Arachchillage DJ, Thachil J, Anderson JAM, Baker P, Poles A, Kitchen S, et al. Diagnosis and management of heparin-induced thrombocytopenia: Third edition. Br J Haematol. 2024;204(2):459-75.
3. Warkentin TE. Platelet-activating anti-PF4 disorders: An overview. Semin Hematol. 2022; 59(2):59-71.
4. Rauova L, Poncz M, McKenzie SE, Reilly MP, Arepally G, Weisel JW, et al. Ultralarge complexes of PF4 and heparin are central to the pathogenesis of heparin-induced thrombocytopenia. Blood. 2005;105(1):131-8.
5. Greinacher A, Warkentin TE. Platelet factor 4 triggers thrombo-inflammation by bridging innate and adaptive immunity. Int J Lab Hematol. 2023;45(S2):11-22.
6. Marchetti M, Zermatten MG, Bertaggia Calderara D, Aliotta A, Alberio L. Heparin-induced thrombocytopenia: A review of new concepts in pathogenesis, diagnosis, and management. J Clin Med. 2021;10(4):683.
7. Zhang Y, Bissola AL, Treverton J, Hack M, Lychacz M, Kwok S, et al. Vaccine-induced immune thrombotic thrombocytopenia: Clinicopathologic features and new perspectives on Anti-PF4 antibody-mediated disorders. J Clin Med. 2024;13(4):1012.
8. Warkentin TE, Greinacher A. Laboratory testing for heparin-induced thrombocytopenia and vaccine-induced immune thrombotic thrombocytopenia antibodies: A narrative review. Semin Thromb Hemost. 2022;49(6):621-33.

CHAPTER 17

Direct Oral Anticoagulants: When to Prescribe and How to Monitor?

Gurpreet Kaur, Renjith Mathew Verghese, Dinesh Chandra

ABSTRACT

Direct oral anticoagulants (DOACs) have are increasing being used as attractive alternatives to vitamin K antagonists. They revolutionized anticoagulant management and are the cornerstone treatment for stroke prevention in atrial fibrillation (AF) and venous thromboembolism (VTE) prophylaxis and treatment, and the list of other usages is fast expanding. Since they were first approved in 2010, DOACs have emerged as leading therapeutic alternatives being effective, safe and convenient to use. While the usage of DOACS increases clinicians are are faced with complex decision as to the usage of an appropriate DOAC, the time duration and the use in certain specific scenarios. This chapter provides an overview of DOACs to optimize DOAC use among common challenging situations and their monitoring as and where needed.

INTRODUCTION

Venous thromboembolism (VTE) includes deep vein thrombosis (DVT) and pulmonary embolism (PE). The incidence estimate is ~2 per 1,000 first events every year in the West, and it is a major cause of morbidity and mortality. Anticoagulant therapy with fast-acting drugs to prevent thrombus extension and its complications is the treatment of choice for acute VTE, followed by extended prophylaxis to prevent recurrence. In current-day practice, we initially use unfractionated heparin (UFH) or low-molecular-weight heparin (LMWH), which is given parenterally. Oral anticoagulants such as vitamin K antagonists (VKAs) provide extended anticoagulation. Newer direct-acting oral anticoagulants have been introduced in recent years, with more under development. These may soon replace VKAs, both for treatment purpose and for prophylaxis. Direct thrombin inhibitors (DTIs) and direct factor Xa inhibitors are two classes of direct oral anticoagulants (DOACs) that block the dominant steps of fibrin clot formation. DOACs such as dabigatran, rivaroxaban, apixaban, edoxaban, and betrixaban are both safe and efficacious. DOACs act in a direct and selective manner, reversibly inhibiting factors IIa or Xa. Their coagulation effect is in sync with the plasma concentration–time profile of the respective anticoagulants. DOACs have a short half-life, and this may be a constraint on daily intake. DOACs do not require monitoring except in specific scenarios due to the predictable pharmacokinetic and pharmacodynamic responses at a fixed dose. Their predictable pharmacokinetic and pharmacodynamic responses at a fixed dose are the reason that monitoring may not be required except in certain scenarios. The knowledge of the individual characteristics, risks, and benefits of DOACs is essential for their appropriate usage.

MECHANISM OF ACTION

Thrombin or factor IIa is the last enzyme of the clotting cascade and results from the proteolytic cleavage of prothrombin by factor Xa. Thrombin cleaves fibrinogen to fibrin and also leads to activation of other coagulation factors, i.e., XI, V, VIII, and XIII and also activates the platelets.

DTIs attach to the active site of the thrombin enzyme. Thrombin is active in both in circulation and its clot-bound form. DTIs inhibit the action of both circulating and clot-bound thrombin as their binding site is not obscured by fibrin, while heparin inactivates only circulating thrombin. Inhibition of factor Xa prevents amplification of the thrombin generation by the thrombin burst as 1,000 molecules of prothrombin are cleaved to thrombin by a single molecule of factor Xa. No cofactor is needed for the binding of direct factor Xa inhibitors to the active site of factor Xa. These drugs also inhibit the activity of both forms of factor Xa, compared to heparin and fondaparinux, which via antithrombin are only able to inactivate circulating factor Xa.

RECENT ICSH RECOMMENDATIONS FOR LABORATORY MEASUREMENT OF DIRECT ORAL ANTICOAGULANTS

The International Council for Standardization in Hematology (ICSH) issued guidelines for laboratory monitoring of DOACs in the year 2018. The key recommendations are as follows:

- Testing on citrated whole blood samples within 4 hours of sample collection for dabigatran and within 8 hours for anti-Xa agents.
- Prothrombin time (PT) and activated partial thromboplastin time (APTT) should not be used routinely to quantify the concentrations of DOACs.
- DOAC levels should be reported in ng/mL units.
- "Therapeutic range" concentrations differ significantly, and monitoring routinely is not recommended due to their wide therapeutic ranges.
- In situations such as bleeding, urgent invasive procedure, thrombolysis, and recurrence of thromboembolism, tests for quantifying DOAC should be performed.

- If nonemergent testing is necessary (elective invasive procedure, overdose without complication, and drug compliance), trough drug level assessment is recommended.
- Liquid chromatography-mass spectrometry/mass spectrometry (LC-MS/MS) is the "gold standard" for measuring DOAC concentration.
- However, due to the several limitations of mass spectrometry, drug-calibrated assays that have shown comparable results are recommended for the quantification of DOACs.
- In an emergency, measuring DOAC levels guides the decisions regarding reversal and optimal timing of interventions.

Indications for monitoring the DOACs are as follows:
- *Outpatient department*: Morbidly obese patients, postbariatric surgery, extremely low body weight, end-stage renal disease (ESRD), and patients on drugs that can potentiate DOACs.
- *Emergency*: Patients needing an invasive procedure are bleeding, with thromboembolism while on therapy or with ischemic stroke intervention.

When monitoring for DOAC levels, consider the time when the patient received the last dose. If assessing absorption, peak levels are important, while trough levels are used to evaluate clearance, such as in older patients, in renal failure, and in liver failure.

QUANTITATIVE ASSAYS FOR ESTIMATING DIRECT ORAL ANTICOAGULANT LEVELS

The important factors to be kept in mind while estimating DOAC effect are: (A) The type of DOAC, (B) patient's kidney and liver function (C) medical records and clinical history, (D) risk of bleeding depending on the procedure to be done, and (E) the timing of last dose of DOAC.

Liquid Chromatography-tandem Mass Spectrometry

Liquid chromatography-mass spectrometry/mass spectrometry and functional assays are used for quantitative estimation of the plasma concentrations of DOACs. LC-MS/MS can asses the drug levels without the need for calibration. It is highly specific and sensitive with the limit of detection (LoD) and a limit of quantitation (LoQ) being 0.025–3 ng/mL. The analytical range varies from 5 to 500 ng/mL for all DOACs, making the quantitation of both the peaks and trough levels. The disadvantages of LC-MS/MS are: It is labor intensive, there are preparatory steps, the technique is complex, and instrument availability may be an issue. Potential problems are: Other substances such as drugs, xenobiotics that may coelute with DOACs, the need for internal standard preparation, and the technique may be unable to detect drug metabolites. A universal calibration standard or international reference is lacking, and this is a potential area of concern.

Functional Assays

Functional assays are recommended and correlate well with the LC-MS/MS assay. The advantage is an easy applicability of these in routine clinical laboratories. Currently in use methods for dabigatran are the ecarin clotting time (ECT) and the ecarin chromogenic assay (ECA), calibration with the appropriate standard is essential in all the mentioned assays. Ecarin venom-based assays are accurate, and here the venom converts prothrombin to meizothrombin that is further neutralized by dabigatran. The endpoint of this tests is detected by a clot-based assay, ECT, where free meizothrombin causes conversion of fibrinogen to a fibrin clot. The caveat is that results are affected by low prothrombin and fibrinogen concentrations in the patient's plasma. The second test, ECA, uses a reagent containing prothrombin. The meizothrombin acts upon a chromogenic substrate giving a color there, and this is unaffected by fibrinogen concentration. Chromogenic anti-FIIa assay and dilute TT have also been used for monitoring dabigatran. Dilute TT-based assays are also very accurate in the measurement of dabigatran concentration. All the above assays use commercially synthesized dabigatran calibrators and controls and have measurable ranges very similar to LC-MS.

Direct factor Xa inhibitors may be assessed using anti-Xa assays calibrated to the particular drug. When a critical surgery is planned, such as neurosurgery, spinal surgery, a routine heparin anti-Xa assay may guide the use of either a specific reversal agent (andexanet) or nonspecific agents such as prothrombin complex concentrate (PCC).

Newer Techniques for Monitoring Direct Oral Anticoagulants

Viscoelastic testing (TEG® and ROTEM®) and thrombin generation assays have been used for DOACs. Viscoelastic tests have variable data for DOAC monitoring and, therefore, are not currently recommended for their monitoring.

■ IMPACT OF DIRECT ORAL ANTICOAGULANTS ON COAGULATION ASSAYS

The screening coagulogram parameters (APTT, PT, and TT) are affected variably depending on the DOACs, as mentioned above. Fibrinogen activity, particularly the Clauss assay, is unaffected by DOACs except sporadically spurious hypofibrinogenemia at very high plasma concentration of dabigatran. Immunoassays for D-dimers remain unaffected by DOACs. Lupus anticoagulant (LA) testing is, however, affected by even low concentrations of DOACs. Both dilute Russell's viper venom time (DRVVT) and APTT-LA assays may yield false-positive LA results as DOACs inhibit FXa or FIIa. Clot-based assays such as protein C, protein S, antithrombin, and activated protein C resistance ratio may also have falsely elevated values, leading to misdiagnosis. Chromogenic assays for measurement of protein C, immunoturbidimetry-based free and total protein S antigens are alternatives that are not affected by DOACs. Molecular assays, enzyme-linked immunosorbent assay (ELISA), or immunoassays are also not influenced by DOACs. Anti-β2 glycoprotein-I, anticardiolipin antibodies for LA, and von Willebrand factor (vWF) antigen levels are also unaffected by DOACs.

STRATEGIES TO MINIMIZE DIRECT ORAL ANTICOAGULANT INTERFERENCE ON THE COAGULATION TEST RESULTS

When using a clot-based assay, it is important that DOAC activity is negated or minimized to avoid false-positive results. The following steps may be taken for the same:

- Discontinue the DOAC at least 48–72 hours prior to testing, depending on the renal function. If there is a patient at a high risk of thrombosis, this may not be feasible, and bridging therapy with heparin is required. LMWH is the drug of choice for patients, requiring bridging on dabigatran. While using an anti-Xa DOAC, this challenge remains as APTT and anti-Xa activity can be prolonged by both the DOAC and LMWH, leading to supratherapeutic levels.
- Testing at expected trough concentration of DOAC.
- DOAC-stop® (Haematex, Hornsby, NSW, Australia) and DOAC-remove® (5-Diagnostics, Quadratech, Switzerland) are options that adsorb DOAC from plasma, thereby nullifying their effects. They have activated charcoal-containing adsorbent compounds. The usage of these agents reduces false-positive LA and interference with clot-based hemostasis assays.

INDICATIONS FOR DIRECT ORAL ANTICOAGULANT USE

In the current era due to major advantages of DOACs over VKAs such as lack of monitorings and stable pharmacology, DOACs have outscored the conventional VKAs in most of the fields except a few. The major indications are VTE prophylaxis and treatment of VTE. Exceptions where DOACs are not the preferred anticoagulants include valvular atrial fibrillation (AF), triple-positive antiphospholipid syndrome, and prosthetic valves.

Atrial Fibrillation and Artificial Heart Valves

Coexistence of valvular heart disease and AF contributes to thromboembolic events and mortality. Valvular AF is the presence of a mechanical prosthetic heart valve or moderate-to-severe mitral stenosis, both of which can increase thromboembolic risk significantly. As per ACCP and ACC/AHA guidelines, VKA remains the preferred agent for this subset of patients. Numerous ongoing studies have shown that the use of DOACs is noninferior to conventional VKAs in patients with bioprosthetic valves.

For secondary prevention of atherosclerotic cardiovascular disease (ASCVD), the use of aspirin is well-established and is widely recommended by major clinical guidelines for indefinite use. Efforts to improve upon the ASCVD risk reduction witnessed with aspirin monotherapy, prior investigations evaluated more potent antiplatelets and VKA therapy as alternatives to aspirin and as add-on therapy with aspirin. This attempt was offset by increased bleeding risk with no major effect on mortality rates. In 2018, the results of the COMPASS trial led to FDA approval of low-dose rivaroxaban with aspirin in patients with acute coronary syndrome (ACS) undergoing percutaneous intervention (PCI), with a significant benefit of the combination in reduction of major cardiovascular events.

Cancer-associated Venous Thromboembolism

Patients with malignancies are at an increased risk for VTE, arterial thrombo-embolic, and bleeding events. Anticoagulating patients with active malignancy are tricky due to multiple issues such as renal failure, deranged liver functions, very high incidence of nausea and vomiting, malnutrition and cachexia, major drug interactions with cytotoxic agents, and targeted therapies which can hamper drug absorption, apart from these listed causes there is high risk of bleeding due to thrombocytopenia, which may be disease or therapy related and patient preferences. Based on the ADAM VTE trial for apixaban revealed no major bleeding events and significant risk reduction of thrombotic events, which led DOACs to become part of the therapeutic armamentarium in active cancer-associated (Ca)-VTE. Patients with gastrointestinal (GI) malignancies and upper or unresected lower GI tumors may have an erratic absorption of DOACs and are at high risk of bleeding; LMWH may be preferred. Due to their obvious benefits, major guidelines now endorse the use of DOACs in Ca-VTE treatment and its prophylaxis in patients.

COMORBIDITIES AFFECTING PHARMACOKINETICS OF DIRECT ORAL ANTICOAGULANTS

Comorbidities that alter the systemic exposure or elimination kinetics lead to the risk of thrombohemorrhagic events. The three most pertinent patient comorbidities are extreme body weights, renal and hepatic impairment.

Extreme Body Weights

In patients with extreme ends of body weight, numerous concerns have cropped up with the use of DOACs, which may lead to alterations in pharmacokinetics and pharmacodynamics. In the landmark trials on DOAC usage, there is a gross underrepresentation of patients with extreme-body-weight populations.

Renal Dysfunction

Patients are at increased risk for thromboembolic and bleeding events. Dabigatran has the most renal excretion, which accounts for 80%, followed by edoxaban, rivaroxaban, apixaban, and betrixaban. The Cockcroft–Gault creatinine clearance (CrCl) equation of renal function is used to derive adjusted doses of most DOACs.

The least renal clearance is exhibited by apixaban; there are uncertain clinical recommendations with varying recommendations regarding dose adjustment, and in severe renal impairment, apixaban is the agent of choice.

Hepatic Impairment

Liver function impairment alters the drug biotransformation to varying extents. Apixaban is heavily dependent on hepatic metabolism for elimination, accounting for more than two-thirds of elimination, which is followed by rivaroxaban, edoxaban, dabigatran, and betrixaban metabolism. All DOACs can be safely used in patients with mild liver dysfunction, and they are contraindicated in patients with severe hepatic dysfunction.

ANTICOAGULANT TRANSITIONING

Clinical scenarios may arise that require transitioning to or off DOACs. The most common two scenarios we encounter in daily practice and require adjustments are as follows:

1. *Switching between anticoagulants*: In daily practice, there can be a transition from one to another anticoagulant because of patient preference, financial constraints, comorbid conditions, concurrent hospitalization, thrombotic and bleeding complications, or emergency or elective procedures.
   The half-life (t1/2) of the VKA guides the transitioning from a VKA to a DOAC. Since warfarin is used widely across the globe, with a t1/2 of 48 hours, warfarin needs to be stopped and international normalized ratio (INR) to be rechecked after 72 hours. Once the INR is <2, DOACs can be initiated. When transitioning from DOAC to VKA, DOACs are to be administered concomitantly with VKAs as VKAs have a slow onset of action ranging from 5 to 10 days. Careful INR monitoring between days 3 and 5 of VKA therapy is recommended.
2. *Procedural management*: Previous guidelines on peri- and postoperative management for patients on DOACs were primarily based on surgical risk, the pharmacokinetic profile of DOACs, concurrent medications, and patient characteristics. Preoperative assessment of hemostasis is useful, especially in high-risk interventions. However, for most patients undergoing elective procedures, interruption of DOAC therapy can be substantiated on a time-based approach with consideration of the procedure's bleeding risk and renal function.

Reversal Agents

With an aging population, an increase in the number of interventions, and device applications, the number of patients requiring long-term oral anticoagulation is increasing. In DOAC-anticoagulated patients, the overall bleeding risk is lower. However, they may develop serious bleeding or need urgent surgery. In principle, reversal can be achieved by specific antidotes such as idarucizumab or andexanet alfa, or unspecific hemostatic agents used to enhance the hemostatic function of the coagulation system, such as PCC, activated PCC (aPCC), or recombinant factor VIIa (rFVIIa).

In resource-limited settings like ours, where the availability and affordability of reversal agent is not feasible, the use of activated charcoal in patients with oral intake within the first 2–4 hours of intake of rivaroxaban, apixaban, and dabigatran is recommended. Hemodialysis can also be considered for patients on dabigatran.

Take Home Points

- Direct oral anticoagulants have revolutionized anticoagulant management and have become the treatment of choice for stroke prevention in AF and VTE prophylaxis and treatment.
- While selecting the appropriate DOAC, comorbidities should be kept in mind, including renal and hepatic function, along with compliance of patient should also be considered.
- Routine laboratory monitoring in DOAC-treated cases is not required, except in certain clinical scenarios.
- It must be remembered that DOACs interfere with clot-based coagulation assays.
- Reversal agents are useful tools to neutralize DOAC anticoagulant activity in case of major bleeding or urgent surgery/invasive procedure.

SUGGESTED READINGS

1. Ansell J, Hirsh J, Hylek E, Jacobson A, Crowther M, Palareti G. Pharmacology and management of the vitamin K antagonists: American College of Chest Physicians Evidence-based Clinical Practice Guidelines (8th edition). Chest. 2008;133:160S-98S.
2. Conway SE, Hwang AY, Ponte CD, Gums JG. Laboratory and clinical monitoring of direct acting oral anticoagulants: What clinicians need to know. Pharmacotherapy. 2017;37(2): 236-48.
3. Ruff CT, Giugliano RP, Braunwald E, Hoffman EB, Deenadayalu N, Ezekowitz MD, et al. Comparison of the Efficacy and Safety of New Oral Anticoagulants with Warfarin in Patients with Atrial Fibrillation: A Meta-analysis of Randomised Trials. Lancet Lond Engl. 2014;383:955-62.
4. Kearon C, Akl EA, Ornelas J, Blaivas A, Jimenez D, Bounameaux H, et al. Antithrombotic Therapy for VTE Disease: CHEST Guideline and Expert Panel Report. Chest. 2016;149: 315-52.
5. Aronis KN, Hylek EM. Evidence Gaps in the Era of Non-Vitamin K Oral Anticoagulants. J Am Heart Assoc. 2018;7:e007338.
6. Perzborn E, Strassburger J, Wilmen A, Pohlmann J, Roehrig S, Schlemmer KH, et al. In Vitro and in Vivo Studies of the Novel Antithrombotic Agent BAY 59-7939—An Oral, Direct Factor Xa Inhibitor. J Thromb Haemost. 2005;3:514-21.
7. Gosselin RC, Adcock DM, Bates SM, Douxfils J, Favaloro EJ, Gouin-Thibault I, et al. International Council for Standardization in Haematology (ICSH) recommendations for laboratory measurement of direct oral anticoagulants. Thromb Haemost. 2018;118(3):437-50.
8. Douxfils J, Ageno W, Samama CM, Lessire S, Ten Cate H, Verhamme P, et al. Laboratory testing in patients treated with direct oral anticoagulants: a practical guide for clinicians. J Thromb Haemost. 2018;16(2):209-19.

9. Cuker A, Siegal DM, Crowther MA, Garcia DA, et al. Laboratory measurement of the anticoagulant activity of the nonvitamin K oral anticoagulants. J Am Coll Cardiol. 2014;64:1128-39.
10. Pfrepper C, Metze M, Siegemund A, Klöter T, Siegemund T, Petros S. Direct oral anticoagulant plasma levels and thrombin generation on ST Genesia system. Res Pract Thromb Haemost. 2020;4(4):619-27.
11. Harenberg J, Schreiner R, Hetjens S, Weiss C. Detecting anti-IIa and anti-Xa direct oral anticoagulant (DOAC) agents in urine using a DOAC dipstick. Semin Thromb Hemost. 2019;4(3):275-84.
12. Tsakiris DA. Direct oral anticoagulants–interference with laboratory tests and mechanism of action. Semin Hematol. 2014;51(2):98-101.
13. Schmitz EMH, Boonen K, van den Heuvel DJA, van Dongen JLJ, Schellings MWM, Emmen JMA, et al. Determination of dabigatran, rivaroxaban and apixaban by ultra-performance liquid chromatography—tandem mass spectrometry (UPLC-MS/MS) and coagulation assays for therapy monitoring of novel direct oral anticoagulants. J Thromb Haemost. 2014;12(10):1636-46.
14. Molenaar PJ, Dinkelaar J, Leyte A. Measuring rivaroxaban in a clinical laboratory setting, using common coagulation assays, Xa inhibition and thrombin generation. Clin Chem Lab Med. 2012;50:1799-807.
15. Samama MM, Martinoli JL, Le Flem L, Guinet C, Plu-Bureau G, Depasse F, et al. Assessment of laboratory assays to measure rivaroxaban, an oral, direct factor Xa inhibitor. Thromb Haemost. 2010;103:815-25.
16. Skeppholm M, Al-Aieshy F, Berndtsson M, Al-Khalili F, Ronquist-Nii Y, Soderblom L. Clinical evaluation of laboratory methods to monitor apixaban treatment in patients with atrial fibrillation. Thromb Res. 2015;136:148-53.
17. Dias JD, Norem K, Doorneweerd DD, Thurer RL, Popovsky MA, Omert LA. Use of thromboelastography (TEG) for detection of new oral anticoagulants. Arch Pathol Lab Med. 2015;139:665-73.
18. Adelmann D, Wiegele M, Wohlgemuth RK, Koch S, Frantal S, Quehenberger P, et al. Measuring the activity of apixaban and rivaroxaban with rotational thromboelastometry. Thromb Res. 2014;134:918-23.
19. Helin TA, Pakkanen A, Lassila R, Joutsi-Korhonen L. Effects of apixaban on prothrombin time, activated partial thromboplastin time and anti-Xa assays: a European survey. Clin Chem Lab Med. 2017;55(8):e178-80.
20. Favresse J, Lardinois B, Sabor L, Devalet B, Vandepapeliere J, Braibant M, et al. Evaluation of the DOAC-stop® procedure to overcome the effect of DOACs on several thrombophilia screening tests. TH open companion. J Thromb Haemost. 2018;2(2):e202-9.
21. Chen A, Stecker E, Warden BA. Direct Oral Anticoagulant Use: A Practical Guide to Common Clinical Challenges. J Am Heart Assoc. 2020;9(13):e017559.
22. Talamo L, Maitland HS, Palkimas S, White D. Safety of DOACs in Patients of Extreme Weight. Blood. 2016;128(22):1450.
23. Rogula S, Gąsecka A, Mazurek T, Navarese EP, Szarpak Ł, Filipiak KJ. Safety and Efficacy of DOACs in Patients with Advanced and End-Stage Renal Disease. Int J Environ Res Public Health. 2022;19(3):1436.
24. Mavrakanas TA. Direct oral anticoagulants: the safer choice in chronic kidney disease? Clin Kidney J. 2024;17(1).
25. Hydes TJ, Lip GYH, Lane DA. Use of Direct-Acting Oral Anticoagulants in Patients with Atrial Fibrillation and Chronic Liver Disease. 2023;147(10):795-7.
26. Tham D, Yu W, Zhao L, Kou R, Kherani J, Li PY, et al. Safety and Efficacy of Direct Oral Anticoagulants in Patients with Liver Cirrhosis: A Systematic Review and Meta-analysis. Blood. 2023;142 (Suppl 1):5534.
27. Wheelock KM, Ross JS, Murugiah K, Lin Z, Krumholz HM, Khera R. Clinician Trends in Prescribing Direct Oral Anticoagulants for US Medicare Beneficiaries. JAMA Netw Open. 2021;4(12):e2137288.

28. Roberti R, Iannone LF, Palleria C, Curcio A, Rossi M, Sciacqua A, et al. Direct Oral Anticoagulants: From Randomized Clinical Trials to Real-world Clinical Practice. Front Pharmacol. 2021;12:684638
29. Levy JH, Shaw JR, Castellucci LA, Connors JM, Douketis J, Lindhoff-Last E, et al. Reversal of direct oral anticoagulants: guidance from the SSC of the ISTH. J Thromb Haemost. 2024;22:2889-99.
30. Milling TJ, Pollack CV. A review of guidelines on anticoagulation reversal across different clinical scenarios – Is there a general consensus? Am J Emerg Med. 2020;38:1890-903.

CHAPTER 18

How to Approach a Case of Microcytic Hypochromic Anemia Not Responding to Iron Therapy

Swetha Palla, Prateek Bhatia

ABSTRACT

Anemic children are frequently encountered in the outpatient clinics and it is a serious public health concern in our country. Its prevalence ranges from 40 to 67% in children < 5 years of age and has increased from 59 to 67% in the National Family Health Survey-5 (NFHS-5). Iron deficiency anemia is the most prevalent subtype, accounting for one-third of all cases. As a result, physicians often initiate a trial of oral iron supplementation and assess the response in patients with microcytic hypochromic anemia, even without a baseline iron profile. A lack of response to oral iron therapy causes apprehension among parents and pediatricians alike. These cases often go neglected due to the absence of a structured testing approach, leading to delays in diagnosis. Consequently, patients receive repeated cycles of iron supplementation without any improvement.

The most common causes of poor response to oral iron include noncompliance, inadequate dosing, intolerance to oral iron, malabsorption, ongoing blood loss, etc. Occasionally, alternative etiologies may arise, such as thalassemia, sideroblastic anemia, and iron refractory iron deficiency anemia (IRIDA). Many of these conditions are misdiagnosed or underdiagnosed in iron-deficient setting due to a lack of awareness among physicians and insufficient testing. This review outlines the approach to anemia in children who fail to respond to oral iron therapy. Practical points in history, examination, investigations, and management are discussed.

INTRODUCTION

Iron is an essential element for numerous physiological processes, serving as a key component of proteins and enzymes. It plays a critical role in oxygen transport through hemoglobin (Hb), catalyzes redox reactions as part of various enzymes, and is vital for neurocognitive development in young children. The human body contains 4–5 g of iron, with approximately 75% (around 3 g) actively utilized—

primarily in Hb (2.5 g) and other proteins (0.5 g). The remaining iron is stored in the form of ferritin and hemosiderin (around 1 g). A small fraction (3–4 mg) circulates in the plasma, bound to transferrin.

Since the human body lacks a mechanism for iron excretion, iron homeostasis is primarily regulated at the level of absorption by duodenal enterocytes. Hepcidin, a peptide hormone secreted by hepatocytes, acts as the master regulator of iron metabolism. It binds to the iron exporter ferroportin on the basolateral membrane of enterocytes and macrophages, triggering its degradation. This process prevents iron release into circulation and limits redistribution from stores. Hepcidin production increases in states of iron overload or inflammation and decreases during iron deficiency, ensuring tight regulation of iron levels.

DEFINITIONS (AS GIVEN BY WORLD HEALTH ORGANIZATION)

- *Anemia*: Defined as Hb of < 110 g/L in children aged 0.5–4.9 years and Hb < 115 g/L in those aged 5–12 years of age.
- *Iron deficiency*: Defined as a ferritin of < 12 μg/L in children < 5 years and < 15 μg/L in those 5–12 years without evidence of any anemia or fall in Hb below normal standard range.
- *Iron deficiency anemia (IDA):* Defined as Hb < 110 g/L with a ferritin < 12 μg/L in children < 5 years and Hb <115 g/L with a ferritin < 15 μg/L in children 5–12 years.

IRON DEFICIENCY ANEMIA

Iron deficiency anemia results from the interplay of three distinct risk factors: increased iron requirements, inadequate intake (due to poor dietary habits, low bioavailability, or malabsorption), and increased blood loss. A complete blood count (CBC) with red blood cell (RBC) indices and a peripheral smear can identify most cases. The condition is typically characterized by microcytic, hypochromic RBCs, along with the presence of anisopoikilocytosis, elliptocytes, and cigar-shaped cells on the smear. Treatment often begins with a trial of 3–4 mg/kg/day of elemental iron, administered in one or two divided doses, with a maximum daily dose of 200 mg. An adequate therapeutic response is indicated by a rise in Hb of at least 1 g/dL after 4 weeks of oral iron therapy.

The most common cause of failure to respond to oral iron therapy is improper dosing, administration errors, or poor compliance. Other common causes of microcytic hypochromic anemia that do not respond to iron therapy are summarized in **Box 1**. These cases represent an important subgroup of patients that require detailed evaluation to establish an accurate diagnosis. Approach to a case of microcytic anemia is shown in **Flowcharts 1 and 2**. Key practical considerations in history, examination, investigations, and management are outlined in the following text.

BOX 1: Common causes of microcytic anemia that fail to respond to oral iron therapy.

- Gastrointestinal (GI) malabsorption states (celiac disease, Crohn's disease, Giardiasis)
- Medications (proton pump inhibitors, histamine type 2 blocking agents)
- Ongoing blood loss (gastrointestinal, respiratory, urinary, and menstrual)
- Thalassemia
- Hereditary pyropoikilocytosis (HPP)
- Sideroblastic anemia
- Iron refractory iron deficiency anemia (IRIDA)
- Other rare hereditary microcytic anemias (aceruloplasminemia, hypotransferrinemia, *DMT1* mutation, and *STEAP3* mutation)
- Lead poisoning, copper deficiency

Q. Does the child have microcytic (MCV < 65 fl), hypochromic (MCH < 20 pg) anemia?

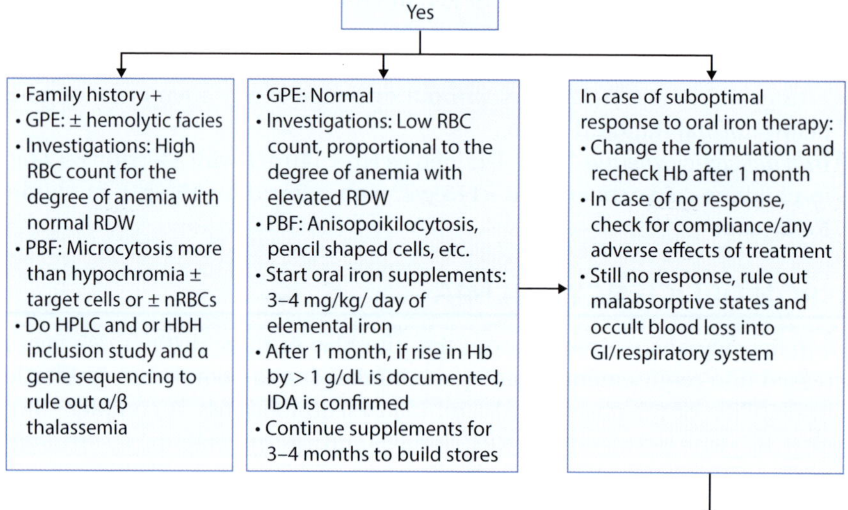

Iron profile—if suggestive of classic IDA with no/suboptimal response to therapy, following conditions need to be ruled out (Hershko et al.):

- Celiac disease—tTG IgA Abs, anti-DGP Abs, endoscopy and biopsy
- *Helicobacter pylori* gastritis—IgG Abs in the serum, urease breath test
- Autoimmune gastritis—antibodies against parietal cells/intrinsic factor
- GI blood loss—stool for occult blood, endoscopy, Meckel scan, RBC scan, CT angiography of abdomen
- Pulmonary blood loss—chest X-ray, CT chest, GL/BAL for hemosiderin laden macrophages

FLOWCHART 1: Approach to a case of microcytic hypochromic anemia.

(BAL: bronchoalveolar lavage; CT: computed tomography; DGP Abs: antideamidated gliadin peptide antibodies; GI: gastrointestinal; HbH: hemoglobin H disease; HPLC: high pressure liquid chromatography; IDA: iron deficiency anemia; MCH: mean corpuscular hemoglobin; MCV: mean corpuscular volume; PBF: peripheral blood film; RBC: red blood cell; RDW: red cell distribution width; tTG IgA Abs: tissue transglutaminase immunoglobulin A antibodies)

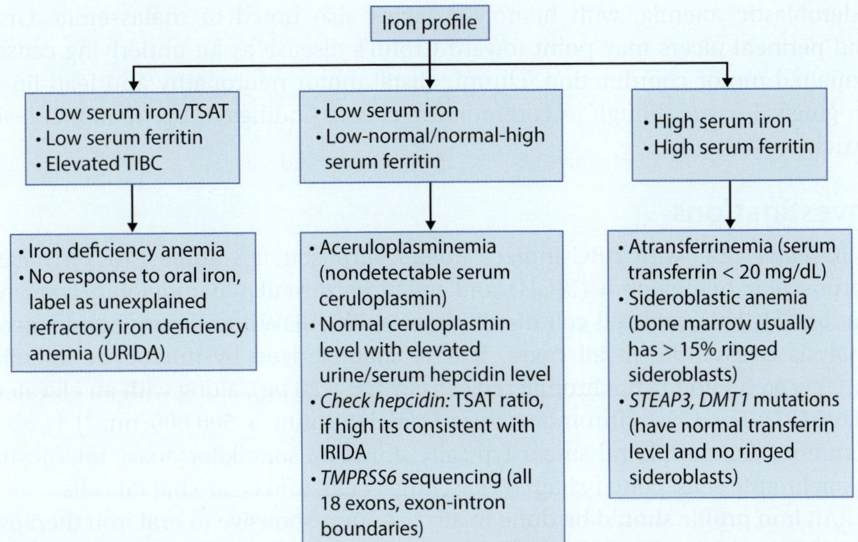

FLOWCHART 2: Approach to a case of microcytic hypochromic anemia based on iron profile.
(IRIDA: iron refractory iron deficiency anemia; TIBC: total iron-binding capacity; TSAT: transferrin saturation)

Patient and Family History

The first step in evaluating nonresponsiveness to oral iron therapy is to confirm true refractoriness. A detailed personal and family history, along with an extended pedigree analysis, can provide valuable insights. Inherited microcytic disorders often have a positive family history, making a CBC with peripheral smear analysis of family members helpful. Many inherited cases exhibit microcytosis from birth, unlike acquired forms, so reviewing previous CBCs is essential.

It is also important to document the history and frequency of transfusions, as this provides information on the amount of iron introduced into the body and helps clarify the clinical phenotype. For instance, patients with IRIDA typically require only 2–3 transfusions per year or fewer in childhood, while those with the autosomal recessive form of sideroblastic anemia (caused by *SLC25A38* mutations) are transfusion-dependent. Notably, the severity of anemia in IRIDA often decreases with age, potentially reducing the need for treatment in adulthood. The presence of additional symptoms, such as altered bowel habits, may indicate a malabsorptive etiology. Endocrine complications resulting from inherent iron overload are often associated with *ALAS2* mutated sideroblastic anemia.

Physical Examination

Apart from pallor, physical examination is typically unremarkable. However, in cases of severe anemia, delayed growth and development may be observed. Hepatosplenomegaly is common in conditions such as thalassemia and sideroblastic anemia, with hemolytic facies also noted in thalassemia. Oral and perineal ulcers may point toward Crohn's disease as an underlying cause. Impaired motor coordination, chronic distal motor neuropathy and lead lines on gingival tissue though uncommon are classic findings in occupational lead toxicity.

Investigations

A baseline CBC with RBC indices [mean corpuscular volume (MCV), mean corpuscular hemoglobin (MCH) and mean corpuscular hemoglobin concentration (MCHC), and red cell distribution width (RDW)] and peripheral smear analysis is essential in all cases. IDA is characterized by microcytic anemia (MCV < 65 fL) and hypochromic red cells (MCH < 20 pg), along with an elevated RDW (RDW > 15%). Thrombocytosis (platelet count > 500,000/mm^3) is also common. The peripheral smear typically shows anisopoikilocytosis, microcytic hypochromic cells, pencil-shaped cells, target cells, and cigar-shaped cells.

An iron profile should be done in all cases unresponsive to oral iron therapy. The classic IDA profile includes low serum iron (< 50 μg/dL), low serum ferritin (< 12 μg/L in children under 5 years, < 15 μg/L in children aged 5–12 years), low transferrin saturation (< 16%), and elevated total iron-binding capacity (TIBC > 350–400 μg/dL).

If the iron profile confirms IDA but there is no response to therapy, occult blood loss from the gastrointestinal (GI) or respiratory tract should be investigated. Additionally, malabsorption disorders must be ruled out. The following step-wise diagnostic approaches can aid in identifying the underlying conditions:

- *Hemoglobinopathy screen:* Mandatory in all cases even if the hematological findings for trait are not evident on CBC and RBC indices (hypochromia is less and microcytosis is more compared to IDA and RBC count is high). This is so, since our country has regions for high endemicity of various hemoglobinopathies including thalassemias. Performing a baseline high pressure liquid chromatography (HPLC) is must and in absence of a raised HbA2 or any other abnormal Hb, attention should be paid to screen for a small early first minute peak suggestive of HbBarts/hemoglobin H disease (HbH) and hence α thalassemia. In such cases, one should subsequently perform parental CBCs, HPLC, and α-gene sequencing studies for confirmation.
- *Inflammatory disorders:* Acute or chronic inflammatory disorders might have associated concomitant ID or IDA and due to relatively higher cytokine levels, block optimal iron absorption via hepcidin axis. Hence, a baseline erythrocyte sedimentation rate (ESR) and or C-reactive protein (CRP) along with correlation to relevant history and clinical findings.
- *Celiac disease:* Common in North India; screen with immunoglobulin (Ig) A tissue transglutaminase (tTG-IgA) antibodies. If positive, confirm with antideamidated gliadin peptide (anti-DGP) antibodies and upper GI endoscopy with biopsy.
- *Helicobacter pylori gastritis:* Screen using serum IgG antibodies and urease breath test (limited pediatric evidence).

- *Autoimmune gastritis:* Diagnose using antiparietal cell and anti-intrinsic factor antibodies (limited pediatric evidence).
- *GI blood loss:* Test stool for occult blood on three consecutive days. If positive, perform upper/lower GI endoscopy to evaluate for inflammatory bowel disease or bleeding polyps, a Meckel scan for Meckel's diverticulum, and an abdominal computed tomography (CT) angiography to identify arteriovenous malformations. A 99m Tc-labeled RBC scan can also help localize bleeding sources.
- *Pulmonary blood loss:* In patients with chronic respiratory symptoms and IDA, perform a chest X-ray/CT chest to detect small nodules or coarse reticular opacities suggestive of pulmonary hemosiderosis, which may be primary or secondary (e.g., due to Goodpasture syndrome or celiac disease). Hemosiderin-laden macrophages can be identified via gastric lavage (GL) or bronchoalveolar lavage (BAL).
- *IRIDA workup:* Refer to section on IRIDA in the following text. Briefly, if iron profile is low (low serum iron and very low or undetectable serum transferrin saturation) similar to IDA except for ferritin which might be in low-normal or high range (due to prior transfusion or treatments), above etiologies are negative and compliance issues ruled out, then hepcidin testing must be done. Hepcidin testing is usually performed by enzyme-linked immunosorbent assay (ELISA) or mass spectrometry (MS) methods with latter being more specific to detect hepcidin-25 active isoform and with levels up to 2–3 times lower than those detected by ELISA methods. ELISA testing is relatively easier to perform and does not require costly instrumentation of MS, but due to lack of international standardized method, levels need to be interpreted with caution after establishing nomograms in healthy population based on age. Generally, adults have higher mean hepcidin levels (20–65 ng/mL) compared to pediatric cases (3–25 ng/mL).

If the iron profile is atypical and does not align with IDA, alternative diagnoses should be explored, as outlined in **Flowchart 2**.

IRON REFRACTORY IRON DEFICIENCY ANEMIA

IRIDA is caused by homozygous or compound heterozygous mutations in the *TMPRSS6* gene, which encodes the transmembrane serine protease matriptase-2. This protease cleaves hemojuvelin, suppressing hepcidin production. Hence, due to biallelic mutations in this gene, hemojuvelin is not cleaved, leaving it free to interact with bone morphogenetic protein receptor-II (BMPR-II) complex to increase hepcidin production. Thus, increased hepcidin levels in turn block iron absorption from the gut and recycling from macrophages.

IRIDA should be suspected in individuals with extreme microcytosis and hypochromia relative to the degree of anemia with a high RBC count and an early onset in life, though typically IRIDA does not present in neonatal or early infancy years. A positive family history may or may not be forthcoming but would require CBC and RBC indices-based screening in all members. The iron profile in IRIDA typically shows low serum iron and very low-undetectable transferrin saturation

(TSAT) with low-normal or elevated ferritin. High serum hepcidin levels with an increased hepcidin-to-TSAT ratio are also characteristic and considered relatively specific for the condition. Diagnosis can be established only through sequencing of all 18 exons and exon-intron boundaries of the *TMPRSS6* gene. Recent evidence does suggest role of monoallelic (heterozygous mutations affecting single *TMPRSS6* allele) pathogenic mutations to be linked with IRIDA phenotype and there are currently many case series as well as systematically evaluated small cohorts which highlight this association.

TMPRSS6 single nucleotide polymorphisms (SNPs) have also been shown to influence Hb and ferritin levels. Wainaina et al. in their systematic review concluded that there is a high frequency of rs855791 and rs4820268 SNPs in Asian population with a stronger negative association with Hb and ferritin. However, isolated SNPs cannot be classified as IRIDA, though they increase susceptibility to iron deficiency. Environmental factors, such as a diet low in bioavailable iron and a high inflammatory state burden, further exacerbate the condition.

As per recommendation guidelines regarding treatment of genetic causes of microcytic hypochromic anemias of iron metabolism, initial management approach in a case of IRIDA should typically involve initiation with high-dose oral iron (6–10 mg/kg/day) along with vitamin C (30–250 mg/day) for 6–8 weeks. Vitamin C is known to modulate iron absorption dynamics by upregulating ferroportin messenger ribonucleic acid (mRNA) synthesis and increased divalent metal-ion transporter-1 (DMT1) expression in enterocytes thereby partially overcoming the oral iron absorption blockage effect created due to high hepcidin levels. However, responses to such combination of oral iron and vitamin C therapy are variable and not usually sustained. The response needs to be monitored at 3–4 weeks with a CBC and a reticulocyte count, though with availability of reticulocyte indices like reticulocyte-Hb equivalent or reticulocyte Hb concentration (Ret-He or CHr), responses can be evaluated much earlier at 1 week as these markers give information on acute bioavailability of iron to bone marrow over past 2–3 days. In severe, nonresponsive cases, regular administration of parenteral iron (e.g., iron sucrose, iron dextran, or ferric carboxymaltose) may be necessary. The parenteral iron dose is calculated as follows—iron intravenous (IV) dose = Body weight in kg × 2.3 (Target Hb – Actual patient Hb) + 500 mg. If IV iron is required to be given, ferric carboxymaltose is usually the initial choice, especially in pediatric patients, at 20 mg/kg IV single dose, repeated at 3 weekly intervals. However, many patients experience a reduction in disease severity over time, potentially alleviating the need for continued iron supplementation, due to reduction in physiological iron requirements with age.

Rarely, certain noniron metabolism genetic disorders can have presentation similar to IRIDA, especially cases with autoimmune polyglandular endocrinopathies (*AIRE* gene mutations), that lead to anemia primarily due to antiparietal cell antibodies. In addition, cases of Ghosal hematodiaphyseal dysplasia (*TBXAS1* gene mutations), present with anemia that can be longstanding along with symptoms of bowing of legs and difficulty in walking. An imaging of long bones reveals dense bones and a bone marrow can show fibrosis. The anemia in this case does not respond to oral iron but to corticosteroids or nonsteroidal anti-inflammatory drugs (NSAIDs).

Take Home Points

- All cases of microcytic hypochromic anemia that do not respond to oral iron require a structured diagnostic approach to avoid delays in diagnosis and ensure appropriate therapy.
- A thorough patient and family history, detailed physical examination, and baseline investigations—including complete blood count (CBC) with red blood cell indices, reticulocyte count, and peripheral smear—provide valuable insights into the underlying etiology.
- Additional investigations required in such cases are outlined in **Flowcharts 1 and 2**.
- Iron-refractory iron deficiency anemia (IRIDA) is a distinct subset that may respond to high-dose oral iron combined with vitamin C. However, some cases are unresponsive to oral therapy and may require blood transfusions, although disease severity often decreases over time, reducing the need for transfusion support.

SUGGESTED READINGS

1. Sarna A, Porwal A, Ramesh S, Agrawal PK, Acharya R, Johnston R, et al. Characterisation of the types of anaemia prevalent among children and adolescents aged 1–19 years in India: a population-based study. Lancet Child Adolesc Health. 2020;4(7):515-25.
2. Singh SK, Lhungdim H, Shekhar C, Dwivedi LK, Pedgaonkar S, James KS. Key drivers of reversal of trend in childhood anaemia in India: evidence from Indian demographic and health surveys, 2016–21. BMC Public Health. 2023;23(1):1574.
3. Tripathi S, Pathak VK, Lahariya C. Key findings from NFHS-5 India report: Observing trends of health indicators between NFHS-4 and NFHS-5. J Family Med Prim Care. 2023;12(9): 1759-63.
4. Kliegman R, Stanton BF, St Geme JW, Schor NF. Nelson Textbook of Pediatrics, 20th edition. Vol. 1. Philadelphia: Elsevier; 2015.
5. WHO Scientific Group on Nutritional Anaemias & World Health Organization. Nutritional anaemias. Report of a WHO scientific group. World Health Organ Tech Rep Ser. 1968;405: 5-37.
6. Hershko C, Camaschella C. How I treat unexplained refractory iron deficiency anemia. Blood. 2014 ;123(3):326-33.
7. Camaschella C. How I manage patients with atypical microcytic anaemia. Br J Haematol. 2013;160(1):12-24.
8. Thappa S, Bhatia P, Jain R, Bharti B. Plasma hepcidin levels in healthy children: Review of current literature highlights limited studies. J Pediatr Hematol Oncol. 2019;41(3):238-42.
9. Bhatia P, Marathe R, Hegde A, Bhardwaj D, Jain R. Plasma hepcidin levels in healthy children from North India. Indian Pediatr. 2017;54(7):599-600.
10. Bhatia P, Jain R, Singh A. A structured approach to iron refractory iron deficiency anemia (IRIDA) diagnosis (SAID): The more is "SAID" about iron, the less it is. Pediatr Hematol Oncol J. 2017;2(2):48-53.
11. Athiyarath R, Shaktivel K, Abraham V, Singh D, Bondu JD, Chapla A, et al. Association of genetic variants with response to iron supplements in pregnancy. Genes Nutr. 2015;10(4):25.
12. Sharma P, Bhatia P, Singh M, Das R, Attri SV, Ghara N, et al. Genomics of iron refractory iron deficiency anemia phenotype reveals a spectrum of novel pathogenic biallelic and monoallelic TMPRSS6 variants and rare overlapping disorders. Gene. 2024;895:147981.

13. Donker AE, Schaap CC, Novotny VM, Smeets R, Peters TM, van den Heuvel BL, et al. Iron refractory iron deficiency anemia: a heterogeneous disease that is not always iron refractory. Am J Hematol. 2016;91(12):E482-E490.
14. Gichohi-Wainaina WN, Towers GW, Swinkels DW, Zimmermann MB, Feskens EJ, Melse-Boonstra A. Inter-ethnic differences in genetic variants within the transmembrane protease, serine 6 (TMPRSS6) gene associated with iron status indicators: a systematic review with meta-analyses. Genes Nutr. 2015;10(1):442.
15. Donker AE, Raymakers RAP, Vlasveld LT, Van Barneveld T, Terink R, Dors N, et al. Practice guidelines for the diagnosis and management of microcytic anemias due to genetic disorders of iron metabolism or heme synthesis. Blood. 2014;123(25):3873-86.
16. De Falco L, Sanchez M, Silvestri L, Kannengiesser C, Muckenthaler MU, Iolascon A, et al. Iron refractory iron deficiency anemia. Haematologica. 2013;98(6):845-53.
17. Sourabh S, Bhatia P, Jain R. Favourable improvement in haematological parameters in response to oral iron and vitamin C combination in children with Iron Refractory Iron Deficiency Anemia (IRIDA) phenotype. Blood Cells Mol Dis. 2019;75:26-9.
18. Khuong-Quang DA, Schwartzentruber J, Westerman M, Lepage P, Finberg KE, Majewski J, et al. Iron refractory iron deficiency anemia: Presentation with hyperferritinemia and response to oral iron therapy. Pediatrics. 2013;131(2):e620-5.

CHAPTER 19

Measurable Residual Disease in B-cell Acute Lymphoblastic Leukemia: What is Known and What is New?

Khaliqur Rahman

ABSTRACT

Measurable residual disease (MRD) assessment has become an indispensable tool in the risk stratification and therapeutic monitoring of B-cell acute lymphoblastic leukemia (B-ALL). It stands as an independent prognostic and prediction tool in B-ALL. Traditionally, flow cytometry and molecular methods, especially the quantitative PCR targeting Ig/TCR rearrangements have been used with a sensitivity ranging from 10^{-4} to 10⁻6. Both these methods have their own advantages and limitations. FCM has a higher applicability and yields a rapid result. On the other hand, the molecular technique has better sensitivities and are better standardised. Recent innovations are reshaping MRD assessment. Availability of better and sensitive instruments, better analysis softwares aided by the identification of newer discriminatory markers had improved the sensitivity of FCM based MRD assessment. Similarly, next-generation sequencing (NGS)-based MRD now allows for deeper sensitivity (up to 10^{-6}), with improved standardization and applicability across diverse B-ALL subtypes. There is also growing interest in cell-free DNA (cfDNA)-based MRD assessment. This offers a non-invasive approach and is particularly useful in cases with difficult marrow access, CNS involvement or the patchy disease distribution. The chapter reviews the established and newer knowledge of the MRD assessment in B-ALL

INTRODUCTION

B-cell acute lymphoblastic leukemia (B-ALL) is the most common immunophenotypic type which accounts for ~75% of ALLs. The estimated incidence worldwide is 1–4.75 cases per 100,000 person-years. There has been a significant advancement in the diagnosis and treatment outcomes of ALL over the past four decades. The 5-year survival rates have improved from ~40 to 50% between 1975 and 1980 to ~70% between 2012 and 2018. The mainstay of treatment still remains the induction, consolidation, and maintenance chemotherapy, with hematopoietic stem cell transplantation (HSCT) reserved for certain high-risk category of patients. Adjunct to these treatment modalities are the tyrosine kinase inhibitors, which has shown efficacy in patients with Ph-positive disease as well as some non-Ph ALLs. Additionally, several targeted therapies have been developed for these patients such as rituximab (anti-CD20), inotuzumab ozogamicin (anti-CD22), blinatumomab (anti-CD19 BiTE), and anti-CD19-chimeric antigen receptor T-cell (CAR-T) therapy. These newer agents have demonstrated a greater effectiveness than salvage chemotherapy in the very high-risk setting of relapsed/refractory ALLs.

In spite of these treatment advancements, a proportion of patients relapse with the disease owing to the persistence of minor submicroscopic residual population of leukemic cells. The presence of this residual population of tumor cells is known as "measurable residual disease (MRD)" and it requires some highly specialized diagnostic modality to identify and quantitate them accurately. MRD assessment has emerged as a crucial prognostic and predictive tools in B-ALL. Its clinical utility has been extensively validated in both pediatric and adult settings, significantly influencing treatment strategies, both in transplant and nontransplant contexts. Both, National Comprehensive Cancer Network (NCCN) and European Society for Medical Oncology (ESMO) clinical practice guidelines recommend the quantification of MRD whenever possible.

CLINICAL IMPLICATIONS OF MEASURABLE RESIDUAL DISEASE ASSESSMENT: WHY DO WE NEED TO PERFORM MEASURABLE RESIDUAL DISEASE?

B-ALL has been the poster boy for MRD assessment and its clinical relevance in hematological neoplasm. It has been found to have a significant prognostic value both in children and adult, in both transplant and nontransplant settings. A study involving 7,430 children enrolled in the Children's Oncology Group (COG) treatment protocol demonstrated the prognostic significance of MRD evaluation by flow cytometry on day 29. 5-year disease-free survival (DFS) was significantly higher in patients who were MRD-negative as compared to those who were MRD-positive (89% vs. 72%). Notably, among MRD-negative patients, the presence or absence of morphologic evidence of disease on a day 14 bone marrow (BM) examination had little impact on outcomes, with 5-year DFS rates being nearly identical (89% vs. 91%). This underscores the importance of MRD status as a robust predictor of long-term outcomes.

A large systematic literature review and meta-analysis performed to elucidate the clinical significance of MRD with respect to relapse-free survival (RFS) and overall survival (OS) in adult B-ALL including 5,979 patients from 23 articles and abstracts, published between 2012 and 2016, revealed improved RFS and OS across all studies for patients who achieved MRD negativity. No difference in the impact of MRD status in subgroups based on disease stage, Ph chromosome status, MRD sensitivity levels, risk group, MRD timing after induction, etc., was noted.

In an Indian study from the Christian Medical College (CMC) Vellore, which included 481 patients undergoing treatment for B-ALL between August 2012 and March 2019, showed that end of induction MRD and baseline karyotype were the strongest predictors of EFS and RFS on multivariate analysis. The EFS was found to be inversely related to the MRD value and patients with MRD ≥ 1.0%

had outcomes similar to those without morphological remission. This finding was similar across the different subgroups of ALL.

Information from MRD testing can help in tailoring the treatment as per the need of the patient. It can help to target highly effective immunotherapies, as well as therapies that are less well tolerated and are associated with increased risk, such as HSCT, to those at high risk of relapse.

In GRALL 2003 and 2005 trial for the Ph-negative ALL patients, HSCT could prolong RFS compared with chemotherapy among those who did not achieve an early MRD response. But there was no apparent benefit in those who did achieve an early MRD response. Similarly, the PETHEMA ALL AR03 trial used MRD to guide treatment decisions at the end of consolidation, and found that HSCT could be avoided in MRD negative patients without adversely affecting their prognosis. Similar studies with smaller cohorts are also available in literature. All these studies prove that MRD assessment can help in sparing patients from the risks associated with transplantation, without negatively affecting survival outcomes for the patients who achieve MRD negative status. Additionally, new systemic targeted therapies like blinatumomab may offer alternatives to HSCT and has been found to induce a complete MRD response in over three-quarters of patients with MRD-positive ALL in first-line treatment.

These above studies provide strong arguments in favor of MRD as a clinical tool for assessing prognosis and guiding treatment decisions in precursor B-cell ALL and this has now become a standard of care in almost all treatment protocols. The National Comprehensive Cancer Network (NCCN) guideline 2017 suggests that MRD should be used as one of the deciding parameters for the further management of patients. Based on the results, patients with elevated levels of MRD should be subjected to treatment escalation, while those having a rapid clearance of tumor cells may be the candidate of treatment deintensification.

The generalization about "Why" MRD is needed in the clinical management of B-ALL can be summarized as follows:

- To provide an objective methodology for the establishment of a deeper remission status.
- To refine outcome prediction and inform postremission treatment.
- To identify impending relapse and enable early intervention.
- To allow more robust post-transplant surveillance.
- To be used as a surrogate endpoint to accelerate drug testing and approval.

TECHNICAL CONSIDERATIONS FOR MEASURABLE RESIDUAL DISEASE ASSESSMENT: HOW TO PERFORM MEASURABLE RESIDUAL DISEASE?

The technology used: The assays targeting MRD have a sensitivity beyond the routine morphological assessment. These assays can be cytogenetics, flow cytometric (FCM) analysis, polymerase chain reaction (PCR)/reverse transcriptase (RT-PCR) based assay and the high throughput/next-generation sequencing (NGS) assays. The choice of methodology to be used, should be a well-balanced approach keeping in view the applicability, availability, sensitivity, specificity, reproducibility, turn-around time (TAT), etc. To be clinically informative, the chosen methods should be providing reliable and reproducible results with a sensitivity of 0.01% or better. However, different disease and different clinical trials may use different methodologies with different clinically relevant cutoffs.

The FCM approach utilizes the presence of protein epitopes (antigens) in the nucleus, cytoplasm, or cell surface, which are acquired during normal cell development. Antigens, differently expressed by B- and T-lymphoblasts, are analyzed using fluorochrome-conjugated monoclonal antibodies (MoAbs). Immunophenotype associated with leukemic cells [leukemia-associated immunophenotypes (LAIP)] and its difference from normal population (DfN) are the two common approaches utilized for identifying the MRD. A set of these marker/antibodies in combination, usually called as "panel" is used, which aims at identification of precursor B cells and differentiation between normal and leukemic precursors. The normal precursors display a series of maturation pattern and expression, while the leukemic blasts do not follow this maturation pattern and frequently show loss/gain/aberrant expression pattern. Initially, a four-color combination tube containing CD10, CD19, CD34, and CD45 was used to identify blasts in mid-induction day 19 BM. This approach, known as "MRD lite," assumed that any cells with this precursor phenotype were abnormal residual blasts, as normal lymphoid precursors are highly sensitive to chemotherapy. However, during subsequent therapy phases, regenerating B-cell precursors (hematogones) complicate the distinction between abnormal blasts and normal precursors. To address this, additional markers and advanced multiparametric analysis using eight or more antibodies in a single tube improve identification accuracy. Commonly used markers include CD45, CD10, CD19, CD34, CD38, CD20, CD73, CD66c, CD33, CD86, CD81, CD58, CD304, and CD123. Core markers (CD10, CD19, CD34, CD45, and CD38) serve as a backbone for the identification of B-cell precursors, while others differentiate abnormal blasts from hematogones. Variations in marker expression—overexpression, underexpression, asynchronous expression, or aberrant expression—are collectively termed LAIP and aid in identifying MRD. Use of other gating markers like CD22 and CD24 is required only in some specialized situation where CD19 expression is either suboptimal or absent. This is encountered with anti-CD19 therapy or CD19 directed CAR-T cell therapy. It is essential to recognize that, although the diagnostic immunophenotype is typically stable, changes in immunophenotype, such as antigenic gain or loss, may sometimes occur. Using bulk lysis protocols and increasing the number of events improves the sensitivity of assay but causes identification of some previously unidentified populations which may mimick the B MRD. These includes populations such as CD19-positive plasmacytoid dendritic cells (pDCs) or CD10/CD73 positive mesenchymal stem cells. Recognizing these mimics and artifacts is critical when performing high-sensitivity MRD analysis, in order to strongly labeling these populations as blasts. A summary of common markers used and their normal expression along with their expression on B-ALL is summarized in **Table 1**. The scatter plots of a representative case of B MRD is shown in **Figure 1**.

Advancements in flow cytometry [multicolor flow cytometry (MFC)] have significantly improved sensitivity and analysis capabilities, now allowing the use of up to 18 colors per cell via innovations such as ultraviolet and violet lasers

TABLE 1: Details of common markers used for B-cell acute lymphoblastic leukemia measurable residual disease analysis.

Marker	Normal expression	Expression in B-ALL	Comments
CD19	A pan B-cell marker	Expressed in almost all B-ALL	Diminished/absent expression may be seen in few BCP ALL (diminished), anti-CD19 therapy (blinatumomab)/CAR-T cell therapy
CD10	Pre-B to immature B-cell precursors, dim to moderate expression on granulocytes	Expressed at bright levels in B-ALLs	Negative in pro-B-ALLs
CD20	Expressed in mature B cells	Expressed only a minority of B-ALLs	Knowledge of expression helpful for anti-CD20 therapy
CD22	Expressed in almost all B cells from pro B-cell onward	Expressed in almost all B-ALLs	Can be used as a gating marker for MRD in cases with anti-CD19 therapy
CD24	Expressed on B cells and on granulocytes	Expressed on most of the B-ALLs	Can be used as a gating marker for MRD in cases with anti-CD19 therapy
CD38	Expressed in B-cell precursors and activated B cells	Downregulated on almost all the B-ALLs (as compared to hematogones)	One of the best and stable marker which is downregulated
CD34	Hematopoietic stem cells, in pro B and pre-B-cells	Expressed in majority of B-ALL	Expression may be absent or heterogeneous
CD81	Highly expressed on B cells and precursors	Underexpressed in majority of B-ALL	
CD73	Expressed in mature B cells, T cells, dendritic cells, mesenchymal stem cells	Overexpressed in majority of B-ALL	Dimmer expression in pro-B-ALL
CD304	Highly expressed on plasmacytoid dendritic cells	Overexpressed in most of B-ALLs	Overexpression associated with certain specific genetic subtypes
CD66c	Not expressed on B cell, expressed on myeloid cells	Aberrantly expressed in a fair proportion of B-ALLs	Overexpression associated with certain specific genetic subtypes
CD13/33	Not expressed on B cell, expressed on myeloid cells	Aberrantly expressed in a fair proportion of B-ALLs	Overexpression associated with certain specific genetic subtypes

(B-ALL; B-cell acute lymphoblastic leukemia; BCP: B-cell precursor; CAR-T: chimeric antigen receptor T-cell; MRD: measurable residual disease)

and quantum dots. Development of advanced analysis softwares such as Kaluza, Cytognos, FlowJo, etc., have also improved the sensitivity of flow cytometry based MRD analysis over time. However, limitations exist, including the need for fresh samples, potential false positives due to normal cell regeneration, and challenges

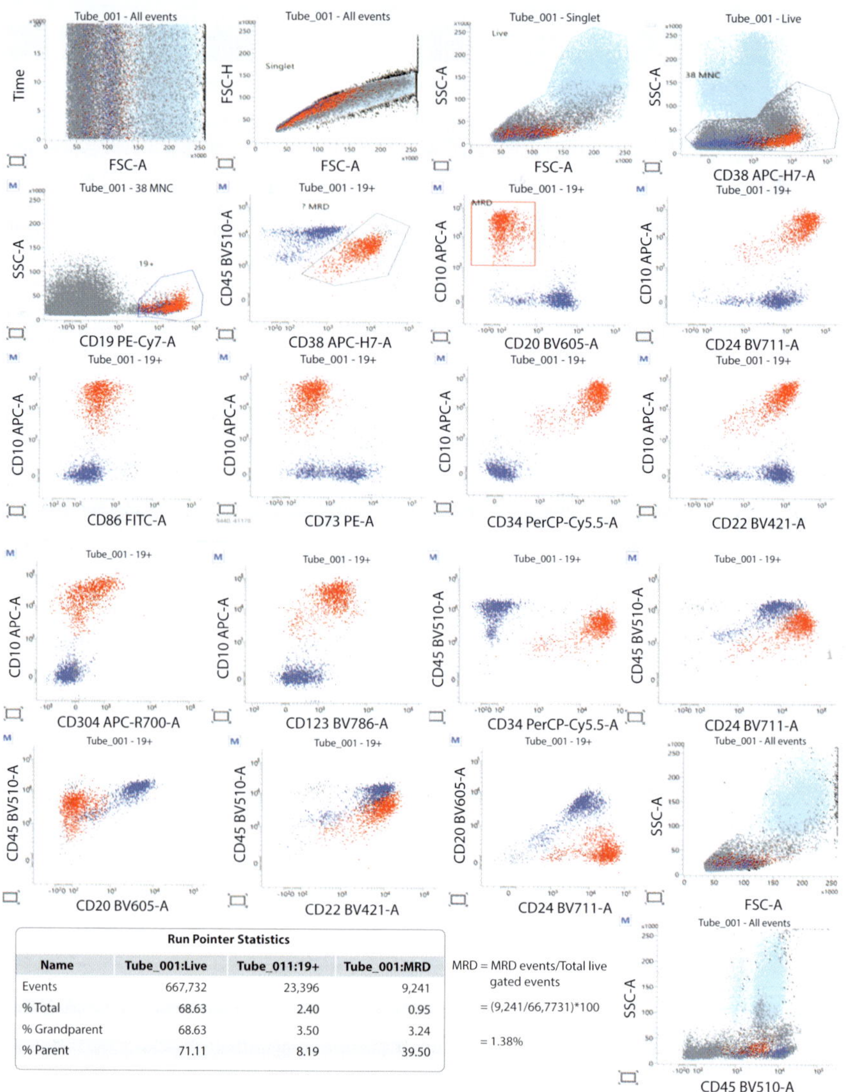

Run Pointer Statistics

Name	Tube_001:Live	Tube_011:19+	Tube_001:MRD
Events	667,732	23,396	9,241
% Total	68.63	2.40	0.95
% Grandparent	68.63	3.50	3.24
% Parent	71.11	8.19	39.50

FIG. 1: Gating strategies and scatter plots from a representative case of B minimal residual disease (MRD).

with BM hypocellularity or phenotypic shifts. The EuroFlow Consortium has standardized protocols for MRD detection, though experienced operators remain essential for accurate interpretation. Next generation flow cytometry (NGF) developed by Euroflow group has higher applicability, better sensitivity, and cost lesser that NGS. The greater sensitivity of NGF-MRD is attributed to the use of standardized approaches, including instrument setting, sample processing with bulk lysis procedure, immunostaining, data acquisition, and data analysis with standardized and sometimes automated gating strategies for differentiating different cell populations. However, the acquisition of a large number of cells is needed to reach the required sensitivity. Several other home developed protocols for high sensitivity assays have been utilized across various labs which are not exactly NGF, but are inspired by it.

The molecular study of antigen-receptor gene rearrangements is a widely used technique for detecting MRD. During B- and T-cell development, immunoglobulin (*IG*) and T-cell receptor (*TR*) genes undergo somatic rearrangement, combining *V*, *D*, and *J* gene segments to create unique receptor sequences for each lymphocyte. In leukemia, all malignant cells share the same clonal *IG/TR* gene rearrangement, enabling detection of leukemic cells among normal lymphocytes. This method is highly sensitive for assessing lymphoid cell clonality. Identification of these markers involves PCR amplification of DNA from leukemic cells, followed by heteroduplex or gene scan analysis to confirm clonality.

Clonal PCR fragments are sequenced to define junctional regions and develop allele-specific primers, facilitating accurate MRD monitoring mostly using the quantitative PCR. This real-time-quantitative-PCR (RQ-PCR) protocol combined with fluorescently labeled probes allow the detection of up to 1 leukemic cell in 100,000 (10^{-5}) normal background cell population.

Antigen-receptor gene rearrangement analysis for MRD detection and has been extensively standardized by the EuroMRD Consortium to ensure consistent application across treatment protocols for childhood and adult ALL. However, around 5–10% of cases, particularly those involving immature cells, lack IG/TR rearrangements or face technical issues, hindering MRD target identification. Clonal evolution during disease progression or relapse, especially in oligoclonal cases, can result in false negatives. Additionally, the need for diagnostic DNA in each MRD experiment poses challenges.

Another method for detecting the MRD is analysis of the fusion transcript analysis. Approximately 30–40% patients harbor these fusion transcript which can be *BCR::ABL1, KMT2A::AFF1,* and *TCF3::PBX1*. Thus, RNA is the optimal starting material to detect these fusion transcript and analyzing them using RQ-PCR. Quantification is achieved by comparing the amplified product to a standard curve derived from the amplification of serial dilutions of a cell line or plasmid DNA (i.e., *BCR::ABL1+).* The sensitivity is similar to that of RQ-PCR of IG/TCR assay. However, the accuracy of this assay is compromised by the variability in the number of RNA transcripts per leukemic cell among different patients as well as different cells from same clone. This technique for the quantification of the fusion gene is well standardized within the EuroMRD Consortium.

Digital droplet PCR (ddPCR), a third-generation PCR, addresses RQ-PCR's limitations by using sample partitioning and Poisson statistics for precise nucleic acid quantification without calibration curves. It offers improved accuracy, higher amplification efficiency, and resistance to inhibitors, with 95% confidence intervals. ddPCR has shown promise in molecular oncology, prenatal diagnostics, and hematologic malignancies, demonstrating superior performance to RQ-PCR in recent studies. It provides a more reliable endpoint measurement and holds potential for widespread application in MRD assessment, improving sensitivity, reproducibility, and clinical decision-making in the coming decade. However, no standard guidelines for the analysis and interpretation of the MRD based on ddPCR has yet been developed.

Next-generation sequencing technologies have proven valuable for MRD detection in both precursor and mature B-cell tumors. NGS enables the identification and quantification of clone-specific IG/TR sequences, allowing clonal sequences detected at diagnosis to be tracked in subsequent samples. Using universal primers, NGS monitors all *IG/TR* gene rearrangements simultaneously, providing insights into both residual leukemia and the normal immune repertoire. Using the same comprehensive panel at the diagnosis and monitoring helps in picking up the new clones during the relapse. NGS can achieve sensitivity levels as high as 10^{-6}, surpassing the 10^{-5} sensitivity of RQ-PCR, especially with larger DNA quantities. Studies have shown NGS to be more specific than RQ-PCR in predicting relapse after induction therapy and allogeneic stem cell transplantation (SCT). Despite its advantages, NGS involves significant complexity and costs. Additionally, standardized, broadly applicable protocols for NGS-based MRD detection remain unavailable in many academic laboratories, limiting widespread implementation. Nonetheless, its potential for precise relapse prediction and improved risk stratification underscores its growing importance in MRD monitoring. Euroclonality—NGS consortium has also published its recommendations for the evaluation of B-cell clonality.

The summary and comparative analysis of all these techniques are mentioned in **Table 2**. The choice of one technique over the other depends on various factors. Some studies or trial may include MRD analysis using more than one technique.

The sample type: It has been debated in past whether peripheral blood (PB) can be preferred over the BM for MRD monitoring. There have been some promising

TABLE 2: Comparison of different techniques for the measurable residual disease (MRD) assessment.

	Input material	Target	Applicability	Sensitivity	Advantage	Disadvantage
Flow cytometry (6–8 colors)	BMA sample in majority cases, PB and FNA sample may also be used	Leukemia-associated immunophenotype (LAIP)/ Different from normal (DfN) antigenic expression	> 90–95%	10^{-4}	Rapid, gives idea about other background cell population, diagnostic sample may not be needed	Sensitivity is lesser as compared to PCR, Less harmonized and standardized across the globe
NGF/HS FCM (10 color or more)	BMA sample in majority cases, PB and FNA sample may also be used	LAIP and DfN	> 95%	10^{-4} -10^{-6}	Rapid, highly sensitive, standardized approach, gives idea about other background cell population	Large number of cells needed, high level of expertise needed, relatively costlier

Continued

Continued

	Input material	Target	Applicability	Sensitivity	Advantage	Disadvantage
RQ-PCR Fusion transcripts	RNA/DNA	Fusion gene	30–40%	10^{-4} -10^{-5}	Rapid, sensitive, relatively easy, stable markers	Applicability is less, Input material RNA is relatively unstable, relatively costlier
RQ-PCR IG/TCR	DNA	IG/TCR	90–95%	10^{-4} -10^{-5}	High sensitivity, applicability, well standardized, consensus guidelines available	Diagnostic material is required, large amount of input DNA, laborious, time consuming, relatively expensive
Digital/ddPCR	DNA	IG/TCR	90–95%	10^{-4} -10^{-5}	High sensitivity, applicability, absolute quantification without standard curves	Diagnostic material is required, no standard guidelines, limited availability, relatively expensive
NGS	DNA	IG/TCR	90–95%	10^{-4} -10^{-6}	High sensitivity, applicability, ability to identify the clonal evolution	Limited availability, standard guidelines are still lacking, high level of bioinformatic support needed

(BMA: bone marrow aspirate; ddPCR: digital droplet polymerase chain reaction; IG/TCR: immunoglobulin/T-cell receptor; HS FCM: high sensitivity flow cytometry; NGF: next generation flow cytometry; NGS: next generation sequencing; PB: peripheral blood; RQ-PCR: real time quantitative polymerase chain reaction)

results with the T-ALL MRD assessment, but in B-ALLs, MRD levels have been found to be 1–3 logs lower in PB than in BM. Hence, regardless of the technique used (MFC or PCR) it is to be accepted that the BM assessments cannot be replaced by blood analyses for the B-cell ALL MRD. To ensure that adequate number of cells are stained and analyzed for FCM or sufficient quantity of representative leukemic nucleic acid is extracted for molecular techniques, hemodilution need to be avoided. This calls for taking the first marrow pull for the MRD analysis. To further enrich the leukocytes during flow cytometry and ensure acquisition and analysis of more than one million cells a bulk lysis-stain-wash protocol is used.

Key time points: WHEN to perform MRD. Although the key time points for MRD analysis depends on treatment protocol, the two most critical junctures are postinduction and postconsolidation. Other time points may be incorporated based on specific treatment protocols. These time points provide critical information for predicting outcomes and guiding therapy adjustments. Other time points include before maintenance therapy, postallogeneic stem cell transplant and any subsequent time points for the disease surveillance. MRD analysis before maintenance therapy provides insight into the durability of remission and risk of relapse during long-term maintenance. MRD assessment post-HSCT evaluates for early signs of relapse and guides post-transplant interventions such as donor lymphocyte infusions or tapering immunosuppression. Additionally, subsequent periodic MRD monitoring during maintenance and follow-up identifies early relapse, even in asymptomatic patients, facilitating timely intervention.

RECENT ADVANCES: WHAT IS NEW?

The assessment of MRD is continually advancing, incorporating innovative markers and highly sensitive technologies to improve diagnostic accuracy. Current research focuses on refining MRD thresholds and harmonizing protocols across institutions to ensure consistency. The integration of flow cytometry with molecular techniques offers enhanced precision in predicting patient outcomes, paving the way for more personalized and effective treatment strategies in B-ALL.

Advancements in flow cytometry (FCM)-based MRD analysis have been driven by the development of more sophisticated and stable cytometers, improved fluorophore-tagged antibodies, and the integration of machine learning and artificial intelligence into data analysis. Modern flow cytometers offer high acquisition rates (> 30,000 events/sec) with minimal carryover and automated PMT-independent compensation settings. This allows for the rapid and accurate acquisition of large datasets, addressing a key limitation of earlier systems. Enhanced fluorophores, such as Q-dots and Sirigen dyes, exhibit sharp emission peaks with reduced spillover, improving signal clarity. Additionally, genetically engineered antibodies now provide more specific epitope binding with minimal nonspecific cellular interactions. Advanced software further streamlines the analysis of large datasets, enabling faster and more precise results. These also have integrated clustering programs such as t-distributed stochastic neighbor embedding (tSNE) and SPADE (spanning-tree progression analysis of density-normalized events) for the supervised as well as unsupervised analysis and helping better discrimination of the rare events clusters automatically.

Spectral cytometry represents a significant advancement in clinical diagnosis and MRD detection for B-AL. Unlike conventional flow cytometry, which uses narrowband filters to detect emission spectra, spectral cytometry captures the entire emission spectrum of fluorophores. This allows for more precise discrimination of fluorophores with overlapping spectra, increasing the number of markers that can be simultaneously analyzed. This technology is particularly valuable in MRD assessment, as it enables highly multiplexed immunophenotyping to differentiate abnormal leukemic blasts from normal regenerating hematogones. Spectral cytometers, such as Cytek Biosciences

(Aurora and Northern Lights models), Sony (ID7000), and Becton Dickinson (BD) (Symphony A5 SE) can analyze 30 or more fluorescent parameters in a single tube, providing a comprehensive immunophenotypic profile. Enhanced resolution and reduced spillover further improve sensitivity and specificity, critical for detecting low levels of residual disease. Spectral cytometry also supports the use of novel fluorochromes and minimizes compensation-related inaccuracies, offering greater reliability in complex MRD panels. Furthermore, its ability to resolve rare cell populations is vital for high-sensitivity MRD detection, especially when leukemic cells exhibit immunophenotypic shifts postchemotherapy.

NGS has revolutionized MRD assessment in B-ALL by offering unparalleled sensitivity and specificity. NGS identifies and quantifies clone-specific *IG* gene rearrangements, detected at diagnosis, in subsequent follow-up samples. This method provides a comprehensive view of residual leukemia and the reconstitution of the normal immune repertoire, making it a robust tool for MRD evaluation. Unlike RQ-PCR, NGS does not rely on calibration curves, reducing variability and improving reproducibility. Owing to the massive parallel sequencing, a broader genetic signature is visible as contrast to other molecular techniques, which essentially have a tubular vision. Thus, NGS also offers insights into clonal evolution, a common occurrence in relapsed B-ALL, by capturing dynamic changes in leukemic clones over time. Among the commercial assay, the LymphoTrack assay was established by combining the basic strategy of BIOMED-2 and NGS technology. Using locus-specific primer sets for IGH-V, -D, and -J rearrangements and an NGS platform, a clonotype was identified, with characterization of the exact V–D–J sequence and their corresponding frequency. The malignant clone with the highest frequency in the baseline sample was named the "index" clone, and it was tracked in the follow-up samples for the MRD measurement. A similar product, ClonoSeq from Adaptive Biotechnologies has already been approved by the FDA for MRD tracking in ALL and multiple myeloma (MM). However, challenges persist, including limited availability, high costs, complex protocols, and the lack of widespread standardization.

Cell-free DNA (cfDNA) from the peripheral blood and cerebrospinal fluid (CSF) is one of the promising input materials for the MRD analysis and predicting relapse and CNS involvement in B-ALLs. Being a noninvasive diagnostic modality, its utility is being explored in various studies. The genetic aberration present in the leukemic cells of the marrow usually mirrors in the cfDNA. These genetic aberrations can be targeted during follow-up using the high sensitivity molecular techniques such as digital droplet (dd) PCR and NGS. The aberrant methylation patterns can also serve as the MRD markers. While cfDNA-based MRD monitoring is not yet a standard of care, it represents a promising adjunct to traditional methods for guiding personalized treatment strategies in B-ALL.

In summary, it has been established through various studies that MRD assessment is one of the most robust and independent prognostic and predictive tools for the appropriate management of B-cell precursor ALL. MRD evaluation have been incorporated as the standard of care in various international treatment protocols. There are two broad methods of MRD analysis which include the FCM approach, including the standardized NGF and the molecular approach including the NGS. These methods vary in their sensitivity and have their own advantages and disadvantages. The choice of these methods depends on the various factors such as availability, applicability, costs, adapted treatment protocols, etc. The two well accepted time points are the postinduction and the postconsolidation period with a clinically relevant sensitivity cutoff being 0.01%. It is continually advancing field with newer methodologies such as spectral cytometry, ddPCR, NGS, and use of cfDNA as noninvasive modality for MRD assessment, coming on board. A continuous cross-talk between a clinical hematologist and hematopathologist is mandatory for making the successful use of these high sensitivity assay into routine clinical practice.

Take Home Points

- MRD assessment is an independent factor which is required for the evaluation of treatment response and predict disease relapse.
- Different methods (like FCM, PCR based or NGS based) can be used which have their own advantages and disadvantages.
- The chosen methods should be sensitive, specific, reproducible and stable and may vary depending upon the availability, applicability, cost and turnaround time (TAT).
- Same methodology should be followed throughout the treatment protocol. Changing the methods may lead to confusion to the treating physician.
- Post-induction and post-consolidation are the two well established time points in routine clinical practice.
- The dynamics of MRD, as assessed by MRD analysis at different time points, provides a better idea about the treatment response, as compared to a single value.

SUGGESTED READINGS

1. Redaelli A, Laskin BL, Stephens JM, Botteman MF, Pashos CL. A systematic literature review of the clinical and epidemiological burden of acute lymphoblastic leukaemia (ALL). Eur J Cancer Care (Engl). 2005;14(1):53-62.
2. Hoelzer D, Bassan R, Dombret H, Fielding A, Ribera JM, Buske C. Acute lymphoblastic leukaemia in adult patients: ESMO Clinical Practice Guidelines for diagnosis, treatment and follow-up. Ann Oncol. 2016;27(Suppl 5):v69-v82.
3. Parikh SA, Litzow MR. Philadelphia chromosome-negative acute lymphoblastic leukemia: therapies under development. Future Oncol. 2014;10(14):2201-12.
4. Zhang H, Gu L, Liu T, Chiang KY, Zhou M. Inhibition of MDM2 by nilotinib con tributes to cytotoxicity in both Philadelphia positive and negative acute lymphoblastic leukemia. PLoS One. 2014;9(6):e100960.
5. Kantarjian H, Stein A, Gokbuget N, Fielding AK, Schuh AC, Ribera JM, et al. Blinatumomab versus chemotherapy for advanced acute lymphoblastic leukemia. N Engl J Med. 2017;376(9):836-47.
6. Brown PA, Shah B, Advani A, Aoun P, Boyer MW, Burke PW, et al. Acute lymphoblastic leukemia. Version I. 2018. NCCN clinical practice guidelines in oncology with NCCN evidence blocks; 2018.
7. Short NJ, Jabbour E, Albitar M, de Lima M, Gore L, Jorgensen J, et al. Recommendations for the assessment and management of measurable residual disease in adults with

acute lymphoblastic leukemia: a consensus of North American experts. Am J Hematol. 2019;94(2):257-65.

8. Borowitz MJ, Wood BL, Devidas M, Loh ML, Raetz EA, Salzer WL, et al. Assessment of end induction minimal residual disease (MRD) in childhood B precursor acute lymphoblastic leukaemia (ALL) to eliminate the need for day 14 marrow examination: A Children's Oncology Group study (abstract 10001). J Clin Oncol. 2013;31:613s.
9. Bassan R, Brüggemann M, Radcliffe HS, Hartfield E, Kreuzbauer G, Wetten S. A systematic literature review and meta-analysis of minimal residual disease as a prognostic indicator in adult B-cell acute lymphoblastic leukemia. Haematologica. 2019;104(10):2028-39.
10. Dhèdin N, Huynh A, Maury S, Tabrizi R, Beldjord K, Asnafi V, et al. Role of allogeneic stem cell transplantation in adult patients with Ph-negative acute lymphoblastic leukemia. Blood. 2015;125(16):2486-96.
11. Ribera JM, Oriol A, Morgades M, Montesinos P, Sarrà J, González-Campos J, et al. Treatment of high-risk Philadelphia chromosome-negative acute lymphoblastic leukemia in adolescents and adults according to early cytologic response and minimal residual disease after consolidation assessed by flow cytometry: final results of the PETHEMA ALL-AR-03 trial. J Clin Oncol. 2014;32(15):1595-604.
12. Bassan R, Masciulli A, Intermesoli T, Spinelli O, Tosi M, Pavoni C, et al. Final results of Northern Italy Leukemia Group (NILG) trial 10/07 combining pediatric-type therapy with minimal residual disease study and risk-oriented hematopoietic cell transplantation in adult acute lymphoblastic leukemia (ALL). Blood. 2016;128(22):176.
13. Gökbuget N, Dombret H, Bonifacio M, Reichle A, Graux C, Faul C, et al. Blinatumomab for minimal residual disease in adults with B-precursor acute lymphoblastic leukemia. Blood. 2018;131(14):1522-31.
14. Coustan-Smith E, Ribeiro RC, Stow P, Zhou Y, Pui CH, Rivera GK, et al. A simplified flow cytometric assay identifies children with acute lymphoblastic leukaemia who have a superior clinical outcome. Blood. 2006;108(1):97-102.
15. Arunachalam AK, Selvarajan S, Mani T, Janet NB, Maddali M, Lionel SA, et al. Clinical significance of end of induction measurable residual disease monitoring in B-cell acute lymphoblastic leukemia: A single center experience. Cytometry B Clin Cytom. 2023;104(6):440-5.
16. Kotrova M, Volland A, Kehden B, Trautmann H, Ritgen M, Wäsch R, et al. Comparison of minimal residual disease levels in bone marrow and peripheral blood in adult acute lymphoblastic leukemia. Leukemia. 2020;34(4):1154-7.
17. Coustan-Smith E, Sancho J, Hancock ML, Razzouk BI, Ribeiro RC, Rivera GK, et al. Use of peripheral blood instead of bone marrow to monitor residual disease in children with acute lymphoblastic leukemia. Blood. 2002;100:2399-402.
18. Brüggemann M, Kotrova M. Minimal residual disease in adult ALL: technical aspects and implications for correct clinical interpretation. Blood Adv. 2017;1(25):2456-66.
19. Borovitz MJ, Devidas M, Hunger SP, Bowman WP, Carroll AJ, Carroll WL, et al.; Children's Oncology Group. Clinical significance of minimal residual disease in childhood acute lymphoblastic leukemia and its relationship to other prognostic factors: a Children's Oncology Group study. Blood. 2008;111(12):5477-85.
20. Pui CH, Pei D, Raimondi SC, Coustan-Smith E, Jeha S, Cheng C, et al. Clinical impact of minimal residual disease in children with different subtypes of acute lymphoblastic leukemia treated with Response-Adapted therapy. Leukemia. 2017;31(2):333-9.
21. Kalina T, Flores-Montero J, van der Velden VH, Martin-Ayuso M, Bottcher S, Ritgen M, et al. EuroFlow standardization of flow cytometer instrument settings and immunophenotyping protocols. Leukemia. 2012;26:1986-2010.
22. Flores-Montero J, Sanoja-Flores L, Paiva B, Puig N, García-Sánchez O, Böttcher S, et al. Next generation flow for highly sensitive and standardized detection of minimal residual disease in multiple myeloma. Leukemia. 2017;31:2094-103.
23. Tembhare PR, Subramanian Pg PG, Ghogale S, Chatterjee G, Patkar NV, Gupta A, et al. A high-sensitivity 10-color flow cytometric minimal residual disease assay in b-lymphoblastic leukemia/lymphoma can easily achieve the sensitivity of 2-in-106 and is superior to

standard minimal residual disease assay: A Study of 622 Patients. Cytometry B Clin Cytom. 2020;98(1):57-67.

24. Germano G, del Giudice L, Palatron S, Giarin E, Cazzaniga G, Biondi A, et al. Clonality profile in relapsed precursor-B-ALL children by GeneScan and sequencing analyses. Consequences on minimal residual disease monitoring. Leukemia. 2003;17:1573-82.
25. Verhagen OJ, Willemse MJ, Breunis WB, Wijkhuijs AJ, Jacobs DC, Joosten SA, et al. Application of germline IGH probes in real-time quantitative PCR for the detection of minimal residual disease in acute lymphoblastic leukemia. Leukemia. 2000;14:1426-35.
26. van der Velden VH, Cazzaniga G, Schrauder A, Hancock J, Bader P, Panzer Grumayer ER, et al. European Study Group on MRD detection in ALL (ESG-MRD-ALL). Analysis of minimal residual disease by Ig/TCR gene rearrangements: Guidelines for interpretation of real-time quantitative PCR data. Leukemia. 2007;21:604-11.
27. Pfeifer H, Cazzaniga G, van der Velden VHJ, Cayuela JM, Schäfer B, Spinelli O, et al. Standardisation and consensus guidelines for minimal residual disease assessment in Philadelphia-positive acute lymphoblastic leukemia (Ph +ALL) by real-time quantitative reverse transcriptase PCR of e1a2 BCR ABL1. Leukemia. 2019;33(8):1910-22.
28. Burmeister T, Marschalek R, Schneider B, Meyer C, Gökbuget N, Schwartz S, et al. Monitoring minimal residual disease by quantification of genomic chromosomal breakpoint sequences in acute leukemias with MLL aberrations. Leukemia. 2006;20:451-7.
29. Vincent ME, Liu W, Haney EB, Ismagilov RF. Microfluidic stochastic confinement enhances analysis of rare cells by isolating cells and creating high density environments for control of diffusible signals. Chem Soc Rev. 2010;39:974-84.
30. van den Brand M, Möbs M, Otto F, Kroeze LI, Gonzalez de Castro D, Stamatopoulos K, et al. EuroClonality-NGS Recommendations for Evaluation of B-Cell Clonality Analysis by Next-Generation Sequencing: A Structured Approach with the DEPART Algorithm. J Mol Diagn. 2023;25(10):729-39.
31. García-Aguilera G, Castillo-Robleda A, Sanz A, Ramírez M. Validation of a spectral flow cytometry single-tube panel for the clinical diagnosis and follow-up of children and adolescents with B-Cell acute lymphoblastic leukemia. Cells. 2024;13(22):1891.
32. Nolan JP. The evolution of spectral cytometry. Cytometry. 2022;101:812-7.
33. Wood B, Wu D, Crossley B, Dai Y, Williamson D, Gawad C, et al. Measurable residual disease detection by high-throughput sequencing improves risk stratification for pediatric B-ALL. Blood. 2018;131(12):1350-9.
34. Cho H, Shin S, Chung H, Jang JE, Kim YR, Cheong JW, et al. Real-world data on prognostic value of measurable residual disease assessment by fragment analysis or next-generation sequencing in multiple myeloma. Br J Haematol. 2022;198:3.
35. Ryan CE, Sahaf B, Logan AC, O'Brien S, Byrd JC, Hillmen P, et al. Ibrutinib efficacy and tolerability in patients with relapsed chronic lymphocytic leukemia following allogeneic HCT. Blood. 2016;128:25.
36. Colmenares R, Álvarez N, Barrio S, Martínez-López J, Ayala R. The minimal residual disease using liquid biopsies in hematological malignancies. Cancers. 2022;14(5):1310.
37. Sampathi S, Chernyavskaya Y, Haney MG, Moore LH, Snyder IA, Cox AH, et al. Nanopore sequencing methods detect cell-free DNA associated with MRD and CNS infiltration in pediatric acute lymphoblastic leukemia. bioRxiv. 2021;09:1-16.

CHAPTER 20

Revisiting B-ALL MRD in CAR-T Cell and Blinatumomab Era

Devasis Panda, Narender Tejwani

ABSTRACT

Monitoring measurable residual disease (MRD) in B-cell acute lymphoblastic leukemia (B-ALL) following anti-CD19 therapy requires strategic gating markers to ensure accurate detection and differentiation of B cells. The challenges in MRD assessment are multifaceted, involving markers such as CD22, CD24, and CD79a, each with specific advantages and limitations. The presence of therapy targeted toward multiple markers, such as anti-CD19 and anti-CD22, can complicate disease identification, making it crucial to combine multiple markers for comprehensive evaluation. Boolean gating strategies, which incorporate multiple markers, offer an improved approach for selecting B cells and ensuring accurate disease detection in patients undergoing targeted therapies.

Furthermore, the possibility of lineage switches posttherapy, particularly in cases of KMT2A rearranged and Philadelphia-positive B-ALL, underscores the importance of incorporating myeloid and T-lineage markers into MRD analysis. These complex scenarios highlight the need for an adaptable and thorough MRD testing strategy to detect CD19-negative disease, ensuring the precise monitoring of treatment efficacy and the identification of emerging disease components.

Ultimately, integrating advanced gating techniques and awareness of potential therapeutic impacts on marker expression will lead to more accurate MRD assessments and better patient management in the era of targeted therapies.

INTRODUCTION

Measurable residual disease (MRD) is a robust prognostic parameter for predicting therapeutic response and relapse in adult and pediatric B-lineage acute lymphoblastic leukemias (B-ALLs). The acceptable cut-off for MRD positivity in B-ALL is defined as the presence of ≥0.01% leukemic B-lineage blasts in a postinduction bone marrow aspirate sample. However, newer modalities, including next-generation flow cytometry (NGF) and next-generation sequencing (NGS), have shown that even a disease burden of <0.01% could adversely affect patient outcomes.

Multiparametric flow cytometry (MFC), polymerase chain reaction (PCR), and NGS are all well-established methods for MRD evaluation in B-ALL and are superior to morphological assessments of remission status. However, the presence of an informative molecular marker is essential for utilizing molecular techniques, which may not be available in every case. Moreover, the turnaround time is also longer than that of MFC. MFC is a very good and cost-effective alternative to molecular methods and can be easily applied in all cases with comparable sensitivity.

Conventionally, two different approaches are used to identify MFC-MRD: The leukemia-associated immunophenotype (LAIP) approach and the different-from-normal (DFN) approach. The LAIP approach identifies cells that recapitulate the initial diagnostic immunophenotype, including expression of lineage infidelity markers such as CD304/CD123/CD73/CD86/CD5/CD13 on B cells. The drawback of this methodology is that knowledge of the diagnostic immunophenotype is necessary, which may not be available in every case. Additionally, leukemic cells may lose some antigens due to immunomodulation, making MRD interpretation difficult. On the other hand, the DFN approach does not require knowledge of the diagnostic immunophenotype and is useful in almost every case. This method studies the normal maturation of B cells and identifies cells exhibiting any deviant or aberrant patterns. The DFN approach is considered the method of choice for B-ALL MRD assessment.

Nonetheless, regardless of the approach, gating all CD19-positive cells is the cornerstone of the gating technique used in MFC-MRD evaluation in B-ALL. CD19 is the defining B-lineage marker universally expressed in all B-ALL cases. Not surprisingly, it serves as the target molecule of choice in relapse/refractory patients. This chapter will focus on the use of MFC-mediated MRD evaluation in B-ALL and the challenges posed by immunotherapy.

CONVENTIONAL APPROACH TO B-ALL MRD IN MFC

As mentioned earlier, the widely used DFN approach involves studying normal B-cell ontogeny and their precursors (hematogones). Broadly, all *B cells* in MFC-MRD evaluation are divided into three groups depending on their maturation and antigen expression patterns. The hematogone 1 population comprises B cells that are CD34+, hematogone 2 consists of B cells that are CD10+/CD38+/CD34–, and mature B cells are CD10–/CD38–/CD34–. Another important population is plasma cells, which are B cells that are CD38++/CD10–/CD34–. The term "B cell" has been highlighted above because the first step in B-MRD assessment is gating all B cells (both normal and malignant) using a sensitive B-cell marker. CD19 has been routinely used for this purpose. **Figures 1A to L** show the normal maturation pattern of normal B cells (10-color panel on BD-FACS Canto with FACS Diva analysis software). **Figures 2A to F** show how the abnormal malignant cells stand out as a population and do not merge with the normal populations.

Figures 2A to F show how MRD appears as a cluster that stands out differently from the normal cell populations.

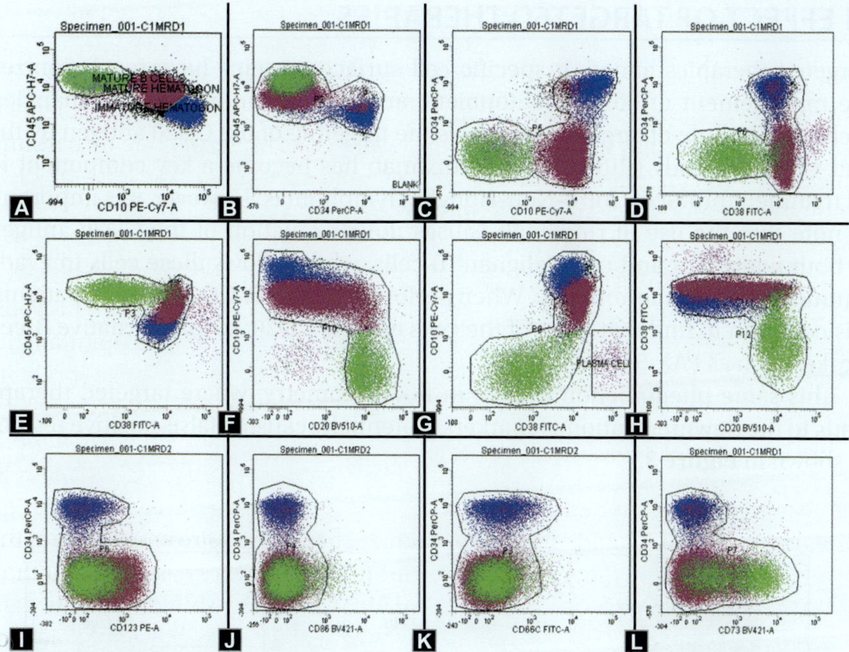

FIGS. 1A TO L: Maturation pattern of normal B-cell components of marrow gated on CD19-positive cells (markers used: CD19, CD45, CD34, CD10, CD38, CD20, CD123, CD86, CD66c, and CD73). Green population = mature B cells; brown population = hematogone 2 (Hg2); blue population = hematogone 1 (Hg1); magenta population = plasma cells. (10-color panel on BD-FACS Canto with FACS Diva analysis software).

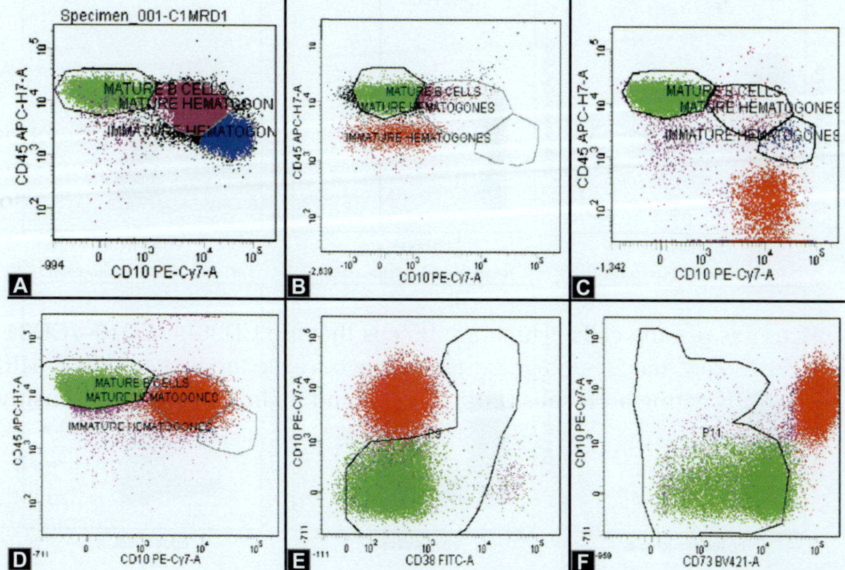

FIGS. 2A TO F: Measurable residual disease (MRD) (red color) appears as a population distinct from normal B cells. The picture shows various plots taken from multiple positive cases.

EFFECT OF TARGETED THERAPIES

Targeted therapies aimed at specific cell surface proteins have revolutionized the management of both hematopoietic and nonhematopoietic malignancies. A classic example of targeted therapy is the targeting of the CD20 antigen by the anti-CD20 antibody (Rituximab®). Rituximab has become a key component in all treatment protocols for B-Non-Hodgkin lymphomas. However, it is important to note that the use of rituximab causes downregulation of the CD20 antigen in both malignant and nonmalignant B cells, which allows these cells to evade immune attack by the antibody. When performing IHC for CD20 in these patients, it is common to find that none of the cells express CD20, so an alternative B-cell marker such as PAX-5 is used.

This same phenomenon is seen in flow cytometry, where targeted therapy leads to the downregulation of markers, potentially causing false-positive results, as shown in **Figure 3**.

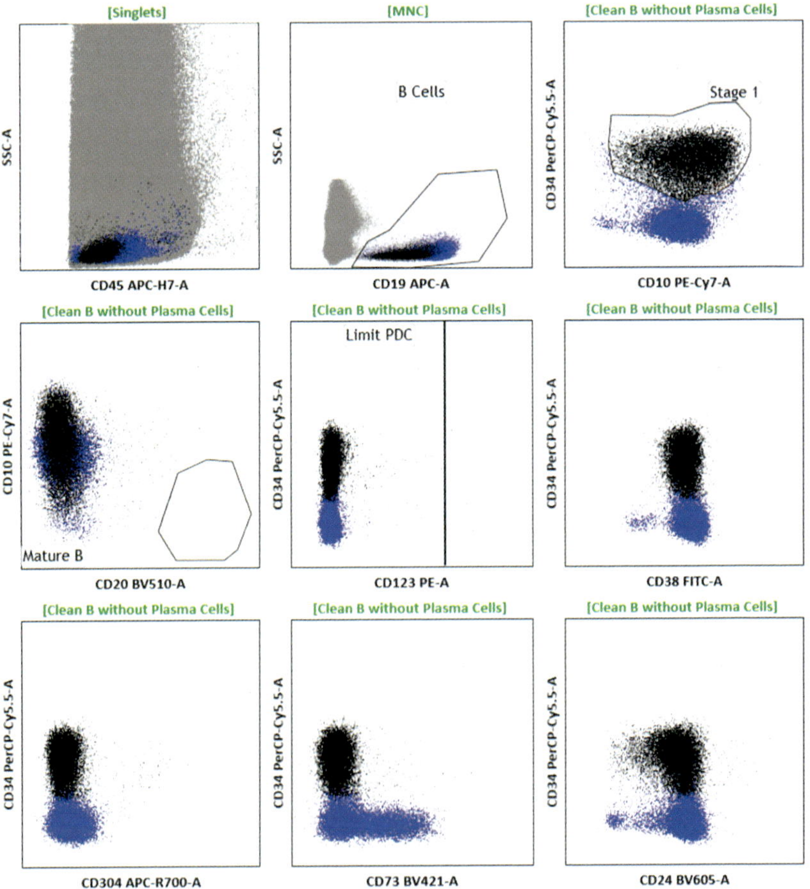

FIG. 3: A B-ALL patient may be labeled measurable residual disease (MRD)-positive after therapy with rituximab. Complete loss of CD20 is observed in hematogone 2 and 3 populations.

THERAPIES DIRECTED TOWARD CD19 AND THEIR EFFECT ON MRD ASSAY

In the current era, two therapeutic approaches target CD19 in B-ALL. One is the 2014 FDA-approved anti-CD19 antibody marketed under the name Blinatumomab®. The advantage of blinatumomab is that it is commercially available for all patients. Though it is more cost-effective than other therapies, such as CAR-T, the overall expenses during the entire therapeutic cycle remain high. A disadvantage is that the therapy's effectiveness depends on its half-life. To overcome this issue, blinatumomab is administered as a continuous intravenous infusion over 28 days per cycle, which can be inconvenient for patients.

The second anti-CD19 therapy approved for B-ALL patients is chimeric antigen receptor T-cell (CAR-T) therapy. This therapy is personalized for each patient and involves the extraction of T cells via apheresis. These T cells are transfected to express a chimeric receptor to recognize the CD19 antigen, and after selection and expansion, they are reinfused into the patient to target and kill CD19-positive cells. The advantages of this therapy include requiring only a single infusion, with the modified T cells continuing to target CD19-positive cells for a long time. Currently, the FDA has approved two CAR-T therapies for relapsed/refractory B-ALL: Tisagenlecleucel (approved for patients up to 25 years old) and brexucabtagene autoleucel (approved for adult patients only). In addition, NexCAR19 has been approved for use in India.

The use of CD19-targeted therapies in B-ALL patients presents significant challenges for MRD detection by MFC. Most laboratories use CD19 as the primary gating marker, but as mentioned earlier, targeted therapies may lead to the downregulation of CD19 on both malignant and nonmalignant cells. As a result, malignant cells may be excluded from analysis, leading to false-negative results if the history of anti-CD19 therapy is unknown. Additionally, distinguishing non-B cells requires a comprehensive panel of markers.

APPROACH TO B-ALL MRD IN PATIENTS TREATED WITH ANTI-CD19 THERAPIES

Almost all B-ALL MRD assays through MFC worldwide rely on gating CD19-positive normal and abnormal B cells. CD19 is highly useful for this purpose for several reasons:

- CD19 is expressed by almost all normal B cells and their precursors. The only exceptions are hematogone zero (Hg0) and, in some cases, a subset of plasma cells. Both conditions may interfere with MRD interpretation, as discussed later in this chapter.
- CD19 is essentially expressed in all B-ALL cases. Routine MRD evaluation involves CD19 expression along with one or two additional markers (depending on the intensity of CD19 expression), such as CD10, CD22, and cytoplasmic CD79a, to identify B-lineage differentiation. Thus, all malignant B cells will be captured by CD19 during MRD evaluation.

- CD19 antigen is almost exclusive to normal and abnormal B-lineage cells, which ensures that non-B cells are not mistakenly labeled as abnormal B cells. The only exceptions are in cases of leukemia of ambiguous lineage or, rarely, a phenomenon called trogocytosis in NK cells.

Since CD19-targeted therapies are associated with the downregulation of this marker, it is possible to mistakenly label an MRD-positive case as negative, as the malignant cells may be gated out in the first step of the gating technique. Moreover, partial loss of CD19 expression may lead to falsely lower MRD estimations, resulting in a negative interpretation **(Fig. 4)**. Approximately 9–25% of B-ALL patients exhibit loss/downregulation of CD19 following CAR-T therapy, and 28% show loss/downregulation after treatment with blinatumomab. This analytical issue can be addressed using alternative, sensitive B-cell gating markers such as

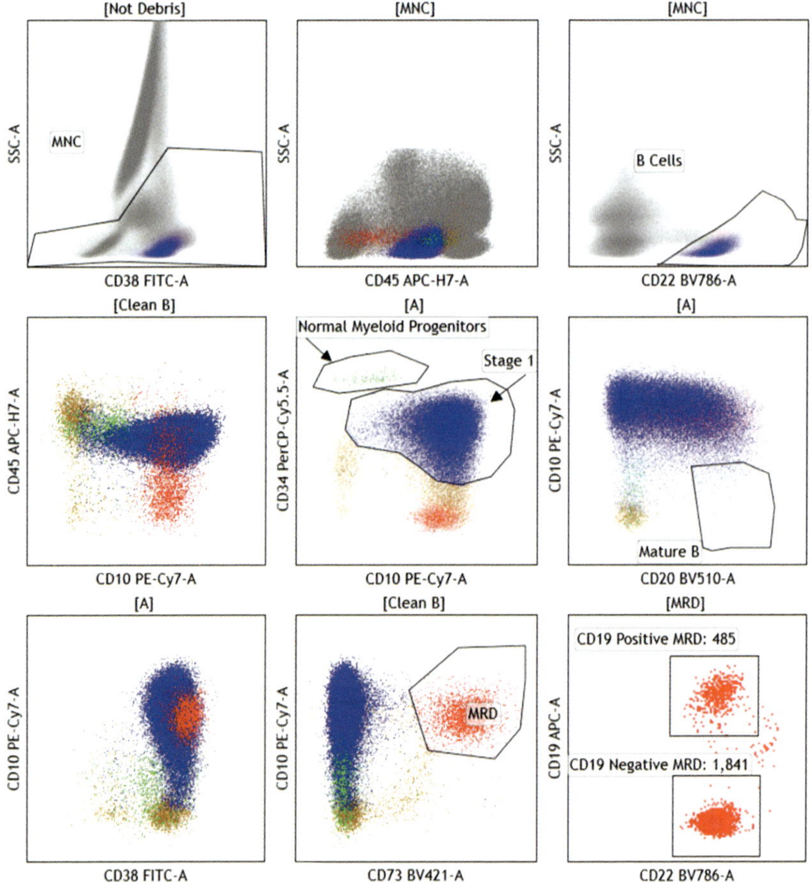

FIG. 4: A significant portion of measurable residual disease (MRD) (red color population) may appear negative after therapy with blinatumomab, leading to underestimation or missing disease if only CD19 is used as the primary gating marker. CD22, however, will help identify hematogone zero and many cells from non-B-cell lineages, such as myeloid progenitors (green), dendritic cells, and mesenchymal stem cells.

CD22, CD24, or cytoplasmic CD79a and employing an MRD exclusion strategy using non-B-cell lineage markers in the panel.

ALTERNATIVE GATING MARKERS IN B-ALL MRD FOLLOWING ANTI-CD19 THERAPY

CD22: This molecule belongs to the lectin family and is a specific B-cell marker present on all B cells, including B-cell precursors and mature B lymphocytes. The intensity of CD22 expression gradually increases as the B-cell precursors mature to B lymphocytes. A few drawbacks exist to using CD22 alone as a primary gating marker. The first and most important is the dim nature of this marker expression in immature cells (both normal and blasts). This makes it impossible to clearly separate the true positive and negative cells in flow cytometry. Thus, identifying the B-cell nature of the cells will often require the support of one or more markers in the panel, such as CD10, CD20, or CD24. The second important drawback is the significant downregulation of this marker in cases with *KMT2A* mutation and, to a lesser extent, in *BCR::ABL1* positive cases. *KMT2A*-rearranged cases are also negative for CD24 and CD10. The gating of B cells may become very difficult in these cases. The third challenge with CD22 is the presence of two normal populations in the marrow that express CD22 but lack CD19 and CD24. These populations represent very early multipotent lymphoid stem cells (CD22+/CD34+/CD38-dim/CD10–/CD20–/CD24–) and Hg0 (CD22+/CD34+/CD38-bright/CD10-heterogeneous/CD20-dim). One should consider these populations when interpreting cases using CD22 for initial gating **(Fig. 5)**. The fourth challenge is the presence of therapy like inotuzumab directed toward CD22. This therapy may cause the disease to be missed if CD22 is used alone as a gating marker **(Fig. 6)**. The advantage of using CD22 and CD24 is that plasma cells are excluded at the initial stage of gating, as they are negative for both markers.

CD24: This marker starts getting expressed at early stages of B-cell development; however, the intensity reduces as the cell prepares to leave the bone marrow. Thus, the Hg1 and Hg2 populations show very bright expression of the marker, while very dim levels are expressed in the mature B-cell population. Plasma cells are negative for CD24, just like CD22. In myeloid cells, CD24 expression is a marker of maturity, and all myeloid cells express this beyond the stage of promyelocytes. The expression pattern closely follows that of CD11b or CD66b. Therefore, when using CD24 as a gating marker, we must ensure that maturing myeloid cells are excluded. This can be done by two methods: One is the use of an additional marker to exclude myeloid cells, such as CD66b or CD11b, and the other is by excluding myeloid cells by selecting only mononuclear cells for analysis by initial gating on SSC versus CD38 or CD45. The drawback of the first method is that we need to use an additional marker for exclusion, and not every laboratory has a vacant channel in their panels to accommodate this. The drawback of the second method is that although granulocytes are effectively excluded, CD24+ monocytes will still be included, affecting our interpretation. The use of CD24 alone is also not advisable, as it is significantly downregulated in cases of *KMT2A*-rearranged B-ALLs **(Fig. 6)**.

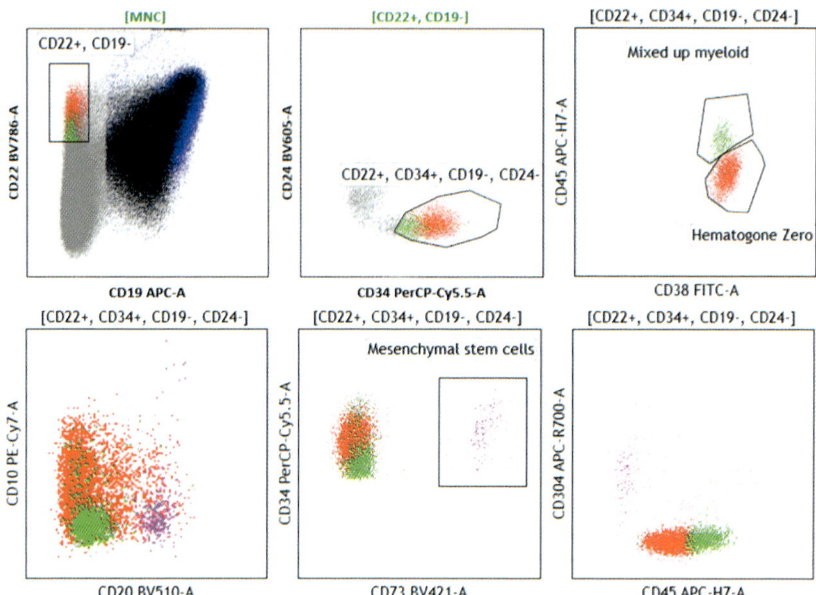

FIG. 5: Hematogone zero (Hg0) population isolated on CD22+ population (red color). Note that the population is negative for CD19 and CD24. This population may be interpreted as disease when CD22-based gating strategy is used in patients receiving anti-CD19 therapy. Note that CD22-based gating may include nonspecific populations such as mesenchymal stem cells (CD73++, CD304+, CD45–) and nonspecific binding on myeloid cells.

Cytoplasmic CD79a: Not much literature is available on the use of cytoplasmic CD79a as a gating marker for selecting B cells for B-ALL MRD evaluation. CD79a has been reported to show 88% specificity and 100% sensitivity for B-lineage differentiation. We have used this marker in our laboratory in occasional cases and found it useful for identifying B cells. This marker is especially useful in patients receiving multiple immunotherapies such as anti-CD19 and anti-CD22, with or without anti-CD38. It is even more useful if the case is negative for CD24 (e.g., *KMT2A*-rearranged cases). However, due to the cytoplasmic nature of the antibody, one needs to have multiple myeloid markers in the panel to clearly segregate the MRD population **(Fig. 7)**.

Use of Boolean gating in MFC: The use of multiple gating markers to select B cells is increasingly being used these days for B-ALL MRD in cases receiving targeted therapies. This method involves gating B cells using CD22, CD24, and CD19, and making a Boolean gate to include all these gated events. These events are then analyzed like a routine B-ALL MRD assay. One should remember that while using these markers (CD22/CD24) for gating, it is essential to exclude the normal myeloid cells from analysis using a sensitive myeloid marker such as CD66b or CD11b, as described in **Figure 7**. Currently, most commercially available software for MFC MRD analysis provides Boolean gating strategies for seamless analysis. This method will, however, require additional antibodies in addition to routine

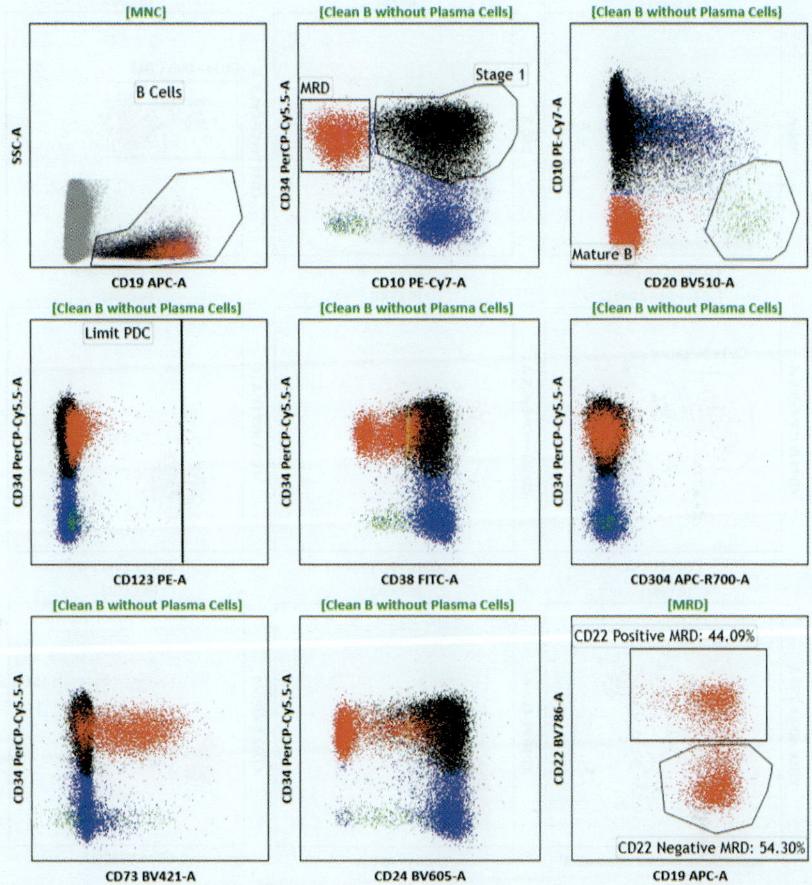

FIG. 6: CD22 used alone may miss a significant proportion of measurable residual disease (MRD) (red color population). This may happen, especially in cases with *KMT2A* gene rearrangement and Ph+ ALL. The case shown above is an *MLL* gene rearranged refractory B-ALL patient on therapy with inotuzumab (anti-CD22). Note the total absence of CD24 (characteristic of *KMT2A* rearrangement), which makes the identification of the B-lineage of the disease very difficult and nearly impossible if the patient has received both anti-CD19 and anti-CD22 therapies **(Fig. 7)**.

markers. This will result in an addition to the cost of the assay and also will require a flow cytometer of higher configuration to accommodate these new markers.

In addition to all the above strategies, we should remember that, despite targeted therapies, CD19+ relapses remain the most common. Therefore, one should always start the analysis as a normal B-ALL MRD using CD19 as the gating marker. However, alternative approaches should always be used in both positive and negative cases. The use of alternative gating is obviously to rule out CD19-negative disease. Positive cases need alternative gating to rule out the underlying CD19-negative component and to correctly measure the exact burden of the underlying disease.

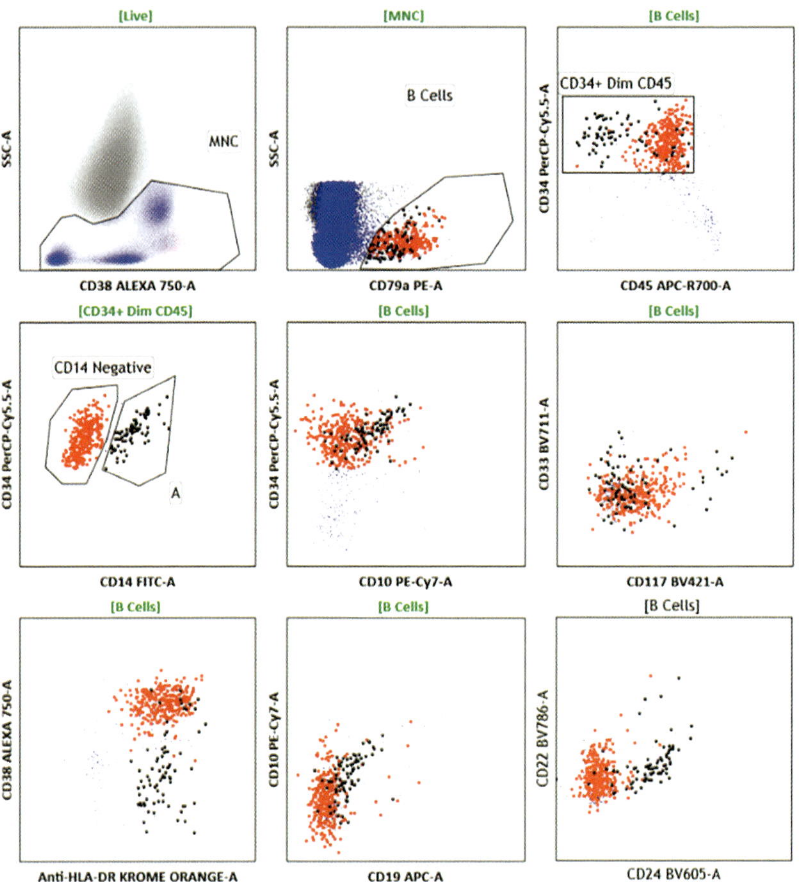

FIG. 7: The same case of *KMT2A*-rearranged B-ALL (as in **Fig. 6**) after therapy with both anti-CD22 and anti-CD19. Note the disease (red color) isolated with cytoplasmic CD79a, which is negative for both CD22 and CD19. The identification of B-lineage here is not completely possible, and these cases are often a diagnosis of exclusion, where we have to show that markers of other lineages, such as CD14, CD33, and CD117, are absent in this case.

CRITICAL POINTS TO REMEMBER

Treatment after CD19-directed therapies can sometimes lead to unforeseen outcomes. Lineage switch following anti-CD19 therapy is a rare but well-documented event that could be missed in MRD assays if myeloid/monocytic or T-lineage markers are not included in the panel. Lineage switch is an uncommon finding often associated with *KMT2A*-rearranged, Philadelphia-positive, and *ZNF384*-rearranged B-ALLs. Additionally, the incidence of this lineage switch is much higher in patients receiving blinatumomab. This is a novel mechanism of resistance to therapy, which may be due to the selective proliferation of a small underlying myeloid clone that has escaped therapy for anti-CD19 or due to leukemic stem cell reprogramming to a different lineage. The clonal selection of a CD19-negative clone following anti-CD19 therapy warrants the suitable combination of gating and key lineage-identifying markers.

Take Home Points

- There are three important B-cell gating markers for B-ALL MRD:
  - i. CD19 is sensitive and specific.
  - ii. CD22 is sensitive; however, not specific as it also includes a lot of other populations such as stem cells (including myeloid precursors) and Hg0 population (CD34+, CD38+, CD10 heterogeneous, CD24 negative, and CD19 negative).
  - iii. CD24-based gating is not sensitive (negative in KMT2A mutation) and not very specific (positive in myeloid cells beyond promyelocyte state).
- Boolean gating is advised and used widely, however, it requires myeloid markers such as CD13, CD11b, and CD66b to exclude myeloid cells.
- Cytoplasmic CD79a-based gating is sensitive however needs more experience and may pick up masqueraders such as Hg0.
- Comparison with diagnostic immunophenotype may be helpful in difficult cases.
- Always keep your senses open to unexpected outcomes such as lineage switch.

SUGGESTED READINGS

1. Saygin C, Cannova J, Stock W, Muffly L. Measurable residual disease in acute lymphoblastic leukemia: methods and clinical context in adult patients. Haematologica. 2022;107(12): 2783-93.
2. Mikhailova E, Illarionova O, Komkov A, Zerkalenkova E, Mamedov I, Shelikhova L, et al. Reliable Flow-Cytometric Approach for Minimal Residual Disease Monitoring in Patients with B-Cell Precursor Acute Lymphoblastic Leukemia after CD19-Targeted Therapy. Cancers (Basel). 2022;14(21):5445.
3. Chen X, Gao Q, Roshal M, Cherian S. Flow cytometric assessment for minimal/measurable residual disease in B lymphoblastic leukemia/lymphoma in the era of immunotherapy. Cytometry Part B: Clinical Cytometry. 2023;104(3):205-23.

CHAPTER 21

Measurable Residual Disease in T-cell Acute Lymphoblastic Leukemia/Lymphoma

Man Updesh Singh Sachdeva

ABSTRACT

T-cell acute lymphoblastic leukemia/lymphoma (T-ALL) is an aggressive hematologic malignancy accounting for 10–15% of pediatric and 20–25% of adult acute lymphoblastic leukemia (ALL) cases. It typically presents with features of hematopoietic failure, mediastinal masses, and central nervous system involvement. Originating from thymus-seeding progenitors, T-ALL is marked by dysregulation in T-cell development, with *NOTCH1* mutations and *FBXW7* loss being key pathogenic drivers. Subtypes of T-ALL—Early T-precursor (ETP), Early Cortical, and Late Cortical—are classified based on gene expression and immunophenotype, each associated with distinct prognoses.

Over recent decades, advancements in multiagent chemotherapy and targeted therapy have significantly improved survival rates in T-ALL. Measurable residual disease (MRD) has emerged as a critical prognostic tool, with its assessment at the end of consolidation therapy providing the strongest predictive value. While end-of-induction MRD assessment has shown prognostic relevance, especially in Western and Indian studies, delayed blast clearance in T-ALL supports the utility of end-of-consolidation MRD as a key timepoint for risk stratification.

MRD detection employs multicolor flow cytometry (MFC) and molecular techniques targeting immunoglobulin/T-cell receptor (Ig/TCR) rearrangements. MFC offers rapid, sensitive (up to 10^{-6}), and cost-effective detection by identifying immunophenotypic aberrancies in T cells. In contrast, molecular techniques like allele-specific oligonucleotide PCR and next-generation sequencing (NGS) provide high sensitivity and broader clonal detection but are technically demanding and affected by clonal evolution.

Pre-analytic variables, including sample quality, bone marrow vs. peripheral blood selection, and timing, critically affect MRD assay reliability. Analytic accuracy hinges on understanding T-cell maturation, using a standardized panel to distinguish leukemic cells from normal T/NK cells and other mimics. Post-analytic considerations emphasize standardized reporting of MRD levels, methodology, and sample parameters to guide clinical decisions.

Overall, MRD assessment in T-ALL integrates clinical, biological, and technical insights to refine prognostication and personalize therapy. With continued standardization and technological advances, MRD will increasingly inform treatment decisions and long-term outcomes in T-ALL management.

INTRODUCTION

The incidence of acute lymphoblastic leukemia (ALL) in the United States of America is 1.8 per constitute 100,000 for all age groups. T-cell acute lymphoblastic leukemia/lymphoma (T-ALL) constitute 10–15% of pediatric and 20–25% of adult ALL. It is twice as prevalent in males as in females. T-ALL is an aggressive disease that frequently presents with hyperleukocytosis accompanied by features of hematopoietic failure such as anemia, neutropenia, and thrombocytopenia. In addition, the patients commonly present with a mediastinal mass due to involvement of the thymus. Meningeal infiltration of the central nervous system and lymph nodes may also be noted at presentation. Patients with infiltration of T-lineage immature tumor cells primarily in the thymus and no or a limited bone marrow infiltration are diagnosed to have T-cell lymphoblastic lymphomas.

The normal hematopoiesis is a tightly regulated process that proceeds through continuous stages of differentiation as well as self-renewal. This is mostly governed by cell–cell interaction and growth/differentiating factors that control the expression of lineage-specific transcription factors. The maturation proceeds through a continuous stage of differentiation to multipotent progenitors that, upon progressive loss of self-renewal capacity, give rise to first oligopotent- and then to lineage-committed precursors. It is important to note that whereas the B- and myeloid-lineage cells mature in bone marrow, the T-lineage cells mature in the thymus. The "Thymus-seeding progenitor (TSP)", possibly residing in special niches of bone marrow, migrates to the thymus via peripheral blood in response to CCL21 and CCL25. These TSPs show expression of CD34, CD7, CD45RA, CCR7, CCR9, CXCR4, PSGL1 (P-selectin glycoprotein ligand-1), and Eph (Ephrin receptor) as they pass through the peripheral blood to reach the thymus. The early differentiation occurs in thymic microenvironment with NOTCH1 pathway playing an important role. NOTCH1 is a transmembrane receptor protein expressed on the lymphoid progenitors and serves as a transcription factor. It is activated by its ligands, i.e., "Jagged" and "delta-like", which are expressed on thymic epithelial cells. Once activated by the ligands, the intracellular domain of NOTCH1 is cleaved by gamma secretase. This cleaved portion then translocates to the nucleus and activates the expression of target genes. Further, FBXW7 directs the intracellular portion of NOTCH1 for degradation, thus terminating NOTCH signaling. Activating mutations of *NOTCH1* gene and loss of function mutations of the *FBXW7* gene lead to constitutive NOTCH signaling in T-ALL.

Notably, the lymphoid precursor cells retain NK- and myeloid-lineage-associated markers. Early thymocytes that lack surface CD4 and CD8 are called double-negative (DN) cells. These progress through four stages of differentiation, i.e., DN1, DN2, DN3, and DN4. DN3 cells express the preT cell receptor (pre-TCR), which is composed of an invariable pre-TCRα chain and a rearranged TCRβ. DN3 cells also have high levels of NOTCH signaling, which induces marked cell proliferation as they become DN4 cells. Cells that successfully rearrange TCRβ chain transform to double-positive (DP) cells expressing CD4 and CD8. At this point, the proliferation stops, and the TCRα chain is rearranged to form a complete TCR. Further, the cells with TCRs capable of recognizing major histocompatibility complex (MHC) survive and finally develop into single-positive CD4 or CD8 cells.

SUBGROUPS OF T-CELL ACUTE LYMPHOBLASTIC LEUKEMIA/LYMPHOMA

The present classification of T-ALL represents different clinically relevant subgroups. Importantly, the entities show an association with a unique gene expression profile and also with a distinct immunophenotype that reflects thymocyte development arrest at different stages of development. These are classified into early T-cell precursor (ETP) leukemia, early cortical, and late cortical subtypes. **Table 1** summarizes the gene expression signature, immunophenotype, and clinical relevance of the three subtypes of T-ALL.

TABLE 1: Gene expression signature, immunophenotype, and clinical relevance of T-cell acute lymphoblastic leukemia/lymphoma (T-ALL) subtypes.

Feature	Early T precursor	Early cortical	Late cortical
Gene signature	• Activating mutations in genes regulating cytokine receptors and RAS signaling such as *NRAS, KRAS, FLT3, IL7R, JAK3, JAK1, SH2B3,* and *BRAF* • Inactivating mutations or deletions of *GATA3, ETV6, RUNX1, IKZF1,* and histone-modifying genes such as *EZH2, EED, SUZ12, SETD2,* and *EP300* • Lower prevalence of *NOTCH1* mutations, very rare *CDKN2A* deletions	• High frequency of *NOTCH1* mutations and *CDKN2A* loss • Activation of homeobox genes *TLX1, TLX3, NKX21* and *NKX22* • Genetic alterations in *WT1, PHF6, PTPN2,* and *NUP214-ABL1* rearrangement	• Frequently show mutations in *NOTCH1* and *CDKN2A* • Higher prevalence of *PTEN* mutations and deletions • Aberrant expression *TAL1, LMO1* or *LMO2*
Immunophenotype	CD1a– and CD8, weakly express CD5 (<75% cells positive), and express one or more myeloid or stem cell markers (at least 25% of blasts) including CD11b, CD13, CD33, CD34, CD65, CD117, and HLADR	Surface CD3–, CD4+, CD8+, and CD1a+	Surface CD3+, CD4+, CD8+, CD1a–
Clinical relevance	High-risk group with reduced overall survival. Recent clinical series have reported better outcomes with intensified treatment strategies	Favorable prognosis	The presence of *PTEN* mutations is generally associated with high-risk disease and poor prognosis

STRATEGIC ADVANCEMENT IN THE MANAGEMENT OF T-CELL ACUTE LYMPHOBLASTIC LEUKEMIA/LYMPHOMA

There has been a steady improvement in the survival of children as well as young adolescents over the past several decades. This has been primarily due to progressive strategic changes in multiagent chemotherapy regimens in children and the adoption of the same for young adults. The 5-year survival of children with T-ALL was approximately 80% by the year 2000. These advancements in regimens include intensification of induction and consolidation, use of dexamethasone instead of prednisolone, omitting routine prophylactic cranial radiation, addition of nelarabine, precision medicine strategies such as use of targeted drugs, i.e., dasatinib, bortezomib, or ruxolitinib, in addition to combination chemotherapy, and use of minimal/measurable residual disease (MRD) assessment to evaluate response to therapy and predict outcomes for better management of the patients.

CLINICAL RELEVANCE AND TIME POINT DURING THERAPY FOR MEASURABLE RESIDUAL DISEASE ASSESSMENT

Introduction of MRD assessment in treatment protocols has played a crucial role in the management of patients of T-ALL. The consensus over time points during the course of therapy for assessment of MRD is lower when compared to that of B-ALL. In B-ALL, the end of induction time point is highly prognostic. In T-ALL, it seems that the blasts take a little longer to clear, and hence an early time point may not have the same impact on outcome. Therefore, for patients of T-ALL, a second time point, i.e., end of consolidation, generally after 2 months of additional therapy, seems to be most critical in terms of clearance and correlation with outcome. More than two decades ago, Willemse et al. showed that at the first 5 follow-up time points, the frequency of MRD-positive patients and the MRD levels were higher in T-ALL than in precursor-B-ALL, indicating a distinctly dynamic response to treatment compared to B-ALL. However, there are several studies over the past few years showing the utility of MRD assessment at the end of the induction phase, especially in context of providing prognostic information for event-free and/or overall survival in treatment naïve freshly diagnosed patients of T-ALL. The Children's Oncology Group phase 3 clinical trial AALL231 showed that the absence of residual leukemic cells (MRD $< 0.1\%$) at the end of induction was associated with a significantly better event-free survival (EFS) than those with detectable leukemic cells (MRD $\geq 0.1\%$). A study by Xue Y et al. on a cohort of 136 pediatric patients of T-ALL revealed similar results. At the end of the induction time point, MRD $< 0.1\%$ was associated with a better EFS as well as overall survival (OS) in comparison to children with detectable residual disease (MRD $\geq 0.1\%$). Some of the Indian studies have revealed comparable data when compared to published Western literature. Tembhare et al. looked into the utility of MRD assessment in their cohort of patients of T-ALL and found end of induction as a useful time point, giving prognostic information for relapse-free survival (RFS), EFS, and OS. Similar results for RFS and EFS were noted by Karthik et al. in their cohort of pediatric patients with T-ALL. Some other studies showed a later time point than the end of induction to be more predictive of outcomes.

Schrappe et al. conducted a multicentric study which included 464 children with T-ALL. The authors analyzed MRD at the end of induction (day 33) and at the end of consolidation (day 78) and found that MRD positivity at the end of induction became irrelevant when MRD at the end of consolidation was negative. They concluded that MRD $\geq 10^{-3}$ at the end of consolidation constituted the most important predictive factor relapse in childhood T-ALL. The study supports the concept of a delayed response to therapy in T-ALL compared to B-ALL and hence indicates that end of consolidation may yield better prognostic information than end of induction for T-ALL. The "Indian Collaborative Childhood Leukemia" (ICiCLe) study group's risk-stratified treatment incorporates MRD assessment for T-ALL both at the end of induction and the end of consolidation, similar to its B-ALL treatment strategy. Overall, assessment at both time points remains prevalent among most institutions routinely treating patients of T-ALL.

TECHNIQUES

Multicolor flow cytometry (MFC), with most assays comprising 8–12 antibody panels, and molecular assays targeting detection of patient-specific V(D) J rearrangements in immunoglobulin/T-cell receptor (*Ig/TCR*) genes are two principal techniques presently in use for high-sensitivity MRD assays.

Multicolor Flow Cytometry

Multicolor flow cytometry is a rapid, directly quantitative, relatively inexpensive, and less laborious technique that is applicable to nearly all cases of acute lymphoblastic leukemia, and the knowledge of the baseline immunophenotype of the leukemic cells may not be necessary. Irrespective of the age of an individual, there is a dynamic and well-orchestrated expression pattern of various markers which upregulate or downregulate as a hematopoietic cell develops from a stem cell to its early immature stage to a mature cell. Notably, unlike B- and myeloid-lineage cells, T-cells do not mature in the bone marrow. Hence, the maturation patterns noted for B- and myeloid-lineage cells in the bone marrow aspirate sample are not seen for T cells. As the maturation occurs in the thymus, the maturation patterns can be elucidated on thymocytes. The early T-precursor cells show expression of CD7, which remains consistently high throughout the stages of maturation. This is closely followed by expression of CD2 and CD5, while CD3, CD4, CD8, and CD1a expression are still absent (precortical stage). The next stage of maturation shows CD3 in the cytoplasm but lack of its surface expression. A dim CD4 expression is seen after this, followed by a dual expression of CD4 and CD8 along with CD1a (cortical stage). Further maturation of thymocytes leads to a surface CD3 expression accompanied by T-cell receptor (TCR), single positivity of CD4 or CD8, and loss of CD1a. In T-ALL, CD7 is highly expressed in nearly all cases, but the expression of other T-lineage-associated markers, such as CD1a, CD2, CD3, CD4, CD5, and CD8, is variable. The expression profile is often related to the maturational state of the blasts and may reasonably well recapitulate the normal stage in T-cell development. No matter how closely the leukemic blasts are immunophenotypically similar to the stage of maturation of the normal counterpart in the thymus, there are variations or aberrancies in expression of more than one marker, which help in distinguishing tumor cells from the normal. MFC utilizes a standardized panel of antibodies against known markers that are known to distinguish leukemic cells from normal hematopoietic cells. This has been conventionally called "different from normal" or "DfN" approach. MFC easily achieves a detection sensitivity of 10^{-4}; however, the technology and handling of samples have evolved over time to reach the sensitivity of 10^{-6}.

Molecular Techniques

The detection of V(D)J rearrangements in *Ig/TCR* genes has traditionally been done by the use of allele-specific oligonucleotide real-time qualitative polymerase chain reaction (ASO-qPCR). The MRD detection requires knowledge of the type of V(D)J rearrangement present in the leukemic blasts at diagnosis, and hence, a "fingerprint"-like leukemic cell-specific V(D)J rearrangement is identified at the time of diagnosis. This characterization of sequence requires a panel of screening PCRs using established primers for the complementarity-determining region 3 (CDR3). CDR3 represents the hypervariable heavy chain region of *Ig/TCR* genes. The PCR is followed by Sanger sequencing of products to identify the clone specific to the case and to develop the "patient-specific primers". The patient-specific primers are then used for MRD detection at the time of assessment of response to therapy. This technique generally has a sensitivity of 10^{-5}. The European BIOMED-2 (now called EuroClonality consortium) worked to standardize a multiplex-PCR assay for nearly all Ig/TCR targets and showed very high rates of detection in most B- and T-cell malignancies. The efforts eventually led to the commercial availability of kits to run these assays and further helped in interpretations, which were much less subjective with the introduction of interpretation algorithms.

The ASO-qPCR has now been gradually taken over by less laborious and higher sensitivity techniques, i.e., next-generation sequencing (NGS). The sensitivity of NGS is as high as 10^{-6}. The assay targets sequencing of V(D)J rearrangements of *Ig/TCR* genes as in ASO-qPCR but has capability to simultaneously amplify multiple combinations of rearranged *Ig/TCR* genes, and hence a single experiment can evaluate the entire *Ig/TCR* gene repertoire. This enables detection of additional clones, besides the main clone, which may exist at lower frequencies at the time of diagnosis but expand during the course of therapy. The analysis of NGS MRD data requires a bioinformatic pipeline. The "EuroClonality-NGS working group" had put efforts in developing and designing the amplicon-based Ig/TCR NGS assay, including bioinformatics, and also validating it for MRD marker identification in acute lymphoblastic leukemia. The results showed that NGS was particularly successful in correctly identifying biallelic rearrangements, which may be challenging for Sanger sequencing. Also, NGS performed better in the presence of a background of polyclonal rearrangements, and it allowed a more comprehensive coverage of rearrangement types. In addition, the presence of oligoclonality in ALL, which hampers conventional Ig/TCR MRD assessment, was better identified by NGS.

The sensitivity of molecular assay depends on the amount of input, i.e., DNA extracted from the sample. The yield, purity, and integrity of extracted nucleic acid remain the utmost important for optimal clonality testing results. The *Ig/TCR* gene rearrangement-based molecular assays are applicable to around 90% of cases of acute lymphoblastic leukemia. Notably, the early T-precursor ALL may arise from a more immature stage of precursor cells, which have not yet undergone TCR rearrangement. This is likely to reduce the sensitivity of these molecular assays. In addition to its laborious and time-consuming methodology, ASO-qPCR may be limited by the loss or emergence of new V(D)J sequences, leading to false negative MRD results.

Preanalytic Considerations

Assays for MRD assessment are high-sensitivity assays meant to detect a single residual leukemic cell among 10 thousand to 1 million normal hematopoietic cells, i.e., a sensitivity of 10^{-4} to 10^{-6}. The prerequisite of sample handling and processing for T-ALL MRD assay are like MRD assay for B-ALL or acute myeloid leukemia or multiple myeloma. Briefly, the bone marrow aspirate sample should be adequate in quantity to yield acquisition of millions of cells and should have no or minimal dilution of peripheral blood. "First-pull" bone marrow aspirate sample is necessary and most crucial for achieving adequate sensitivity of the assay. The initial pull is recommended to be not >3 mL to provide sufficient cellularity and avoid hemodilution. Bone marrow aspirate remains the sample of choice for MRD detection; however, in contrast to B-ALL, the peripheral blood sample has been shown to yield MRD results similar to the bone marrow aspirate sample. Most institutes still prefer bone marrow aspirates for MRD testing. The sample needs to be kept and transported at room temperature. It is best to process and acquire the sample as soon as possible and preferably within 48 hours of withdrawal. For the flow cytometry-based assays, the EuroFlow Consortium recommends "erythrocyte bulk lysis" procedure for the preparation of the sample for acquisition. This has been shown to increase the cell yield for carrying out a "high sensitivity" assay. Acquisition of above 4 million events may yield sensitivity of 10^{-5}, which is similar to that of PCR-based assays. Other studies have shown even higher sensitivity to the tune of 10^{-6} similar to NGS-based assays.

Quality control remains a central pillar for MRD assays, which includes appropriate checks on instrument settings as well as reagents, especially the fluorochrome-conjugated antibodies. Pretitration and cocktailing of the antibody panel is preferred for reducing errors and maintaining robustness of the assay. Another very crucial component is the determination of sensitivity, which is primarily done by establishing a limit of detection (LOD) and lower limit of quantification (LLOQ). LOD and LLOQ measurements can be obtained by "spiking experiments". In the context of T-ALL, it is advised to use non-T-ALL bone marrow aspirate samples, which preferably include bone marrow samples from patients of B-ALL under treatment. Other bone marrow aspirates, like staging marrows of lymphoma patients, may also be used. This sample is divided into four to five equal portions, and each tube is "spiked" by bone marrow aspirate from a diagnostic sample of a known T-ALL patient with a known percentage of T-lineage blasts. The spiking is undertaken in a way to achieve serial dilutions of leukemic cells across the four or five tubes of the non-T-ALL sample. The number of cells per microliter of bone marrow aspirate sample of T-ALL and that of non-T-ALL aspirate is prerequisite to calculate the volume of sample to be spiked for obtaining each dilution. Four or five serial dilutions of leukemic cells are usually achieved at low levels of positivity. For example, serial dilutions of 0.1%, 0.01%, 0.001%, and 0.0001% leukemic cells in a non-T-ALL bone marrow sample. Each tube is acquired in replicates of four or five, and the list mode files are analyzed for detection of the "spiked" leukemic cells in each replica of each tube of the sample. The percentage positivity obtained (observed positivity) is correlated with calculated (actual) positivity, and a coefficient of variation (CV) is also obtained for each dilution. LLOQ is usually determined as the percentage positivity (or the number of leukemic cell events) at which the CV is around ≤10%. Definite events detected as leukemic cells but with a higher CV, indicating a lesser precision in the quantification of MRD, represent LOD. In order to establish the sensitivity of MRD assay, it is recommended to carry out "spiking experiments" in around four to five separate non-T-ALL bone marrow samples, dividing each sample into four to five parts for obtaining serial dilutions of leukemic cells, and acquiring four to five replicates of these tubes.

Analytic Considerations

Measurable residual disease analysis by multicolor flow cytometry requires knowledge, training, and experience of "normal" to detect "different from normal". The marker-panel for T-ALL MRD analysis usually comprises CD2, CD3 (both surface and cytoplasmic), CD4, CD5, CD7, CD8, CD56 ± CD16, CD34, CD38, and CD45. Other markers commonly used are CD1a, CD48, CD99, and TdT. The key in the analysis is to utilize differential expression of cell-surface CD3, which is brightly expressed on normal T cells and in contrast is usually absent or dim on leukemic cells, whereas cytoplasmic expression of CD3 is noted both in normal and leukemic T cells, though the expression may vary in intensity in the blasts. In addition, CD7 expression is retained in nearly all T-ALL cases, which is in contrast to the mature T-cell neoplasms where downregulation of CD7 is often seen. Its persistence at bright levels makes CD7 a good candidate marker for initial gating of T cells. The principal task in the analysis is to discriminate residual leukemic cells from normal T and NK cells. CD56 ± CD16, along with CD38, helps in the identification of NK cells, which may be the most crucial cells to delineate before confirmation of residual leukemic cells. The over- or underexpression of other markers such as CD2 and CD5 compared to the expression levels on normal T and NK cells, and also the dual positive or dual negative expression of CD4 and CD8, assist in discriminating leukemic cells from normal T and NK cells. The expression of immaturity such as CD1a, CD34, and TdT on gated T-lineage cells indicates the presence of residual leukemic cells, as normal bone marrow does not show identifiable immature T cells. However, it is important to note that there may be downregulation of expression of one or more of these markers as a result of post-therapy immunophenotypic modifications, when compared to the expression levels on blasts at the time of diagnosis. CD48 is another promising marker which can be used to assess leukemic T cells. It has a lower expression in immature cells and shows a rise in expression levels with maturation. This marker has been shown to be useful for discriminating T-cell blasts from mature T and

NK cells and has shown stability and even enhanced ability to discriminate blasts after therapy.

The denominator for quantification of MRD requires filtering of viable cells from all acquired events. **Figure 1** depicts gating of viable cells for further analysis based on forward scatter (FSC) and side scatter (SSC) properties; however, many centers prefer to use a cell membrane permeable nucleic acid binding dye, like "Syto dyes" which fluoresce brightly after binding to nucleic acids and provide a denominator comprising all "nucleated cells". The sample may be assessed for hemodilution by quantifying cells which mostly reside in bone marrow and are either absent or in very low numbers in peripheral blood, such as erythroid precursors, myeloid precursors, hematogones, plasma cells, mast cells, and plasmacytoid dendritic cells. One or more of these cells may be assessed depending on the markers available in the antibody panel to evaluate these cells. Conversely, a larger proportion of neutrophils in a bone marrow sample would indicate the possibility of hemodilution.

The primary gate for T-ALL MRD analysis is based on the fact that CD7 is expressed in nearly all T-ALL cases and remains stable post-therapy. Hence, a gate based on CD7 positivity is very unlikely to exclude any residual leukemic cells from analysis. It is important to note that events included in SSC low and CD7 dim to bright positive gate **(Fig. 2)** is likely to show presence of not only mature T lymphocytes (both TCRαβ and TCRγδ types), NK cells (both mature and immature), TNK cells, and residual leukemic cells (if present), but also shows presence of a subset of plasmacytoid dendritic cells and a small proportion of myeloid precursors . Although a small proportion of mature T lymphocytes may be CD7 negative, this does not affect T-ALL MRD analysis. The residual leukemic cells are likely to be surface CD3 (sCD3) negative and hence are required to be discriminated from NK cells, which also lack sCD3 expression. These can be distinguished by the presence of cytoplasmic CD3 (cCD3) expression in leukemic T cells but absent in NK cells. However, a small proportion of NK cells may show the presence of cCD3, and adding to the complexity is the fact that cCD3

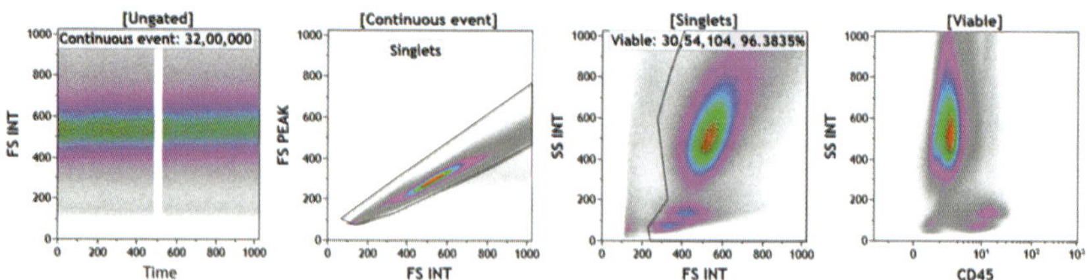

FIG. 1: Representative panel of plots from bone marrow aspirate sample of a case of T-ALL evaluated for treatment response. The first plot shows the gating of continuous events noted in FSC channel and acquired over a specific time duration. The second plot shows events gated from the continuous events, labeled as "Singlets". This is a "doublet discrimination" gate which selects "single cells" and removes any cell aggregates. The third plot shows the "single cells" on the FSC versus SSC plot with a viability gate placed to exclude any events smaller than the size of lymphocytes. A total number of viable events is depicted on the plot and shows 96.38% viable cells in the sample. The fourth plot shows all viable events depicted on the CD45 versus SSC plot.

(FSC: forward scatter; FS INT: forward-scatter integral; SSC: side scatter)

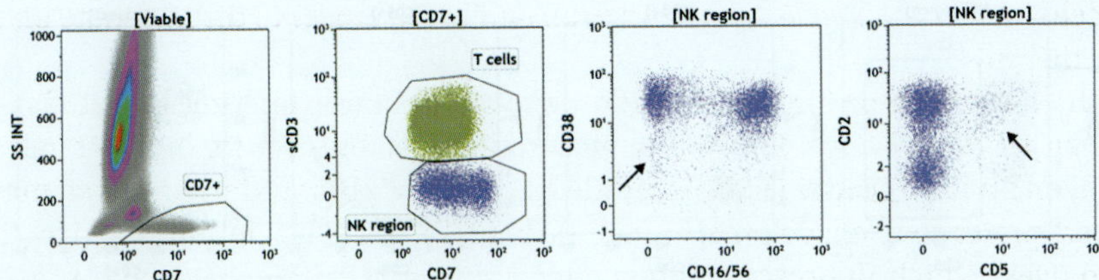

FIG. 2: The first plot shows gating of CD7+ and low SSC events. The second plot shows CD7+ events on CD7 versus surface CD3 (sCD3) plot. The residual leukemic cells are usually negative for sCD3; hence, analysis of the "NK region" gate (blue color) is important. Notably, an upregulation of sCD3 on leukemic cells may occur post-therapy, which implies that the "T cells" gate (green color) should always be analyzed (not shown in the figure) for the presence of any abnormal cells. The third plot shows the distribution of NK cells, which are either CD56/CD16 bright and are also present among CD38 bright and CD56/CD16 negative cluster. The black arrow indicates CD38 dim to negative and CD56/CD16 negative events and is a "suspicious" population. The fourth plot shows "NK region" events on CD2 versus CD5 plot. Normal NK cells have heterogenous CD2 expression and are mostly negative for CD5. The black arrow indicates a "suspicious" population showing a bright CD2 and CD5 expression.

on leukemic cells may be heterogenous and at times dim enough to make their discrete separation difficult. The surface marker profile of commonly used T/NK cell markers, such as CD56/CD16, CD38, CD2, CD5, CD4, and CD8, assists in separating NK cells from any residual leukemic cells **(Figs. 2 and 3)**.

The "NK region" depicted in **Figure 2** (comprising blue color events) may also contain a few mature T cells which have a downregulated sCD3. It is generally seen as a "shower" from above and can be identified as true T cells by their bright expression of CD2 and CD5 with a split in single positive CD4 and CD8 cells, and absence of NK cell marker profile **(Fig. 3)**. This "NK region" gate is also likely to have a few plasmacytoid dendritic cells and a few myeloid precursors, which can express heterogenous levels of CD7 (not shown in figures).

Overall, the residual leukemic cells may be demarcated and identified using a "different from normal" immunophenotypic profile with a background knowledge of all normal cells likely to be present in CD7+ gate. The MRD population (red color) from a case of T-ALL on therapy is depicted with normal mature T cells (green color) and NK cells (blue color) in **Figure 4**, to appreciate its distinct immunophenotypic profile in the index case.

Postanalytic Considerations

In the present era of risk-based management strategies of acute lymphoblastic leukemia, MRD results have crucial and distinct implications in treatment decisions at different time points and scenarios during the course of therapy. The general considerations and quality checks at the time of dispatch of the report remain similar to the reporting of most other laboratory tests, but a focus on components of the MRD-report format is necessary.

Patient Identifiers

The top first page details should include patient identifiers, which generally include name, age, gender, and medical record number.

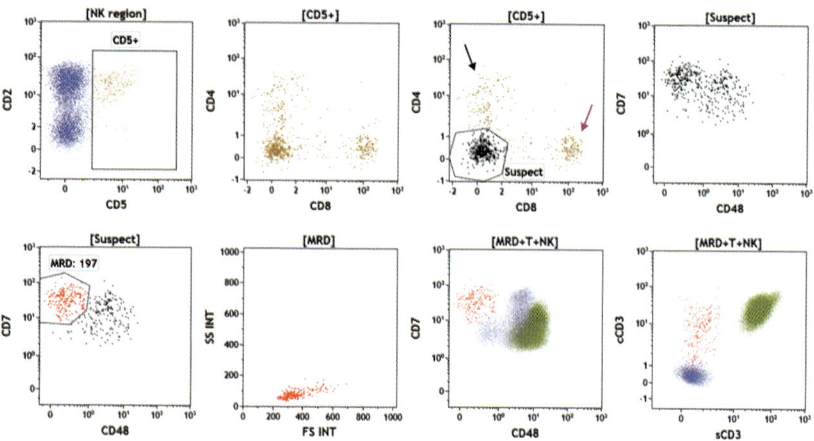

FIG. 3: The upper row first plot shows gating of CD5+ events, unlikely to be NK cells. The upper row second plot shows CD5+ events on a CD4 versus CD8 plot, and three discrete clusters are noted. The upper row third plot is same as the second plot and depicts CD4+CD8– (black arrow) and the CD4–CD8+ (pink arrow) populations which represent normal mature T cells with loss of sCD3 expression, whereas the third cluster of CD4–CD8–labeled as "suspect" (black color) does not have immunophenotype of mature T cells or NK cells (i.e., CD7+ sCD3– CD2+ CD5+ CD4– CD8–). The upper row fourth plot shows the "suspect" population in CD7 versus CD48 plot. The "suspect" population splits in two clusters, i.e., CD7bright + CD48dim and CD7 + CD48+. The lower row first plot shows gating of CD7bright + CD48dim cells labeled as "MRD" (red color) and depicts the definite residual leukemic cells, amounting to 197 events. The lower row second plot depicts "MRD" population in FSC versus SSC plot and shows these to be nicely clustered events. The lower row third and fourth plots depict three distinct cell populations together, i.e., mature T cells (green color), NK cells (blue color), and residual leukemic cells (red color). The residual leukemic cells are CD7bright+, CD48dim, sCD3 negative, and cCD3 heterogeneously positive. Also, note that the "NK cell events" (blue color) may include a subset of plasmacytoid dendritic cells and/or myeloid precursors which exhibit heterogeneous levels of CD7 positivity (not shown).

Measurable Residual Disease Results

It is good to provide and highlight the percentage of MRD detected prominently at the first page itself, preferably with a mention of "MRD-negative" or "MRD-positive" results, depending on the limit of detection (LOD) of the assay. For the flow cytometric assay, it is also advised to provide the absolute number of "MRD" events (numerator) and the number of viable cells (denominator) in the sample, along with the sensitivity of the assay achieved.

Patient's Medical History

Patient's medical history should be mentioned on the first page, which includes initial diagnosis (e.g., early T-precursor acute lymphoblastic leukemia), a mention of immunophenotype of blasts at the time of diagnosis and any major immunophenotypic shifts during post-therapy assessments. Any important molecular-assay results should be provided. There should be mention of current disease status (e.g., in complete morphological remission), followed by current phase of treatment (e.g., induction completed), and possibly the day of therapy (e.g., day 35). Medical history should include mention and details of hematopoietic stem cell transplant (if done) and details of any "targeted therapy" given.

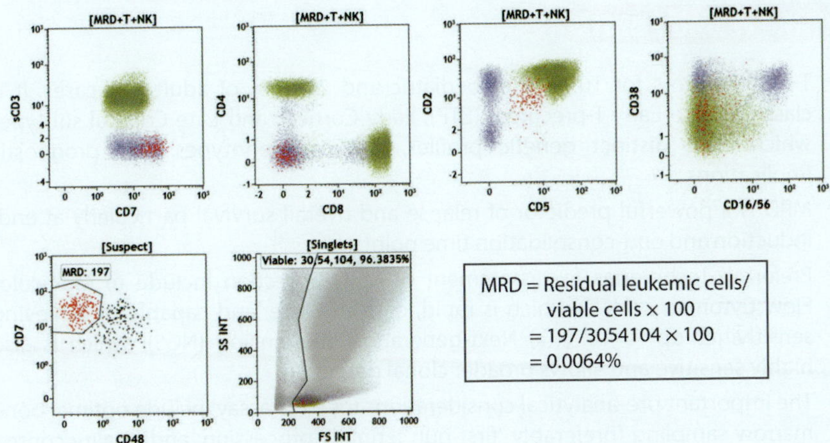

FIG. 4: The upper row plots depict three distinct cell populations together, i.e., mature T cells (green color), NK cells (blue color), and residual leukemic cells (red color). The residual leukemic cells are CD7bright+, sCD3–, CD4–, CD8–, CD2dim+, CD5dim+, CD56/16– and CD38–to dim+. The lower row shows the calculation of MRD. The lower row first plot shows MRD gate with a total of 197 events (numerator), and the second plot shows total viable events based on FSC and SSC properties and amounts to 3,054,104 events (denominator). The text box shows the actual calculation of MRD, which is "total MRD events" divided by "total viable events" multiplied by 100 to give the percentage of residual disease, amounting to 0.0064%, for the index case.

Sample Details

The first page should include sample details such as the source (e.g., bone marrow aspirate), sample volume, date and time of withdrawal of the sample to get information about the "sample age", and a mention of sample quality (optimal or not). In case of bone marrow aspirate, it is good to know if the aspirate for MRD assay is a "first-pull" sample or not.

Methodology Details

Method for assessment of MRD should be provided (e.g., multicolor flow cytometry with details of flow cytometer used for assessment), followed by the assay details (e.g., single tube, 10-color assay, comprising sCD3, cCD3, CD4, CD5, CD7, CD8, CD56/CD16, CD38, CD45, and CD48). The assay sensitivity should be mentioned in the methodology section of the report.

Summary of Results

The results should be mentioned in detail in this section, which includes a statement whether MRD is detected or not, the levels of MRD (in percentage), and a description of the immunophenotype of residual blasts. A section of comments may be added as per the requirements (e.g., comment on quality of sample, especially if inadequate events or hemodilution is noted, any major shifts of immunophenotype of blasts from diagnostic and/or previous immunophenotype). This section may also include a summary of any previous MRD results of the patient, if possible, in a graphical format, showing a trend of MRD results.

Take Home Points

- T-ALL accounts for 10–15% of pediatric and 20–25% of adult ALL cases. It is classified into Early T-precursor (ETP), Early Cortical, and Late Cortical subtypes which have distinct genetic profiles, immunophenotypes, and prognostic implications.
- MRD is a powerful predictor of relapse and overall survival particularly at end-induction and end-consolidation time points.
- Preferred techniques for assessment of MRD detection include (i) Multicolor Flow Cytometry (MFC) which is rapid, cost-effective, and capable of achieving sensitivities up to 10^{-6}; (ii) Next-generation Sequencing (NGS), which is also highly sensitive and allows broader clonal detection.
- The important pre-analytical considerations for MRD assay include optimal bone marrow sampling (preferably "first-pull"), timely processing, and quality control are crucial for high assay sensitivity.
- The analytical strategies for accurate MRD detection by MFC rely on recognizing aberrant immunophenotypes and distinguishing leukemic cells from normal T, NK, dendritic, and myeloid cells. CD7 is a stable and useful gating marker; CD3, CD4, CD8, CD5, CD2, CD48 assist in analysis and identification of MRD.
- The post-analytical reporting should include patient identifiers, sample details, methodology, MRD levels, assay sensitivity, and interpretative comments.
- Integration of MRD with risk-adapted protocols supports personalized therapy in T-ALL.

SUGGESTED READINGS

1. SEER Database. (2021). [online] Available from https://seer.cancer.gov/statfacts/html/alyl.html [Last accessed May, 2025].
2. Belver L, Ferrando A. The genetics and mechanisms of T cell acute lymphoblastic leukaemia. Nat Rev Cancer. 2016;16(8):494-507.
3. Vadillo E, Dorantes-Acosta E, Pelayo R, Schnoor M. T cell acute lymphoblastic leukemia (T-ALL): New insights into the cellular origins and infiltration mechanisms common and unique among hematologic malignancies. Blood Rev. 2018;32(1):36-51.
4. Shiraz P, Jehangir W, Agrawal V. T-Cell Acute Lymphoblastic Leukemia-Current Concepts in Molecular Biology and Management. Biomedicines. 2021;9(11).
5. Willemse MJ, Seriu T, Hettinger K, d'Aniello E, Hop WCJ, Panzer-Grümayer ER, et al. Detection of minimal residual disease identifies differences in treatment response between T-ALL and precursor B-ALL. Blood. 2002;99(12):4386-93.
6. Hayashi RJ, Hermiston ML, Wood BL, Teachey DT, Devidas M, Chen Z, et al. MRD at the end of induction and EFS in T-cell lymphoblastic lymphoma: Children's Oncology Group trial AALL1231. Blood. 2024;143(20):2053-8.
7. Xue YJ, Wang Y, Lu AD, Jia YP, Zuo YX, Ding MM, et al. Clinical Analysis of Pediatric T-Cell Acute Lymphoblastic Leukemia Using the MRD-Oriented Strategy System. Clin Lymphoma Myeloma Leuk. 2023;23(7):477-83.
8. Tembhare PR, Narula G, Khanka T, Ghogale S, Chatterjee G, Patkar NV, et al. Post-induction Measurable Residual Disease Using Multicolor Flow Cytometry Is Strongly Predictive of Inferior Clinical Outcome in the Real-Life Management of Childhood T-Cell Acute Lymphoblastic Leukemia: A Study of 256 Patients. Front Oncol. 2020;10:577.
9. Bommannan K, Arumugam JR, Radhakrishnan V, Kalaiyarasi JP, Karunakaran P, Mehra N, et al. Relevance of flow cytometric categorization and end-of-induction measurable

residual disease assessment in pediatric and adult T-lymphoblastic leukemia patients. Blood Res. 2022;57(3):175-96.

10. Schrappe M, Valsecchi MG, Bartram CR, Schrauder A, Panzer-Grümayer R, Möricke A, et al. Late MRD response determines relapse risk overall and in subsets of childhood T-cell ALL: results of the AIEOP-BFM-ALL 2000 study. Blood. 2011;118(8):2077-84.
11. Das N, Banavali S, Bakhshi S, Trehan A, Radhakrishnan V, Seth R, et al. Protocol for ICiCLe-ALL-14 (InPOG-ALL-15-01): a prospective, risk stratified, randomised, multicentre, open label, controlled therapeutic trial for newly diagnosed childhood acute lymphoblastic leukaemia in India. Trials. 2022;23(1):102.
12. DiGiuseppe JA, Wood BL. Applications of Flow Cytometric Immunophenotyping in the Diagnosis and Posttreatment Monitoring of B and T Lymphoblastic Leukemia/Lymphoma. Cytometry B Clin Cytom. 2019;96(4):256-65.
13. Saygin C, Cannova J, Stock W, Muffly L. Measurable residual disease in acute lymphoblastic leukemia: methods and clinical context in adult patients. Haematologica. 2022;107(12): 2783-93.
14. Flores-Montero J, Grigore G, Fluxá R, Hernández J, Fernandez P, Almeida J, et al. EuroFlow Lymphoid Screening Tube (LST) database for automated identification of blood lymphocyte subsets. J Immunol Methods. 2019;475:112662.
15. Langerak AW, Groenen PJTA, Brüggemann M, Beldjord K, Bellan C, Bonello L, et al. EuroClonality/BIOMED-2 guidelines for interpretation and reporting of Ig/TCR clonality testing in suspected lymphoproliferations. Leukemia. 2012;26(10):2159-71.
16. Brüggemann M, Kotrová M, Knecht H, Bartram J, Boudjogrha M, Bystry V, et al. Standardized next-generation sequencing of immunoglobulin and T-cell receptor gene recombinations for MRD marker identification in acute lymphoblastic leukaemia; a EuroClonality-NGS validation study. Leukemia. 2019;33(9):2241-53.
17. Kotrova M, Volland A, Kehden B, Trautmann H, Ritgen M, Wäsch R, et al. Comparison of minimal residual disease levels in bone marrow and peripheral blood in adult acute lymphoblastic leukemia. Leukemia. 2020;34(4):1154-7.
18. van der Velden VHJ, Jacobs DCH, Wijkhuijs AJM, Comans-Bitter WM, Willemse MJ, Hählen K, et al. Minimal residual disease levels in bone marrow and peripheral blood are comparable in children with T cell acute lymphoblastic leukemia (ALL), but not in precursor-B-ALL. Leukemia. 2002;16(8):1432-6.
19. Theunissen P, Mejstrikova E, Sedek L, van der Sluijs-Gelling AJ, Gaipa G, Bartels M, et al. Standardized flow cytometry for highly sensitive MRD measurements in B-cell acute lymphoblastic leukemia. Blood. 2017;129(3):347-57.
20. Tembhare PR, Subramanian PG, Ghogale S, Chatterjee G, Patkar NV, Gupta A, et al. A High-Sensitivity 10-Color Flow Cytometric Minimal Residual Disease Assay in B-Lymphoblastic Leukemia/Lymphoma Can Easily Achieve the Sensitivity of 2-in-10(6) and Is Superior to Standard Minimal Residual Disease Assay: A Study of 622 Patients. Cytometry B Clin Cytom. 2020;98(1):57-67.
21. Wood B, Jevremovic D, Béné MC, Yan M, Jacobs P, Litwin V. Validation of cell-based fluorescence assays: practice guidelines from the ICSH and ICCS - part V - assay performance criteria. Cytometry B Clin Cytom. 2013;84(5):315-23.
22. Wood BL, Levin G, Wilson M, Winter SS, Dunsmore K, Loh ML, et al. High-Throughput Screening by Flow Cytometry Identifies Reduced Expression of CD48 As a Universal Characteristic of T-ALL and a Suitable Target for Minimal Residual Disease (MRD) Detection. Blood. 2011;118(21):2547.
23. El Hussein S, Wang W. Flow Cytometry Profiling of Plasmacytoid Dendritic Cell Neoplasms. Cancers (Basel). 2024;16(11).
24. Kriegsmann K, Löffler H, Eckstein V, Schulz R, Kräker S, Braun U, et al. CD7 is expressed on a subset of normal CD34-positive myeloid precursors. Eur J Haematol. 2018;101(3):318-25.
25. De Smedt M, Taghon T, Van de Walle I, De Smet G, Leclercq G, Plum J. Notch signaling induces cytoplasmic CD3ε expression in human differentiating NK cells. Blood. 2007;110(7): 2696-703.

CHAPTER 22

Setting Up a Diagnostic Laboratory: Costing and Inventory Management

Ananthvikas Jayaram, Sujay Ramaprasad

ABSTRACT

Costing and inventory management are crucial for hematopathology laboratories to ensure efficient operations and financial sustainability. Effective costing involves understanding direct, indirect, fixed, and variable costs, as well as utilizing cost accounting and break-even analysis. Key components of laboratory costs include consumables and reagents, equipment and maintenance, staffing and training, and overhead costs. Efficient inventory management is essential to balance availability and cost, involving principles such as optimal stock levels, timely reordering, and usage pattern tracking. Challenges in inventory management include tracking items with varying shelf lives and predicting demand fluctuations.

Strategies for cost optimization include lean laboratory practices, automation, vendor negotiations, and standardization of protocols. Various inventory control techniques, such as activity-based costing (ABC) analysis, just-in-time inventory management, and first in, first out (FIFO), help maintain efficient operations. Technology plays a significant role in inventory management, with laboratory information systems, barcode and radio frequency identification (RFID) tracking, and integrated inventory management software enhancing accuracy and streamlining workflows. Quality management is closely linked to inventory management, ensuring the availability of high-quality reagents and proper expiry management.

Costing models such as ABC and per-test costing help laboratories understand and manage expenses effectively. Resource-limited settings face unique economic challenges, requiring cost-effective practices and innovative solutions. Regulatory and ethical considerations are crucial in cost and inventory management, ensuring compliance and patient-focused decision-making. Future trends include advances in inventory management technologies, predictive analytics for cost forecasting, and the impact of telepathology and remote diagnostics.

Costing and inventory management are pivotal to the efficient functioning of hematopathology laboratories. Hematopathology, as a diagnostic and research field, requires adequate resources and infrastructure to deliver accurate results. Managing costs and inventory effectively ensures not only the sustainability of laboratory operations but also the timely accessibility of advanced diagnostic tools to patients.

The importance of these practices lies in their ability to optimize resources, reduce waste, and enhance laboratory efficiency. Proper costing allows laboratories to determine the true expense of tests and services, enabling informed decisions on pricing and budgeting. Meanwhile, efficient inventory management minimizes stockouts and overstocking of reagents and consumables, ensuring uninterrupted operations and the prevention of expired or unused inventory. It helps in laboratory tests being competitively priced in the market.

The impact of effective costing and inventory management extends beyond operational efficiency. Timely availability of diagnostic tools improves turnaround times, directly influencing patient outcomes. By controlling costs, laboratories can maintain affordability for patients while adhering to high standards of care.

This chapter aims to explore the principles, strategies, and tools for effective costing and inventory management in hematopathology. It will provide insights into optimizing laboratory processes, balancing quality with cost constraints, and adopting innovative solutions to meet the evolving demands of this dynamic field.

INTRODUCTION

Costing and inventory management form the backbone of efficient hematopathology laboratory operations. They help balance resource utilization with financial prudence, ensuring high-quality diagnostics remain accessible. This chapter introduces the essential concepts, challenges, and tools involved in managing costs and supplies. It also highlight strategies to streamline processes while upholding clinical and ethical standards.

FUNDAMENTALS OF COSTING IN HEMATOPATHOLOGY

Understanding the fundamentals of costing is essential for efficient financial management in hematopathology laboratories. Accurate costing ensures that laboratory services remain sustainable while maintaining high standards of diagnostic care.

Direct costs include expenses directly tied to performing a test, such as reagents, consumables, and technician salaries. In contrast, *indirect costs* are shared expenses, including utilities, administrative support, and equipment depreciation. Identifying and allocating these costs correctly is critical for accurate test pricing and financial planning.

Fixed costs, such as rent and equipment maintenance, remain constant regardless of test volume, while *variable costs*, such as consumables and utilities, fluctuate with the number of tests performed. Analyzing these cost categories helps laboratories optimize operations, especially when scaling services or managing fluctuating workloads.

Cost accounting plays a pivotal role in providing a detailed understanding of expenses. It helps laboratories allocate costs appropriately, set competitive prices, and identify inefficiencies. Tools such as *break-even analysis* further aid decision-making by identifying the point at which revenue equals total costs. This helps determine whether a new test or service is financially viable.

By mastering these costing fundamentals, hematopathology laboratories can ensure fiscal responsibility, improve decision-making, and enhance the affordability and accessibility of their services. This chapter will delve deeper into these concepts, providing actionable strategies for laboratory management.

COMPONENTS OF LABORATORY COSTS

The cost structure of a hematopathology laboratory encompasses various components, each of which plays a critical role in maintaining operational efficiency and diagnostic accuracy. Understanding these components allows laboratories to optimize expenditures without compromising service quality.

Consumables and reagents are among the most significant direct costs. These include test-specific items such as reagents, slides, pipettes, and disposable gloves. Proper inventory management is essential to prevent stockouts and minimize wastage due to expired products. *Equipment and maintenance* are substantial capital and operational expenses. High-performance analyzers, microscopes, and hematology-specific instruments are necessary for precise diagnostics. Regular maintenance and calibration are crucial to ensure reliable results and prolong the lifespan of these costly assets.

Staffing and training represent another significant cost. Qualified pathologists, laboratory technicians, and support staff are vital to laboratory operations. Continuous professional development and training ensure the workforce is equipped with the latest skills and knowledge to handle complex tests and technologies.

Overhead costs include utilities such as electricity and water, software for laboratory management, and administrative expenses such as recordkeeping and regulatory compliance. These costs, while indirect, are essential to sustaining operations and maintaining quality standards.

By analyzing these cost components, laboratories can allocate resources effectively, streamline operations, and achieve a balance between quality, efficiency, and cost-effectiveness.

INVENTORY MANAGEMENT BASICS

Inventory management is a systematic process of overseeing and controlling the procurement, storage, and utilization of materials to ensure their availability while minimizing costs and waste. In a hematopathology laboratory, effective inventory management is vital for uninterrupted operations, cost efficiency, and maintaining diagnostic quality.

The principles of inventory management include ensuring optimal stock levels, timely reordering, and tracking usage patterns. These principles aim to strike a balance between availability and cost, avoiding both stockouts and overstocking. Hematopathology laboratories handle diverse inventory types, including reagents, consumables such as slides and pipettes, equipment spare parts, and quality control materials. Each category requires distinct handling protocols, shelf-life considerations, and storage conditions. Inventory turnover, which measures how often inventory is used and replenished, is a critical metric.

High turnover indicates efficient inventory use and minimal waste, while low turnover may signal overstocking or underutilization. Proper turnover ensures fresh reagents and consumables are always available, directly impacting test reliability. Managing laboratory inventory comes with challenges, such as tracking items with varying shelf lives, predicting demand fluctuations, and ensuring compatibility with evolving equipment and protocols. Overcoming these challenges requires robust systems, such as laboratory information systems (LIS) and automated inventory tracking, coupled with strategic planning and staff training to ensure seamless operations.

STRATEGIES FOR COST OPTIMIZATION

Cost optimization in hematopathology laboratories is critical for maintaining financial sustainability while delivering high-quality diagnostic services. Several strategies can help laboratories streamline operations and reduce expenses.

- *Lean laboratory practices* focus on eliminating waste, improving workflows, and maximizing resource utilization. Techniques such as process mapping, continuous quality improvement, and minimizing non-value-added activities help optimize test processing, reduce turnaround times, and lower costs.
- *Automation* plays a transformative role in cost-efficiency. Automated systems reduce human errors, increase throughput, and enhance precision, leading to long-term savings. For example, robotic sample handling and digital pathology solutions streamline operations and allow staff to focus on higher-value tasks, further driving efficiency.
- *Vendor negotiations and bulk purchasing* are key to reducing procurement costs. Establishing long-term partnerships with suppliers and leveraging economies of scale can result in significant discounts on reagents, consumables, and equipment. Additionally, aligning contracts with laboratory needs—such as flexible delivery schedules—ensures optimal inventory management and cost control.
- *Standardization of protocols and test panels* minimizes variability, improves efficiency, and simplifies inventory requirements. By consolidating similar tests into standardized workflows, laboratories can reduce the need for specialized reagents, decrease training costs, and enhance operational consistency.

Together, these strategies empower laboratories to optimize costs without compromising diagnostic quality, ensuring sustainability and accessibility.

INVENTORY CONTROL TECHNIQUES

Effective inventory control is crucial for hematopathology laboratories to maintain uninterrupted operations, minimize waste, and optimize costs. Various techniques provide frameworks for managing inventory efficiently. A few examples are listed here:

- *Activity-based costing (ABC) analysis* is a categorization method that classifies inventory into three groups based on usage and value. Group A includes high-value, low-quantity items requiring tight control (e.g., specific reagents or rare quality control materials). Group B includes moderately important items, while Group C contains low-value, high-quantity items (e.g., general consumables such as gloves). This categorization helps prioritize resources and focus management efforts on critical items.

- *Just-in-time (JIT) inventory management* minimizes stock levels by ordering materials only when needed. This technique reduces storage costs and waste due to expired items. However, it requires a reliable supply chain and precise demand forecasting to avoid stockouts.
- *First in, first out (FIFO)* ensures older inventory is used first, reducing the risk of expired or outdated stock, especially for time-sensitive reagents. Conversely, *LIFO* may be used in specific scenarios where newer stock is prioritized, though it is less common in laboratories.
- *Safety stock and reorder point calculations* help maintain a buffer for unexpected demand or supply chain disruptions. Safety stock ensures continuity during delays, while reorder points trigger timely procurement to prevent stockouts.

These techniques collectively enhance inventory control, ensuring efficient and cost-effective laboratory operations.

TECHNOLOGY IN INVENTORY MANAGEMENT

Advancements in technology have revolutionized inventory management in hematopathology laboratories, enabling precise tracking, streamlined workflows, and cost efficiency. Implementing robust technological solutions is essential for maintaining accurate inventory and meeting the high standards required in diagnostics.

Laboratory information systems play a pivotal role in inventory management. They facilitate real-time tracking of inventory levels, consumption rates, and expiration dates. Integration with procurement systems ensures automated reordering when stock reaches critical levels, reducing the risk of stockouts or overstocking. LIS also enhances traceability by linking inventory data to specific tests and patient records, ensuring compliance with quality standards and regulatory requirements. Barcode and RFID tracking add another layer of precision. Barcode systems streamline the recording of incoming and outgoing inventory, reducing manual errors and improving accountability. Radio frequency identification (RFID) technology further enhances tracking by allowing instant scanning and real-time location updates, even for large inventories. These tools enable fast inventory audits, saving time and improving accuracy. The integration of inventory management software consolidates all inventory-related data into a single platform. This integration allows seamless communication between storage, procurement, and usage data, providing comprehensive insights into inventory trends. Advanced analytics and reporting features in these systems support demand forecasting, cost control, and informed decision-making.

QUALITY MANAGEMENT AND INVENTORY

Effective inventory management is a cornerstone of quality control in hematopathology laboratories, directly influencing diagnostic accuracy and patient outcomes. A robust relationship between inventory and quality management ensures that laboratory operations are reliable, efficient, and compliant with industry standards.

Proper inventory management supports quality control by ensuring the availability of high-quality reagents and consumables. A well-maintained inventory system prevents stockouts and ensures that all materials used in testing meet the required standards, thereby reducing errors and enhancing test consistency. By integrating inventory tracking with quality management processes, laboratories can ensure compliance with accreditation and regulatory requirements.

Expiry management is a critical component of quality control. Reagents and consumables must be monitored for expiration dates to avoid using degraded materials that could compromise test results. Automated tracking systems and regular inventory audits are essential to manage expiration effectively, reducing waste and maintaining reliability. Calibration and preventive maintenance schedules for equipment are vital to both inventory and quality management. Spare parts and calibration kits must be readily available to minimize downtime and ensure that instruments function optimally. Preventive maintenance reduces the risk of unexpected failures, supporting consistent and accurate testing.

COSTING MODELS FOR HEMATOPATHOLOGY LABORATORIES

Costing models are critical tools for understanding and managing expenses in hematopathology laboratories. They enable accurate pricing, resource optimization, and informed decision-making, ensuring both financial sustainability and high-quality patient care.

Activity-based costing is a detailed approach that assigns costs to specific activities within the laboratory. It identifies the resources consumed at each step of a test process, from sample preparation to reporting. By linking costs directly to activities, ABC provides a clearer picture of where resources are being utilized and highlights areas for improvement. This model is especially useful for complex tests, requiring multiple steps and significant resource allocation.

Per-test costing approaches focus on calculating the total cost of individual tests. This involves aggregating direct costs, such as reagents and consumables, and allocating a portion of indirect costs, such as equipment depreciation and staff salaries. Per-test costing helps laboratories determine pricing strategies and assess the financial feasibility of introducing new tests or services.

Cost allocation in multidepartment laboratories involves distributing shared costs, such as utilities, administrative expenses, and common equipment, across various departments. Accurate allocation ensures that each department bears its fair share of expenses, fostering transparency and accountability.

ECONOMIC CHALLENGES IN RESOURCE-LIMITED SETTINGS

Hematopathology laboratories in resource-limited settings face unique economic challenges that demand innovative and cost-effective solutions to ensure quality diagnostic services. These laboratories must balance financial constraints while meeting the growing demand for accurate and timely diagnostics.

Cost-effective practices are essential for such settings. These include bulk purchasing of reagents and consumables to benefit from economies of scale, reusing certain laboratory items (where safe and permissible), and adopting open-source software for LIS. Collaboration with government initiatives or nonprofit organizations can also provide access to subsidized equipment or testing materials.

Balancing cost constraints with quality is a constant challenge. Laboratories must avoid compromising diagnostic accuracy due to budgetary pressures. Implementing standardized protocols and lean laboratory practices can optimize resource utilization while maintaining high-quality standards. Training staff to perform multiple roles and maintaining equipment through regular preventive maintenance can further enhance efficiency.

Public health laboratories provide inspiring examples of overcoming resource limitations. For instance, centralized testing hubs reduce costs by consolidating services for multiple smaller laboratories. Additionally, partnerships with international organizations have facilitated access to affordable testing kits and training programs.

REGULATORY AND ETHICAL CONSIDERATIONS

Regulatory and ethical considerations are integral to cost and inventory management in hematopathology laboratories, ensuring compliance, transparency, and a patient-focused approach to decision-making. Adherence to these principles fosters trust, minimizes risks, and enhances the overall quality of diagnostic services.

Compliance with financial and inventory regulations is essential for laboratory operations. Laboratories must adhere to local and international guidelines for financial reporting, procurement practices, and inventory control. Accurate documentation of expenses and inventory levels ensures accountability and facilitates audits. Compliance with storage and usage standards for reagents and equipment, as defined by regulatory authorities, is critical to maintaining the reliability and safety of diagnostic procedures.

Ethical issues in cost containment often arise when financial constraints impact decision-making. Laboratories must avoid compromising the quality of diagnostics for cost-saving measures. This includes using substandard reagents, deferring equipment maintenance, or limiting essential testing. Ethical practices involve prioritizing patient safety and ensuring that cost-cutting strategies do not jeopardize diagnostic accuracy or accessibility. A patient-centric approach in resource allocation emphasizes equity and fairness. Resources should be

TABLE 1: A sample table to aid in capturing all the required inputs for performing a test and to calculate the cost per reportable result.

Particulars	Total	Input 1	Input 2	Input 3	Input 4
Vendor					
Name of reagent/control/ calibrator/accessory	xx				
Cost per kit	xx				
GST%	xx	12%	12%	12%	12%
Cost per kit inclusive of GST	xx	–	–	–	–
No. of tests/kit	xx	15.00	1.00	1.00	1.00
Cost per test	–	–	–	–	–
QA/QC @ 20%	–	–	–	–	–
Cost per reportable test (CPRT)	–	–	–	–	–

allocated to maximize patient benefit, particularly in resource-limited settings. Balancing cost efficiency with the need to provide affordable, high-quality care is a fundamental ethical obligation for laboratories, ensuring positive outcomes for all stakeholders.

SAMPLE PROCESS OF CALCULATING COST PER REPORTABLE RESULT FROM THE AUTHOR'S LABORATORY

When calculating the cost of a test to the laboratory, a variety of entry data points are captured, including reagents and consumables, to derive the cost per test. To this, a variable percentage is added to account for the cost of quality control measures (internal and external) and to account for repeat testing in special circumstances. The third component that is added to the mix is the cost of overheads, which are predetermined per department based on the annual expenses on fixed components, including facility, staff salary, and utilities. These components, when added up, provide the *cost per reportable result*. The cost per reportable test (CPRR) is used as the basis on which test pricing is decided. A sample of a table used to calculate these is shown in **Table 1**.

FUTURE TRENDS

The future of cost and inventory management in hematopathology laboratories is being shaped by technological advancements, data-driven decision-making, and evolving diagnostic approaches. These trends promise to enhance efficiency, reduce costs, and improve patient outcomes.

Advances in inventory management technologies are transforming laboratory operations. Automation tools, such as RFID tracking, barcode systems, and integrated inventory management software, enable real-time monitoring of stock levels, expiration dates, and usage patterns. These technologies improve accuracy, reduce waste, and streamline procurement processes. Cloud-based solutions further enhance scalability and allow laboratories to centralize inventory management across multiple locations. Predictive analytics for cost forecasting is a game changer in financial planning. By leveraging historical data and machine learning algorithms, laboratories can predict future inventory requirements and associated costs with high accuracy. This enables proactive budgeting, optimal resource allocation, and the prevention of overstocking or stockouts. Predictive tools also help identify trends in test volumes and reagent usage, allowing laboratories to align their operations with anticipated demand. The impact of telepathology and remote diagnostics on costs is profound. These technologies reduce the need for physical infrastructure and allow centralized laboratories to support remote locations, significantly lowering operational expenses. Digital pathology systems and cloud-based diagnostics also minimize transportation costs and enhance accessibility, making high-quality diagnostics more affordable and widespread. These innovations are paving the way for more sustainable and efficient hematopathology practices.

CONCLUSION

Costing and inventory management are vital aspects of hematopathology laboratory operations, directly influencing financial sustainability, diagnostic quality, and patient outcomes. This chapter has explored key principles and practices essential for efficient resource utilization and cost control, providing a roadmap for laboratories to achieve operational excellence.

A well-structured approach to costing enables laboratories to identify and manage direct and indirect expenses, allocate resources effectively, and price services appropriately. Techniques such as ABC and per-test cost analysis provide valuable insights into financial operations, allowing laboratories to make informed decisions. Similarly, robust inventory management practices, including real-time tracking, predictive analytics, and inventory control techniques such as ABC analysis and JIT minimize waste and ensure the uninterrupted availability of critical resources.

Integrating these practices into laboratory management is not just a financial necessity but also a quality imperative. By adopting advanced technologies, standardizing protocols, and balancing cost constraints with ethical considerations, laboratories can deliver affordable, high-quality care while maintaining compliance with regulatory standards.

This chapter calls upon laboratory managers and stakeholders to prioritize sustainable and efficient practices in resource management. Embracing innovation, continuous improvement, and a patient-centric approach will ensure that hematopathology laboratories remain resilient, reliable, and prepared to meet the demands of an evolving healthcare landscape.

Declaration: The authors used a large language model for the outline of this chapter, which was then reviewed, formatted, edited, and verified by the authors.

Take Home Points

- Effective costing and inventory management are essential for hematopathology laboratories to ensure efficient operations and financial sustainability.
- Key components of laboratory costs include consumables and reagents, equipment and maintenance, staffing and training, and overhead costs.
- Efficient inventory management involves balancing availability and cost, utilizing techniques such as ABC analysis and just-in-time inventory management.
- Technology plays a significant role in enhancing inventory management, with LIS, barcode and RFID tracking, and integrated software solutions.
- Costing models such as ABC and per-test costing help laboratories understand and manage expenses effectively, while regulatory and ethical considerations are crucial in ensuring compliance and patient-focused decision-making.

SUGGESTED READINGS

1. World Health Organization. Laboratory Quality Management System: Handbook. WHO Press; 2011.
2. Clinical and Laboratory Standards Institute. Managing and Controlling Laboratory Inventory: Guidelines and Best Practices. CLSI Document QMS20-A2; 2020.
3. Kaplan RS, Anderson SR. Time-Driven Activity-Based Costing: A Simpler and More Powerful Path to Higher Profits. Harvard Business School Press; 2007.
4. International Organization for Standardization. ISO 15189:2022 Medical laboratories – Requirements for quality and competence. [online] Available from https://www.iso.org/obp/ui/#iso:std:iso:15189:ed-4:v1:en [Last accessed May, 2025].
5. College of American Pathologists. Laboratory Accreditation Program: Inventory Control and Cost Management Tools. [online] Available from https://www.cap.org/laboratory-improvement/accreditation/laboratory-accreditation-program [Last accessed May, 2025].

CHAPTER 23

How to Set Up a Molecular Hematology Laboratory?

Sweta Rajpal, Anumeha Chaturvedi, Papagudi Subramanian

ABSTRACT

This chapter outlines the essential requirements and guiding principles for setting up a diagnostic molecular laboratory, emphasizing that while specific equipment needs may vary based on the tests performed, the core principles of laboratory design and workflow remain constant. The importance of unidirectional workflows, physical segregation of Pre-PCR, PCR and Post-PCR and post-PCR areas, and robust contamination control measures is emphasized to ensure accurate and reliable results. The chapter also highlights the significance of independent verification and validation of molecular tests, ensuring the accuracy and reliability of results. Adherence to quality protocols, including accreditation to international standards and participation in external quality assessments, is vital for maintaining laboratory credibility and diagnostic precision. By integrating molecular diagnostics into a broader diagnostic framework, laboratories can achieve a holistic understanding of patient conditions, ultimately improving patient care.

INTRODUCTION

The understanding of molecular biology in hematology has revolutionized diagnostics by enabling precise disease characterization, risk stratification, and personalized therapy. Sickle cell disease, which is the first molecularly defined human disease, started the trend of diseases having a molecular definition. In the current era, more and more inherited diseases, as well as cancers in hematology, are getting a molecular definition. This results in the molecular laboratory being an essential component of diagnostic hematology. Like any medical laboratory, establishing a molecular laboratory relies on appropriate planning after assessing requirements and allocation of resources in terms of space, manpower, machines, and logistical support.

To ensure accuracy and clinical benefit for patients, molecular tests have to be interpreted in the context of clinical information and conventional hematological tests. Hence, a molecular laboratory for hematology should preferably be integrated or associated with a comprehensive diagnostic setup. Molecular laboratories that function as a standalone entity should work in consultation and close cooperation with a clinical service and a conventional hematological testing facility. For example, the detection of the *JAK2* V617F mutation alone is insufficient to diagnose polycythemia vera. Integrating molecular findings with complete blood counts (CBC), bone marrow aspirates, and biopsy results is crucial to accurately differentiate between conditions where *JAK2* V617F mutations are known to occur like polycythemia vera, essential thrombocythemia, primary myelofibrosis, myelodysplastic/myeloproliferative neoplasm with *SF3B1,* and thrombocytosis or acute myeloid leukemia (AML). Such an approach enhances the utility of molecular tests in patient care.

STRATEGIC PLANNING

Setting up a molecular hematology laboratory begins with:

- Assessment of requirements of the patient population who would be utilizing the laboratory
- Assessment of clinical needs of the projected test volume and the turnaround time

A phased setup of a molecular laboratory is recommended, starting with conventional molecular tests and then advancing to more complex technologies such as next-generation sequencing (NGS). It is to be noted that the availability of advanced modalities such as NGS does not eliminate the need for conventional methods, as they take less time to perform, are more sensitive and cost-effective in many scenarios and are essential for validation of many NGS results. Many high frequency, recurrent and clinically significant specific molecular variants can be detected rapidly using conventional PCR and quantitative PCR (qPCR).

ISSUES PECULIAR TO MOLECULAR LABORATORY

Contamination

Contamination control has to be overemphasized when designing a molecular laboratory. PCR forms the backbone of molecular testing, enabling the amplification of target sequences from nucleic acid templates for detection. Standard PCR can amplify a single molecule of template DNA up to 10^{12} times, making the process highly sensitive but also vulnerable to contamination. Even minute aerosol or droplet contamination can be amplified, potentially leading to false-positive or false-negative results. Sources of contamination and measures that can be used to prevent contamination are given in **Table 1**.

To mitigate these risks, molecular laboratories must implement the measures given in **Table 1** rigorously. One of the most critical strategies is the physical separation of different workflow areas, coupled with regular and thorough decontamination of workspaces and liquid handling systems. Ideally, these workflow areas should be housed in separate rooms, each dedicated to a specific stage of the process. These designated areas include the pre-PCR (also referred

TABLE 1: Sources of contamination and measures to prevent contamination.

Source of contamination	Measures to reduce the contamination
Other samples	Use vials with airtight lids and open only one vial at a time
Other polymerase chain reaction (PCR) products	Separate post-PCR areas from other areas
From operator/technologist	Proper training and systematic work practices
Unclean surfaces	Alcohol wiping of surfaces
Reuse of improperly washed instruments or tips	Avoid reuse of tips and use only filter tips, wipe pipette tips with alcohol, and do not move pipettes between work areas
Aerosol contamination	Use of PCR hoods and separation of work areas

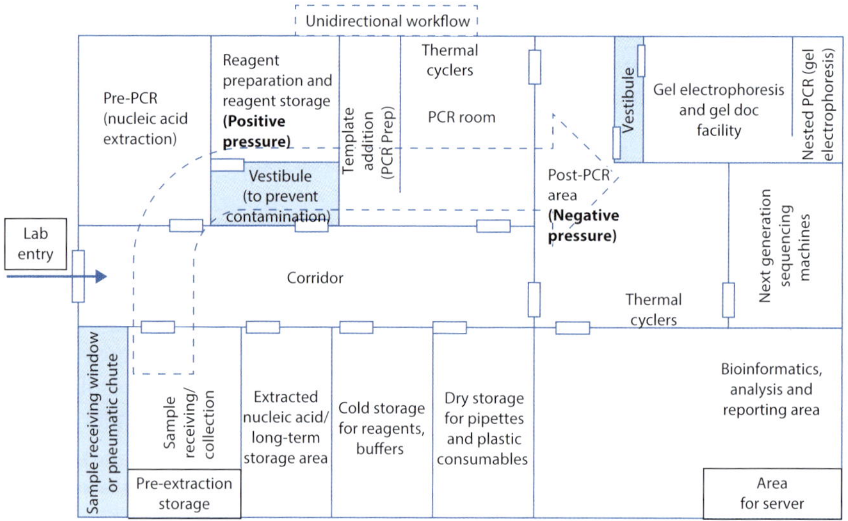

FIG. 1: Schematic layout of a molecular laboratory, illustrating the designated workflow zones, pressure-controlled areas, and equipment placement for optimized contamination control and efficiency. The dotted lines represent the direction of a unidirectional workflow.

to as the "clean" or "low-copy" room), the PCR setup room, and the post-PCR (also known as the "amplification" or "high-copy" room). Each area should have its own set of equipment, reagents, and consumables, including separate refrigerators, centrifuges, vortex mixers, pipettes, pipette tips, and water baths, to prevent cross-contamination. **Figure 1** presents the floor plan of a molecular laboratory, outlining designated workflow areas. It is advisable to have slightly positive pressure in pre-PCR rooms in order to avoid the inflow of air from contaminated areas. The post-PCR rooms should have slight negative pressure to contain and prevent the escape of aerosols of the amplicons from completed PCR reactions. If pressure areas are unavailable, the processing should be done in laminar flow hoods. The ventilation of pre-PCR and post-PCR laboratories should be separate and opened out from different locations.

Generation and Usage of Secondary, Tertiary, and Quaternary Samples from Primary Samples

Unlike routine laboratories, molecular workflows involve primary sample processing—RBC lysis and cell pellet preparation—before further processing as a secondary sample, which may be stored or directly converted to DNA/RNA. Each step involves sample transfer to different tubes, necessitating meticulous labeling and stringent contamination control. Adherence to standardized protocols is critical, underscoring the importance of rigorous personnel training. It is also important to make procedures for maintaining traceability of secondary, tertiary, and quaternary samples to primary samples.

PERSONNEL

A molecular laboratory requires personnel for both the technical and interpretative aspects of testing. Technicians are responsible for performing the assays, while qualified experts handle result interpretation and reporting. To ensure accuracy and efficiency, all personnel should possess the necessary qualifications and undergo periodic training to stay updated with evolving methodologies and quality standards.

EQUIPMENT

- *Installation*: Instruments such as PCR machines, qPCR systems, and sequencers should be installed by certified professionals following the manufacturer's guidelines to prevent technical issues and ensure optimal performance.
- *Calibration*: Routine calibration of pipettes, spectrophotometers, centrifuges, and thermal cyclers is essential to maintain precision in molecular assays.
- *Documentation*: To comply with accreditation standards, laboratories must maintain detailed logs of calibration, servicing, and performance verification. A structured approach to instrument maintenance not only ensures data accuracy but also prolongs equipment lifespan and minimizes workflow disruptions.

The laboratory equipment essential and desirable for setting up a molecular laboratory is listed in **Table 2**.

STORAGE

Storage is essential at various stages of molecular testing:

- *Storage of samples*:
  - Short-term storage of samples received is at 4°C before it undergoes processing into a cell pellet.
  - Long-term storage of samples processed: WBC pellets can be stored at −70°C in phosphate buffered saline (PBS) for DNA extraction or TRIzol or other solutions containing chaotropic agents for RNA extraction. NABL recommends a 10-year storage period for molecular diagnostic samples.

TABLE 2: List of essential and desirable equipment for molecular techniques.

Area	Essential equipment	Desirable equipment
Pre-PCR		
Nucleic acid extraction	• Laminar flow hood and biosafety cabinet (BSL2) • Refrigerator • Test tube racks • Ice box • Microcentrifuge • Microcentrifuge tube • Centrifuge • Refrigerator (4°C), –20°C freezer • Spectrophotometer • Pipettes	• Automated DNA/RNA extraction system • Magnetic stirrer • Falcon tube • Refrigerated centrifuge • –80°C freezer
Reagent preparation and storage	• pH meter • Weighing balance • Microwave/Hot plate • Measuring cylinder	Water purification system
PCR	• Laminar flow hood and biosafety cabinet (BSL2) • Thermal cycler (PCR machine) • Micro-spin • Vortex mixer • Refrigerator (4°C), –20°C freezer • Pipettes	• Real-time qPCR system • Droplet digital PCR system
Post-PCR	• High throughput sequencer* • Thermal cycler (PCR machine) • Gel electrophoresis system • Pipettes (single channel) • 96-well plates* • PCR setup rack • Ice bucket • Ultraclear sealing film* • Magnetic bead separator* • High-performance computing system* • Dedicated NGS workstations* • Refrigerator (4°C), –20°C freezer • Waste container	• Capillary sequencer • Pipettes (multichannel) • Tape station*

*Instruments required for next-generation sequencing.

- It is important to know total leukocyte count (TLC) estimated using a cell counter, either of a blood/bone marrow sample or a cell pellet after red cell lysis in order to have 1 million cells in each aliquot after lysis. For instance, in a case of CML with a TLC of 100,000/μL, even 1 μL of the sample would yield 100,000 cells, whereas in a case of pancytopenia with a TLC of 500/μL, 200 μL of the sample would be required to achieve the same cell count. Silica column-based kits can effectively process up to 1000,000 cells, but exceeding this limit may clog the column and compromise nucleic acid yield. Additionally, repeated freezing and thawing of samples can lead to degradation of nucleic acids. In order to mitigate this, it is advisable to prepare and store multiple aliquots with appropriate WBC counts rather than storing the entire WBC pellet as a single unit.

- *Storage of reagents and consumables*: The reagents used in molecular laboratory including various master mixes, oligonucleotides, nucleic acid extraction kits, flow cells, and buffers require precise storage conditions. These should be stored in a dedicated refrigerator or freezer according to its temperature requirements specified by the manufacturer.
- *Dry storage for plastic wares and consumables*: The plastic wares, including pipette tips, PCR plates, microcentrifuge tubes, gloves, etc., form a bulk of consumables required for a molecular laboratory and should have a dedicated storage area.

INVENTORY MANAGEMENT

Inventory in a molecular laboratory should be maintained for both reagents as well as the sample/extracted nucleic acid.

- *Reagents*: The use of inventory management software is recommended for real-time tracking of stock levels, enabling laboratories to prevent shortages and overstocking. Regular audits, following first in first out policy of usage of reagents and expiration date monitoring, help ensure that reagents and kits are utilized before their expiration, thereby reducing errors and financial losses. Additionally, establishing strong relationships with reliable vendors and anticipating lead times helps maintain a steady supply chain. To mitigate unexpected procurement delays, maintaining a buffer stock of critical reagents is essential.
- *Sample/nucleic acid*: Storage of samples/nucleic acids should be done in an organized and catalogued manner with careful indexing and proper accession logs to avoid misidentification of the samples during testing. Implementing inventory management for stored aliquots helps track sample usage and determine availability for further testing.

PREEXAMINATION PROCESSES

- *Sample collection*:
  - Peripheral blood, body fluid, or bone marrow samples should be collected in ethylenediamine tetraacetic acid (EDTA) tubes. Heparin tubes should be avoided as heparin is a PCR inhibitor.
  - The tubes should be labeled neatly, preferably barcoded, and should have at least two patient identifiers, e.g., full name, registration number, or test requisition number, etc.
  - Other samples such as tissues or chorionic villus should be taken in appropriate transport media such as Ham F-10 supplemented with gentamycin and sodium heparin.

- *Sample transport*:
  - For DNA based tests, samples should be sent to a laboratory within 24 hours of collection at room temperature or within 72 hours of collection at 2–8°C.
  - For RNA-based tests, samples should be sent to the laboratory within 48 hours of collection at 2–8°C so that it can be processed by 72 hours.
  - Body fluids should be chilled immediately on wet ice and transported to the laboratory.
- *Sample receiving and accession*:
  - Samples should be accompanied by requisition forms having sufficient relevant clinical information.
  - The temperature at which samples are being received in the laboratory should be documented.
  - Use of barcode-labeled samples and requisitions should be encouraged.
  - Sample accessioning and allotment of a laboratory ID should be done immediately after sample receiving. The date and time of sample receiving should be recorded.
  - The laboratory should define sample rejection criteria. Unlabeled or wrongly labeled samples should be rejected if it is not an invasive sample. For precious and invasive samples, every effort should be made to correctly identify the sample.

EXAMINATION PROCESSES

Nucleic Acid Extraction

- The choice of nucleic acid extraction technique (manual vs. automated) may differ among various laboratories based on workload, manpower availability, and infrastructure. It is advised to use CE-marked in vitro diagnostic approved kits and reagents for extractions.
- The extraction should be done using validated and documented protocols.
- DNA extraction from blood samples should be done within 14 days if the sample is stored at room temperature. If stored at 2–8°C, the extraction should be done before 28 days.
- RNA extraction should be done within 72 hours of sample collection. To prevent RNA from degradation, considering the ubiquitous presence of RNase, gloves, sterile plasticware, barrier tips, and diethyl pyrocarbonate (DEPC)-treated glassware should be used to minimize RNase contamination.
- RNA should be converted to complementary DNA (cDNA) as soon as possible, as RNA is unstable.
- There are various metrics for checking the quality of extracted nucleic acid, including spectrophotometer, fluorometer, and bioanalyzer.
- Spectrophotometer may give a spuriously high quantity of RNA due to contamination of DNA. The utility of spectrophotometer is rather in the determination of the purity of extracted nucleic acid.
- Fluorometer uses dye that binds to the nucleic acid and quantitates nucleic acid with accuracy.

- Bioanalyzer uses electrophoresis and is accurate in providing RNA integrity index, however is expensive.
- Simple method to look at the quality of RNA is by doing agarose gel electrophoresis and looking at 18s and 28s rRNA bands **(Fig. 2)**.
- The best indicator of RNA and cDNA quality is copy number/microliter of housekeeping genes such as *ABL1*.

Choosing the Correct Molecular Test

The choice of molecular tests plays a critical role in the examination process, as it must align with the clinical context and morphological findings to ensure accurate and efficient diagnosis. In addition, detailed protocols should be documented in standard operating procedures (SOPs) prior to use.

In time-sensitive scenarios, such as those involving targeted therapies, conventional PCR provides a faster turnaround time, enabling earlier clinical intervention. Reverse transcription PCR (RT-PCR) for *BCR::ABL1* in chronic myeloid leukemia (CML) or *PML::RARA* in acute promyelocytic leukemia (APL) provides rapid and reliable confirmation of these diseases. Similarly, fragment analysis for *BRAF* V600E in hairy cell leukemia (HCL) or *MYD88* L265P in lymphoplasmacytic lymphoma (LPL) serves as an effective diagnostic tool.

Additionally, understanding the strengths and limitations of different techniques is critical for effective test selection. For instance, *FLT3* internal tandem duplication (ITD) mutations in AML can vary widely in size, from a few base pairs to over 200 base pairs. While short-read NGS efficiently identifies small insertions (up to 50 base pairs), larger insertions are more reliably detected using conventional PCR followed by capillary electrophoresis.

In contrast, high-throughput sequencing assays, such as NGS, are indispensable for cases requiring multigene testing such as AML, myelodysplastic

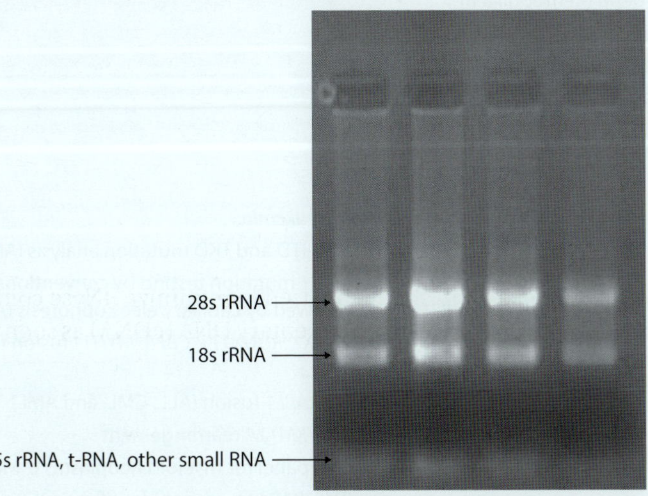

FIG. 2: Agarose gel electrophoresis (1% gel) showing distinct bands of 28s and 18s rRNA, along with other small RNA species. High-quality RNA is characterized by sharp and well-defined bands, whereas degraded or poor-quality RNA exhibits a smeared pattern with the loss of crisp band definition.

syndromes, etc. It should be remembered that as NGS library preparations involve multiplex PCR, there may be dropout of reads in areas of high GC content. These advanced techniques enable precise disease classification and provide comprehensive diagnostic, prognostic, and therapeutic insights. A suggested list of tests for a molecular hematology laboratory, categorized into nonneoplastic and neoplastic disorders, is provided in **Table 3**.

TABLE 3: A comprehensive list of molecular diagnostic tests performed in a hematology laboratory, organized by nonneoplastic and neoplastic disorders.

Non-neoplastic hematology	Neoplastic hematology
Hemoglobinopathies and thalassemia: • Dot blot test/PCR for common variants in the *HBB* gene (sickle cell disease and β-thalassemia) • *HBB* gene sequencing (for rarer variants) • Gap PCR for common deletions (α-thalassemia) • *HBA1/HBA2* gene deletion analysis (α-thalassemia)	*Myeloproliferative neoplasms (MPNs)*: • *BCR::ABL1* transcript identification by PCR • *BCR::ABL1* quantitative PCR (CML) • *JAK2* V617F mutation by PCR • *CALR* mutation by PCR followed by capillary electrophoresis • *MPL* mutation testing by PCR • NGS panel for myeloid neoplasms • Kinase domain mutation analysis by sanger sequencing/NGS
Inherited bleeding disorders: • Screening for intron 1/22 inversion of F8 (hemophilia A) • Sequencing of the *F8* gene (hemophilia A) • Restriction fragment length polymorphism for common variants in the *F9* gene (hemophilia B) • Sequencing of the *F9* gene (hemophilia B) factor • von Willebrand (*vWF*) gene sequencing • Next-generation sequencing (NGS) panel for rare bleeding disorders	*Myelodysplastic syndromes (MDS):* • Comprehensive NGS panel for myeloid neoplasms • Screening for *NPM1* gene mutation by PCR followed by capillary electrophoresis
Inherited platelet function defects: • Whole-exome sequencing/targeted gene sequencing to identify inherited platelets disorders such as Bernard–Soulier syndrome, platelet type vWF, Glanzmann thrombasthenia, platelet secretion, storage pool deficiency, etc.	*Acute leukemia:* • *FLT3*-ITD and TKD mutation analysis (AML) • *NPM1* mutation testing by conventional PCR followed by capillary electrophoresis (AML) • *RUNX1::RUNX1T1*, *CBFB::MYH11* fusion testing (AML) • *BCR::ABL1* fusion (ALL, CML, and AML) • MLL/*KMT2A* rearrangement • NGS panel for myeloid neoplasms (AML) • *PML::RARA* transcript identification • Testing for common fusions in B ALL like *ETV6::RUNX1, TCF3::PBX1, BCR::ABL1, KMT2A::AFF1*

Continued

Continued

Non-neoplastic hematology	Neoplastic hematology
	• Targeted RNA/DNA sequencing for genes implicated in B-ALL • *IKZF1* deletion testing by PCR/MLPA (B-ALL) • MLPA for detection of copy number alterations (B-ALL) • Targeted DNA/RNA sequencing (T-ALL) • Whole transcriptomic sequencing (ALL)
Inherited thrombophilia: • Factor V Leiden (*F5*) mutation analysis • Prothrombin (*F2*) G20210A mutation • *MTHFR* C677T and A1298C variants • *SERPINC1*, *PROC*, and *PROS1* gene analysis (antithrombin, protein C/S deficiencies)	*Myeloid/lymphoid neoplasms with eosinophilia and tyrosine kinase gene fusions:* • Screening PCR for *FIP1L1::PDGFRA* • Targeted RNA sequencing to identify fusion partners implicated including *PDGFRA*, *PDGFRB*, *FGFR1*, *JAK2*, *ABL1*, and *FLT3*
Bone marrow failure syndromes: • Fanconi anemia (*FANC* genes) comprehensive panel • Dyskeratosis congenita (*DKC1*, *TERT*, and *TERC* genes) • Diamond–Blackfan anemia (*RPS* and *RPL* genes) • *GATA1* mutation	*Lymphoma:* • IGHV mutation analysis (CLL) • *TP53* mutation and deletion (CLL) • *MYD88* L265P mutation (lymphoplasmacytic lymphoma) • *BRAF* V600E mutation (hairy cell leukemia) • T-cell clonality testing • B-cell clonality testing • Comprehensive NGS panel for lymphomas
Other disorders: • Glucose-6-phosphate dehydrogenase (*G6PD*) mutation testing • Pyruvate kinase (*PKLR* gene) deficiency analysis • Hereditary spherocytosis panel (*ANK1*, *SPTA1*, *SPTB*, etc.) • Thrombotic thrombocytopenic purpura (*ADAMTS13*) • Targeted NGS or whole-exome sequencing with other causes of inherited hemolytic anemias • Hemochromatosis (sequencing to identify variants in the common genes implicated including *HFE*, *HJV*, *HAMP*, *TFR2*, and *SLC40A1*) • Congenital dyserythropoietic anemia (*CDAN1*, *C15orf41*, *SEC23B*, *KIF23*, and *KLF1*)	*Plasma cell disorders:* • *TP53* mutation • NGS panel for plasma cell disorders including the genes that are commonly implicated *KRAS*, *NRAS*, *FAM46C*, *BRAF*, *TP53*, and *DIS3*

Continued

Continued

Non-neoplastic hematology	Neoplastic hematology
Prenatal testing: Case-specific genetic testing for prenatal diagnostics	
Transplant related: • Chimerism testing using variable number of tandem repeats (VNTR)/ short-tandem repeats (STR)/variants in certain points • HLA typing (sequence-specific probe hybridization, sequence-specific primer amplification, and sequencing-based typing)	

Verification of Molecular Tests

Validated tests without any modifications, for example, the use of a validated kit for detection of *BCR::ABL1*, should undergo independent verification within the laboratory before being implemented for clinical reporting.

Validation of Molecular Tests

For most molecular tests that use nonstandard methods, laboratory-developed or modifications of a validated method should undergo validation before being implemented for clinical reporting.

QUALITY CONTROL

Accreditation of the laboratory to various international standards (ISO 15189, CLIA, CAP, etc.) or their national equivalents (NABL), adequate internal quality assurance (IQA) measures, regular internal audits, and registering in interlaboratory comparison programs (ILCP) or EQAS can help in maintaining good intra- and interlaboratory standards and thereby establishing the credibility of the laboratory. Adequate training of staff, scheduled periodic competency evaluation of the staff, and having a documented SOP (based on ISO15189) for the workflow helps in establishing good laboratory practices.

Internal Quality Assurance

The quality of the starting material is a critical determinant of the reliability of molecular diagnostic results. Laboratories should implement policies to perform quality checks at every step of the workflow. For instance, the quality of cDNA can be assessed by amplifying housekeeping genes such as *ABL1* or *GUSB* using PCR. Laboratories should establish thresholds for acceptable copy numbers of housekeeping genes, below which repeat testing is mandated. This ensures that only high-quality starting material is used for downstream analyses.

To verify the quality of testing, the inclusion of positive, negative, and no-template controls in each batch run is essential. Positive controls, derived from known positive cases or commercial standards, verify the efficiency and accuracy of the assay. Negative controls serve as indicators of effective contamination control, while no-template controls, in which no nucleic acid is added, ensure that the master mix is free of contamination. The detection of any amplification in the no-template control indicates contamination and necessitates corrective measures. Laboratories should incorporate controls to identify potential sources of contamination at each step of the workflow. For example, elution buffers used for RNA extraction or RLT buffer should be included as controls to detect any contamination.

For quantitative methods, standards representing the range of testing including the level of expected sensitivity should be included in every run to monitor assay performance to ensure reliability and reproducibility of molecular testing.

For NGS-based assays, cell lines can be used with known mutations, which are diluted to the lower level of detection of the assay with every run. The quality control measures needed for each kind of molecular tests are summarized in **Table 4**.

TABLE 4: Key considerations for quality control of molecular tests.

Test type	Target analyte	Limit of detection (LOD)	Quality control measures
DNA extraction	-	-	Quantitation should be performed using a fluorometer to ensure accurate measurement during validation
RNA extraction	-	-	Quantitation should be performed using a fluorometer to ensure accurate measurement during validation
cDNA	-	-	The copy number of a housekeeping gene helps determine the success of cDNA synthesis. For example, a copy number >10,000 for the *ABL* gene indicates good-quality cDNA. For measuring deeper response, at least 45,000 copies of *ABL* are required
Qualitative reverse transcription PCR (RT-PCR)	Gene fusions (e.g., *PML::RARA*)	-	Each RT-PCR run should include a positive control, a negative control, and a no-template control. The presence of a band in the no-template control indicates master mix contamination

Continued

Continued

Test type	Target analyte	Limit of detection (LOD)	Quality control measures
Quantitative PCR (qPCR)	Fusion genes (e.g., *BCR::ABL1*)	10^4–10^5 copies	Each run should include low- and high-precision level positive controls, buffers from each extraction step, cDNA synthesis controls, and a reaction master mix without reverse transcriptase
Allele-specific PCR	Point mutations	1% variant allele frequency (VAF)	In addition to standard positive, negative, and no-template controls, a precision control with 1% VAF should be included
Droplet digital PCR (ddPCR)	Mutations, fusion genes	1–10 copies	Control wells should include wild-type, mutant, and no-template controls. Poisson distribution should be applied for the accurate quantification of rare variants
Conventional PCR followed by fragment length analysis	Detection of deletion and insertion of the gene	-	LIZ size standard controls should be used for accurate determination of fragment size
Next-generation sequencing (NGS)	Mutations, gene panels, fusions	Depends on the depth of reads being given to samples. For diagnostics, it is usually 5% and for measurable residual disease it can go up to 0.001%	Cell lines with known mutations should be used to verify mutation detection. For MRD assessment, dilution experiments must be conducted to determine the limit of detection
Sanger sequencing	Point mutations (e.g., *TP53*, *FLT3*)	10–20% VAF	Bidirectional sequencing should be performed for confirmation. Positive and negative controls must be included. Sequencing chromatograms should be reviewed for base-calling accuracy, and a minimum signal-to-noise ratio should be established

External Quality Assurance/Proficiency Testing/ Interlaboratory Comparison Program

Enrollment in external quality assurance (EQA)/proficiency testing (PT) allows verification of test and reporting standards of the laboratory periodically. The tests for which EQA/PT is unavailable, signing up for ILCP can be an alternative approach for EQA.

POSTEXAMINATION PROCESSES

Reporting of Results

Accurate and comprehensive reporting is crucial in molecular diagnostics, as it directly impacts patient care and clinical decision-making. The following elements must be included in the report:

- *Patient and sample information*:
  - Patient identifiers (e.g., name and unique ID)
  - Date and time of sample collection and receipt
  - Type and quality of the sample received
- *Methodology*: Detailed description of the test performed, including the disease locus analyzed and the technology or platform used (e.g., PCR and NGS)
- *Results and interpretation*: Clear presentation of findings with appropriate nomenclature for somatic or germline variants
- *References to standard databases or guidelines (e.g., HGVS and ClinVar)*: Comprehensive interpretation linking the results to potential clinical implications, where applicable
- *Personnel details*: Names and roles of the technical and medical personnel involved in testing and report validation

To ensure clarity and clinical utility, reports should use standardized terminology such as HUGO nomenclature and the version of the human genome used and adhere to structured templates that facilitate consistency and ease of interpretation. They should include actionable insights derived from current evidence and guidelines, ensuring that the results are clinically meaningful. Additionally, any limitations of the test must be clearly outlined to provide context to the findings. Where appropriate, complementary diagnostic tests should be suggested to address potential gaps or to confirm results.

Take Home Points

- *Integrated approach*: A molecular hematology laboratory should be part of a comprehensive diagnostic setup to ensure appropriate test utilization and accurate interpretation of results.
- A *unidirectional workflow* and stringent contamination control are essential for reliable molecular diagnostics.
- Advanced molecular techniques, such as NGS, offer comprehensive insights but require careful planning, significant resources, and bioinformatics support.
- A phased approach, starting with high-demand, cost-effective tests and gradually expanding to advanced techniques, ensures sustainable and impactful laboratory development.
- Adherence to *quality assurance standards* and accreditation protocols is critical for ensuring diagnostic accuracy and laboratory credibility.
- Real-time inventory tracking, buffer stock maintenance, and routine instrument calibration help prevent disruptions and maintain efficiency.

SUGGESTED READINGS

1. Mifflin TE. Setting up a PCR laboratory. CSH Protoc. 2007:pdb.top14.
2. Cree IA, Cree IA, Deans Z, Ligtenberg MJL, Groenen P, Van Krieken JH, et al. Guidance for laboratories performing molecular pathology for cancer patients. J Clin Pathol. 2014;67(11):923-31.
3. Foroni L, Wilson G, Gerrard G, Mason J, Grimwade D, White HE, et al. Guidelines for the measurement of BCR-ABL1 transcripts in chronic myeloid leukaemia. Br J Haematol. 2011;153(2):179-90.
4. Aysal A, Pehlivanoğlu B, Ekmekci S, Gündoğdu B. How to Set Up a Molecular Pathology Lab: A Guide for Pathologists. Turk Patoloji Derg. 2020;36(3):179-87.
5. Chatterjee G, He R, Patkar N, Viswanatha D, Langerak AW. Molecular techniques in haematopathology: what and how? Histopathology. 2025;86(1).

CHAPTER 24

Optical Genome Mapping: Introduction of New Era of Cytogenomics in Hematological Malignancies

Barun Kumar Chakrabarty

ABSTRACT

Hematological malignancies such as myeloma, lymphoma, and leukemia pose challenging diagnostic, prognostic, and management issues because of advances in therapeutics and our growing understanding of the molecular basis of disease. Traditional cytogenetic techniques, such as chromosomal microarray, karyotyping, and fluorescence in situ hybridization (FISH), have been effective in detecting genomic abnormalities. However, these methods have limitations in terms of resolution, throughput, and the capacity to identify complex structural changes. However, despite its significant advancements in genetic profiling of malignant cancers, next-generation sequencing (NGS) technology has drawbacks of its own. These challenges are addressed by a novel method called optical genome mapping (OGM), which provides a comprehensive and complete image of genomic alterations. OGM eliminates the necessity for sequence-based amplification by using high-molecular-weight DNA molecules to create an optical map of the entire genome. With great resolution and accuracy, OGM can detect structural variations, intricate rearrangements, and copy number variations that conventional approaches could overlook. OGM can solve the drawbacks of NGS because it does not require DNA fragmentation or polymerase chain reaction (PCR) amplification, unlike sequencing, and preserves native structural information. OGM assays have the potential to streamline the diagnostic workflow and save costs by replacing several conventional cytogenetic procedures with a single assay. OGM helps with targeted therapy selection and risk stratification by providing a comprehensive genetic landscape. Integration with NGS is anticipated to yield even more accurate diagnosis as OGM technology develops. Hematological oncology could undergo a revolution if OGM is incorporated into standard therapeutic practice.

INTRODUCTION

Existing clinical guidelines highlighted the critical utility of characteristic recurrent genetic abnormalities in many hematologic neoplasms. These genetic anomalies are investigated using various molecular and cytogenetic techniques either in isolation or amalgamation as part of the genetic diagnostic, prognostic, or predictive workup in routine clinical use. The use of karyotyping in clinical practice has increased over the past four decades, and it is now regarded as the "gold standard" test for evaluating chromosomal alterations in a variety of hematologic malignancies. In many hematologic neoplasms, karyotyping is still the accepted method since it offers a comprehensive picture of the genome and finds structural and numerical anomalies. Currently, cytogenetic analysis uses a variety of conventional methods crippled with major limiting factors **(Table 1)**. Thus, our existing standard-of-care (SOC) methods are unable to handle more clinically important data.

On the other hand, next-generation sequencing (NGS) technology has made substantial strides in the molecular profiling of these tumors. Despite various intrinsic limitations of NGS, in detecting structural variations (SVs), it has been studied extensively as a method to detect cytogenetic anomalies **(Table 2)**.

ONE STOP FASTER AND DEEPER SOLUTION

The OGM is currently being considered as a technique that may soon either take the place of or enhance conventional cytogenetic testing. Schwartz et al. first developed the OGM technology in 1993. Bionano Genomics® has since modified it, developing the chemistry and imaging capture technology to use the Saphyr® whole-genome imaging platform to reach the current levels of productivity and

TABLE 1: Comparison of optical genome mapping (OGM) and standard-of-care (SOC) cytogenomic techniques.

	Karyotyping	FISH	CMA	OGM
Coverage	Genome wide	Targeted	Genome wide	Genome wide
Type of specimen	Viable cell sample	Viable/fixed cell sample	Viable/fixed cell sample	Viable/frozen cell sample
Culture artefacts	Yes	Yes: for metaphase FISH	No	No
Nature of analysis	Single cell genomics	Single cell genomics	Multiple specimen	Multiple specimen
Level of resolution	≥5–10 MB	>100–200 kbp	≥5 for LOH, 200 kb for gain or losses	≥500 bp–5 MB for SVs, 500 kb for CNVs
Sensitivity (%VAF)	10%	2–5%	10–15%	5–10%
Structural variant types	CNV + SV	CNV + SV	CNV ± AOH/ CN – LOH	CNV + AOH + SV
Subjectivity of analysis	Biased	Biased	Unbiased	Unbiased
Average TAT	1–2 weeks	1–3 days	<1 week	<1 week
Detection bias	Unbiased	Targeted probe	Design bias	Unbiased

(AOH: absence of heterozygosity; CNV: copy number variations; CMA: chromosomal microarray analysis; FISH: fluorescence in situ hybridization; LOH: loss of heterozygosity)

TABLE 2: Comparison of optical genome mapping (OGM) as a complement to next-generation sequencing (NGS) in hematological malignancies.

Technique	NGS		OGM
	Short read	**Long read/WGS**	
Resolution of SV detection	150 bp	10–20 kbp	500 kbp
Mutations	Detect	Detect	Cannot detect
SVs	Can detect (by indirect inference)	Can detect (by high confidence)	Can detect (by high confidence and sensitivity)
Limitations	Sensitivity is low	High rate of error	Lack base level resolution
Time and cost	Time consuming, costly		Faster, less expensive
Subjectivity of analysis	Analysis pipeline bias		Unbiased
Detection bias	PCR bias/sequence bias		Unbiased
Sample preparation automation	Available		Not available
Bioinformatics	Separate extensive services required		Complete bioinformatic and analysis process is covered
Interpretation of results	Complicated		Less complicated

(PCR: polymerase chain reaction; WHO: whole genome sequencing)

resolution. Numerous hematologic neoplasms have been successfully analyzed cytogenomically using OGM technology. In a recent study, Sahajpal et al. analyzed 69 well-characterized samples of unique hematological neoplasms using OGM, achieving a high concordance rate of 99.2% accuracy, 100% specificity, and 98.7% sensitivity, along with a positive predictive value of 100% and a negative predictive value of 98% compared to classical methods.

TECHNICAL CONSIDERATIONS

Preanalytical Requirements

Sample collection: The OGM approach's main prerequisite is the extraction of ultra-high molecular weight (UHMW) DNA (≥150 kb). For hematological malignancies it is recommended to collect bone marrow (BM) aspirate or peripheral blood samples in EDTA tubes. Sample viability is crucial, and processing needs to be finished within the first 24 hours of aspiration. For longer storage, sample should be frozen at 80°C or cryopreserved with DNA stabilizer. OGM cannot use DNA that has previously been retrieved using other techniques.

Sample adequacy: Sample must contain at least 1–1.5 million cells, best ascertained by an automated cell counter. Maintaining a critical level of >50% cell viability is recommended particularly in cryopreserved samples. Selective enrichment of the target population is recommended wherever possible.

Steps of Optical Genome Mapping

There are three steps to the OGM technical protocol **(Fig. 1A)**:

1. *UHMW DNA extraction:* This is most crucial stage of the process. The extraction process employ paramagnetic nanodiscs, which prevent fragmentation and enable the recovery of DNA >150 kb. Careful pipetting is required throughout the process to avoid fragmentation. Because the isolated DNA is so fragile, transport should be avoided.

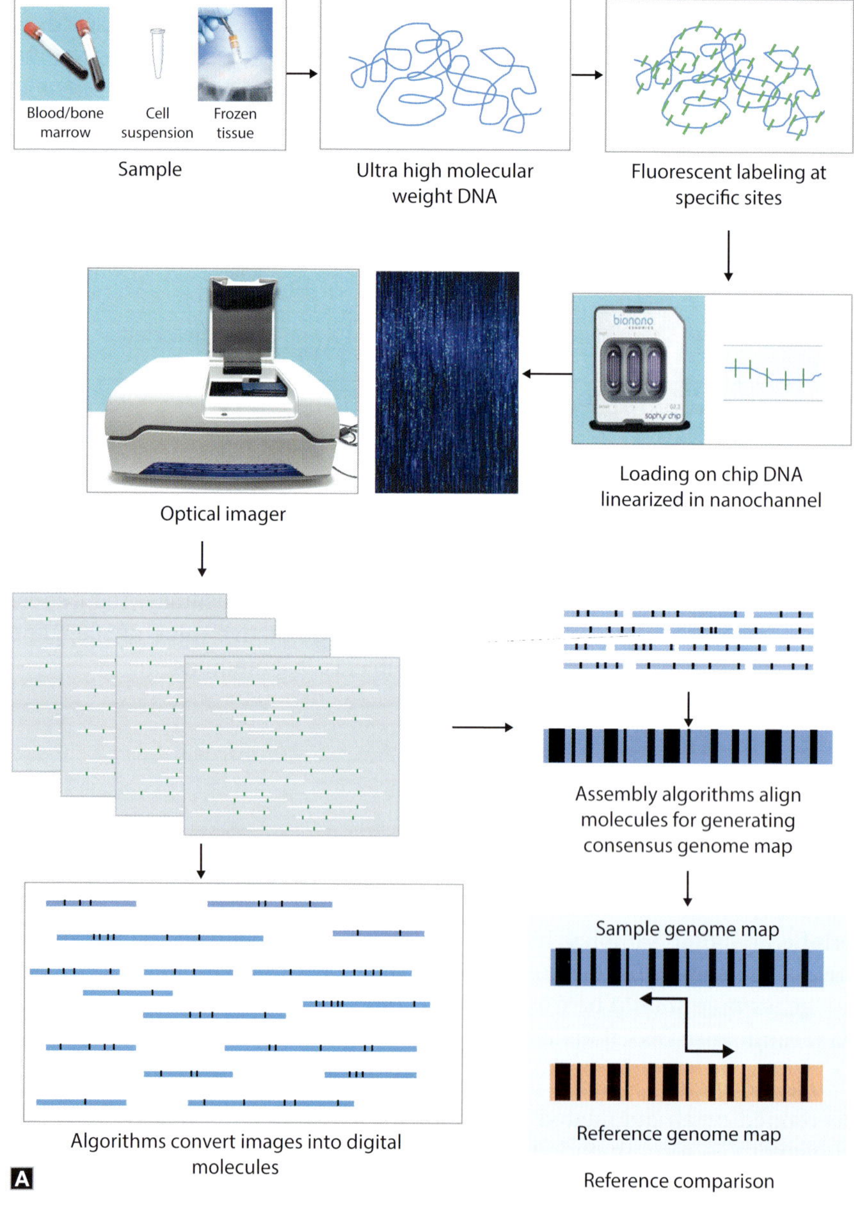

FIGS. 1A AND B: *Continued*

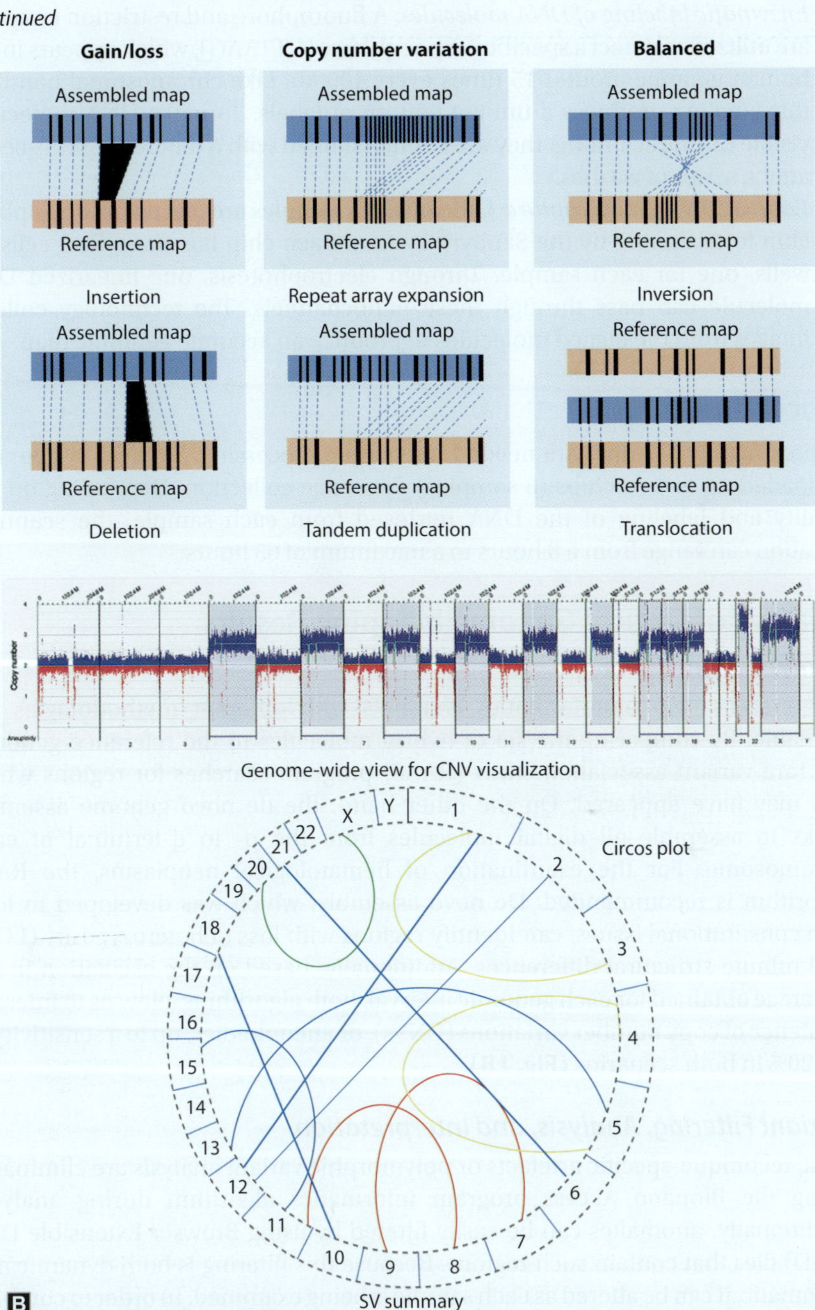

FIGS. 1A AND B: (A) Optical genome mapping (OGM) technical protocol: Basic steps: Ultra high molecular weight DNA extraction, enzymatic attachment of fluorescent tags to specific sequence motifs across the genome, utilization of nanochannel system for stretching and immobilization of labeled DNA molecule, detection of fluorescently labeled DNA molecules using a high-resolution imaging system, and generation of a genome-wide structural map. (B) Analysis and interpretation of OGM results: By comparing the genome map to a reference genome, structural variations (e.g., duplications, deletions, translocations, and inversions) can be found. Bioinformatics pipelines are used to interpret detected variations to provide insights into genomic alterations.

2. *Enzymatic labeling of DNA molecules:* A fluorophore and restriction enzymes are utilized to detect a specific 6-bp sequence (CTTAAG), which appears in the human genome around 15 times every 100 kb. Like chromosomal banding, this labeling produces a unique pattern of labels. To make DNA molecules visible during scanning, they are counterstained with a different fluorescence after a series of washes.
3. *Labeled DNA image capture:* Labeled DNA samples are placed onto a Saphyr® chip for scanning by the Saphyr® system. Each chip has three flow cells, or wells, one for each sample. Through electrophoresis, one linearized DNA molecule can pass through these nanochannels. The technology collects images from the tagged molecules to produce an accurate genomic map.

Processing Time

Approximately 3–7 days are needed for sample processing. Saphyr® system can be loaded up to two chips (6 samples) for image collection. Depending on the quality and labeling of the DNA retrieved from each sample, the scanning duration can range from a 8 hours to a maximum of 65 hours.

Analysis of Optical Genome Mapping Results

Analysis Algorithms

For analysis, two bioinformatics channels with different methodologies are available. By comparing the set of hybrid molecules to the reference genome, the rare variant association study (RAAS) program searches for regions where SVs may have appeared. On the other hand, the de novo genome assembly seeks to assemble all digital molecules from the p- to q-terminal of each chromosome. For the examination of hematological neoplasms, the RAAS algorithm is recommended. De novo assembly, which was developed to look into constitutional issues, can identify regions with loss of heterozygosity (LOH) and minute structural differences. Additionally, based on the oscillation in the coverage obtained for each genomic interval, both algorithms allow us to infer the existence of copy number variations (CNVs), or aneuploidies, up to a sensitivity of 15–20% in both scenarios **(Fig. 1B)**.

Variant Filtering, Analysis, and Interpretation

First, technique-specific artefacts or polymorphic variant analysis are eliminated using the Bionano Access program informatics algorithm during analysis. Additionally, anomalies can be easily filtered by using Browser Extensible Data (BED) files that contain such regions. Because this filtering is both dynamic and automatic, it can be altered as each sample is being examined. In order to combine fragmented CNV alterations, eliminate duplicates, and rule out any false positives, a visual inspection of the abnormalities is required in a subsequent stage. OGM data should be reported along with any clinically significant alterations of each hematological neoplasm, as is the case with other cytogenomic and molecular techniques.

Quality Controls

- A minimum of two sample aliquots recommended for storage whenever feasible to avoid quality or reagent issue while processing.
- Generally, it is recommended that hematological samples collect 1,500 Gb of data coverage to detect anomalies with a variable allele frequency (VAF) of up to 5%.
- Inbuilt quality control system of Bionano Access program analyze images from the Saphyr system with a reference genome.

OPTICAL GENOME MAPPING: WHERE ARE WE NOW?

The OGM is an excellent substitute as a first-line test to identify chromosomal abnormalities in a range of hematological neoplasms, particularly in acute myeloid leukemia (AML), myelodysplastic syndromes (MDS), acute lymphoblastic leukemia (ALL), and chronic lymphocytic leukemia (CLL), according to a number of recent publications **(Table 3)**. Virtual customized "heme malignancy panel" can be created based on disease subtype using inbuilt bioinformatics setup to quickly analyze the actionable targets. Nevertheless, there are currently no published society guidelines for OGM use in hematological malignancies.

TABLE 3: Summary of optical genome mapping (OGM) clinical validation studies in hematological malignancies.

Reference	Clinical diagnosis	Cohort size	Number of abnormalities included	Concordance with reference cytogenomic results
Neveling et al., 2021	Hematological malignancies (AML, MDS, CML, CLL, ALL, MM, MPN, T-PLL, LYBM)	48	112	100%
Lestringant et al., 2021	ALL (6 B-cell ALL and 4 T-cell ALL)	10	78	97%
Levy B et al., 2023	AML	100	190	98.4%
Yang H et al., 2022	MDS	101	194	99%
Kriegova E et al., 2021	MM	11	172	98%
Valkama A et al., 2023	CLL	18	86	100%
Stinnett V et al., 2022	Leukemia/Lymphoma and solid tumors	5	30	100%
Sahajpal NS et al., 2022	CLL, AML, MDS, MM, lymphoma, PCM, CML, ET and others	69	164	99%

(ALL: acute lymphoblastic leukemia; AML: acute myeloid leukemia; CLL: chronic lymphocytic leukemia; CML: chronic myeloid leukemia; ET: essential thrombocytosis; LYBM: bone marrow sample in which lymphoma cells; MM: multiple myeloma; MDS: myelodysplastic syndrome; MPN: myeloproliferative neoplasm; PCM: plasma cell myeloma; T-PLL: T-cell prolymphocytic leukemia)

In their 2024 guidelines, the Standing Committee for the International System for Human Cytogenomic Nomenclature (ISCN) now recognizes the need for a consistent nomenclature for genome mapping commiserating the growing amount of genome mapping data.

Myeloid Neoplasms

Varied cytogenetic abnormalities in AML are found in roughly 76% of pediatric AML cases and 55% of adult AML cases. The OGM research on AML patients has shown that the method is helpful for both identifying known abnormalities such as DEK::NUP214, RBM15::MRTFA, BCR::ABL1, etc., and detecting cryptic abnormalities in the karyotype, such as NUP98 or MECOM rearrangements, and characterizing gene rearrangement pairs, such as KMT2A. OGM is particularly helpful for complex karyotypes, which are present in 10–12% of AML samples.

In myelodysplastic syndrome (MDS) patients finding recurrent genetic anomalies, clonality assessment, and detection of structural anomalies, such as 5q deletion or biallelic TP53 inactivation are essential requirement for determining their diagnosis, prognosis, and course of treatment. But unfortunately >50% of cases a normal karyotype is present and many times culture yields no definable metaphases resulting in call for further fluorescence in situ hybridization (FISH) or genomic microarray analysis. OGM research to far has shown that its application raises the proportion of individuals having useful cytogenetic findings.

OGM has great potential in the study of typical myeloproliferative neoplasms, despite the limited experience published to date. 50% of BM karyotype in primary myelofibrosis are uninformative due to the presence of BM fibrosis.

Myeloid/lymphoid tumors with eosinophilia requires analysis by karyotyping or multiple FISH probes. However, OGM could detect or rule out in a single test clonal eosinophilia linked to tyrosine kinase gene fusion.

Lymphoid Neoplasms

Currently, strategy-based techniques that use karyotyping and FISH can detect recurrent genetic abnormalities, such as translocations t(9;22)(q34;q11.2) [BCR::ABL1], iAMP21, and other cryptic abnormalities (like CRLF2 gene rearrangements). Abnormalities with poor prognosis (such IKZF1region) can be found using the single nucleotide polymorphism (SNP)-array technique. Additionally, it can precisely identify B-cell ALL (B-ALL) subgroups with aneuploidies. This method is expensive and time-consuming. OGM is the perfect time-and money-efficient a single test tool reducing turnaround time and better risk stratification.

T-cell acute lymphoblastic leukemia (T-ALL) also has a significant level of genetic heterogeneity. A significant portion of patients with uninformative karyotypes (30%) or normal findings (30%) that may include hidden abnormalities are frequently seen in conventional cytogenetics. Compared to traditional cytogenomic methods, OGM confirms that it offers a lot more information. It is useful for demonstrating fusion genes with significant clinical potential, such as TRA::LMO2, TRB::MYC, IGH::TAL1, etc.

Whether examined SOC cytogenetics, the true significance of genomic complexity in CLL is still constrained by methodological considerations. In this regard, OGM in CLL enables us to better define cytogenetic abnormalities in addition to identifying anomalies that are presently being investigated by FISH.

Plasma Cell Neoplasms

At the cytogenetic level, multiple myeloma (MM) is a very diverse illness, with 90% of patients having chromosomal abnormalities. It is very difficult to extract metaphases from mature plasma cells therefore targeted FISH is the standard method for identifying high-risk anomalies in isolated CD138+ cells.

But utilizing FISH it is impossible to investigate how other chromosomal abnormalities affect prognosis or patient outcomes because the full genetic variability of MM is unknown. Therefore, even though OGM is still being standardized in a few CD138+ cells, it is a very promising method in the management of MM.

Reclassifying Patients and Determining New Therapeutic Targets

The OGM also help to explain the phenomenon of "mimicking," in which certain cytogenetic anomalies identified by G-banding may not hold up at the molecular level upon closer examination. t(9;22)(q34;q11.2), which does not include BCR::ABL1, and t(4;12)(q12;p13), which has a claimed ETV6::PDGFRA rearrangement that does not actually affect PDGFRA, are two examples that are discussed in the medical literature. In these cases, OGM made it possible to identify these aberrations at a higher resolution and provided an explanation for the resistance to tyrosine kinase inhibitors.

The clinical care of patients is directly impacted by OGM, which enables patient categorization with improved identification of cryptic rearrangements [such as MECOM (3q26) rearrangements, or deletions of TP53] or identifying genes that have multiple partners for rearrangements, such KMT2A for which specialized FISH probes are not accessible or characterize complex abnormalities involving genes crucial to leukemogenesis, like JAK2. All these will help into creating new diagnostic categories and into various prognostic or predictive response groups potential for clinical trials.

Defining Complex Karyotype

They differ in the number of anomalies needed to classify a case as complex karyotype (CK): ≥3, ≥4, and ≥5. The number of abnormalities needed to classify a case as CK utilizing the OGM technique will need to be reevaluated because it enables the discovery of more cytogenomic abnormalities.

Characterization of Chromoanagenesis and its Clinical Consequences

The concept of chromoanagenesis encompasses a variety of catastrophic events named as chromoplexy, chromothripsis, and chromoanasynthesis that cause chromosomal rearrangements and various genetic disorders. Up until now, these phenomena could only be identified using whole genome sequencing techniques or genomic microarrays, which provided biased information by only providing data on CNVs. With the OGM technique, we can obtain much more comprehensive and detailed information on these phenomena.

Strength

Various advantages of OGM techniques are tabulated in **Tables 1, 2, and 4**. In addition to having a far higher sensitivity than KT (×10,000 resolution), OGM also gives the variant allele fraction (VAF) of each variation, which helps identify the different abnormalities in these somatic samples. Another unique feature of the OGM assay that allows process standardization and scalability for one or more hematologic malignancy subtypes is the standard preanalytical and analytical protocols, which are independent of disease subtype. The inclusion of guideline-driven, illness subtype-specific target variations into the analytical

TABLE 4: Structural variants: Comparison of available techniques.

Structural variants class	Karyotype	FISH	CMA	NGS	OGM
Aneuploidy	Detect	Targeted detection	Detect	Detect	Detect (detection limited to monosomy and trisomy)
Deletion	Can detect; Detection limited by size	Targeted detection	Detect	Detect	Detect
Duplication	Can detect; Detection limited by size	Targeted detection	Detect	Detect	Detect
Inversion	Can detect; Detection limited by size	Targeted detection	Cannot detect	Cannot detect	Detect
AOH	Cannot detect	Cannot detect	Detect	Detect	Detect; germ line
Repeat expansion (macrosatellite/ microsatellite)	Cannot detect	Cannot detect	Cannot detect	Detect; Limited to short repeats	Detect; Limited to large repeats
Repeat contraction	Cannot detect	Cannot detect	Cannot detect	Cannot detect	Detect
Sequence variants (SNV/ INDELs)	Cannot detect	Cannot detect	Cannot detect	Detect	Cannot detect
Translocation	Can detect; Detection limited by size	Targeted detection	Cannot detect	Detect; Restricted targets	Detect

(AOH: absence of heterozygosity; SNV: single nucleotide variants; FISH: fluorescence in situ hybridization; CMA: chromosomal microarray analysis; NGS: next-generation sequencing; OGM: optical genome mapping)

process enables semiautomated and straightforward variant categorization and reporting. Furthermore, if the clinical symptoms of a heme malignancy subtype are unclear at the time of the doctor's consultation, a "pan-heme" genomic analysis can still be conducted concurrently in a disease-agnostic manner.

Limitations

- Requires specific equipment and reagents and costlier than traditional cytogenetic methods.
- OGM is incapable to identify individual clonal architecture and identify loss of heterozygosity (LOH) regions.
- It shows only 15–20% sensitivity to anomalies in copy number gain and loss. This restriction may apply to CLL and myeloma patients, which is currently detected by FISH and linked to a poor prognosis.
- OGM is insensitive to tiny indels (<500 bp) and single nucleotide variant (SNVs).
- OGM technology does not adequately cover repetitive regions such as (peri) centromeric, telomeric, short arms of acrocentric chromosomes, or heterochromatin segments areas.
- Sample's ploidy allocation is not always precise. This is especially important when analyzing patients who have B-cell ALL.
- Not suitable for paraffin-embedded tissue, formaldehyde-fixed tissue, or DNA extracted using conventional techniques.

CONCLUSION

In conclusion, OGM is a very promising technique for cytogenomic analysis of hematologic neoplasms that might be added to the list of current techniques. It is anticipated that the combination of OGM and NGS would aid in the diagnosis and therapy decisions for these patients. Before it may be utilized in regular diagnostics, standardization of analytical criteria, result validation, and prospective comparative studies are required to determine under what situations and circumstances it can complement or replace the already recognized cytogenomic techniques.

CASE-BASED DISCUSSION

Case 1

A 50-year-old male diagnosed as a case of AML with 50% blasts. Karyotype showed derivative chromosome 21 with unknown partner. FISH performed with dual color dual fusion t(8;21) probe showed no fusion abnormalities but presence of three copies RUNX1 gene signals (two of them are dim intensity signals). Chromosomal microarray analysis (CMA) showed normal results. Please elaborate how OGM can resolve the mystery.

Ans: Karyotype and FISH result indicate the presence of translocation between chromosome 21 and unknown partner chromosome and CMA normal result hinted that the translocation is balanced. But due to low resolution of karyotype and targeted approach in FISH we cannot get the details of the partner chromosome. OGM can easily resolve this case by identifying the unknown partner.

Case 2

A 36-year-old man diagnosed as a case of AML with 9% CD34+ myeloid blasts and 54% blast equivalents (promonocytes, monoblasts). Karyotype initially reported as an add(6)(p21), add(9)(q34), add(14)(q22) in 16 metaphases with four metaphases showing normal karyotype. Metaphase FISH showed a fusion of the *DEK* and *NUP214* signals on the derivative 6. How OGM can help in this case?

Ans: The karyotype revealed that there are structural abnormalities involving three chromosomes. Metaphase FISH confirmed the presence of DEK::NUP 214 suggesting likely fusion and thereby hinting three way translocation. But due to low resolution of karyotype and targeted approach in FISH we cannot get the details of three way translocation. OGM can easily resolve this case by identifying the translocation partners.

Take Home Points

- The OGM is a brand-new, cutting-edge method for analyzing all structural variation classes and copy number variants found in the human genome.
- A shorter TAT makes it possible to identify clinically significant genetic abnormalities early.
- In several investigations, hematological cancers were found to be 100% consistent with conventional cytogenetic techniques.
- In the case of hematological cancers, the combination of OGM and NGS may eventually replace all other methods.

SUGGESTED READINGS

1. Moore S, McGowan-Jordan J, Smith AC, Rack K, Koehler U, Stevens-Kroef M, et al. ISCN standing committee. Genome Mapping Nomenclature. Cytogenet Genome Res. 2024;163 (5-6):236-46.
2. Sahajpal NS, Mondal AK, Tvrdik T, Hauenstein J, Shi H, Deeb KK, et al. Clinical validation and diagnostic utility of optical genome mapping for enhanced cytogenomic analysis of hematological neoplasms. J Mol Diagn. 2022;24(12):1279-91.
3. Neveling K, Mantere T, Vermeulen S, Oorsprong M, van Beek R, Kater-Baats E, et al. Next-generation cytogenetics: Comprehensive assessment of 52 hematological malignancy genomes by optical genome mapping. Am J Hum Genet. 2021;108(8):1423-35.
4. Balducci E, Kaltenbach S, Villarese P, Duroyon E, Zalmai L, Friedrich C, et al. Optical genome mapping refines cytogenetic diagnostics, prognostic stratification and provides new molecular insights in adult MDS/AML patients. Blood Cancer J. 2022;12(9):126.
5. Yang H, Garcia-Manero G, Sasaki K, Montalban-Bravo G, Tang Z, Wei Y, et al. High-resolution structural variant profiling of myelodysplastic syndromes by optical genome mapping uncovers cryptic aberrations of prognostic and therapeutic significance. Leukemia. 2022;36(9):2306-16.
6. Lestringant V, Duployez N, Penther D, Luquet I, Derrieux C, Lutun A, et al. Optical genome mapping, a promising alternative to gold standard cytogenetic approaches in a series of acute lymphoblastic leukemias. Genes, Chromosomes, and Cancer. 2021;60(10):657-67.

7. Levy B, Kanagal-Shamanna R, Sahajpal NS, Neveling K, Rack K, Dewaele B, et al. A framework for the clinical implementation of optical genome mapping in hematologic malignancies. Am J Hematol. 2024;99(4):642-61.
8. Kriegova E, Fillerova R, Minarik J, Savara J, Manakova J, Petrackova A, et al. Whole-genome optical mapping of bone-marrow myeloma cells reveals association of extramedullary multiple myeloma with chromosome 1 abnormalities. Sci Rep. 2021;11(1):14671.
9. Valkama A, Vorimo S, Kumpula TA, Räsänen H, Savolainen ER, Pylkäs K, et al. Optical genome mapping as an alternative to FISH-based cytogenetic assessment in chronic lymphocytic leukemia. Cancers. 2023;15(4):1294.
10. Stinnett V, Jiang L, Haley L, Ament C, Hardy M, Morsberger L, et al. Adoption of optical genome mapping in clinical cancer cytogenetic laboratory: A stepwise approach. Cancer Genet. 2022;6(2):260-1:3.

CHAPTER 25

Hemoglobin Fraction Analysis in the Diagnosis of Hemoglobinopathies—Methods, Advantages, Pitfalls and Updates

P Lalita Jyotsna, Sunita Sharma, Shailaja Shukla

ABSTRACT

Hemoglobinopathies constitute the most common genetic disorders in the world. In India, the prevalence of the different hemoglobinopathies varies with geographic location (region) and ethnicity. They comprise of quantitative and structural hemoglobin variants and an accurate diagnosis is essential for management. Hemoglobin fraction analysis has become an important modality for hemoglobinopathy screening and presumptive diagnosis.

INTRODUCTION

A hemoglobin (Hb) molecule is a tetramer of four globins chains, each containing a heme group with an iron ion in the center. In adults, the main Hb is HbA0 with 2α and 2β globin chains constituting 96–98% of total Hb and a minor fraction of HbA2 with 2α and 2δ chains which constitutes 2–3.5% of the total Hb. Fetal Hb (HbF—α2γ2), a major Hb in fetal and neonatal life (60–90%), reaches the adult level (<1%) by the age of 1 year. There are many genes coding for the globin chains, clustering on either chromosome 11 (β-globin cluster) or chromosome 16 (α-globin cluster).

Hemoglobinopathies are inherited disorders of globin chains of Hb. They can be:

- *Quantitative defects:* These include thalassemia syndromes due to deletions or point mutations leading to the absence or reduction in amount of one or more globin chains, e.g., α-thalassemia or β-thalassemia. According to the transfusion requirement, the thalassemias form a spectrum and are classified as transfusion-dependent thalassemia (TDT) which needs regular transfusions for survival (β-thalassemia major, α-thalassemia, severe Hb E/β-thalassemia, Hb Bart's, Hb constant spring) and nontransfusion dependent thalassemia (NTDT) which intermittently or rarely require

transfusion (β-thalassemia trait, HbH disease, α-thalassemia trait, mild/moderate HbE/β-thalassemia).
- *Qualitative defects:* Include the structural Hb variants or abnormal hemoglobins resulting from point mutations in globin gene causing the substitution of one or more amino acids in the globin chains of Hb molecule. These include HbS, HbE, HbC, Hb D-Punjab, and Hb D-Iran. Clinical manifestations usually occur in the homozygous state.
- Compound heterozygous states, δ-β thalassemias and hereditary persistence of fetal hemoglobin (HPFH).

WHY IS THERE A NEED FOR HEMOGLOBINOPATHY TESTING?

According to an Indian Council of Medical Research (ICMR) study, the incidence of hemoglobinopathies in India's general population is 1.44%. While thalassemia belt extends from Punjab to Odisha, sickle cell anemia is prevalent in the tribal population of Central India (Maharashtra, Chhattisgarh, Madhya Pradesh, Odisha, and Jharkhand). HbE disease is seen more commonly in the Eastern and Northeastern states. HbD variants are seen in Punjab region. Every year 10,000–15,000 children are born with thalassemias and other hemoglobinopathies leading to significant morbidity and mortality. The huge burden of transfusion requirements and management warrants efforts toward primary prevention and early diagnosis.

WHEN AND WHOM TO TEST AND DIAGNOSE FOR HEMOGLOBINOPATHY?

The ICMR has advocated carrier testing (especially universal antenatal screening) and early diagnosis of hemoglobinopathies to reduce their burden in the country. These tests are essential for decisions related to timely partner analysis, genetic counseling, termination of pregnancy, and management [supportive treatments, transfusions, and hematopoietic stem cell transplantation (HSCT)].

Early diagnosis:
- Neonatal screening
- All infants and children (6 months–6 years) with severe anemia Hb < 7g/dL.

Carrier screening:
- Adolescent screening
- Premarital screening
- Preconception screening
- Antenatal screening in first trimester
- Cascade screening of partner/spouse or family (parents and siblings)

It can help in timely partner analysis, genetic counseling, and primary prevention.

HOW TO SCREEN AND DIAGNOSE HEMOGLOBINOPATHY?

The workup of hemoglobinopathy involves:

- Detailed clinical history with family history.
- Complete blood counts with peripheral smear, reticulocyte count, and iron profile.
- Preliminary screening with NESTROFT (N-ethyl-S-thio-L-cysteine-3,4-dihydro-O-methanesulfonamide), sickling test, sickle cell solubility test, 2,6-dichloroindophenol (DCIP), and reticulocyte preparation.
- *First line tests:* Primary screening is done using Hb fraction analysis by various methods. These include traditional methods such as isoelectric focusing, cellulose acetate, and citrate agar electrophoresis and automated methods such as cation exchange high-performance liquid chromatography (CE-HPLC) and capillary zonal electrophoresis (CZE). These tests detect and quantify HbF, HbA, HbA2, as well as common and rare variant hemoglobins, based on which a provisional diagnosis can be given.
- *Second-line tests:* For a presumptive diagnosis, the findings of a first-line test must be confirmed by a different but complementary second method. For example, CE—HPLC can be combined with CZE to arrive at a diagnosis.
- *Confirmatory tests:* Definitive diagnosis is done by genetic testing using amplification-refractory mutation system (ARMS)-polymerase chain reaction (PCR), Gap PCR, multiplex ligation-dependent probe amplification (MLPA), DNA sequencing of the affected globin gene or by amino acid sequencing using mass spectrometry.

WHAT IS THE TYPE OF SPECIMEN?

Whole blood in ethylenediaminetetraacetic acid (EDTA) 2. Dried blood spot in neonatal screening.

METHODS USED FOR SCREENING AND PRESUMPTIVE DIAGNOSIS OF HEMOGLOBINOPATHY BY HEMOGLOBIN FRACTION ANALYSIS

These methods utilize the relative differences in *surface electric charges* due to amino acid substitutions, to separate normal and variant Hb molecules.

Traditionally, electrophoretic methods such as cellulose acetate membrane (pH—8.4, solid electrophoresis) and citrate agar (pH—6.0, gel electrophoresis) have been used for Hb fraction analysis. At alkaline pH, the Hb molecules are negatively charged and move from their point of application at the cathode toward the anode at a rate directly proportional to their charge. In citrate agar electrophoresis, the point of application is in the center and hemoglobins comigrating in cellulose acetate method can be separated.

Isoelectric focusing (IEF): Gel contains molecular-weight molecules that allow for a pH gradient. The hemoglobins migrate in an electric field to their isoelectric points, where the net charge is zero.

CE-HPLC: Equipment uses programs such as β-thalassemia-short, sickle cell, and HbA1c for Hb fraction analysis. However, dedicated hemoglobinopathy testing methods are more reliable than machines evaluating HbA1c (like Bio-Rad D10).

CZE: Hb fraction separation and analysis occur by migration of Hb molecules in the liquid buffer within a capillary.

Point of care testing (POCT): Rapid testing methods such as lateral flow immunoassays which are antibody-based POCT and portable equipment like modified cellulose acetate electrophoresis can be used for screening. These are of particular use in screening programs for hemoglobinopathies in remote areas.

Currently, the most commonly used methods for screening and diagnosis of hemoglobinopathies are CE-HPLC and CZE. At alkaline pH, the Hb molecule is negatively charged. Here we discuss these two methods of Hb fraction analysis by three commonly used devices:

1. CE-HPLC by Bio-Rad Variant-II (HPLC method 1)
2. Tosoh HLC-723G11 (HPLC method 2)
3. CZE by Sebia minicap flex piercing

Cation Exchange High-performance Liquid Chromatography

Separation of hemoglobins occurs in a column comprising of a *stationary phase* of cation exchange cartridge while the buffers of different ionic strengths constitute the *mobile phase.* While Bio-Rad uses a porous resin column, Tosoh employs a nonporous column for surface adsorption. Negatively charged carboxyl groups are attached to a resin base in the column **(Fig. 1A)**. When a hemolysate containing a mixture of hemoglobins in the test sample is injected at high pressure into the column, positively charged Hb fragments in the hemolysate attach to the carboxyl groups at varying strengths, depending on their relative positive charge **(Fig. 1B)**. This is followed by passage of buffers containing cations in increasing concentrations, into the column. These cations compete with the adsorbed hemoglobins, leading to their elution **(Fig. 1C)**.

The Hb fractions therefore appear in the eluate at a rate depending on their affinity for the stationary phase. For example, the relatively more positively charged HbS and HbC are retained longer in the column, and hence, eluted later. The separated fractions are then consecutively detected in a flow cell, where absorbance is measured. A chromatogram of absorbance versus time is generated, with each Hb having a peak at a particular retention time (RT) in a defined window. The RT is the time from the injection of hemolysate to the appearance of the particular Hb in the eluate. The area under each peak quantifies the Hb fragment. The most common hemoglobins and their variants can thus by identified and quantified based on RT, percentage and peak-characteristics. Hemoglobins without predetermined RTs appear as unknown peaks. Characteristic windows **(Table 1)** like HbF, HbA, HbA2, HbS, HbC, and HbD have been defined, based on RT ranges.

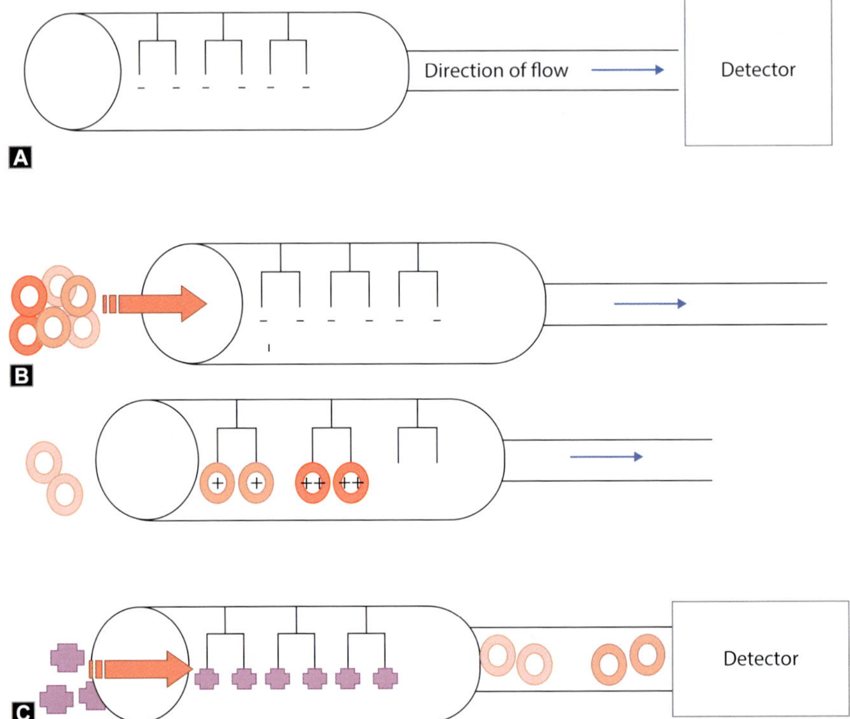

FIGS. 1A TO C: Hemoglobin analysis by cation-exchange high-pressure liquid chromatography. (A) Analytical cartridge contains negatively charged carboxyl groups. (B) Positively charged hemoglobins in injected hemolysate bind to the carboxyl groups. (C) Passage of cations in buffers elutes the hemoglobins at a rate inversely proportionate to their affinity and absorbance is measured at 415 nm and 690 nm.

TABLE 1: Retention time of various peaks and their interpretation (Bio-Rad Variant II).

Region/window	Window period (minutes)	Interpretation
Preintegration region	<1	Bilirubin, HbH, Hb Barts, modified HbF
P1 peak	0.75	Very small peak
F window	0.98–1.22	HbF
P2 window	1.28–1.5	Glycosylated HbA
P3 window	1.5–1.9	Aged samples, HbJ–Meerut
A0 window	1.9–3.1	HbA, Glycated HbS
A2 window	3.3–3.9	HbA2, HbE, HbD-Iran, Hb Lepore
D window	3.9–4.3	HbD-Punjab
S window	4.3–4.7	HbS, HbQ-Thailand, HbA2′
C window	4.9–5.3	HbC, Hb Constant Spring, Hb Agenogi

Note: Hemoglobin variants with RTs in the unknown window (4.70–4.90 minutes)—HbQ India and other less frequent hemoglobins.

Capillary Zone Electrophoresis

It separates ionic species based on their charge and size by applying an electric field across a capillary tube filled with an electrolyte. Two primary forces play crucial roles in CZE: *electroosmotic force (EOF)* and *electrophoretic force (ELP)*.

1. *EOF:* Electroosmotic flow is the bulk movement of liquid caused by applying an electric field to a capillary with charged walls. The inner wall of the capillary has sialanol groups, which are negatively charged (deprotonated) at the buffer pH of 9.4. The cations in the buffer coat the sialanol groups, forming an electrical double layer, also known as a fixed layer. However, not all cations at the wall-electrolyte interface coat the negative sialanol groups and the free cations form the diffuse layer. When voltage is applied from anode to cathode, the cations in the diffuse layer move toward the cathode dragging along the bulk solution toward the cathode **(Fig. 2A)**.
2. *ELP:* Electrophoretic force is the movement of charged particles relative to the solvent under the influence of an electric field. Each Hb fraction in the solution experiences a force proportional to its charge and the strength of the electric field **(Fig. 2B)**, causing it to migrate toward the electrode of the opposite charge.

Overall migration: The observed migration velocity of an ion is the sum of the electroosmotic flow velocity and the electrophoretic velocity **(Fig. 2C)**. For cations, the electroosmotic flow and electrophoretic movement are typically in the same direction (toward the cathode). For anions, the electrophoretic movement is toward the anode. However, if the electroosmotic flow is strong enough, it can overcome the electrophoretic force, causing anions to move toward the cathode as well, albeit at a slower velocity than the cations.

Identification of Hb fractions and variants by CZE is related to their migration positions on the electrophoretogram with HbA2 and HbF as references. Hb fractions are directly detected at the specific absorbance of 415 nm **(Fig. 3)**. The pattern is divided into 15 zones (12 zones for cord blood). Each zone displays a drop-down library of possible variants migrating within this zone. More than 300 variants are listed.

Hemoglobin Fractions and Their Role in Hemoglobinopathy Diagnosis

Apart from HbF, HbA, and HbA2, many α-, β-, and δ-variant hemoglobins can be determined by HPLC and CZE. It is important to use age-appropriate reference ranges for normal hemoglobins.

HbF

It is the main Hb in fetal life and at birth, constitutes almost 80% of total Hb. It gradually decreases in infancy and values are <1% after the second year of life. In severely anemic neonates, presence of predominantly HbF with nearly absent HbA could be seen due to transfusion-dependent β-thalassemia and sickle cell anemia **(Figs. 4B and F)**. By 4–6 months of life, raised HbF for age with minimal HbA and normal or raised HbA2 are seen in transfusion-dependent

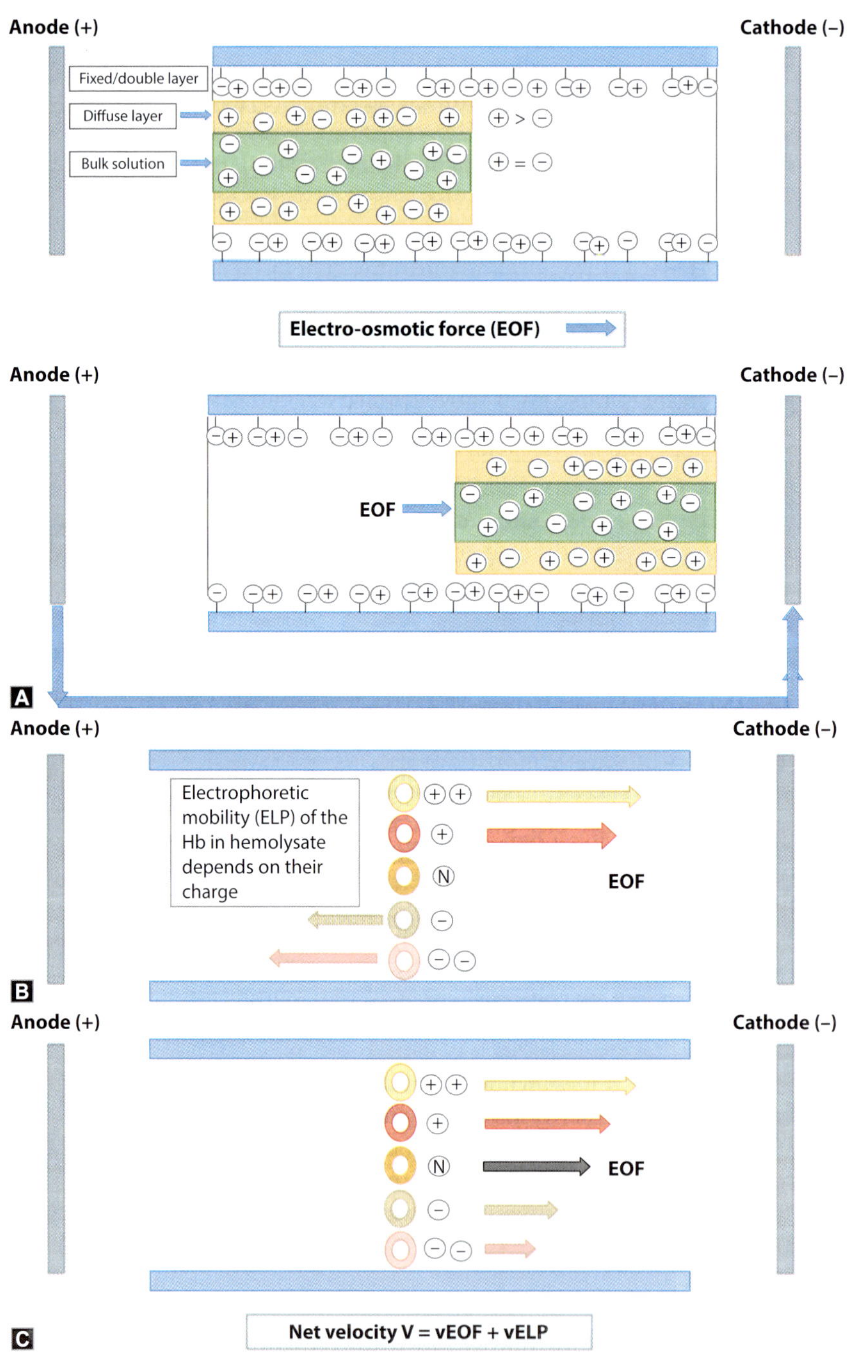

FIGS. 2A TO C: Hemoglobin analysis by capillary zonal electrophoresis. (A) Electroosmotic force causes movement of bulk solution from anode to cathode. (B) Electrophoretic mobility of the Hb in hemolysate depends on their electrical charge. (C) The net mobility of each Hb is the sum of electroosmotic force and the electrophoretic mobility.

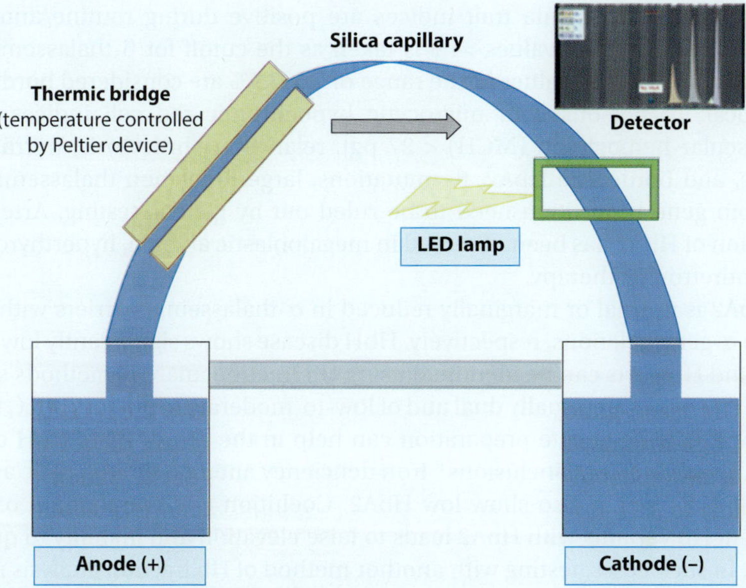

FIG. 3: Capillary zonal electrophoresis technique.

thalassemia (TDT) while raised HbF with HbS are seen in sickle cell anemia, in a nontransfused infant. HbF is also raised in compound heterozygous states such as HbE/β-thalassemia and HbS/β-thalassemia.

Persistence of HbF into adult life with normal hematological parameters may be seen in hereditary persistence of fetal hemoglobin (HPFH). Elevated HbF (5–20%) with anemia is observed in δβ-thalassemia. In equivocal cases, a Kleihauer–Betke test is done, which reveals a pancellular distribution pattern of HbF in red cells, while in δβ-thalassemia, the distribution is heterocellular. Molecular testing is needed for confirmation. HbF measurement has been utilized to monitor sickle cell anemia treatment.

Mild increase in HbF is seen in pregnancy and megaloblastic anemia (HbF—1–3%). However, a value of 5–10% is equivocal and >10% is suspicious, requiring close follow-up and further testing for hemoglobinopathy, respectively. Other congenital or acquired anemias such as bone marrow failure syndromes and sideroblastic anemias can show elevated HbF. Hematopoietic neoplasms, characteristically juvenile myelomonocytic leukemia also show increased fetal Hb. In presence of microcytic hypochromic or normocytic anemia with a leukoerythroblastic blood picture with no blasts in peripheral blood, they may sometimes present as a diagnostic dilemma.

HbA2

HbA2 is postnatally detected at 6–8 months of life. Normal values have a narrow range of 2.2–3.5%. HbA2 estimation is important for detection of β-thalassemia carrier when thalassemia trait indices are positive during routine/antenatal/cascade testing. HbA2 values >4% is taken as the cutoff for β-thalassemia trait (range—4–8%), while values in the range of 3.5–3.9% are considered borderline/equivocal. In persons with microcytic hypochromic red cell indices [mean corpuscular hemoglobin (MCH) < 27 pg], relative erythrocytosis, normal iron profile, and borderline HbA2, β+ mutations, large β deletion thalassemia, and α-globin gene triplication need to be ruled out by genetic testing. Artefactual elevation of HbA2 has been observed in megaloblastic anemia, hyperthyroidism, and antiretroviral therapy.

HbA2 is normal or marginally reduced in α-thalassemia carriers with single or two α-gene deletions, respectively. HbH disease shows significantly low HbA2. HbH and Hb Barts can be identified using Hb fraction analysis methods such as CZE. HbH peaks are usually dual and of low-to-moderate height on HPLC by Bio-Rad. Simple reticulocyte preparation can help in the diagnosis of HbH disease which shows "golf ball inclusions." Iron deficiency anemia, sideroblastic anemia, and δβ-thalassemia also show low HbA2. Coelution and comigration of many different Hb variants with HbA2 leads to false elevation and inability to quantify HbA2. In such cases, testing with another method of Hb fraction analysis may be utilized for accurate quantification. Also, due to the narrow reference interval of HbA2 and its significance in carrier screening, use of calibrators and controls with every run is essential for its precise and accurate measurement.

Hemoglobin Variants

HPLC and CZE can be used to presumptively identify and quantify α- and β-chain variant hemoglobins such as HbS, HbD, HbC, HbE, HbJ, Hb O-Arab, and Hb Constant Spring in heterozygous as well as homozygous states. Many of these may not present with changes in red cell indices, and hence, Hb fraction analysis is essential for carrier and patient diagnosis. Their charge differences lead to their separation and appearance in characteristic windows and zones after elution/migration in an electric field. Compound heterozygous states can also be detected using these methods. Some rare variants can also be identified by pattern analysis. Confirmatory diagnosis is by genetic testing. In case of sickle cell disease, sickling test confirms HbS noted on HPLC/CZE **(Figs. 4A to I)**.

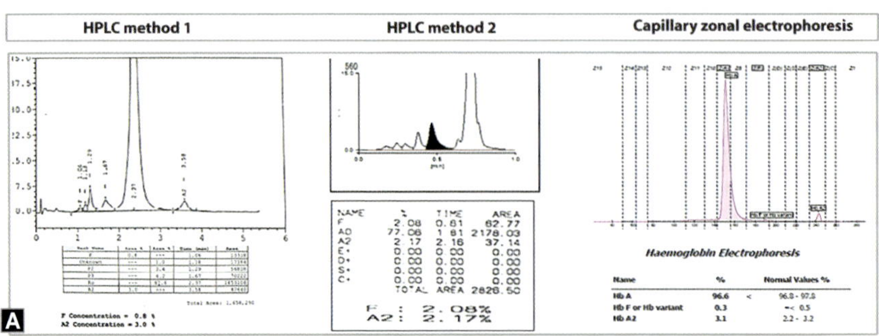

FIGS. 4A TO I: *Continued*

Continued

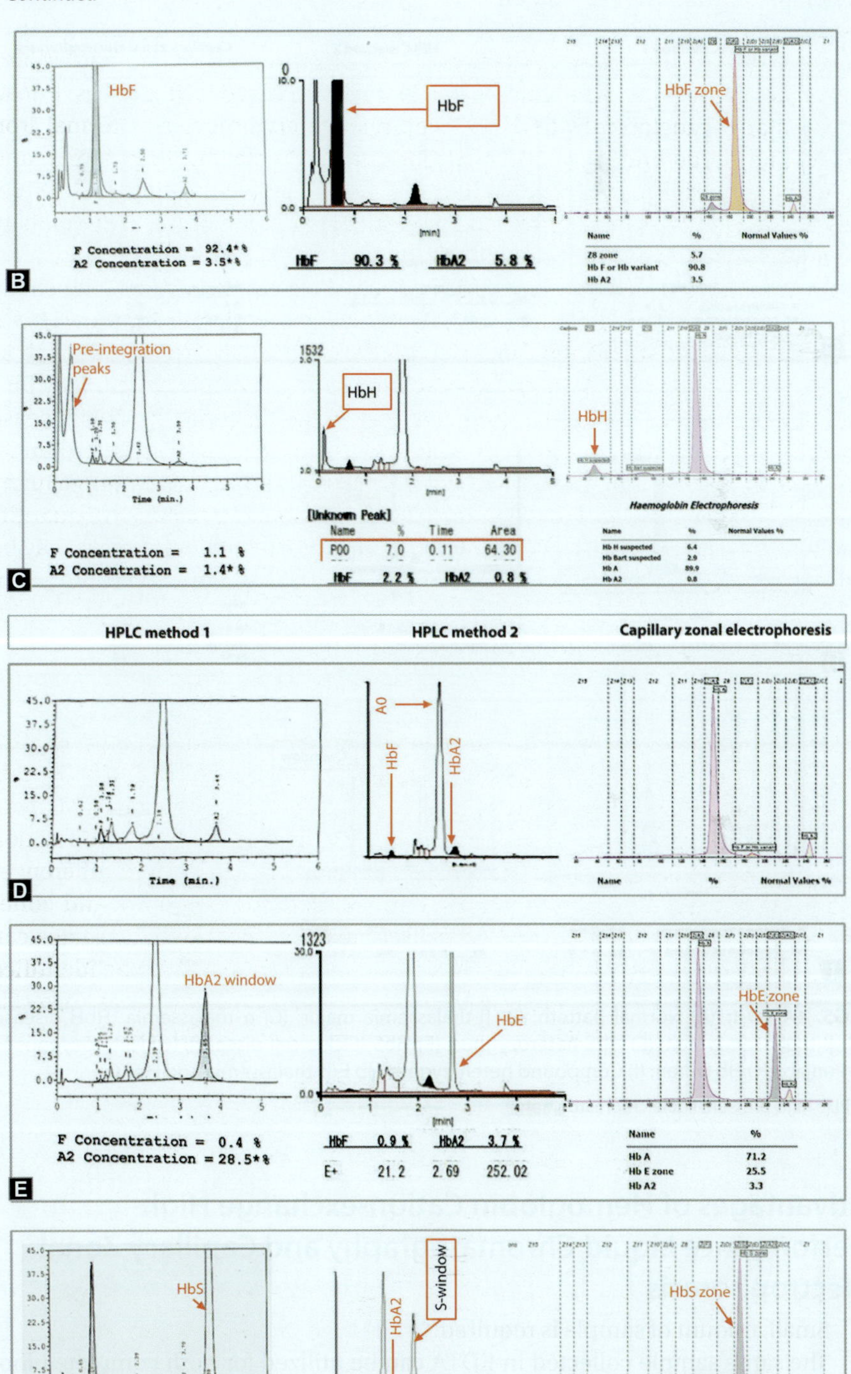

FIGS. 4A TO I: *Continued*

Continued

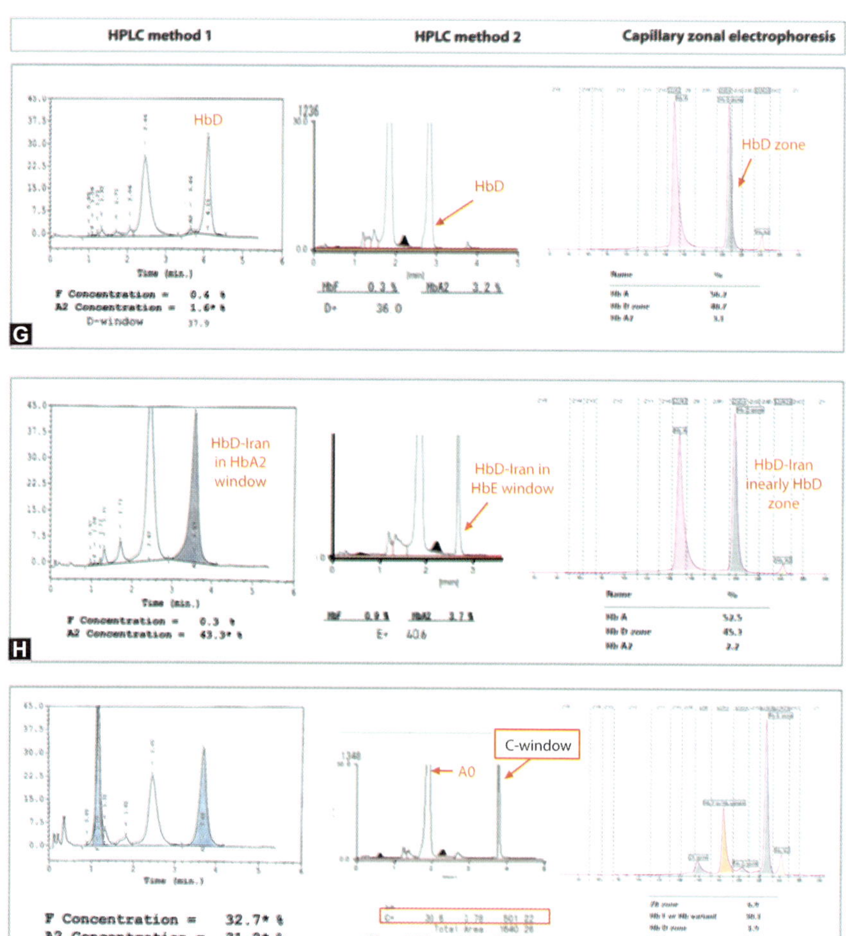

FIGS. 4A TO I: (A) Normal pattern; (B) β-thalassemia major; (C) α-thalassemia (HbH disease); (D) β-thalassemia trait; (E) HbE heterozygous; (F) HbS (Sickle cell disease); (G) Heterozygous Hb D-Punjab; (H) Hb D-Iran; (I) Compound heterozygous Hb E/β-thalassemia and HbAC.

(HPLC: high-pressure liquid chromatography)

Advantages of Hemoglobin Cation-exchange High-performance Liquid Chromatography and Capillary Zonal Electrophoresis

- Small amount of sample is required.
- The same sample collected in EDTA can be utilized for both complete blood count (CBC) and HPLC/CZE.
- Thalassemias, common Hb variants and compound heterozygous states are presumptively identified and quantified.

- High throughput—can be used for rapid screening and diagnosis.
- Automated, rapid, less labor-intensive methods, separate and quantitate the common hemoglobins and variants with high resolution and reproducibility. The graphical representation of results with the availability of extensive libraries, makes interpretation and identification easy.

Pitfalls

- Hemoglobin fraction analysis by HPLC and CZE cannot be performed in transfused patients. In such cases, this analysis should be performed in parents to rule out hemoglobinopathy. Genetic testing provides confirmatory diagnosis in such cases.
- HbA2 value of >4% is recommended for identifying β-thalassemia trait, however, borderline values of 3.5–3.9% or normal values may be seen in some β-thalassemia mutations due to α-gene triplication/quadruplication, even in the presence of microcytosis with erythrocytosis and normal iron profile. Low HbA2 values can occur in α-thalassemia carriers and in nutritional anemias like iron deficiency. Again, gene analysis is required for the correct diagnosis.
- HbE, Hb Lepore, HbD—Iran elute in HbA2 window in Bio-Rad Variant II. RTs and quantity of Hb in HbA2 window may help in arriving at a provisional diagnosis **(Table 2)**.
- HbA2 and HbE are separated from each other showing two different peaks in Tosoh G11 and Sebia CZE. Hb Lepore appears in P08 window in Tosoh and in zone 6 in Sebia CZE. However, HbD-Iran coelutes in E-window in Tosoh G11 **(Fig. 4E)**.
- Similar HbF values may be noted in heterozygous HPFH and δβ thalassemias, requiring further testing. HbF may be overestimated by HPLC in the presence of glycated hemoglobins, however, this does not interfere with the diagnosis.
- HbH and Hb Bart's elute as preintegration peaks in Bio-Rad as the software in usual settings is unable to integrate elution peaks with RT < 0.63. HbH elutes at P00 window in Tosoh G11 and migrates in zone 15 in CZE and are quantified as well. Supravital staining done in such cases shows golf-ball HbH inclusions.

TABLE 2: Hemoglobins eluting in HbA2 window (Bio-Rad Variant II).

	Hb% in HbA2 window	Retention time (min)	Additional remarks
Hb Lepore	7–15	~3.5	Hump on downward slope
HbD Iran	36–45	~3.54–3.62	
β-thalassemia trait	4–9	3.65–3.68	
HbE/β-thalassemia		~3.67	HbE + HbA2, raised HbF
HbE heterozygous	20–40	~3.72	Represents HbE + HbA2
HbE homozygous	70–90	~3.72	Represents HbE + HbA2
HbE/α-thalassemia	<25	~3.72	

- Other preintegration peaks that are seen in Bio-Rad include the early, sharp bilirubin peak and multiple peaks of acetylated HbF.
- Underestimation of HbA2 occurs in Bio-Rad due to baseline elevation in case of HbD Punjab while overestimation occurs in HbS disease due to formation of HbS adducts, however, it is accurately estimated with Tosoh and Sebia CZE.
- Fractions due to post-translational modification of hemoglobins A, S, C, and other hemoglobins are not separated from the unmodified Hb in CZE, leading to accurate estimation while their separation in HPLC leads to imprecision.
- Compound heterozygous HbS/D elute separately in HPLC, however, may migrate together showing a single peak.
- Others—HbQ India is eluted as a sharp peak at RT-4.71 just before C-window in Bio-Rad while in Tosoh it appears in C-window. Variants eluting in the A0 window show a characteristic hump in HPLC, however, show no separation in CZE. HbO-Arab comigrates with HbA2 in CZE **(Table 3)**.

Coelution and comigration of hemoglobins in both methodologies and other causes of under and overestimation or nondetection therefore mandate that any two of these be used in tandem to arrive at a presumptive diagnosis. These findings of Hb fraction analysis should be correlated with clinical features, family studies, red cell indices, peripheral smear findings such as target cells, sickle cells, crystals, and ancillary tests such as sickling test and supravital staining for HbH inclusions.

TABLE 3: Comparison of different methods of hemoglobin fraction analysis (Figs. 4A to I).

	HPLC method 1 (Bio-Rad variant 2 β-thalassemia program)	**HPLC method 2 (Tosoh HLC G11)**	**Capillary zonal electrophoresis (Sebia Minicap Flex piercing)**
Technology	*CE-HPLC:* Stationary phase and mobile phase in column	*CE-HPLC:* Stationary phase and mobile phase in column	Electroosmotic force and electrophoresis-based liquid separation in capillary
Point of detection	Retention time (RT)	Retention time (RT)	Migration time (Tm)
Graphical representation	Chromatogram	Chromatogram	Electropherogram
Peaks and bands	Broader bands	Sharp peaks, bands narrower than method 1	Sharp peaks, narrow bands with high resolution
Flow profile	• Pressure-induced flow • Parabolic profile	• Pressure-induced flow • Parabolic profile	• Electroosmotic flow • Flat profile
Important areas	Windows F, A0, A2, S, C, D, peaks P2, P3	• Windows F, A0, A2, S, C, D, E • Peaks P001, P08	Zones 1–15
HbE	Coelutes with HbA2	HbE window	HbE zone

Continued

Continued

	HPLC method 1 (Bio-Rad variant 2 β-thalassemia program)	HPLC method 2 (Tosoh HLC G11)	Capillary zonal electrophoresis (Sebia Minicap Flex piercing)
HbS	HbS window. False high HbA2 in the presence of HbS adducts	HbS window. No effect on HbA2	HbS zone. No effect on HbA2
HbD-Punjab	False low HbA2 in presence of HbD Punjab	HbA2 is accurately quantified	HbA2 is accurately quantified
HbD-Iran	Coelutes with HbA2	Coelutes in E-window	Early area of HbD zone
HbS/D	HbS and HbD windows	HbS and HbD windows	May show a single peak
Hb Lepore	Coelute in HbA2 window	Elutes in P08 window	Separate zone
HbH and Hb Barts estimation	Preintegration peak	Detected and quantified in P00 window	Separate zone of detection
α variants	HbQ India elutes as a sharp peak at RT 4.74 in S-window, Hb J-Meerut appears as P3 peak	HbQ India elutes in C-window, Hb J-Meerut elutes in unknown window RT—1.4–1.5	HbQ India appears in zone 1, Hb J-Meerut appears as a peak in zone 12

(CE-HPLC: cation exchange high-performance liquid chromatography)

Take Home Points

- HPLC and CZE are widely used methods for hemoglobinopathy testing and presumptive diagnosis.
- These methods utilize the relative differences in surface charge of variant hemoglobins in separating and quantifying the Hb fragments.
- CZE can separate HbE from HbA2 and thus allows more accurate measurement of HbA2 in the presence of HbE (but not so in HbC).
- While a single method of Hb fraction analysis can be used for screening, presumptive diagnosis requires testing by at least two of these complementary methods and definitive diagnosis is by genetic testing.

SUGGESTED READINGS

1. Bain BJ, Daniel Y, Henthorn J, de la Salle B, Hogan A, Roy NBA, et al. The BSH Committee. Significant haemoglobinopathies: A guideline for screening and diagnosis. Br J Haematol. 2023;201(6):1047-65.
2. Mandrile G, Barella S, Giambona A, Gigante A, Grosso M, Perrotta S, et al. First and second level haemoglobinopathies diagnosis: Best practices of the Italian Society of Thalassemia and Haemoglobinopathies (SITE). J Clin Med. 2022;11(18):5426.

3. Bain BJ. Haemoglobinopathy diagnosis. Chapter 2, 3rd edition. Oxford: Wiley Blackwell; 2020.
4. Sharma P, Das R. Cation-exchange high-performance liquid chromatography for variant hemoglobins and HbF/A2: What must hematopathologists know about methodology? World J Methodol. 2016;6(1):20-4.
5. Giordano PC. Universal screening for hemoglobinopathies in today's multi-ethnic societies: How and when. World J Obstet Gynecol. 2015;4(4):86-94.
6. Colah RB, Surve R, Sawant P, D'Souza E, Italia K, Phanasgaonkar S, et al. HPLC studies in hemoglobinopathies. Indian J Pediatr. 2007;74(7):657-62.

CHAPTER 26

Approach to Monocytosis

Aastha Gupta, Sarjana Tiwari

ABSTRACT

Monocytosis is a common hematological entity encountered in routine clinical practice and is caused by a wide spectrum of benign and malignant conditions. To reach to the underlying etiology which is still a challenging area of hematology, a comprehensive and integrated approach with appropriate clinical assessment and relevant laboratory investigations is must. In this chapter we provide a step-wise systemic approach to a patient presenting with monocytosis.

INTRODUCTION

Monocytes and their tissue-specific counterparts, macrophages, are important components of the mononuclear phagocyte system and play an important part in innate and adaptive immunity. In the healthy adult and child, monocytes typically comprise between 1 and 9% of total peripheral blood leukocytes. Normal range of absolute monocyte count (AMC) varies with age. At 24 weeks gestation, monocytes are 0.7×10^9/L (range 0.1–2.5×10^9/L) and gradually increase until the third week following birth where they reach 1.5×10^9/L (0.3–3.0×10^9/L). After that count gradually decreases to below 1.0×10^9/L. No significant difference is seen in the monocyte count by race and gender. The World Health Organization defines persistent monocytosis as an AMC $> 1 \times 10^9$/L with monocytes accounting for ≥10% of leukocytes persisting for ≥3 months.

Recent developments in laboratory technology have made the intricate biology of neoplastic monocytosis well understood. These developments have also improved our understanding of the molecular and biological relationships that underlie distinct phenotypic manifestations and clinical presentations.

DIFFERENTIAL DIAGNOSIS OF MONOCYTOSIS

The etiology of monocytosis range from benign to malignant neoplastic diseases. Comprehending the fundamental cause of monocytosis is essential for proper diagnosis and treatment.

Reactive Monocytosis

In majority of cases, peripheral blood monocytosis is usually a transient response to acute and chronic infections, bone marrow regeneration, medications, acute and chronic stress **(Table 1)**.

Neoplastic/Clonal Monocytosis

Neoplastic causes of monocytosis include both acute and chronic hematological neoplasms. The acute hematological neoplasms with monocytosis include acute myeloid leukemia (AML) with monocytic differentiation defined by the presence of ≥20% blasts and blasts equivalent (i.e., promonocytes and monoblasts). The common genetic abnormalities associated with prominent monocytosis include inv(16) (p13.1q22) or t(16;16)(p13.1;q22); CBFβ-MYH11, t(9;11)(p21.3;q23.3); KMT2A-MLLT3, or other rearrangements involving KMT2A.

Chronic conditions with monocytosis include myeloproliferative neoplasms (MPN) such as chronic myeloid leukemia (CML) with monocytosis, BCR::ABL1 negative MPNs, myelodysplastic/MPN, and myeloid/lymphoid neoplasms with

TABLE 1: Causes of monocytosis.

Reactive causes	Clonal causes
Infections: • *Acute:* Leptospirosis, listeriosis, SARS CoV • *Chronic:* Brucellosis, tuberculosis, malaria, visceral leishmaniasis, syphilis	Acute leukemia with monocytic differentiation-acute monocytic leukemia, acute monoblastic leukemia, acute myelomonocytic leukemia
Bone marrow regeneration after chemotherapy	Chronic myelomonocytic leukemia
Autoimmune and autoinflammatory disorders, e.g., rheumatoid arthritis, systemic lupus erythematosus (SLE), ulcerative colitis, sarcoidosis	Juvenile myelomonocytic leukemia
Medications—steroids, G-CSF, ATG, postradiation	Myeloproliferative neoplasm with monocytosis-chronic myeloid leukemia, polycythemia vera, essential thrombocythemia and primary myelofibrosis
Postsplenectomy	Systemic mastocytosis
Myocardial infarction	Dendritic cell neoplasms
Exercise	Solid tumors
Hemolytic anemias	B- and T-cell malignancies

(G-CSF: granulocytes-colony stimulating factor; ATG: antithymocyte globulin; SARS-CoV: severe acute respiratory syndrome coronavirus)

platelet derived growth factor receptor α and β (*PDGFRA, PDGFRB*), or fibroblast growth factor receptor 1 (*FGFR1*) rearrangement or *PCM1-JAK2* fusions.

Chronic myelomonocytic leukemia (CMML) is the most common neoplastic condition with monocytosis in adults. This entity is defined by the presence of essential criteria:

- Persistent absolute (≥0.5 × 10^9/L) and relative (≥10%) peripheral blood monocytosis.
- Blasts constituting <20% of the cells in the peripheral blood and bone marrow.
- Not meeting diagnostic criteria of chronic myeloid leukemia or other MPN.
- Not meeting the diagnostic criteria of myeloid/lymphoid neoplasms with eosinophilia and tyrosine kinase gene fusions (e.g., *PDGFRA, PDGFRB, FGFR1,* or *JAK2*).

The desirable criteria for diagnosis includes:

- Presence of dysplasia involving ≥1 myeloid lineage.
- Acquired clonal cytogenetic or molecular abnormality.
- Abnormal partitioning of peripheral blood monocyte subsets.

For fulfilment of the WHO diagnostic criteria the essential criteria must be present in all cases. If monocytosis is ≥1 × 10^9/L, one or more desirable criteria must be met and if monocytosis is <1 × 10^9/L, both the desirable criteria must be met. The requirement of ≥10% monocytes adds specificity by excluding patients who may meet the absolute monocytosis criterion because of a high white blood cell count even though the percentage of monocytosis is low. Systemic mastocytosis with an associated hematologic neoplasm (SM-AHN) should carefully be looked for as CMML is one of the commonly associated neoplasms seen with this entity.

Myeloproliferative neoplasms like *BCR-ABL1*-positive CML can present with absolute monocytosis at the time of diagnosis and is more commonly seen with a p190 *BCR-ABL1* fusion protein. Absolute monocytosis has been reported in up to 21% of patients with polycythemia vera associated with older age, leukocytosis, *TET2/SRSF2* mutations, shorter overall survival, and shorter myelofibrosis-free survival. Monocytosis of primary myelofibrosis is associated with features of higher dynamic international prognostic scoring system (DIPPS) risk status and increased frequency of ASXL1 mutations. The identification of driver mutations in *JAK2, CALR,* or *MPL* along with morphological assessment for features of myeloproliferative neoplasm confirm the diagnosis of MPNs.

Concurrent monocytosis and eosinophilia require further evaluation for the possibility of myeloid/lymphoid neoplasms associated with rearrangements of *PDGFRA, PDGFRB, FGFR1,* and *PCM1-JAK2* fusion. Identification of any of these alterations excludes a diagnosis of CMML. Cases with *PDGRFB* (5q32) rearrangement most commonly mimic monocytosis. Diseases linked to *PDGFRA* or *PDGFRB* rearrangements respond well to *tyrosine kinase inhibitor* (TKI) therapy, underscoring the need for molecular testing for effective treatment planning.

Any child presenting with sustained monocytosis with or without other lineage cytopenias after exclusion of reactive causes should be thoroughly evaluated for the possibility of Juvenile myelomonocytic leukemia (JMML).

Diagnostic criteria include presence of peripheral blood monocyte count ≥1 × 10^9/L, blast/blasts equivalents <20% in peripheral blood/bone marrow, clinical evidence of organ infiltration, most commonly splenomegaly, no Philadelphia (Ph) chromosome or *BCR::ABL1* fusion or *KMT2A* (*MLL1*) gene rearrangement along with identification of one or more mutations involving the RAS pathway (*PTPN11, CBL, NRAS, KRAS*, and *NF1*).

Monocytosis can be a manifestation of unrelated malignant diseases such as Hodgkin and non-Hodgkin lymphoma, plasma cell myeloma, and solid tumors.

APPROACH TO MONOCYTOSIS

Peripheral blood monocytosis should be evaluated by a comprehensive clinical assessment and laboratory investigations including complete blood count (CBC), meticulous peripheral blood examination, and bone marrow examination along with ancillary tests such as flow cytometry, cytogenetics, and molecular studies to determine an underlying cause for early initiation of treatment **(Flowchart 1)**.

Clinical Assessment

The duration of monocytosis needs to be ascertained and evaluated in context with the clinical findings. Signs and symptoms of acute infections or autoimmune

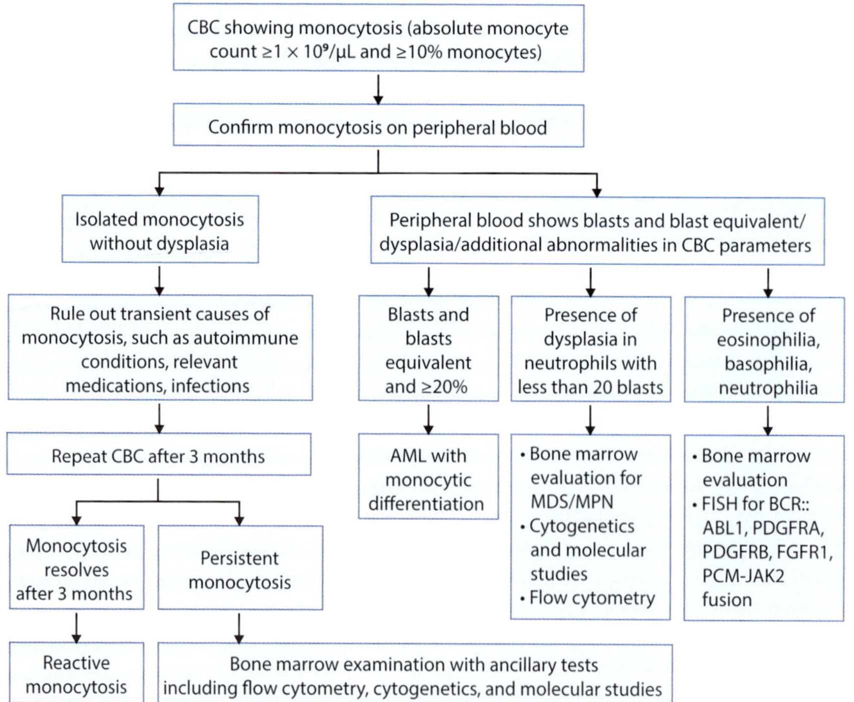

FLOWCHART 1: Diagnostic algorithm for approach to monocytosis.

(AML: acute myeloid leukemia; CBC: complete blood count; FISH: fluorescence in situ hybridization; MDS: myelodysplastic syndrome; MPN: myeloproliferative neoplasms)

disorders such as recent onset fever, joint pains, swelling, early morning stiffness, skin rashes, or recent travel history point toward reactive causes of monocytosis. History of medications such as steroids, growth factors chemotherapy, and radiotherapy along with the duration of intake of these drugs and indications for these medications needs to be documented as it may point toward bone marrow recovery. Acute onset monocytosis with anemia or thrombocytopenia, organomegaly or lymphadenopathy, bony pains, significant weight loss, easy bruising, and fatigue should be promptly evaluated for AML. An unexplained and persistent monocytosis with or without other cytopenias in elderly should be evaluated extensively for the possibility of myelodysplastic syndrome (MDS)/ MPN, MPN or underlying nonhematological neoplasms.

Laboratory Evaluation

Complete Blood Count and Peripheral Blood Examination

Monocytosis flagged by an automated hematology analyzer needs to be confirmed by peripheral smear examination as cells other than monocytes (e.g., blasts, abnormal lymphoid cells, hairy cells, and Sezary cells) may get counted by under monocytes based on size and granularity. Monocytes must be differentiated from these close morphological mimics. After confirmation, monocyte morphology must be evaluated for one of the four forms—mature monocytes, abnormal monocytes, promonocytes, and monoblasts. A common challenge faced by hematopathologists is the interobserver variability and poor reproducibility in identifying various stages especially differentiating promonocytes from abnormal monocytes and hypogranular abnormal promyelocytes. Morphology of accompanying leukocytes, hemoglobin, red blood cell (RBC) morphology, platelet count, and platelet morphology is essential. Neutrophils showing toxic changes or reactive lymphocytes point toward reactive causes of monocytosis. Cytopenias such as neutropenia, thrombocytopenia, or cytosis such as eosinophilia, basophilia, neutrophilia, or lymphocytosis warrant the need for further specific testing for hematological neoplasms. Neutrophilic dysplasia (≥10%) such as hypolobation and hypogranularity favor hematological neoplasm like CMML. Leukoerythroblastic blood picture might suggest a possibility of bone marrow infiltration by metastasis. Peripheral smear should also be evaluated for hemoparasites. Isolated monocytosis with the absence of any dysplasia or clinical suspicion of malignancy should be again evaluated after three months for the possibility of transient monocytosis.

Bone Marrow Examination

Any clinical or peripheral blood findings suggestive or suspicious of a hematological neoplasm needs to be further evaluated by bone marrow examination. Bone marrow examination helps in assessing trilineage hematopoiesis, blast percentage, dysplasia, cellularity, or any fibrosis. It is also important for ruling out/confirming other causes such as lymphoma infiltration, metastasis, or microorganisms such as visceral leishmaniasis and histoplasmosis.

Cytochemistry with myeloperoxidase (MPO) and nonspecific esterase (NSE) helps in differentiating cases of diagnostic dilemma based on morphology like the hypogranular variant of acute promyelocytic leukemia (APML) versus AML with monocytic differentiation. Monocytes exhibit strong, diffuse cytoplasmic positivity for NSE with dim MPO.

Samples of bone marrow can be used for ancillary tests such as flow cytometry, cytogenetics, and molecular genetic studies for further categorization of the hematological neoplasms.

Role of Flow Cytometry

Monocytes are a part of mononuclear phagocytic system, and hence, they express receptors for lipopolysaccharides (CD14) and Fc gamma III receptors (CD16). In humans three types of monocytes have been identified based on their expression patterns and this phenomenon has been called as flowcytometric monocytic repartition (FMR) **(Flowchart 2)**.

An addition of pan-monocytic markers like human leukocyte antigen (HLA)-DR or CD68 can help to clearly differentiate monocytes from CD16 expressing monocytes or natural killer cells. After exclusion of doublets and debris, gating is done on CD45-SSC for total nucleated cells, further gated with CD45–CD33 to look for bright CD33 monocytes and exclusion of granulocytes.

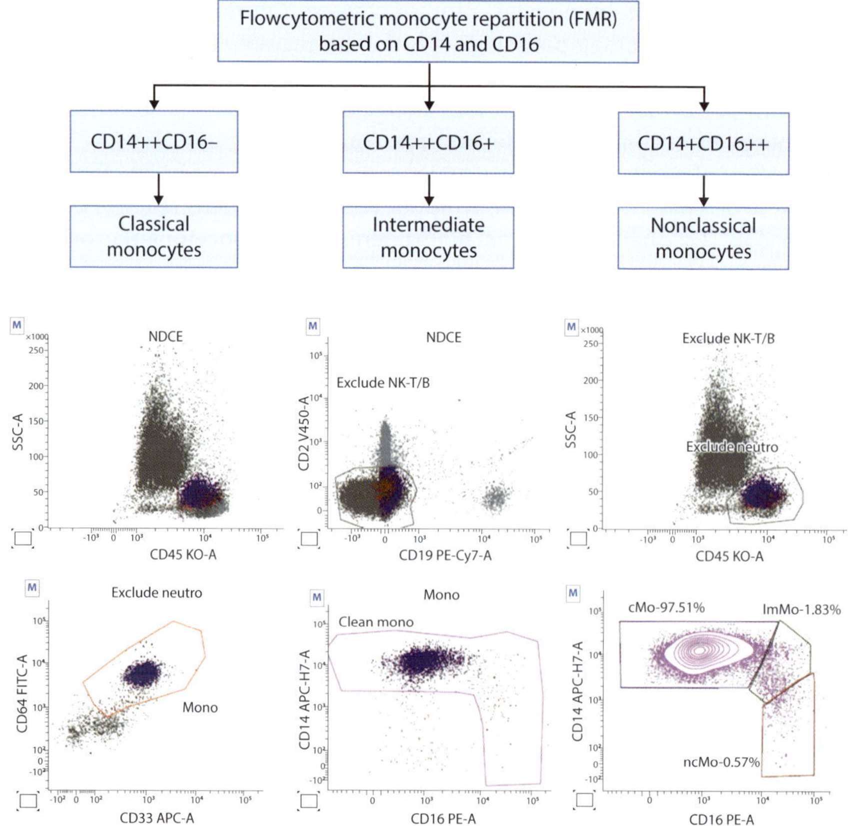

FLOWCHART 2: Flow cytometry based repartioning of monocytes subsets.

In healthy state, classical monocytes (cMo) comprises 85 ± 6%, intermediate monocytes (iMo) 5 ± 2%, and nonclassical monocytes (ncMo) 9 ± 4%.

The most important utility of this information is in distinguishing CMML from other causes of monocytosis. Studies have demonstrated that cMo are significantly higher (>94%) and ncMo are <1.13% in CMML versus other causes. Another group has studies classical and intermediate threshold by FMR on bone marrow samples, to distinguish between CMML, other myeloid neoplasms and normal cohort. These cutoffs may be different when compared to peripheral blood cutoffs. An increase in ncMo to >50% is usually associated with sepsis.

Cytogenetics and Molecular Genetics

Chromosomal analysis should be performed when a bone marrow is obtained in a suspected hematological neoplasm. Cytogenetics and fluorescence in situ hybridization (FISH) studies are warranted to confirm or exclude the AML/CML defining genetic abnormalities, i.e., RUNX1::RUNX1T1, inv (16), PML::RARA, and BCR::ABL1. Monocytosis with eosinophilia must be evaluated for PDGFRA, PDGFRB, FGFR mutation and PCM1::JAK2 fusion abnormalities. 25–40% CMML have been associated with chromosomal abnormalities with the most common being trisomy 8 and most characteristic being monosomy 7. A Spanish group has risk stratified CMML based on the cytogenetic abnormalities into high risk, intermediate risk, and low risk. The 5-year overall survival was found to be 4%, 26%, and 35% in each of these groups, respectively. Mayo-French group have found the lowest median survival of 3 months in high-risk group compared to 41 months in low risk group **(Table 2)**.

Molecular studies by polymerase chain reaction (PCR) and next-generation sequencing (NGS) is paving its way in approaching the diagnosis of monocytosis. Identification of driver mutations such as *NPM1, JAK2V617F, MPL, and CALR* are essential to diagnose AML with even blast <20% or MPN with monocytosis and exclusion of CMML. Several mutations have been identified on CMML that can be divided into five categories.

1. Mutations in epigenetic control of transcription—further subdivided into mutations in histone modification genes (*EZH2, ASXL1*) and DNA methylation genes (*DNMT3A, TET2, IDH1*, and *IDH2*)
2. Spliceosome mutations (*F3B1, SRSF2, U2AF1*)
3. Cell signaling pathway mutations (*JAK2, KRAS, NRAS, CBL, FLT3*)
4. Transcription factors and nucleosome assembly mutations (*SETBP1, RUNX1*)
5. Mutations in DNA damage response genes (*TP53, PHF6*)

Out of all these mutations, *TET2* mutations are most frequent followed by mutations involving *SRSF2, ASXL1*, and *RAS*.

With advent of sequencing, on one hand we can establish the underlying clonal process, however, certain concerns do remain as to how to utilize this

TABLE 2: Risk stratification according to cytogenetics.

High risk	Complex karyotype, trisomy 8, monosomy 7, or del 7q
Low risk	-Y, normal karyotype
Intermediate risk	All other chromosomal abnormalities except those included in high risk and low risk

immense data generated. For example, monocytosis lacking dysplasia and other key diagnostic features of CMML, identification of somatic mutations such as *ASXL2, DNMT3A,* and *TET2* should be interpreted with caution as these are also the mutations of clonal hematopoiesis of indeterminate potential (CHIP). Also, all these mutations described are not specific to CMML and can be found in other myeloid neoplasms. Hence, a good morphological examination remains the cornerstone in primary diagnosis and classification.

CASE-BASED APPROACH

Case 1

A 60-year old woman during her routine health check got CBC done showing hemoglobin of 10.2 g/dL, white blood cell (WBC) count 3.2 × 10^9/L with 25% monocytes (AMC 0.8 × 10^9/L). No previous reports were available. Peripheral smear showed presence of mature monocytes with ~35% dysplasia in neutrophils in form of hypolobation and hypogranulation. After exclusion of reactive causes of dysplasia and monocytosis a bone marrow procedure was performed which showed ~7% blasts along with significant dysplasia in megakaryocytes (~60%) and myeloid lineages (~25%). Biopsy was hypercellular for age (75%). Samples were sent for flow cytometry for evaluation of monocyte subsets which showed CD14 + CD16—subset in ~95% monocytes. NGS done in bone marrow showed *TET2* mutation with a variant allele frequency (VAF) of ~45% **(Fig. 1)**.

Diagnosis: CMML

Case 2

A 30-year-old male presented with history of fever off and on with generalized weakness for 2 weeks. CBC showed bicytopenia with monocytosis [hemoglobin (Hb)-9.2 g/dL, total leukocyte count (TLC) 4.1 × 10^9/μL, DLC:N 47, L 23,

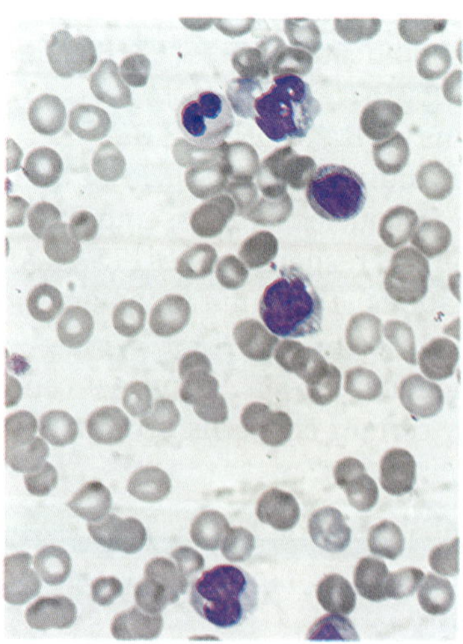

FIG. 1: Peripheral smear shows presence of monocytes with dysplastic neutrophils.

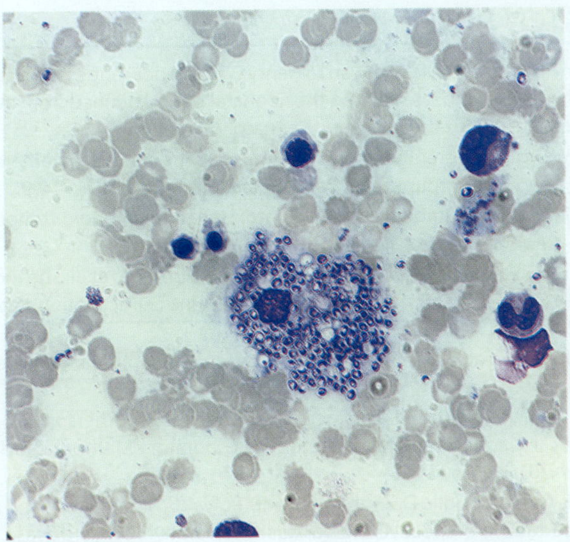

FIG. 2: Bone marrow aspirate shows intracellular and extracellular histoplasma capsulatum (Giemsa stain, 100×).

M 30, platelets (Plts)–82 × 10^3/μL]. Peripheral smear showed monocytosis with no dysplasia, blasts, or hemoparasite. Bone marrow examination for further evaluation showed increase in macrophages with presence of intracellular as well as extracellular histoplasma **(Fig. 2)**.

Take Home Points

- Monocytosis is a hematological abnormality commonly encountered on CBC with wide range of underlying causes.
- Although monocytosis is a nonspecific phenomenon that is most commonly caused by reactive conditions, certain clues such as persistent monocytosis, cytopenias in other lineages, the presence of dysplasia, and organomegaly are indicators that point to neoplastic origins.
- Morphology on peripheral smear and bone marrow must never be undermined as it is the key factory in diagnosing the underlying causes. If any CBC, peripheral smear, or clinical findings raise a suspicion of hematological malignancy, a thorough investigation including bone marrow examination with ancillary techniques is mandatory to reach to a precise diagnosis.
- Ancillary techniques such as flow cytometry, cytogenetics, and molecular studies extremely helpful in certain morphologically challenging cases to establish the clonal process.
- A systematic and methodical approach helps to reach to a definite conclusion and early initiation of effective treatment strategies.
- The success of combining molecular data with monocyte partitioning to accurately assess the reason of persistent monocytosis may be enhanced by more sensitive techniques such as microarray analysis and/or gene expression profiling.

SUGGESTED READINGS

1. Christensen RD, Jensen J, Maheshwari A, Henry E. Reference ranges for blood concentrations of eosinophils and monocytes during the neonatal period defined from over 63 000 records in a multihospital health-care system. J Perinatol. 2010;30(8):540-5.
2. Saxena S, Wong ET. Heterogeneity of common hematologic parameters among racial, ethnic, and gender subgroups. Arch Pathol Lab Med. 1990;114(7):715-9.
3. WHO Classification of Tumours Editorial Board. Haematolymphoid tumours. Lyon (France): International Agency for Research on Cancer; 2024.
4. Raffray L, Giry C, Vandroux D, Fayeulle S, Moiton MP, Gerber A, et al. The monocytosis during human leptospirosis is associated with modest immune cell activation states. Med Microbiol Immunol. 2019;208(5):667-78.
5. Whitelock-Jones L, Carswell J, Rasmussen KC. Listeria pneumonia. A casereport. S Afr Med J. 1989;75(4):188-9.
6. Hutchison RE, Schexneider KI. Leukocytic disorders. In: McPherson RA, Pincus MR (Eds). Henry's Clinical Diagnosis and Management by Laboratory Methods, 23rd edition. St. Louis, MO: Elsevier; 2017. pp. 606-58.
7. Cherfane CE, Gessel L, Cirillo D, Zimmerman MB, Polyak S. Monocytosis and a low lymphocyte to monocyte ratio are effective biomarkers of ulcerative colitis disease activity. Inflamm Bowel Dis. 2015;21(8):1769-75.
8. Wurm K, Lohr G. Immunocytological blood tests in cases of sarcoidosis. Sarcoidosis. 1986;3(1):52-9.
9. Barker S, Scott M, Chan GT. Corticosteroids and monocytosis. NZ Med J. 2012;125:76-8.
10. Thone J, Kessler E. Monocytosis subsequent to ziprasidone treatment: a possible side effect. Prim Care Companion J Clin Psychiatry. 2007;9(6):465-6.
11. Rajadurai VS, Chambers HM, Vigneswaran R, Gardiner AA. Monocytosis in preterm infants. Early Hum Dev. 1992;28(3):223-9.
12. Rotman M, Ansley H, Rogow L, Stowe S. Monocytosis: a new observation during radiotherapy. Int J Radiat Oncol Biol Phys. 1977;2(1-2):117-21.
13. Bearman RM, Kjeldsberg CR, Pangalis GA, Rappaport H. Chronic monocytic leukemia in adults. Cancer. 1981;48(10):2239-55.
14. Liebetrau C, Hoffmann J, Dörr O, Gaede L, Blumenstein J, Biermann H, et al. Release kinetics of inflammatory biomarkers in a clinical model of acute myocardial infarction. Circ Res. 2015;116(5):867-75.
15. Shin YO, Lee JB. Leukocyte chemotactic cytokine and leukocyte subset responses during ultra-marathon running. Cytokine. 2013;61(2):364-9.
16. Wongtong N, Jones S, Deng Y, Cai J, Ataga KI. Monocytosis is associated with hemolysis in sickle cell disease. Hematology. 2015;20(10):593-7.
17. Puigvi L, Baumann T, Fernandez S, Castro P, Pereira A, Merino A. Massive erythrophagocytosis by peripheral monocytes and neutrophils in parvovirus-B19 autoimmune hemolytic anemia. Ann Hematol. 2017;96:881-2.
18. Boiocchi L, Espinal-Witter R, Geyer JT, Steinhilber J, Bonzheim I, Knowles DM, et al. Development of monocytosis in patients with primary myelofibrosis indicates an accelerated phase of the disease. Mod Pathol. 2013;26(2):204-12.
19. Wang SA, Hutchinson L, Tang G, Chen SS, Miron PM, Huh YO, et al. Systemic mastocytosis with associated clonal hematological non-mast cell lineage disease: clinical significance and comparison. Am J Hematol. 2013;88(3):219-24.
20. Hu Z, Sun T. Blastic plasmacytoid dendritic cell neoplasm associated with chronic myelomonocytic leukemia. Blood. 2016;128(12):1664.
21. Barrett O Jr. Monocytosis in malignant disease. Ann Intern Med. 1970;73(6):991-2.

22. Bari A, Tadmor T, Sacchi S, Marcheselli L, Liardo EV, Pozzi S, et al. Monocytosis has adverse prognostic significance and impacts survival in patients with T-cell lymphomas. Leuk Res. 2013;37(6):619-623.39.
23. Tadmor T, Fell R, Polliack A, Attias D. Absolute monocytosis at diagnosis correlates with survival in diffuse large B-cell lymphoma-possible link with monocytic myeloid-derived suppressor cells. Hematol Oncol. 2013;31(2):65-71.
24. Wong KL, Tai JJ, Wong WC, Han H, Sem X, Yeap WH, et al. Gene expression profiling reveals the defining features of the classical, intermediate, and nonclassical human monocyte subsets. Blood. 2011;118(5):e16-31.
25. Barge L, Gooch M, Hendle M, Simleit E. Real world implementation of flow cytometric monocyte subset partitioning for distinguishing chronic myelomonocytic leukaemia from other causes of monocytosis. Pathology. 2023;55(6):827-34.
26. Talati C, Zhang L, Shaheen G, Kuykendall A, Ball M, Zhang Q, Lancet JE, et al. Monocyte subset analysis accurately distinguishes CMML from MDS and is associated with a favorable MDS prognosis. Blood. 2017;129(13):1881-3.
27. Wagner-Ballon O, Bettelheim P, Lauf J, Bellos F, Della Porta M, Travaglino E, et al; European LeukemiaNet International MDS-Flow Cytometry Working Group (ELN iMDS-Flow). ELN iMDS flow working group validation of the monocyte assay for chronic myelomonocytic leukemia diagnosis by flow cytometry. Cytometry B Clin Cytom. 2023;104(1):66-76.
28. Allen SA, Ng E, Hahn UH, Banovic T, Ross DM. Flow cytometric monocyte repartition demonstrates overlap between chronic myelomonocytic leukaemia and myeloid neoplasms with monocytosis. Pathology. 2022;54(7):953-5.
29. Kiefer J, Zeller J, Bogner B, Hörbrand IA, Lang F, Deiss E, et al. An unbiased flow cytometry-based approach to assess subset-specific circulating monocyte activation and cytokine profile in whole blood. Front Immunol. 2021;12:641224.
30. Patnaik MM, Tefferi A. Chronic Myelomonocytic leukemia: 2020 update on diagnosis, risk stratification and management. Am J Hematol. 2020;95(1):97-115.
31. Wassie EA, Itzykson R, Lasho TL, Kosmider O, Finke CM, Hanson CA, et al. Molecular and prognostic correlates of cytogenetic abnormalities in chronic myelomonocytic leukemia: a Mayo Clinic-French Consortium Study. Am J Hematol. 2014;89(12):1111-5.
32. Onida F, Kantarjian HM, Smith TL, Ball G, Keating MJ, Estey EH, et al. Prognostic factors and scoring systems in chronic myelomonocytic leukemia: a retrospective analysis of 213 patients. Blood. 2002;99(3):840-9.
33. Kwon J. Diagnosis and treatment of chronic myelomonocytic leukemia. Blood Res. 2021;56(S1):S5-S16.
34. Such E, Cervera J, Costa D, Solé F, Vallespí T, Luño E, et al. Cytogenetic risk stratification in chronic myelomonocytic leukemia. Haematologica. 2011;96(3):375-83.
35. Wassie EA, Itzykson R, Lasho TL, Kosmider O, Finke CM, Hanson CA, et al. Molecular and prognostic correlates of cytogenetic abnormalities in chronic myelomonocytic leukemia: a Mayo Clinic-French Consortium Study. Am J Hematol. 2014;89(12):1111-5.
36. Abdel-Wahab O, Pardanani A, Patel J, Wadleigh M, Lasho T, Heguy A, et al. Concomitant analysis of EZH2 and ASXL1 mutations in myelofibrosis, chronic myelomonocytic leukemia and blast-phase myeloproliferative neoplasms. Leukemia. 2011;25(7):1200-2.
37. Patnaik MM, Lasho TL, Finke CM, Hanson CA, Hodnefield JM, Knudson RA, et al. Spliceosome mutations involving SRSF2, SF3B1, and U2AF35 in chronic myelomonocytic leukemia: prevalence, clinical correlates, and prognostic relevance. Am J Hematol. 2013;88(3):201-6.
38. Gelsi-Boyer V, Trouplin V, Adelaide J, Aceto N, Remy V, Pinson S, et al. Genome profiling of chronic myelomonocytic leukemia: frequent alterations of RAS and RUNX1 genes. BMC Cancer. 2008;8:299.

39. Kohlmann A, Grossmann V, Klein HU, Schindela S, Weiss T, Kazak B, et al. Next-generation sequencing technology reveals a characteristic pattern of molecular mutations in 72.8% of chronic myelomonocytic leukemia by detecting frequent alterations in TET2, CBL, RAS, and RUNX1. J Clin Oncol. 2010;28(24):3858-65.
40. Itzykson R, Solary E. An evolutionary perspective on chronic myelomonocytic leukemia. Leukemia. 2013;27(7):1441-50.
41. Itzykson R, Kosmider O, Renneville A, Gelsi-Boyer V, Meggendorfer M, Morabito M, et al. Prognostic score including gene mutations in chronic myelomonocytic leukemia. J Clin Oncol. 2013;31(19):2428-36.
42. Lynch DT, Hall J, Foucar K. How I investigate monocytosis. Int J Lab Hematol. 2018;40(2): 107-14.

CHAPTER 27

Juvenile Myelomonocytic Leukemia—Recent Updates

Aditya Kumar Gupta, Anita Chopra, Jagdish Prasad Meena

ABSTRACT

Juvenile myelomonocytic leukemia (JMML) is a rare clonal hematopoietic disorder of infancy and early childhood, driven by oncogenic mutations in genes associated with the RAS signaling pathway. Given its often aggressive clinical course, prompt diagnosis and timely initiation of treatment are crucial for improving patient outcomes. This chapter provides an overview of epidemiology, current diagnostic approaches, and treatment strategies for JMML, with a focus on the latest advancements in therapeutic interventions.

Currently, allogeneic hematopoietic stem cell transplantation (HSCT) is the only potential curative therapy for JMML, achieving a cure in over 50% of patients. Prompt HSCT is recommended for children with *NF1*, somatic *PTPN11* and *KRAS* mutations, and for most children with somatic *NRAS* mutations. On the other hand, a "watch and wait" approach may be suitable for children with germline *CBL* mutations, specific somatic/germline *NRAS* mutations, and those with Noonan syndrome, as spontaneous resolution has been observed in some cases. Chemotherapeutic agents are often used as a bridge to HSCT in JMML. One such agent is 5-azacytidine, a DNA-hypomethylating agent, which has been reported to induce remission in some children with JMML, helping to stabilize the disease and prepare the patient for the transplant procedure.

INTRODUCTION

Juvenile myelomonocytic leukemia (JMML) is a rare clonal hematopoietic disorder primarily affecting young children. It is characterized by abnormal proliferation, primarily of the granulocytic and monocytic lineages, and frequent infiltration of organs such as the liver, spleen, and lymph nodes. Initially included under the myelodysplastic syndrome/myeloproliferative neoplasm (MDS/MPN) category in the revised 4th edition of the World Health Organization (WHO) classification of hematolymphoid tumors [4th edition of the World Health Organization classification of hematolymphoid tumors (R4th WHO-Hem)], JMML has since been reclassified as MPN in the 5th edition of the World Health Organization classification of hematolymphoid tumors (R5th WHO-Hem). This reclassification emphasizes its distinct clinical and biological identity by reflecting its unique molecular pathogenesis and lack of myelodysplastic neoplasm hallmarks.

JMML is widely recognized as a classic example of a RASopathy—a group of disorders driven by mutations that constitutively hyperactivate the RAS-mitogen-activated protein kinase (MAPK) pathway, which is essential for cell growth and differentiation. This molecular signature places JMML at the intersection of oncology, genetic syndromes, and developmental biology. To understand JMML, it is important to consider its clinical characteristics, genetic basis, and the pathway dysregulation underlying its pathogenesis. Its classification as a RASopathy expands our understanding of potential targeted treatments and prognostic indicators, while also underscoring the complexities involved in its diagnosis and management. This chapter examines the distinctive features of JMML, including its genetic profile, pathophysiology, and wider ramifications of JMML's classification as a RASopathy within pediatric hematological illnesses.

EPIDEMIOLOGY

JMML is a rare hematologic malignancy, with an estimated annual incidence of 1–2 cases per million children (aged 0–14 years). It primarily affects infants and young children, with majority of diagnoses occurring before the age of 4. Approximately 9% of JMML patients are diagnosed before the age of 4 months, while only 5% are diagnosed after the age of 4 years. JMML shows a slight male predominance, with a male-to-female ratio of approximately 2:1.

Genetic predispositions play a significant role in the epidemiology of JMML. Approximately 10–15% of cases are associated with predisposing genetic conditions such as neurofibromatosis type 1 (*NF1*), Noonan syndrome (NS), and Casitas B-lineage lymphoma *(CBL)* syndromes, that affect the RAS-MAPK pathway (RASopathies). The presence of these genetic factors highlights the overlap between congenital syndromes and acquired mutations in driving the development of JMML.

PATHOGENESIS

JMML is a bonafide example of RAS-driven malignancy. It is associated with RAS pathway genes mutations in >90% cases (*NRAS* in 15–25%; *KRAS* in 15–20%; *PTPN11* in 35–40%; *NF1* in 5–10%; or *CBL* in 12–15%; rarely *RRAS*, *RRAS2*, or *RIT1*). This leads to constitutive activation of RAS signaling pathway and increasing sensitivity of myeloid progenitors to granulocyte-monocyte colony stimulating factors (GM-CSF).

Intriguingly, RAS-activating mutations found in JMML are mutually exclusive and are associated with distinct clinical and hematological presentations. Secondary mutations (including second hits in one or other RAS pathway genes or other target genes) may emerge during the course of the disease, influencing its severity and progression. Aberrant methylation of promoter regions in certain genes (hypermethylation) contributes to disease progression.

CLINICAL FEATURES

Most patients of JMML are diagnosed before 24 months of age, presenting with symptoms such as pallor, abdominal distension, bleeding, and respiratory issues. Common physical signs include fever, pallor, cutaneous lesions, lymphadenopathy, hepatomegaly, splenomegaly, and bleeding manifestations. Cutaneous lesions include eczema, xanthogranulomas, leukemia cutis, and café-au-lait spots. Splenomegaly is present in all cases of JMML and is considered a prerequisite for its diagnosis. Leukemic infiltration into the lungs or gastrointestinal tract (GIT) may cause respiratory and GIT symptoms. Respiratory symptoms often include cough, difficulty breathing, and wheezing, while diarrhea is a predominant GIT finding. Malnutrition and poor weight gain are also frequently observed. These findings are relatively nonspecific and may resemble those seen in disseminated microbial infections during infancy; hence, these infections should be excluded.

DIAGNOSIS OF JUVENILE MYELOMONOCYTIC LEUKEMIA

The diagnosis of JMML required all five clinical, hematological, and laboratory criteria to be fulfilled, plus one molecular criterion or at least two of the other nonmolecular "other criteria" **(Box 1)**. The workflow followed for the diagnosis of JMML is summarized in **Flowchart 1**.

JMML is diagnosed using a combination of clinical, hematological, laboratory, and genetic criteria. The R5th WHO-Hem has revised the diagnostic guidelines for JMML **(Box 1)**. The key changes in these criteria include: (1) the absence of *KMT2A* rearrangements as one of the required diagnostic criteria; (2) the exclusion of monosomy 7 as a cytogenetic criterion; (3) combining hypersensitivity to granulocyte-macrophage colony-stimulating factor (GM-CSF) in a colony assay and STAT5 hyperphosphorylation as a single minor criterion; and (4) the addition of thrombocytopenia with hypercellular bone marrow (BM) as a minor criterion.

Morphology

Peripheral Blood Smears

In JMML, peripheral blood smears (PBS) examination reveals distinct abnormalities that aid in diagnosis. They typically show leukocytosis with monocytosis $\geq 1 \times 10^9$/L **(Fig. 1A)**. Monocytes often have atypical morphology. The smears often show leukoerythroblastic blood picture. This has been now mentioned as the "other criteria" in the R5th WHO-Hem criteria for JMML diagnosis **(Box 1)**. Eosinophilia and basophilia may be occasionally seen. Blasts and promonocytes are usually <2% of white blood cells. Dysplastic features in myeloid cells may be seen in the form of abnormal nuclear segmentation and pseudo-Pelger–Huët

BOX 1: 5th WHO-Hem diagnostic criteria for JMML.

Clinical, hematological, and laboratory criteria (all five criteria are mandatory):

- Peripheral blood monocyte count $\geq 1 \times 10^9$/L
- Blast and promonocyte percentage of <20% in peripheral blood and bone marrow
- Clinical evidence of organ infiltration, most commonly splenomegaly
- No Philadelphia (Ph) chromosome or *BCR::ABL1* fusion
- No *KMT2A* (*MLL1*) gene rearrangement

Genetic criteria (one criterion is required):

- Mutation in a component or a regulator of the canonical RAS pathway:
    - Clonal somatic mutation in *PTPN11*, *KRAS*, or *NRAS*, or
    - Clonal somatic or germline *NF1* mutation and loss of heterozygosity or compound heterozygosity of *NF1*, or
    - Clonal somatic or germline *CBL* mutation and loss of heterozygosity of *CBL*
- Noncanonical clonal RAS pathway pathogenic variant (*RRAS* or *RRAS2*) or fusions causing activation of genes upstream of the RAS pathway, such as *ALK*, *PDGRB*, and *ROS1*

Other criteria: Cases that do not meet any of the genetic criteria listed earlier (or for which genetic testing is not available) must meet at least two of the following criteria in addition to the aforementioned clinical, hematological, and laboratory criteria.

- Increased hemoglobin F for age
- Myeloid (promyelocytes, myelocytes, and metamyelocytes) and erythroid precursors on peripheral blood smear
- Thrombocytopenia with hypercellular marrow often showing a decreased number of megakaryocytes; dysplastic features may or may not be evident
- Hypersensitivity of myeloid progenitors to GM-CSF as tested in clonogenic assays in methylcellulose or by measuring STAT5 phosphorylation in the absence of or with a low dose of exogenous GM-CSF

(GM-CSF: granulocyte-macrophage colony-stimulating factor; JMML: juvenile myelomonocytic leukemia; R5th WHO-Hem: 5th edition of the World Health Organization classification of hematolymphoid tumors)

forms. Anemia is commonly observed, usually normocytic. Macrocytic red blood cells may be seen in some patients with monosomy 7. Microcytosis may be seen in children with concomitant iron deficiency anemia or thalassemia. Thrombocytopenia is another consistent finding, with the exception of *NF1* syndromic JMML, where platelets can be normal.

Bone Marrow

Bone marrow morphology alone is not diagnostic of JMML. BM aspirates typically show hypercellularity with granulocytic hyperplasia and complete maturation of myeloid progenitors **(Fig. 1B)**. In contrast to prominent peripheral blood (PB) monocytosis, BM shows a limited monocytic infiltration (5–10% of cells). Blasts and promonocytes constitute <20% of all nucleated cells. Mild dysplasia may be seen in any of the three hematopoietic lineages. Auer rods are typically absent. A predominance of erythroid precursors may be seen in patients with monosomy 7. They may also show megaloblastic features. BM often shows a decreased number of megakaryocytes. Reticulin fibrosis is also occasionally noted.

Immunophenotypic Analysis

Flow cytometry is often useful at diagnosis to exclude other leukemias but plays a limited role afterward unless there is clinical suspicion about progression

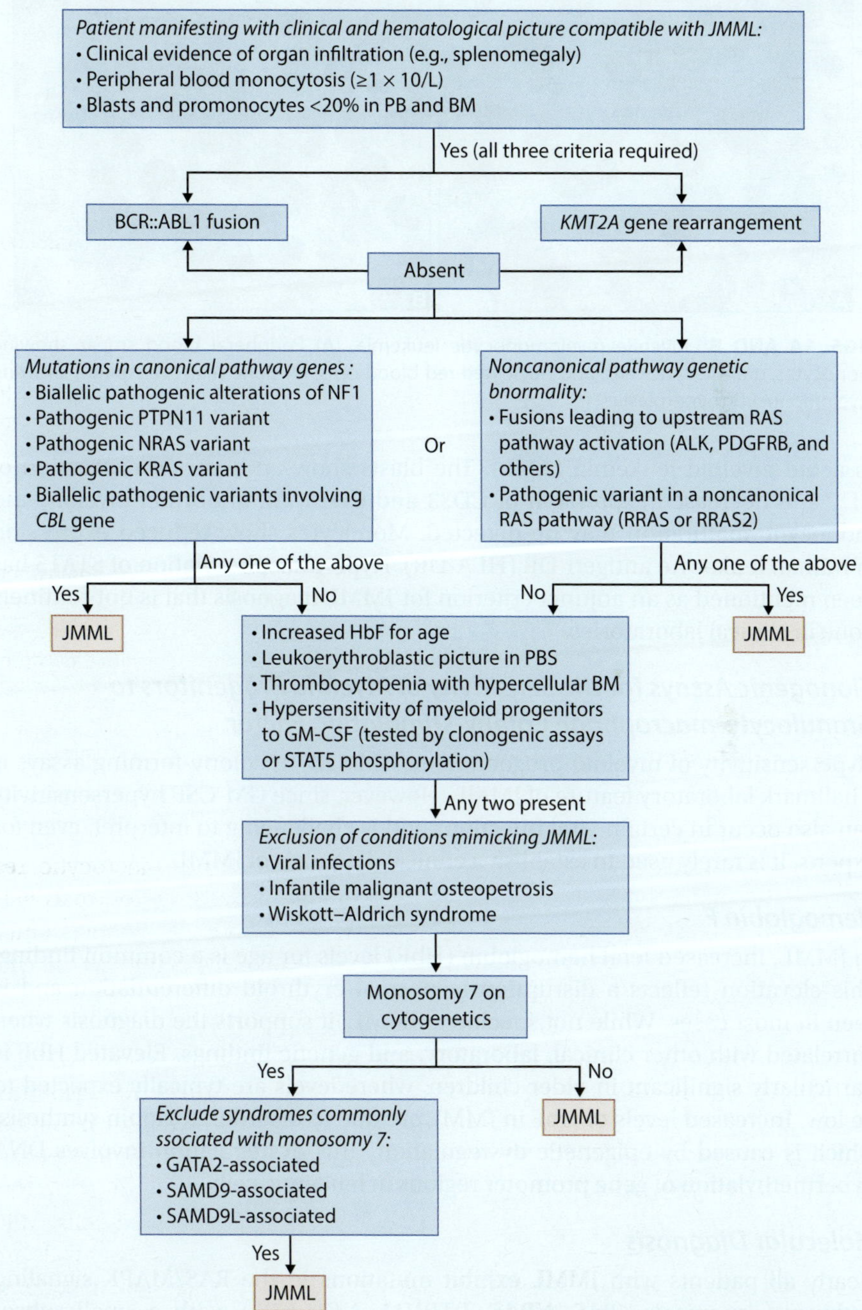

FLOWCHART 1: Workflow for the diagnosis of juvenile myelomonocytic leukemia (JMML).

(BM: bone marrow; GM-CSF: granulocyte-macrophage colony-stimulating factor; PB: peripheral blood)

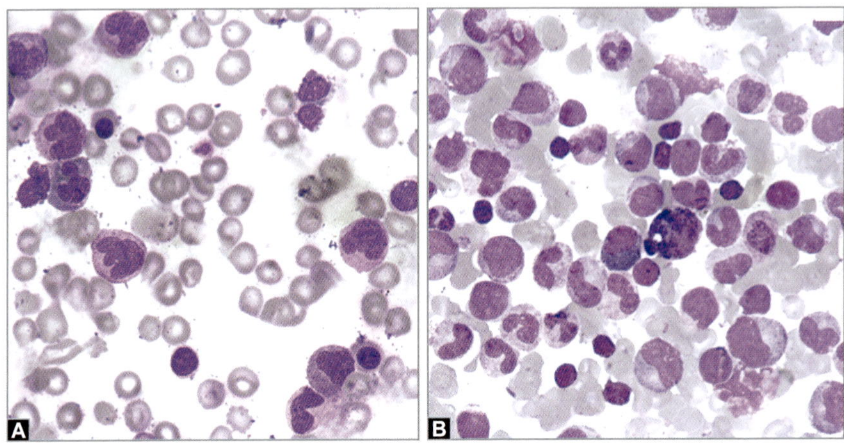

FIGS. 1A AND B: Juvenile myelomonocytic leukemia. (A) Peripheral blood smear showing monocytes, granulocytic cells, and nucleated red blood cells; (B) Bone marrow aspirate showing myelomonocytic hyperplasia.

to acute myeloid leukemia (AML). The blasts show an aberrant expression of CD7 and decreased expression of CD33 and CD13. An abnormal myeloid and monocytic maturation may be detected. Monocytes show reduced expression of human leukocyte antigen-DR (HLA-DR). Hyperphosphorylation of STAT5 has been mentioned as an adjunct criterion for JMML diagnosis that is not routinely done in clinical laboratories.

Clonogenic Assays for the Sensitivity of Myeloid Progenitors to Granulocyte-macrophage Colony-stimulating Factor

Hypersensitivity of myeloid progenitors to GM-CSF in colony-forming assays is a hallmark laboratory feature of JMML. However, since GM-CSF hypersensitivity can also occur in certain viral infections and is challenging to interpret, even for experts, it is rarely used to establish a clinical diagnosis of JMML.

Hemoglobin F

In JMML, increased fetal hemoglobin (HbF) levels for age is a common finding. This elevation reflects a disruption in normal erythroid differentiation and is seen in most cases. While not specific to JMML, it supports the diagnosis when correlated with other clinical, laboratory, and genetic findings. Elevated HbF is particularly significant in older children, where levels are typically expected to be low. Increased levels of HbF in JMML are due to disordered globin synthesis, which is caused by epigenetic dysregulation. This dysregulation involves DNA hypermethylation of gene promoter regions in leukemic cells.

Molecular Diagnosis

Nearly all patients with JMML exhibit mutations in the RAS/MAPK signaling pathway (*canonical: KRAS, NRAS, PTPN11, NF1, CBL*), with a small subset carrying translocations or mutations upstream of this pathway. Mutations in

JMML-associated genes can be either germline or somatic. It is recommended to screen all suspected JMML cases using next-generation sequencing (NGS) with both tumor (BM or blood) and nonhematopoietic tissues. Buccal swabs are typically used as the germline sample at diagnosis, despite potential contamination with leukemia cells, as germline mutations generally display a variant allele frequency near 50%. The gold standard for confirming germline mutations is sequencing skin fibroblasts, though this process can be challenging. If mosaicism is suspected, repeating Sanger sequencing on a buccal swab after treatment, when circulating monocytes are absent, may help clarify results.

Up to 30% of patients present with secondary mutations at diagnosis, often subclonal, with approximately 10% showing compound RAS pathway mutations (one clonal and one subclonal). Quantitative sequencing panels are recommended to distinguish driver mutations from secondary ones. For rare cases lacking RAS pathway mutations, RNA sequencing or targeted RNA sequencing is advised to identify targetable fusions. Routine cytogenetic testing, including fluorescence in situ hybridization (FISH) for monosomy 7 and trisomy 8, is performed at diagnosis. About 30% of JMML patients have cytogenetic abnormalities, with monosomy 7 being the most common (observed in 20% of patients) and frequently associated with *KRAS*-mutant JMML.

DIFFERENTIAL DIAGNOSES MIMICKING JUVENILE MYELOMONOCYTIC LEUKEMIA

Malignant Disorders Mimicking Juvenile Myelomonocytic Leukemia

The NGS now enables molecular confirmation of JMML in nearly all patients. However, when RAS pathway mutations are absent, it is essential to exclude other conditions that mimic JMML. The differential diagnosis includes rare myeloproliferative malignancies characterized by receptor tyrosine kinase translocations. Identifying these cases is essential, as patients may benefit from receptor tyrosine kinase-targeted inhibitors. Additionally, RAS pathway mutation-negative JMML with increased eosinophils should be distinguished from MPNs with eosinophilia caused by constitutively activated platelet-derived growth factor receptor α or β, or fibroblast growth factor receptor 1. Additionally, infants with *KMT2A*-rearranged acute leukemia may occasionally present with low blast counts, resembling JMML.

Nonmalignant Disorders Mimicking Juvenile Myelomonocytic Leukemia

It is also critical to differentiate JMML from non-neoplastic disorders such as viral infections, Wiskott–Aldrich syndrome, and infantile malignant osteopetrosis, to ensure accurate diagnosis and management. It is essential to exclude nonmalignant disorders that can mimic JMML in clinically suspected cases. Viral infections such as cytomegalovirus (CMV), Epstein–Barr virus (EBV), human herpesvirus-6 (HHV-6), and parvovirus B19 can present with overlapping features, including cytopenias, lymphadenopathy, and hepatosplenomegaly. Congenital intrauterine infections are also important differentials. Differentiating JMML from viral infections often necessitates the identification of chromosomal and/or genetic aberrations, with the detection of RAS pathway mutations serving as a key factor in establishing a definitive diagnosis of JMML.

NATURAL COURSE OF JUVENILE MYELOMONOCYTIC LEUKEMIA

The course of JMML is highly variable. While some patients may rarely experience a relatively indolent disease with prolonged survival, the majority progress to death due to infections, complications of BM failure, or transformation to AML. Favorable prognostic factors at diagnosis include a platelet count greater than 33×10^9/L and a lower HbF level (<15%). The median overall survival (OS) for patients with JMML who do not undergo hematopoietic stem cell transplantation (HSCT) is <1 year. Prognosis varies with age at diagnosis; infants may survive better than older children, who typically do not survive without HSCT.

Spontaneous resolution has been reported in infants with NS, *CBL* syndrome, and in some patients with specific somatic/germline *NRAS* mutations presenting in early infancy. In contrast, the presence of multiple mutations at diagnosis is associated with older age and confers an extremely poor prognosis.

Genotype-phenotype Associations in Juvenile Myelomonocytic Leukemia

Many patients with NS and germline *PTPN11* mutations who present with a JMML-like MPN in the neonatal period will spontaneously resolve within the first year of life, similar to the transient myeloproliferative disorder seen in Down syndrome (DS). However, unlike DS patients, those with NS/MPN do not appear to have an increased risk of developing myeloid malignancies later in childhood.

TREATMENT OF JUVENILE MYELOMONOCYTIC LEUKEMIA

Supportive Care

In patients with JMML, hydroxyurea at a dose of 25–30 mg/m^2/day, can be tried for a short duration. It is particularly beneficial when the total leukocyte count (TLC) exceeds 100×10^9/L, helping to prevent end-organ damage caused by leukocytosis. Supportive care measures include maintaining hemoglobin levels above 8 g/dL and platelet counts above 20×10^9/L. Additional interventions such as oxygen support, antibiotics, and adequate pain management should be provided when required. Nutritional rehabilitation, strict hygiene practices, and supportive care also play a crucial role in patient management.

Chemotherapy

JMML is a life-threatening condition if left untreated, with very few spontaneous remissions, observed in cases with specific genetic mutations. The median survival duration for patients with JMML who do not undergo HSCT is approximately 12 months. The role of traditional cytotoxic chemotherapy in JMML remains debatable. Oral 6-mercaptopurine alone or combined with subcutaneous cytarabine has provided symptomatic relief in some patients. In other instances, intensive multiagent chemotherapy (typically used for AML) has induced clinical remissions lasting >24 months. Other chemotherapy agents, such as fludarabine and high-dose cytarabine combinations, have been utilized to induce remission in cases of aggressive JMML or when massive pulmonary infiltration is present.

Azacitidine monotherapy (a DNA-hypomethylating agent) has been a promising treatment option for children with JMML, offering effective disease control with a favorable safety profile [azacitidine (AZA)-JMML-001 trial]. This agent works by reactivating tumor suppressor genes through DNA demethylation, offering a potential therapeutic option to manage the disease before proceeding with HSCT. Reducing the pre-HSCT allele burden to <1% predicts excellent disease-free survival (DFS) post-transplant. Additionally, response to therapy may serve as a marker of chemosensitivity, which could help tailor further treatment.

Hematopoietic Stem Cell Transplant

To date, allogeneic HSCT is the only curative treatment for JMML. Only a few patients with a favorable genotype and a clinically indolent phenotype could be candidates for a wait-and-watch strategy. Response to chemotherapy is generally transient in majority of cases. The common cause of death is lung infiltration with JMML and post-HSCT relapse is the most common cause of death.

The preferred donors for HSCT are matched sibling donors (MSD) and matched family donors (MFD). In conditions such as NF-1, it is important to assess the carrier/disease status of the donor and such donors should not be used. Matched unrelated donors (MUD) and umbilical cord blood (UCB) stem cells can also be used. UCB HSCT is an option if there is an urgent need for HSCT and the patient has a low body weight.

HSCT can cure approximately 50% of patients. Most conditioning regimens have now done away with total body irradiation (TBI) in the conditioning. Using myeloablative conditioning with cyclophosphamide, busulfan, and melphalan, a 5-year event-free survival (EFS) of 55% and 49% was shown by the European Society for Blood and Marrow Transplantation (EBMT) group for MUD and MFD, respectively. Females and older children did poorly and most deaths post-HSCT were due to relapses. Busulfan is the most commonly employed agent in association with other chemotherapeutic agents and the use of multiple alkylating agents with non-cell-cycle-specific action may help in cure as JMML is a stem cell disorder characterized by cell dormancy.

Cyclosporin A and methotrexate are the most commonly used agents for graft versus host disease (GVHD) prophylaxis. With unrelated donors antithymocyte globulin (ATG) has also been used. The intensity of GVHD prophylaxis should be tailored to the risk of the disease. High risk diseases such as NF-1, *NRAS* mutation, somatic *PTPN-11*, older age or high blast counts should receive less intense GVHD prophylaxis to allow for graft versus leukemia effect to occur. With grade I–II GVHD, better survival has been seen, possibly due to a graft versus leukemic (GVL) effect. By day 60–180 the GVHD prophylaxis should be stopped in absence of any GVHD.

Post-HSCT monitoring of disease status and chimerism should be done routinely. In the presence of a falling chimerism, rapid withdrawal of the immunosuppression can be attempted along with donor lymphocyte infusions (DLI). Persistent disease and relapse even after HSCT can occur in 26–58% of patients. A second allogeneic HSCT from a different donor or the same donor using a less aggressive GVHD prophylaxis can be attempted in case of an overt relapse. A second transplant can salvage 33% of the patients.

Novel and Targeted Approaches to the Treatment of Juvenile Myelomonocytic Leukemia

Although HSCT cures about 50% of JMML patients, the limited cure rate combined with significant morbidities and late effects in this population has prompted the search for more effective and less toxic treatment options. They have been summarized in **Table 1**.

TABLE 1: Summary of novel and targeted approaches to the treatment of juvenile myelomonocytic leukemia (JMML).

Approach	Mechanism
GM-CSF analogs with a point mutation at the receptor-binding site	Inhibit JMML cell growth in mice model by causing a dose and time-dependent apoptosis
Zoledronic acid	Post-translational modifications of RAS protein through inhibition of the enzyme farnesyltransferase
Trametinib (MEK-inhibitor)	MEK inhibition has been proven to restore normal hematopoiesis in *NF-1* and *KRAS* mutant mice. Clinical trials are underway
Rapamycin (mTOR inhibitor)	Rapamycin resulted in the mitigation of the JMML phenotype in *PTPN11* mutated mice and corrected the hypersensitivity to GM-CSF of bone marrow (BM) cells in culture
Dasatinib/Ruxolitinib	Both have been known to stabilize the disease in a few of the patients in which they have been tried. Combined inhibition of the pathways is more effective in preclinical models
SH2-containing inositol 5-phosphatase 1 (SHIP-1)	Negatively regulates the GM-CSF signaling. Retroviral-mediated transduction of *SHIP-1* into $CD34^+$ cells from JMML patients with *KRAS* or *PTPN11* mutations led to a reduction in myeloid proliferation

(GM-CSF: granulocyte-monocyte colony stimulating factors; mTOR: mammalian target of rapamycin; MEK: mitogen-activated protein kinase)

Take Home Points

- JMML presents with a wide range of clinical manifestations and poor outcomes. In some cases, a "watch and wait" approach may be appropriate, especially in children with specific genetic mutations or conditions like NS, where spontaneous remission has been observed. However, for others, the prognosis remains poor, even with advanced therapeutic interventions, underscoring the aggressive nature of the disease and the importance of early diagnosis and timely treatment.
- Currently, allogeneic HSCT remains the only potentially curative therapy for JMML, with cure rates of approximately 50%. This underscores the critical role of HSCT in the management of JMML and should be done at the earliest, particularly for patients with high-risk genetic mutations or disease progression.
- Chemotherapeutic agents are commonly used as a bridge to HSCT in JMML, helping to induce remission and stabilize the disease before the transplant procedure.
- 5-azacytidine, which has been reported to induce remission in some children with JMML. This agent works by reactivating tumor suppressor genes through DNA demethylation.

SUGGESTED READINGS

1. Lasho T, Patnaik MM. Juvenile myelomonocytic leukemia: A bona fide RASopathy syndrome. Best Pract Res Clin Haematol. 2020;33(2):101171.
2. Swerdlow SH, Campo E, Harris NL, Jaffe ES, Pileri SA, Stein H, et al. WHO Classification of Tumours of Haematopoietic and Lymphoid Tissues. [Online] Available from https://publications.iarc.fr/Book-And-Report-Series/Who-Classification-Of-Tumours/WHO-Classification-Of-Tumours-Of-Haematopoietic-And-Lymphoid-Tissues-2017 [Last accessed May, 2025].
3. Board WC of TE. Haematolymphoid Tumours. [Online] Available from https://publications.iarc.fr/Book-And-Report-Series/Who-Classification-Of-Tumours/Haematolymphoid-Tumours-2024 [Last accessed May, 2025].
4. Khoury JD, Solary E, Abla O, Akkari Y, Alaggio R, Apperley JF, et al. The 5th edition of the World Health Organization Classification of Haematolymphoid Tumours: Myeloid and Histiocytic/Dendritic Neoplasms. Leukemia. 2022;36(7):1703-19.
5. Fiñana C, Gómez-Molina N, Alonso-Moreno S, Belver L. Genomic and epigenomic landscape of juvenile myelomonocytic leukemia. Cancers. 2022;14(5):1335.
6. Gupta AK, Meena JP, Chopra A, Tanwar P, Seth R. Juvenile myelomonocytic leukemia-A comprehensive review and recent advances in management. Am J Blood Res. 2021;11(1): 1-21.
7. Niemeyer CM, Flotho C. Juvenile myelomonocytic leukemia: who's the driver at the wheel? Blood. 2019;133(10):1060-70.
8. Wintering A, Dvorak CC, Stieglitz E, Loh ML. Juvenile myelomonocytic leukemia in the molecular era: a clinician's guide to diagnosis, risk stratification, and treatment. Blood Adv. 2021;5(22):4783-93.
9. Fluhr S, Krombholz CF, Meier A, Epting T, Mücke O, Plass C, et al. Epigenetic dysregulation of the erythropoietic transcription factor KLF1 and the β-like globin locus in juvenile myelomonocytic leukemia. Epigenetics. 2017;12(8):715-23.
10. Li W. The 5th Edition of the World Health Organization Classification of Hematolymphoid Tumors In: Li W (Ed). Leukemia. Brisbane (AU): Exon Publications; 2022.

11. Blaney SM, Helman LJ, Adamson PC. Pizzo and Poplack's Pediatric Oncology, 8th edition. Philadelphia: Wolters Kluwer; 2020.
12. Wajid MA, Gupta AK, Das G, Sahoo D, Meena JP, Seth R. Outcomes of juvenile myelomonocytic leukemia patients after sequential therapy with cytarabine and 6-mercaptopurine. Pediatr Hematol Oncol. 2020;37(7):573-81.
13. Niemeyer CM, Flotho C, Lipka DB, Starý J, Rössig C, Baruchel A, et al. Response to upfront azacitidine in juvenile myelomonocytic leukemia in the AZA-JMML-001 trial. Blood Adv. 2021;5(14):2901-28.
14. Chan RJ, Cooper T, Kratz CP, Weiss B, Loh ML. Juvenile myelomonocytic leukemia: a report from the 2nd International JMML Symposium. Leuk Res. 2009;33(3):355-62.
15. Smith FO, King R, Nelson G, Wagner JE, Robertson KA, Sanders JE, et al.; National Marrow Donor Program. Unrelated donor bone marrow transplantation for children with juvenile myelomonocytic leukaemia. Br J Haematol. 2002;116(3):716-24.
16. Locatelli F, Algeri M, Merli P, Strocchio L. Novel approaches to diagnosis and treatment of Juvenile Myelomonocytic Leukemia. Expert Rev Hematol. 2018;11(2):129-43.
17. Locatelli F, Niemeyer CM. How I treat juvenile myelomonocytic leukemia. Blood. 2015;125(7):1083-90.
18. Patel SA, Coulter DW, Grovas AC, Gordon BG, Harper JL, Warkentin PI, et al. Cytosine arabinoside and mitoxantrone followed by second allogeneic transplant for the treatment of children with refractory juvenile myelomonocytic leukemia. J Pediatr Hematol Oncol. 2014;36(6):491-4.
19. Bernard F, Thomas C, Emile JF, Hercus T, Cassinat B, Chomienne C, et al. Transient hematologic and clinical effect of E21R in a child with end-stage juvenile myelomonocytic leukemia. Blood. 2002;99(7):2615-26.
20. Ohtsuka Y, Manabe A, Kawasaki H, Hasegawa D, Zaike Y, Watanabe S, et al. RAS-blocking bisphosphonate zoledronic acid inhibits the abnormal proliferation and differentiation of juvenile myelomonocytic leukemia cells in vitro. Blood. 2005;106(9):3134-41.
21. Liu W, Yu W-M, Zhang J, Chan RJ, Loh ML, Zhang Z, et al. Inhibition of the Gab2/PI3K/mTOR signaling ameliorates myeloid malignancy caused by Ptpn11 (Shp2) gain-of-function mutations. Leukemia. 2017;31(6):1415-22.
22. Loh ML, Tasian SK, Rabin KR, Brown P, Magoon D, Reid JM, et al. A phase 1 dosing study of ruxolitinib in children with relapsed or refractory solid tumors, leukemias, or myeloproliferative neoplasms: A Children's Oncology Group phase 1 consortium study (ADVL1011). Pediatr Blood Cancer. 2015;62(10):1717-24.
23. Koike K, Matsuda K. Recent advances in the pathogenesis and management of juvenile myelomonocytic leukaemia. Br J Haematol. 2008;141(5):567-75.

CHAPTER 28

Case-based Approach to Eosinophilia

Sreejesh Sreedharanunni, Praveen Sharma

ABSTRACT

This chapter outlines a comprehensive approach to hypereosinophilic syndrome (HES), emphasizing systematic evaluation. Initial workup comprises careful exclusion of secondary/reactive causes based on clinical history, physical examination, and serological and other basic investigations. Any suspicion of clonal disorder based on preliminary evaluation or absence of significant findings in the initial screening or imminent organ failure necessitates detailed evaluation by bone marrow examination, cytogenetics, flow cytometry, and molecular tests. We highlight the morphological findings that need to be stressed while performing bone marrow or peripheral blood film examination, the purpose of immunohistochemistry and flow cytometry, the pitfalls in depending purely on karyotyping, the panel to be used in fluorescence in situ hybridization (FISH) testing, and the role of molecular testing including next-generation sequencing (NGS). We highlight the newer molecular markers described, such as *JAK2*, *FLT3*, and *ETV6* rearrangements, and *STAT5b* N642H mutation. Further, we explain how to reach a diagnosis of chronic eosinophilic leukemia (CEL) or idiopathic HES. Finally, a brief overview of advances in targeted therapies is given. The paper emphasizes that genetic profiling remains essential for selecting optimal therapy, particularly with emerging targeted treatments.

INTRODUCTION

Peripheral blood and tissue eosinophilia represent a diverse spectrum of hematological and non-hematological conditions. In healthy individuals, eosinophils constitute 1–5% of peripheral blood leukocytes, with an absolute eosinophil count (AEC) normally $<0.5 \times 10^9$/L. The bone marrow typically maintains eosinophils between 1 and 6% of nucleated cells.

Eosinophilia, defined as an AEC exceeding 0.5×10^9/L, can be categorized based on severity into mild ($0.5–1.5 \times 10^9$/L), moderate ($1.5–5.0 \times 10^9$/L), and severe ($>5.0 \times 10^9$/L) forms. The temporal pattern of eosinophilia also carries clinical significance, with cases classified as transient, episodic, or persistent. Persistent eosinophilia, documented on at least two occasions separated by a minimum of 4 weeks, carries particular importance due to the increased risk of end-organ damage from prolonged exposure to eosinophil-derived mediators.

Mild eosinophilia affects approximately 10% of the general population, most commonly due to allergic conditions, medication effects, or parasitic infections. When moderate-to-severe eosinophilia persists ($>1.5 \times 10^9$/L) or significant tissue eosinophilia is present, the condition is termed hypereosinophilia (HE). The progression from HE to hypereosinophilic syndrome (HES) occurs when organ dysfunction develops, manifesting as cardiac failure, pulmonary impairment, neurological deficits, or gastrointestinal dysfunction.

The complexity and diversity of eosinophilic disorders can be best understood through clinical cases that illustrate various presentations and diagnostic challenges. Let us begin with a series of illustrative cases, highlighting different aspects of this sometimes difficult-to-diagnose disorder.

CLINICAL VIGNETTES

Case 1: A 16-year-old male presented with a persistent dry cough and moderate eosinophilia for 1 month. He was otherwise healthy with no significant past medical history. The physical examination was unremarkable, and there was no lymphadenopathy or organomegaly. His hemogram showed hemoglobin 13.8 g/dL, total leukocyte count 14.2×10^9/L with AEC of 3.8×10^9/L (27%), and platelet count 285×10^9/L. Peripheral blood film examination showed mature eosinophils without any dysplastic features and no microfilariae. Multiple stool examinations were negative for ova and parasites. Further workup revealed elevated serum immunoglobulin E (IgE) (600 IU/mL; normal <100 IU/mL), but aspergillus-specific IgE was normal. Autoimmune workup, including antinuclear antibody (ANA) and antineutrophil cytoplasmic antibody (ANCA), was negative. A trial of albendazole did not result in improvement. He was empirically treated with diethylcarbamazine for 14 days. His symptoms resolved completely with normalization of eosinophil count (AEC 0.4×10^9/L) by day 14 of therapy, suggesting a diagnosis of tropical pulmonary eosinophilia. This case demonstrates the importance of considering parasitic infections, particularly in endemic regions, even when initial screening tests are negative.

Case 2: A 43-year-old male presented with a 2-year history of easy fatiguability, anemia, and recent onset of pruritis with shortness of breath for 4 months. On examination, he had pallor and moderate splenomegaly. The hemogram showed hemoglobin of 7.2 g/dL with marked leukocytosis (TLC 43.2×10^9/L) and significant eosinophilia (AEC 25.8×10^9/L). The patient also had a history of extrapulmonary tuberculosis, and stool examination revealed roundworm infestation. The eosinophilia did not respond to a course of albendazole and diethylcarbamazine. Bone marrow examination revealed a hypercellular marrow with significant eosinophilia and grade 1+ reticulin fibrosis. Molecular studies using fluorescence in situ hybridization (FISH) analysis detected the *FIP1L1::PDGFRA* rearrangement **(Fig. 1A)**, confirming the diagnosis of myeloid/

lymphoid neoplasm with eosinophilia and *PDGFRA* rearrangement (MLN-TK fusions with *PDGFRA*-r). The patient responded very well to 100 mg of imatinib therapy. However, he left treatment on his own accord. In the next few weeks, his leukocyte count increased with recurrent eosinophilia, suggesting disease relapse. This case illustrates the importance of molecular testing in eosinophilia, the effectiveness of targeted therapy, and the challenges of ensuring treatment compliance.

Case 3: A 55-year-old gentleman presented with acute onset right upper limb weakness upon waking one morning. His condition rapidly progressed to include right-sided hemiparesis and altered sensorium. Initial workup revealed marked eosinophilia with an AEC of 13.1 × 10^9/L. Physical examination showed moderate hepatosplenomegaly but no lymphadenopathy. Imaging revealed multiple ill-defined subcapsular hypodense lesions in the spleen, bronchiectasis with bronchial wall thickening and nodules in the right upper lobe, and most significantly, multiple discrete bilateral T2 FLAIR DWI restricting hyperintensities in watershed regions with bilateral cerebellar and cerebral hemisphere white matter changes. Given the severity of presentation with eosinophilia and thrombosis, high-dose steroids were initiated immediately after collecting samples for a comprehensive workup, including autoimmune markers, biochemistry, parasitic serology, bone marrow examination, cytogenetics, flow cytometry, and molecular studies. Despite steroid therapy, the patient showed no improvement. Empiric imatinib was then initiated, considering the possibility of a tyrosine kinase-driven process, but again without response. The bone marrow examination revealed hypercellularity with eosinophilia but notably showed no excess blasts, evidence of mastocytosis, or fibrosis. Initial FISH studies were negative for commonly tested rearrangements, including *FIP1L1::PDGFRA, PDGFRB, FGFR1,* and *JAK2*. *ETV6* rearrangement was present **(Fig. 1B)**; however, the partner was not identified. RNA sequencing identified this as an *ETV6::FLT3*

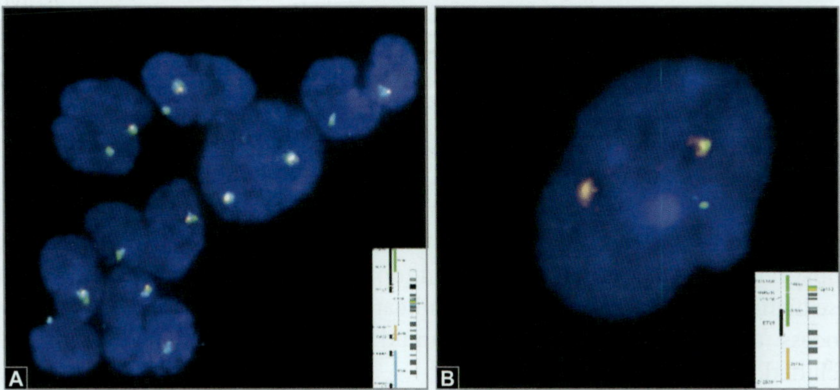

FIGS. 1A AND B: (A) Fluorescence in situ hybridization (FISH) using a tricolor probe (*PDGFRA*—aqua; *CHIC2*—orange; and *FIP1L1*—green) showing deletion of one copy of *CHIC2* resulting in *PDGFRA::F1P1L1* rearrangement; (B) FISH using a dual-color break-apart probe showing rearrangement of the *ETV6* gene.

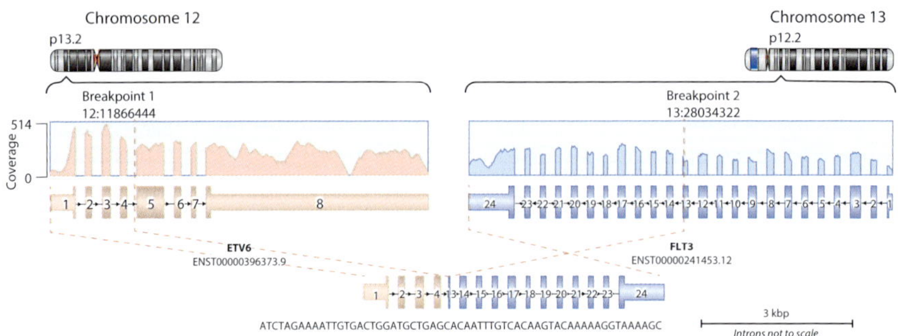

FIG. 2: Visualization generated by Arriba bioinformatics tool showing *ETV6::FLT3* gene rearrangement by RNA sequencing in a case of hypereosinophilic syndrome (HES).

rearrangement **(Figs. 1B and 2)**, a rare fusion associated with aggressive disease. The patient's clinical course was refractory to multiple therapeutic interventions. He developed numerous complications, including myocardial infarction and multiple thrombotic events. This case demonstrates the importance of comprehensive molecular testing in HE with thrombosis, as rare molecular alterations may drive particularly aggressive disease phenotypes that prove resistant to conventional therapies. Targeted therapy with *FLT3* inhibitors may aid these patients in achieving clinical response and improved outcomes.

Case 4: A 26-year-old male presented with neck swelling and progressive weakness. Initial workup revealed severe anemia (hemoglobin 3.2 g/dL) with marked eosinophilic leukocytosis (AEC 134.2 × 10^9/L). Peripheral blood smear showed prominent red cell agglutination with microspherocytes. The reticulocyte percentage was surprisingly low despite severe anemia. The peripheral blood film also showed morphological changes in eosinophils, including dysplastic forms with mono- and hyperlobation and cytoplasmic vacuoles. Bone marrow examination revealed marked erythroblastopenia (1% erythroid precursors) and significant eosinophilia (48% eosinophils and precursors). His serum IgE was elevated, while autoimmune markers (ANA, ANCA) and parasitic serology were negative. Direct Coombs test was positive. Flow cytometry revealed a small but significant population (0.4%) of abnormal clonal T cells with a distinctive immunophenotype (CD3-dim/neg, CD4-positive) **(Figs. 3A and B)**. Based on these findings, a lymphocytic variant of HES (L-HES) was diagnosed. The patient showed a good initial response to corticosteroid therapy. However, 6 months later, the patient presented with significant lymphadenopathy. A lymph node biopsy revealed a diagnosis of angioimmunoblastic T-cell lymphoma (AITL). This case highlights that eosinophilia may indicate an underlying lymphoproliferative process, and a diagnosis of L-HES should not be offered till lymphomas are excluded.

Case 5: A 10-year-old male presented with abdominal pain and a history of exposure to pet pigeons at home. Initial workup revealed mild anemia and moderate eosinophilia. Physical examination showed mild splenomegaly and

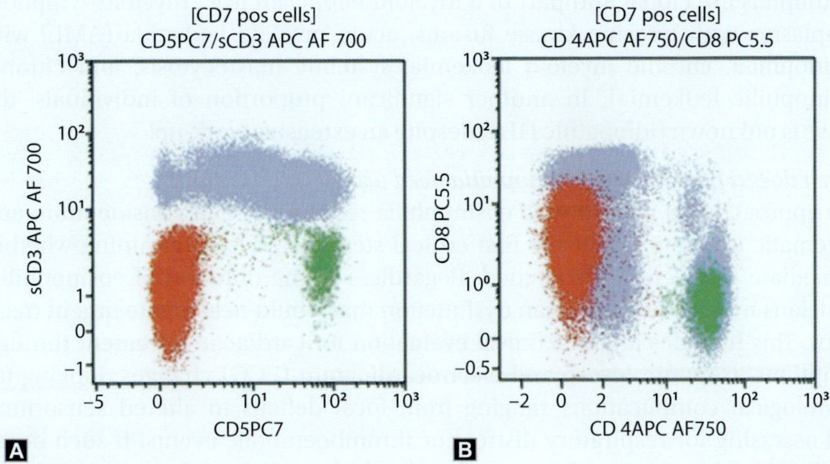

FIGS. 3A AND B: Flow cytometry shows an abnormal clone of T cells (target population—green) with CD7posCD5posCD4posCD3neg immunophenotype.

abdominal tenderness. His hemogram demonstrated mild anemia with moderate eosinophilia. Comprehensive infectious disease workup was negative, including stool examination for ova and parasites. Autoimmune markers (ANA and ANCA) were negative, and there was no response to empirical antihelminthic therapy. Bone marrow examination showed increased eosinophils and precursors. FISH was negative for all tyrosine kinase rearrangements. Flow cytometry showed no evidence of T-cell clones. Next-generation sequencing was negative for myeloid mutations. A bladder biopsy, performed due to urinary symptoms, revealed eosinophilic cystitis. The patient showed excellent response to corticosteroid therapy but experienced disease flares whenever steroids were tapered or stopped. After 2 years of recurring symptoms and extensive negative workup for secondary causes, clonal disorders, and lymphocytic variant, a diagnosis of idiopathic HES (iHES) was established. The patient is currently being treated with mepolizumab as a steroid-sparing agent. This case illustrates the importance of systematic work-up and the complexities of identifying a cause in some cases.

APPROACH TO EOSINOPHILIA

What causes eosinophilia?

Eosinophilia can result from a wide range of causes. In the majority of cases, eosinophilia is secondary to another disorder ranging from infections (e.g., fungal infections such as aspergillus), infestations (e.g., helminths), drugs [e.g., drug rash with eosinophilia and systemic symptoms (DRESS) associated with phenytoin], allergies (e.g., bronchial asthma), autoimmune [e.g., eosinophilic granulomatosis with polyangiitis (EGPA)], connective tissue disorders (e.g., rheumatoid arthritis), hematological (e.g., T-cell non-Hodgkin lymphoma) or solid malignancies (e.g., paraneoplastic eosinophilia) among many others. In a minor proportion, eosinophils are clonal and part of a myeloid neoplasm [e.g., myeloid/lymphoid neoplasms with tyrosine kinase fusions, acute myeloid leukemia (AML) with eosinophilia, chronic myeloid leukemia, systemic mastocytosis, and chronic eosinophilic leukemia]. In another significant proportion of individuals, the cause is unknown (idiopathic HES) despite an extensive work-up.

When does a patient with eosinophilia need urgent intervention?

The approach to a patient with eosinophilia requires careful consideration and systematic evaluation, but the first critical step is always determining whether immediate intervention is needed. Regardless of the duration of eosinophilia, clinicians must assess for organ dysfunction that would necessitate urgent treatment. This includes a good clinical evaluation for cardiac involvement through symptoms, troponin levels, and electrocardiogram (ECG) changes; looking for neurological complications ranging from focal deficits to altered sensorium; and assessing for respiratory distress or thromboembolic events. If such organ involvement is present, while samples should be collected for comprehensive testing, treatment (typically with high-dose corticosteroids) should be started on time while awaiting results.

What essential aspects should be included in the patient's medical history?

A comprehensive assessment of the patient's current and past medical history is crucial, as meticulous inquiry can often uncover the underlying cause of symptoms. History should focus on allergic conditions, familial predispositions, and socioeconomic factors that may influence exposure to parasites or infectious agents. A detailed environmental history is essential, covering aspects such as recent travel to tropical or endemic regions, pet ownership, and dietary habits, especially the consumption of undercooked meat or exotic foods. Medication history, including prescription drugs, traditional medicines, and dietary supplements, should be thoroughly reviewed. In children and occasionally in adults, accidental exposure to pet or insect excreta should be considered. Recurrent infections, particularly in pediatric patients, may indicate an underlying immunodeficiency, while rheumatological symptoms could point toward connective tissue diseases as a potential cause.

What are the critical physical examination findings to consider when evaluating eosinophilia?

Physical examination is pivotal in complementing medical history by providing critical diagnostic insights. Pallor may indicate an underlying helminthic infection, especially in children with eosinophilia. Organomegaly is particularly informative: Moderate-to-massive splenomegaly often suggests a clonal process or myeloproliferative neoplasm (MPN), whereas significant lymphadenopathy may point to a lymphoproliferative disorder or leukemia. Skin findings warrant careful attention—eczematous changes may reflect an allergic etiology, while plaques or nodules could signify lymphoma. Pulmonary findings, such as wheezing or crepitations, might suggest conditions such as allergic bronchopulmonary aspergillosis or tropical pulmonary eosinophilia, though they can also signal end-organ damage directly caused by eosinophilia.

What initial laboratory investigations are crucial for the evaluation of eosinophilia?

Laboratory evaluation begins with a detailed examination of the peripheral blood film, often providing critical early diagnostic insights. While no single morphological feature definitively differentiates clonal from reactive eosinophilia, specific findings such as monolobated or hypersegmented forms, vacuolization, and variations in granulation should be carefully noted. The presence of blasts, significant basophilia, erythrocytosis, granulocytic dysplasia, or a leucoerythroblastic picture warrants prompt investigation for an underlying hematological malignancy. The blood film should also be assessed for evidence of parasites, particularly microfilariae.

A basic laboratory workup includes a complete blood count with differential, renal, and liver function tests, inflammatory markers, and lactate dehydrogenase (LDH) levels. Elevated LDH may suggest a lymphoproliferative disorder, while increased vitamin B12 levels can indicate a myeloproliferative condition. Serum IgE levels, although not diagnostic in isolation, provide valuable context, with marked elevations suggesting allergic or parasitic etiologies. Further targeted investigations should be guided by clinical suspicion, such as stool analysis for ova and parasites, serological testing for specific infections, and autoimmune markers where relevant. ANA and ANCA should be performed in all cases to exclude autoimmune disorders such as EGPA, though ANCA-negative EGPA exists and can cause eosinophil-mediated organ damage.

What is the role of imaging?

Imaging studies generally begin with chest radiography in all cases, followed by additional targeted imaging based on symptoms and physical findings. Cardiac imaging becomes essential when heart involvement is suspected, while contrast-enhanced chest CT (CECT) or high-resolution CT (HRCT) is used to assess respiratory involvement. Imaging can also reveal organ damage, extramedullary disease, and underlying conditions such as lymphoma, solid tumors, or parasitic infections such as cysticercosis or hydatid.

When is a bone marrow examination necessary, and what ancillary tests should it include?

The decision to perform a bone marrow examination is guided by clinical history and other laboratory findings. It becomes necessary when initial investigations fail to identify an obvious cause, when blood film results suggest a possible hematologic disorder, or when eosinophilia persists without a clear explanation. Bone marrow examination is also advised in all patients with significant organomegaly, extramedullary disease, or cytopenias. A comprehensive bone marrow evaluation is required, which includes a detailed morphological examination of both aspirate and biopsy. Key aspects to assess include overall cellularity, blast percentage, and the presence of mastocytosis or fibrosis **(Figs. 4A to E)**. If mastocytosis is present, evaluating the pattern of infiltration—both in terms of quantity (with >25% suggesting systemic mastocytosis) and distribution (loose versus tight clusters)—provides crucial diagnostic insight. Clonal eosinophilia should be highly suspected in cases with myelodysplasia, excess or blasts, fibrosis, or mastocytosis. Morphological findings should be complemented by flow cytometry, cytogenetic analysis, and molecular testing for a thorough assessment.

What is the role of flow cytometry and immunohistochemistry in evaluating eosinophilia?

While flow cytometry cannot differentiate clonal from reactive eosinophils, it is crucial for identifying abnormal T-cell populations, particularly the CD3-negative and CD4-positive cells associated with L-HES. High-sensitivity flow cytometry can also assist in detecting occult T-cell lymphomas linked to eosinophilia. Additionally, it is essential for diagnosing occult B-cell acute lymphoblastic leukemia (B-ALL) associated with eosinophilia, as B-ALL with *IGH::IL3* translocations may present with low blast counts. In cases of eosinophilia with mastocytosis, flow cytometry helps identify the clonal nature of mast cells through the expression of CD2, CD25, and CD30. Immunohistochemistry of the bone marrow biopsy adds vital information about mast cell patterns and lymphoid infiltrates.

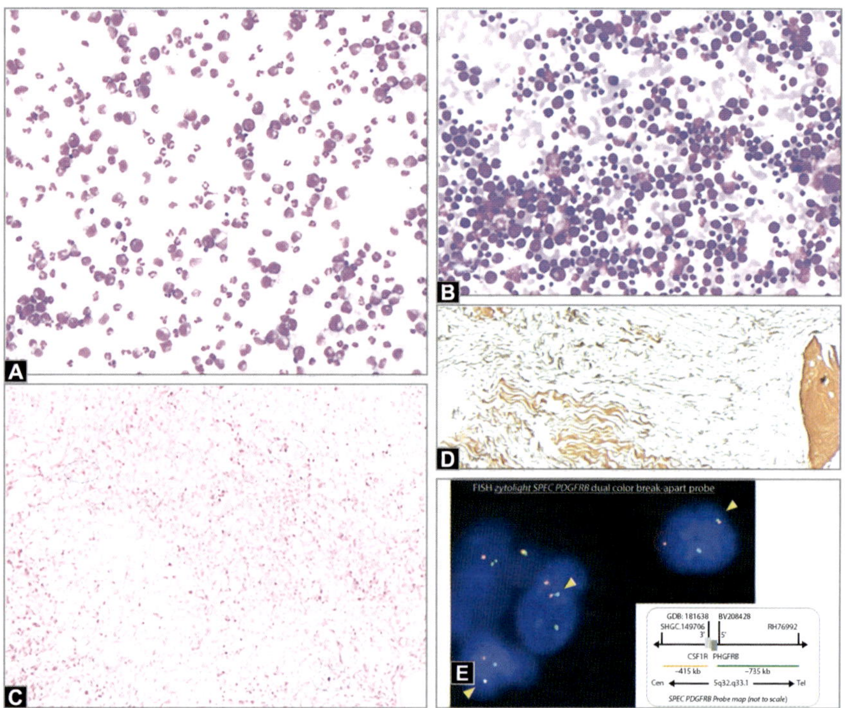

FIGS. 4A TO E: (A) Peripheral blood showing increased leukocyte count, eosinophilia, and leucoerythroblastic picture (May–Grünwald Giemsa), 400×; (B and C). Hypercellular bone marrow aspirate (May-Grünwald Giemsa stain, 400×) and biopsy (hematoxylin and eosin, 400×) with increased eosinophils and its precursors; (D) Reticulin stain demonstrating grade 3 fibrosis (reticulin stain, 400×); (E) FISH showing *PDGFRB* rearrangement on a break-apart probe (DAPI, 600×).

What is the role of cytogenetic testing in eosinophilia?

Cytogenetic studies, particularly FISH, are essential for detecting chromosomal rearrangements involving *PDGFRA, PDGFRB, FGFR1*, and other tyrosine kinase genes. Abnormalities in genes such as *FLT3, JAK2, ETV6*, and others have also been associated with eosinophilia. These genetic evaluations are crucial as they directly influence treatment decisions and help predict prognosis in patients with eosinophilia.

Does a normal karyotype exclude eosinophilia associated with cytogenetic abnormalities?

More than 50% of these genetic abnormalities are cryptic and cannot be detected by conventional karyotyping. As such, FISH or RNA sequencing (RNA-seq) is mandatory for identifying these hidden rearrangements. For example, using *FIP1L1/CHIC2/PDGFRA* tri-color probes to detect the *CHIC2* deletion is crucial in cases of eosinophilia associated with *FIP1L1::PDGFRA*. Break-apart probes in FISH testing have become the standard of care for detecting genetic abnormalities that would otherwise go unnoticed by traditional cytogenetic methods.

Does a lower AEC of <1,500/μL preclude the need for cytogenetic and molecular testing?

The presence of a lower AEC (<1,500/μL) does not prevent the need for comprehensive cytogenetic and molecular evaluation. Genetic abnormalities associated with eosinophilia can manifest with varying levels of eosinophil counts. These abnormalities may be related to pure eosinophilia, or they might be found in conjunction with other hematologic conditions such as lymphoma, acute lymphoblastic leukemia (ALL), chronic myelomonocytic leukemia (CMML), MPNs, or mixed MPN/MDS (myelodysplastic syndrome). Therefore, ideally, genetic testing should be considered in all cases of eosinophilia.

What is the role of next-generation sequencing in evaluating eosinophilia?

Next-generation sequencing has significantly advanced our understanding of eosinophilia by identifying previously unknown genetic alterations, particularly in cases where the cause seemed idiopathic. This technology allows for a more detailed assessment of genetic mutations and has helped refine diagnoses, especially in complex or unclear cases. However, the interpretation of molecular findings requires careful contextual analysis, including considering factors such as variant allele frequency and the potential for age-related clonal hematopoiesis of indeterminate potential (CHIP). The documentation of a clonal cytogenetic or molecular abnormality is essential for diagnosing chronic eosinophilic leukemia. These abnormalities include mutations in *ASXL1, TET2, EZH2, DNMT3A, SRSF2, TP53, SETBP1* and various genes of JAK/STAT pathway such as *JAK1, JAK2, STAT5A*, and *STAT5B*. One of the mutations, i.e., STAT5B N642H, has been recurrently found in cases of myeloid neoplasms associated with eosinophilia, and these cases can have heterogeneous presentation varying from MDS/MPN, MPN, or CML-like pictures.

When to call a case idiopathic HES?

Despite several advances, a definitive cause has not been identified in many HES cases. In these cases, eosinophilia remains persistent for >6 months or at least 4 months in the presence of organ dysfunction. Common secondary causes, including infections, drugs, malignancies, and autoimmune disorders, are excluded. There is no evidence of L-HES or clonal cytogenetic/molecular abnormalities, and bone marrow is morphologically normal except for eosinophil hyperplasia. These cases often show fluctuating clinical course, usually respond to steroids, and become steroid dependent, creating significant issues for the patient and treating clinician. The approach to diagnosis is summarized in **Flowchart 1**.

TREATMENT OF EOSINOPHILIA

The treatment approach varies significantly based on the underlying cause and complications. Emergency situations require immediate intervention with high-dose steroids, cytoreductive agents such as hydroxyurea, and appropriate organ support. Once a specific diagnosis is established, targeted therapy can be initiated. While some conditions have readily available targeted treatments, others have limited therapeutic options due to numerous factors, including clinical trial restrictions, drug availability, prohibitive costs, or limited clinical experience. These treatments range from antiparasitic agents for helminthic infections to tyrosine kinase inhibitors (particularly imatinib at specific doses for *PDGFRA*/*PDGFRB* rearrangements) and other-directed therapies. In refractory cases, particularly those with *FGFR1* rearrangements or certain complex molecular profiles, hematopoietic stem cell transplantation might need consideration.

For specific molecular abnormalities, targeted therapies have shown significant efficacy. *PDGFRA* and *PDGFRB* rearrangements typically respond well to imatinib. In cases of *PDGFRA* with resistance mutations such as T674I, ponatinib is preferred, while those with D842V mutations respond better to avapritinib. *FGFR1*-rearranged cases may benefit from pemigatinib or futibatinib, typically followed by bone marrow transplantation. *PCM1::JAK2* cases often require ruxolitinib followed by bone marrow transplant (BMT). For *ETV6::FLT3* rearrangements, multiple options exist, including sorafenib, sunitinib, midostaurin, and gilteritinib. *ETV6::ABL1* cases usually show resistance to imatinib and may require nilotinib or ponatinib.

CEL treatment options include steroids, hydroxyurea, pegylated interferon alpha (PEG-IFN alpha), imatinib, and potentially bone marrow transplantation. L-HES typically responds to steroids and steroid-sparing agents. For idiopathic HES, the treatment paradigm includes steroids as initial therapy, other immunomodulators and cyclophosphamide. Several biological agents are available as additional options, including mepolizumab, benralizumab, depemokimab, and reslizumab. Other therapeutic options include dexpramipexole and lirentelimab. The choice of therapy should be individualized based on disease severity, organ involvement, and treatment availability.

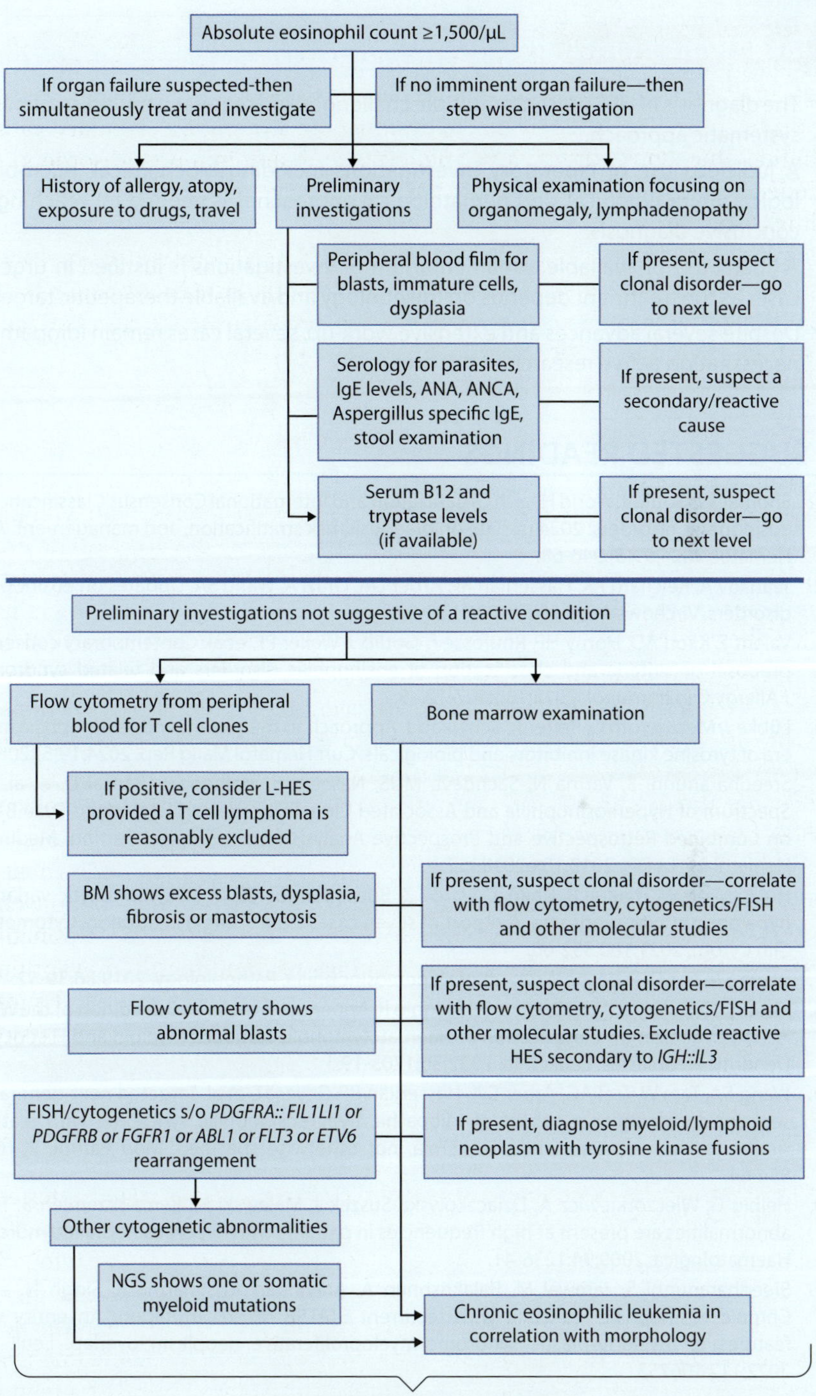

FLOWCHART 1: Algorithm summarizing the approach to a case of hypereosinophilia.

(ANA: antinuclear antibody; ANCA: antineutrophil cytoplasmic antibody; HES: hypereosinophilic syndrome; IgE: immunoglobulin E)

Take Home Points

- The diagnosis of HES presents multiple challenges and requires a multidisciplinary, systematic approach.
- A judicious use of laboratory investigations including biochemical, microbiological, immunological, and hematological approaches is needed for reaching a conclusive diagnosis.
- A liberal use of available armamentarium of investigations is justified in urgent cases as the treatment depends on the etiology and available therapeutic targets.
- Despite several advances and extensive work-up, several cases remain idiopathic, necessitating active research in this area.

SUGGESTED READINGS

1. Shomali W, Gotlib J. World Health Organization and International Consensus Classification of eosinophilic disorders: 2024 update on diagnosis, risk stratification, and management. Am J Hematol. 2024;99(5):946-68.
2. Tzankov A, Reichard KK, Hasserjian RP, Arber DA, Orazi A, Wang SA. Updates on eosinophilic disorders. Virchows Arch. 2023;482(1):85-97.
3. Valent P, Klion AD, Horny HP, Roufosse F, Gotlib J, Weller PF, et al. Contemporary consensus proposal on criteria and classification of eosinophilic disorders and related syndromes. J Allergy Clin Immunol. 2012;130:607-12.e9.
4. Lübke J, Metzgeroth G, Reiter A, Schwaab J. Approach to the patient with eosinophilia in the era of tyrosine kinase inhibitors and biologicals. Curr Hematol Malig Rep. 2024;19(5):208-22.
5. Sreedharanunni S, Varma N, Sachdeva MUS, Naseem S, Malhotra P, Bansal D, et al. The Spectrum of Hypereosinophilia and Associated Clonal Disorders: A Real-World Data Based on Combined Retrospective and Prospective Analysis from a Tropical Setting. Mediterr J Hematol Infect Dis. 2018;10:e2018052.
6. Hu Z, Wang W, Thakral B, Chen Z, Estrov Z, Bueso-Ramos CE, et al. Lymphocytic variant of hypereosinophilic syndrome: A report of seven cases from a single institution. Cytometry B Clin Cytom. 2021;100:352-60.
7. Wang SA. The Diagnostic Work-up of Hypereosinophilia. Pathobiology. 2019;86:39-52.
8. Khoury JD, Solary E, Abla O, Akkari Y, Alaggio R, Apperley JF, et al. The 5th edition of the World Health Organization Classification of Haematolymphoid Tumours: Myeloid and Histiocytic/Dendritic Neoplasms. Leukemia. 2022;36:1703-19.
9. Wang SA, Tam W, Tsai AG, Arber DA, Hasserjian RP, Geyer JT, et al. Targeted next-generation sequencing identifies a subset of idiopathic hypereosinophilic syndrome with features similar to chronic eosinophilic leukemia, not otherwise specified. Mod Pathol. 2016;29:854-64.
10. Helbig G, Wieczorkiewicz A, Dziaczkowska-Suszek J, Majewski M, Kyrcz-Krzemien S. T-cell abnormalities are present at high frequencies in patients with hypereosinophilic syndrome. Haematologica. 2009;94:1236-41.
11. Sreedharanunni S, Jamwal M, Balakrishnan A, Aravindan AV, Sharma R, Singh N, et al. Chronic eosinophilic leukemia with recurrent STAT5B N642H mutation: An entity with features of myelodysplastic syndrome/myeloproliferative neoplasm overlap. Leuk Res. 2022;112:106753.

CHAPTER 29

Monitoring and Follow-up of Chronic Myeloid Leukemia Including Tyrosine Kinase Domain Mutation Assessment

Shivangi Harankhedkar, Rahul Naithani

ABSTRACT

Chronic myeloid leukemia (CML) is a myeloproliferative neoplasm (MPN) characterized by the presence of a distinct reciprocal translocation between chromosomes 9 and 22, involving the *ABL1* (Abelson murine leukemia viral oncogene homolog 1) and breakpoint cluster region (*BCR)* genes, respectively. Depth of the response, stability of remission, and treatment-free remission (TFR) are now the current treatment goals in patients with CML. Routine molecular methods for monitoring include real-time quantitative polymerase chain reaction (RT-qPCR) and the tyrosine kinase domain (TKD) mutation assessment using Sanger sequencing. Newer definitions of response, including early molecular response (EMR) along with newer monitoring methods, including digital PCR (RT-dPCR) and next-generation sequencing (NGS), have found ways into the current guidelines. The recommendations given by European Leukemia Net (ELN) and the National Comprehensive Cancer Network (NCCN) are the most widely accessed documents for monitoring of CML. This chapter discusses the overall monitoring of CML in light of newer definitions and monitoring methods, including TKD mutation analysis.

INTRODUCTION

Chronic myeloid leukemia (CML) is a myeloproliferative neoplasm (MPN) characterized by the presence of a distinct reciprocal translocation between chromosomes 9 and 22, involving the *ABL1* (Abelson murine leukemia viral oncogene homolog 1) and breakpoint cluster region (*BCR)* genes, respectively. The early 21st century was a remarkable milestone in the management of CML as tyrosine kinase inhibitors (TKI) emerged as a targeted treatment. Molecular monitoring of response has been an integral part of CML management for over the last 3 decades. The presence of a signature abnormality in the form of BCR::ABL1 fusion forms the basis of molecular monitoring of the disease burden and therefore assessment of response. With targeted therapy in the form of four generations of currently available TKIs, the goal of treatment in CML has now evolved from survival outcomes to the attainment of depth and stability of response and even treatment-free remission (TFR). Resistance to TKIs, the emergence of additional cytogenetic abnormalities (ACA), particularly i(17)(q10)-7/del7q, and 3q26.2 rearrangements, and myeloid mutations may contribute to inadequate response, loss of response, and progression of the disease. All these factors make monitoring crucial. Broadly, the disease can be detected by (1) Demonstration of the chromosomal translocation on conventional karyotyping (CK), (2) Detection of BCR::ABL1 fusion on fluorescence in-situ hybridization (FISH) using dual-color dual-fusion probes, or (3) Quantification of the fusion transcript by a real-time quantitative polymerase chain reaction (RT-qPCR) or RT digital PCR (RT-dPCR), using messenger ribonucleic acid (mRNA) as the starting material. Owing to the lower sensitivities of CK and FISH, disease monitoring is most commonly performed using RT-qPCR.

DEFINITIONS OF RESPONSE

The three main categories of response in CML are complete hematological response (CHR), cytogenetic response, and molecular response, depending on the respective methods used. The CHR is defined when total leucocyte count (TLC) is $<10 \times 10^3/\mu L$, platelet count is $<450 \times 10^3/\mu L$, absence of immature myeloid cells on peripheral smear, resolution of clinical symptoms, and palpable splenomegaly. Complete cytogenetic response (CCyR) is defined when no Philadelphia (Ph) chromosome-positive metaphases are encountered. The molecular responses are defined based on the BCR::ABL1, International Scale (IS) values, or log reduction from patient baselines as determined by RT-qPCR. The IS scale values are in comparison with the original baseline in the IRIS trial. For example, a value of 1% defines 2 log reduction (MR2: 100 → 10 → 1), a value of 0.1% defines 3 log reduction (MR3: 100 → 10 → 1 → 0.1), and so on. A BCR::ABL1 IS value of ≤0.1% (MR3) or ≥3 log reduction from standardized baseline (if IS is not available) defines a "major molecular response" (MMR). Deep molecular response (DMR) is defined as ≤0.01% (MR4). These responses whether achieved or not at specific milestones (3 months, 6 months, etc.) define the optimal responses, warnings, or failures **(Fig. 1)**. The recent ELN and NCCN guidelines have newer milestones like an early molecular response (EMR) defined by BCR::ABL1 value of <10% IS at 3 and 6 months, and later molecular milestones (MR2 at 12+ months, MMR at 36–48 months).

Relapse is defined as a loss of hematologic response or CCyR or MR2 (equivalent to BCR::ABL1 IS >1%) or 1 log increase in the BCR::ABL1 levels with loss of MMR.

PREREQUISITES FOR MONITORING

Diagnosis of CML is established either by conventional karyotyping, FISH, or RT-PCR. Each of these tests has its advantages and limitations. The choice of an initial screening test may differ from center to center. As RT-qPCR is the most sensitive and widely used test for monitoring, the knowledge of the BCR::ABL1

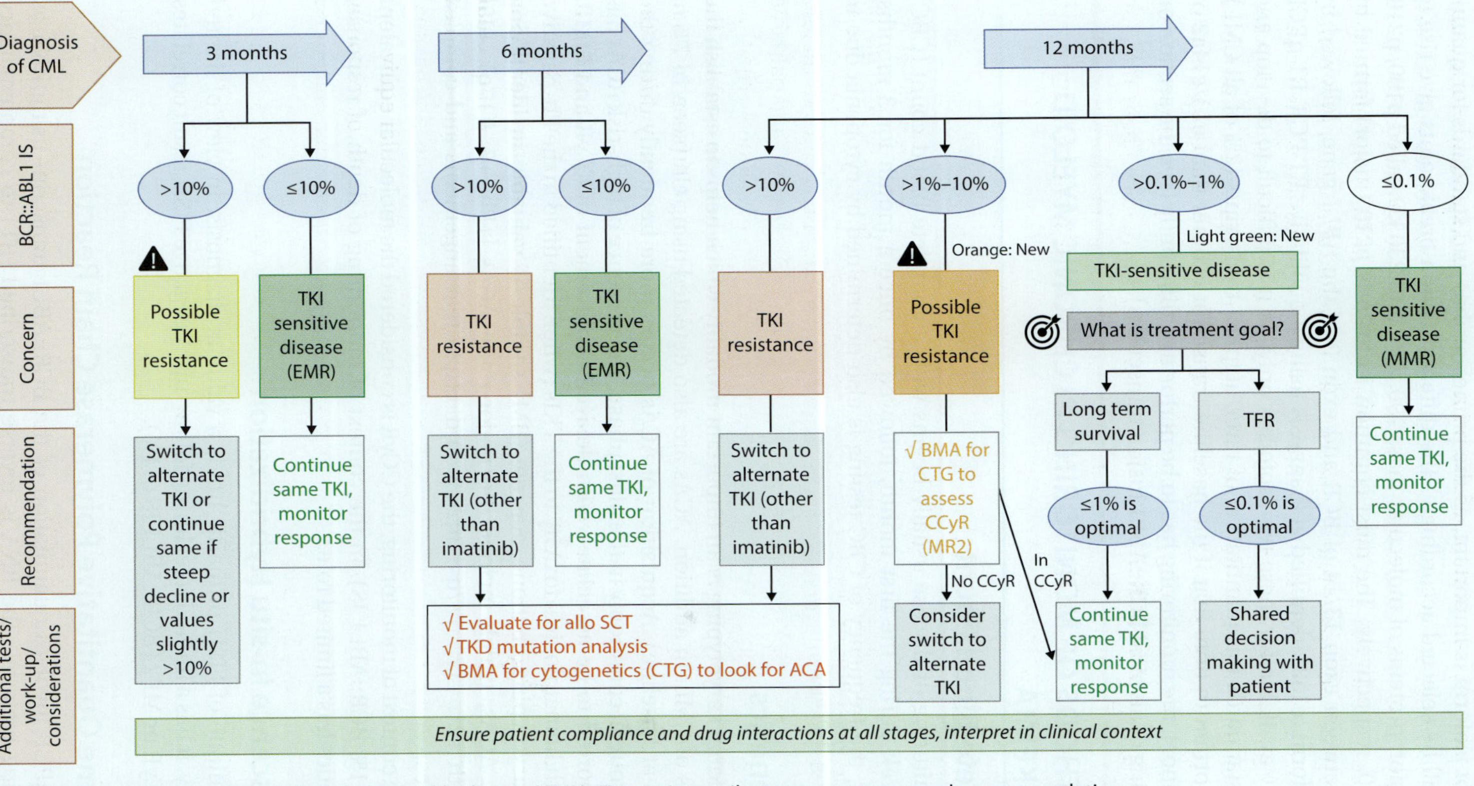

FIG. 1: Molecular monitoring of chronic myeloid leukemia (CML): Timepoints, milestones, concerns, and recommendations.

(EMR: early molecular response; MMR: major molecular response; TKI: tyrosine kinase inhibitor)

Source: Adapted from NCCN v3.2025.

transcript isoform is important, as the primer-probes and standards for quantitation will be selected accordingly. The different fusion breakpoints give rise to three fusion proteins of molecular mass 190, 210, and 230 kD called p190, p210, and p230, respectively. The most common isoform is p210 (major) formed by fusion between exon 13/14 of BCR and exon 2 of the *ABL1* gene, followed by p190 isoform (e1a2) identified at diagnosis using a qualitative RT-PCR. RT-qPCR is usually available for these two isoforms only, as it is difficult to develop and sustain standards for quantitation of rarer/atypical transcripts (2% of all CML). It is important to note that if the baseline transcript is other than e13/e14a2 or e1a2 (minor), the monitoring has to be performed differently (see the section on monitoring of atypical BCR::ABL1 fusion transcripts).

METHODS OF MONITORING IN CHRONIC MYELOID LEUKEMIA

Complete Blood Count

The monitoring of disease usually begins with a complete blood count (CBC) every week during the first month, followed by once a month for 3 months. However, the frequency of CBC testing is also determined by cytopenia due to TKI during therapy.

Cytogenetics

Conventional karyotyping is an important modality which helps to establish the diagnosis of CML. In addition, ACAs are also detected using CK (seen in 7% of CML-CP at baseline). Acquisition of ACAs occurs more frequently during the disease course, commonly in the blast phase. The presence of high-risk ACAs has been reported to be associated with delayed achievement of CCyR and MMR, along with hematological toxicity to the TKIs (when identified in the Ph-negative cells). Karyotyping on bone marrow (BM) sample is valuable in identifying high-risk ACAs, which include the major-route ACAs [+Ph, +8, i(17q), +19] along with +21, +17, –7/7q–, 3q26.2, and 11q23 rearrangements and complex karyotypes.

In the context of monitoring, the CCyR is considered the molecular equivalent of MR2 (1% BCR::ABL1 IS). In the context of monitoring of depth of response, cytogenetics has a limited role.

Fluorescence In-situ Hybridization

The technique of FISH primarily holds a value at diagnosis. In view of limited sensitivity, it has a limited role during follow-up. A negative FISH result correlates with a CCyR or MR2 (BCR::ABL1 IS of 1%).

Real-time Quantitative Polymerase Chain Reaction

The RT-qPCR involves quantitation of the BCR::ABL1 transcript using RNA as the starting material. The RNA is reverse transcribed (RT) to complementary deoxyribonucleic acid (cDNA), followed by a quantitative real-time PCR (qPCR) using the standard curve method. The *BCR* and *ABL1* primer-probes flanking the BCR::ABL1 region are used for amplification. In the same PCR, a housekeeping gene (e.g., *ABL1, GUSB,* and *BCR)* is also simultaneously amplified, which helps in the normalization and derivation of normalized copy number (NCN). The housekeeping genes also serve as an indicator that the desired sensitivity is obtained. The NCN is converted to IS-NCN using conversion factors provided with the kit or derived by the laboratory following proper validation.

To ensure the accuracy of results and uniformity of results across different laboratories in the world, a lot of technical considerations go into performing RT-qPCR in the laboratories. Following are some of the important considerations:

- The tests should be optimized to detect a response of MR^4 to $MR^{4.5}$ so that DMR can be assessed. A sensitivity of MR4 is ensured by achieving a minimum 10,000 copies of *ABL1* (32,000 for $MR^{4.5}$) and 24,000 for *GUSB* (77,000 for $MR^{4.5}$).
- The limit of detection (LoD) must be obtained using clinical samples.
- Tests can be performed using a commercial international scale (IS) calibrated kits, preferably, or complex laboratory-developed tests (LDT) following proper validation for IS.
- For LDTs, the conversion factors (CF) for IS should be revalidated annually using sample exchange with reference laboratories or calibration using secondary reagents or stored samples with known IS values.
- RNA extraction from the peripheral blood [ethylenediaminetetraacetic acid (EDTA)] should be completed within 24 hours (not after 48 hours) as RNA starts to degrade outside the body once drawn.
- The amplification efficiencies of BCR::ABL1 and housekeeping genes may vary according to the quantity of input material. This can be checked using plasmids such as ERM-AD623, which harbor both targets together in them.

Real-time Digital Polymerase Chain Reaction

Digital PCR involves direct absolute quantification of the BCR::ABL1 copies, without the use of standards. Unlike RT-qPCR, it is less susceptible to differences in amplification efficiency. It is a highly sensitive and specific technique, especially valuable in the monitoring of the TFR setting. The Food and Drug Administration (FDA) cleared the first digital droplet PCR (ddPCR) assay for BCR::ABL1 monitoring in CML in 2022. A detection limit of $MR^{4.7}$ (0.002%) was met in this assay.

RNA Sequencing-based Minimal Residual Disease

Improved sensitivity can be obtained using RNA-based targeted next-generation sequencing (NGS) for the detection of BCR::ABL1 fusion. This is, however, presently not in routine use or recommendations.

DNA-based Minimal Residual Disease

Theoretically, DNA-based monitoring (qPCR/dPCR/NGS) is easy to standardize, and results can be extrapolated to cell numbers (like flowcytometry-based MRD for acute leukemias). However, as the exact genomic breakpoints differ from patient to patient, the implementation would require the designing of patient-specific primers adding to the cost. Currently, these methods are being used to study the biology of TFR and are not done in routine practice.

MONITORING OF ATYPICAL BCR::ABL1 FUSION TRANSCRIPTS

Atypical BCR::ABL1 fusions involve breakpoints other than the common e13/14a2 (p210) and e1a2 (p190). It is important that whenever an atypical transcript of BCR::ABL1 is encountered at diagnosis, the monitoring method is also selected accordingly. This is important to avoid false negative results if routine RT-qPCR for BCR::ABL (e13/e14 a2) is blindly performed. The fusion-specific RT-qPCR is recommended. Although not validated for IS, the RT-qPCR should achieve the detection of low-level responses. The *ABL1* and *GUSB* gene copy numbers should be ≥10,000 (ideally ≥32,000) and 24,000 (ideally ≥77,000), respectively. The IS scale and monitoring milestones cannot be applied in these cases.

TYROSINE KINASE DOMAIN MUTATION ANALYSIS

Mutations, mostly single-nucleotide variants (SNVs) in the kinase domain of BCR::ABL1 fusion, are among the reasons for failure to attain an expected response to TKIs or a loss of response. The presence of specific SNVs leads to resistance to specific drugs, which can be stopped/avoided, and the drugs effective against that particular SNV can be employed in the management. The knowledge of which drug is resistant or sensitive comes from the IC50 data performed in cell lines and is widely reported. Following are some of the important mutations and the respective drugs they are contraindicated in:

- For asciminib, the contraindicated mutations are A337T, P465S, M244V, or F359V/I/C.
- For bosutinib, the contraindicated mutations are T315I, V299L, G250E, or F317L.
- For dasatinib, the contraindicated mutations are T315I/A, F317L/V/I/C, or V299L.
- For nilotinib, the contraindicated mutations are T315I, Y235H, E255K/V, or F359V/C/I.
- For ponatinib or allogeneic stem cell transplant, there are no contraindicated mutations.

When is TKD mutation testing indicated?

The mutations in the KD arise under stress encountered during the TKI therapy and are not found during the diagnosis. Hence, testing should not be performed at the beginning of the chronic phase of CML. Current recommendations (ELN and NCCN) advise performing TKD mutation analysis in the following scenarios:

- Suboptimal response (failure to attain milestones) or loss of response to TKIs
- Relapse following allogeneic hematopoietic stem cell transplant (≥0.1% BCR::ABL1 IS), if the mutation was present before the transplant

- Loss of hematologic response or cytogenetic response (or equivalent molecular response, i.e, MR2 or 1% IS BCR::ABL1)
- Disease progression (blast phase)
- No improvement after 3–6 months or worsening of response when using third-line TKI.

How is TKD mutation testing initiated?

As the test is targeted to look for mutations in the kinase domain contained within the BCR::ABL1 transcript, amplification of the BCR::ABL1 transcript is usually the first step (1st PCR), with RNA as the starting material. This is followed by amplification of the ABL1 kinase domain (2nd PCR) for sequencing (Sanger sequencing or NGS). The two important practical considerations arise here: (1) The patient sample being tested should have an "amplifiable" BCR::ABL1 transcript. The value usually stated is >0.1% IS, with levels >1% giving more reliable results. This suggests that testing of patients in MMR or deeper responses is futile and wasteful. (2) The baseline transcript type/isoform of the patient is essential before proceeding to the subsequent steps, as appropriate primers need to be used in the first PCR for amplifying the particular BCR::ABL1 isoform.

What are the methods of testing?

- Sanger sequencing is considered the gold standard of kinase domain mutation (KDM) testing. It can detect all known as well as unknown variants spanning the KD region. While it is easier to perform than other assays, it has a shorter turnaround time (TAT) and is cost-effective, the main drawback is the lower sensitivity. The sensitivity is 20–25% (meaning that out of say 100 BCR::ABL1 transcripts, at least 20–25 need to harbor the mutation for it to be detectable). Also, if two or more mutations are detected in one patient, it is not possible to tell if they are on the same transcripts or different (cis vs. trans).
- NGS is the emerging and newly recommended method for KDM testing. The major advantage of NGS over Sanger sequencing is the higher sensitivity (2–5%). A higher frequency of TKD mutations is encountered when NGS is used (40–50% of failure, 30–40% of warning cases) compared to when Sanger sequencing is used for testing (20–35% of failure, 10–20% of warning cases). Studies have shown that the detection of smaller clones with mutated BCR::ABL1 KD is important, as these clones can escape the drug effect, expand, and lead to an inadequate response. Secondly, the presence of compound mutations (two mutations in cis on the same transcript) is shown to have inferior outcomes and can only be detected by NGS in contrast to Sanger sequencing. Higher cost, throughput requirement, and false calls (need for stringent assay performance) are some of the challenges involved in KDM NGS. It is important to note that sequential monitoring can be important when low-level mutations or mutations with unknown significance are encountered. Also, a mutation with a variant allele frequency (VAF) of <15% not previously known as clinically actionable should be confirmed on an independent sample (to see if it is expanding) before considering it as potentially actionable. Only recurrent variants and novel variants above

VAF of 15% should be considered for immediate clinical decision making. Previously reported 35 ins (between exon 8 and 9) is now known to be a result of alternative splicing and should not be reported.

- Digital droplet PCR is also being performed for KDM testing. While it could result in higher sensitivity than NGS, only known mutations against whom the assay is developed can be detected. A four-tube method of ddPCR is studied, each tube run directed against testing mutations causing resistance to the respective drug.
- *Mass spectrometry*: This is a relatively new mutation-specific approach, more sensitive (0.05–0.5%), and less error-prone, however, currently less employed.
- Multiplex PCR is an old method involving the detection of known mutations by PCR. It is less frequently performed and not recommended owing to the sensitivity and limited number of detectable mutations.

MYELOID MUTATION ANALYSIS

In addition to the role of TKD mutation analysis, the presence of BCR::ABL1 independent mechanisms plays an important role. Mutations in the genes associated with myeloid malignancies (e.g., *ASXL1*, *RUNX1*, *BCOR*, *IKZF1*, etc.), especially epigenetic mutations, have been reported to influence the course of chronic-phase CML. In the absence of KDM, NGS for these myeloid mutations is recommended, especially where inadequate response or unexplained cytopenias develop, although data pertaining to their relevance is currently limited. In cases with persistent thrombocytosis while in remission, the *JAK2* V617F mutation should be looked for as the BCR::ABL1 and JAK2 V617F are known to co-occur.

Figure 2 summarizes the overview of molecular methods in CML monitoring.

PRACTICAL TIPS

- It is advised to do all serial investigations at the same laboratory only. More so when TFR is attempted.
- It is important for clinicians not to react to just one rise in BCR::ABL1 numbers.
- Reports need to be generated in IS format for cross-laboratory comparisons.
- Before doing KD mutation, it is important to realize that yield is better if BCR::ABL1 transcripts are 0.1% or above.
- Peripheral blood is sufficient for these samples. A bone marrow sample is not required except for cytogenetics.

Take Home Points

- Monitoring of CML performed for response assessment is performed using molecular assays such as RT-qPCR. New assays such as digital PCR also find a place in the recent guidelines.
- Newer response definitions such as EMR have been included in the latest recommendations.

Conventional karyotyping

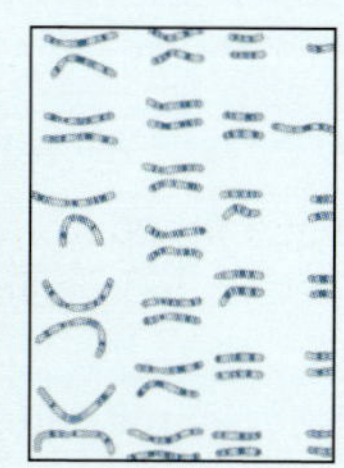

- Significant in detection of additional chromosomal abnormalities (ACA) at diagnosis, relapse, failure, progression, abnormal counts in remission
- Limited role in assessing depth of response
- Complete cytogenetic response (CCyR) corresponds to MR2

Digital droplet PCR

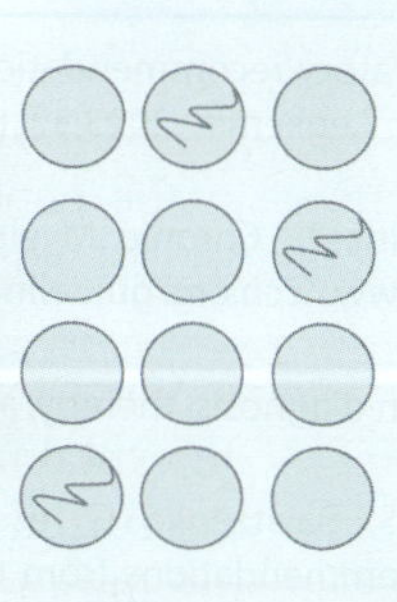

- Absolute quantification of the targets
- RT-dPCR (or else RT-qPCR) mandatory in monitoring of depth of response, esp in TFR setting
- Also studied for kinase domain mutation (KDM) testing: Only known important mutations targeted

Fluorescence in situ hybridization (FISH)

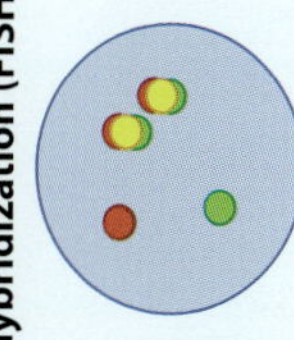

- Not recommended for monitoring of response in view of limited sensitivity
- Role at diagnosis only

Sanger sequencing

- No role in monitoring the depth of response
- Widely used for detection of KDM: Can detect both known, unknown variants: Sensitivity is limited

Reverse transcriptase PCR (RT-PCR)

- RT-qualitative PCR not recommended for monitoring
- RT-quantitative PCR (or else RT-dPCR) mandatory and most widely used for assessment of depth of response
- IS scale applicable for only e13/e14a2 (major, p210) isoform
- Multiplex PCR for KDM detects only known variants, not recommended

Next generation sequencing (NGS)

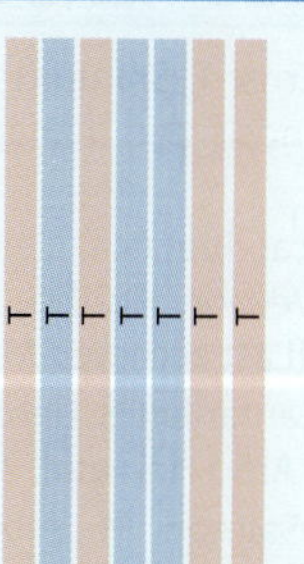

- No role in monitoring the depth of response currently
- Increasingly being used for detection of TKD mutations as low level mutations (known, unknown) can be detected. Technically challenging: Artefacts and errors possible (VAF cut off of 15% important)
- NGS for myeloid mutations recommended in hematological relapse, disease progression and when KDM is not detected

FIG. 2: Spectrum of molecular tests and their role in monitoring of chronic myeloid leukemia (CML).

- Knowledge about mechanisms of inadequate response such as KDM is valuable to tailor therapy based on the type of mutation detected. NGS is the recommended method because of its ability to detect small clones of actionable mutations (higher sensitivity).
- Preanalytical factors and performance of molecular testing according to the recommended protocols are essential for reliable results and achievement of the desired sensitivity for deeper response assessments.
- The challenges in monitoring CML involve the translation of information arising out of increasingly sensitive tests into patient decisions such as stopping the therapy, changing the drugs, dose modifications, etc., while taking into account the patient-related factors such as comorbidities, drug interactions, and costs.

SUGGESTED READINGS

1. Cross NCP, Ernst T, Branford S, et al. European LeukemiaNet laboratory recommendations for the diagnosis and management of chronic myeloid leukemia. Leukemia. 2023;37(11): 2150-67.
2. NCCN Clinical Practice Guidelines in Oncology (NCCN Guidelines®). Chronic Myeloid Leukemia Version 3.2025. [online] Available from https://www.nccn.org/guidelines/category_1 [Last accessed May, 2025].
3. Jabbour E, Kantarjian H. Chronic myeloid leukemia: 2025 update on diagnosis, therapy, and monitoring. Am J Hematol. 2024;99(11):2191-212.
4. White HE, Salmon M, Albano F, Andersen CSA, Balabanov S, Balatzenko G, et al. Standardization of molecular monitoring of CML: results and recommendations from the European treatment and outcome study. Leukemia. 2022;36(7):1834-42.
5. Branford S, Apperley JF. Measurable residual disease in chronic myeloid leukemia. Haematologica. 2022;107(12):2794-809.
6. Shelton DN, Bhagavatula P, Sepulveda N, et al. Performance characteristics of the first Food and Drug Administration (FDA)-cleared digital droplet PCR (ddPCR) assay for BCR::ABL1 monitoring in chronic myelogenous leukemia. PLoS One. 2022;17(3):e0265278.
7. Soverini S. Resistance mutations in CML and how we approach them. Hematol Am Soc Hematol Educ Program. 2023;2023(1):469-75.

CHAPTER 30

Primary Immunodeficiency Disorders: Approach to Diagnosis and Treatment

Umair Ahmed Nazir Ahmed Bargir, Mukesh Desai, Manisha Rajan Madkaikar

ABSTRACT

Primary immunodeficiency disorders (PIDs), now referred to as inborn errors of immunity (IEI), are a diverse group of inherited conditions affecting the immune system. These disorders predispose individuals to recurrent infections, immune dysregulation, autoimmunity, lymphoproliferation, and malignancies due to underlying genetic defects. With over 555 IEIs and 17 phenotypic defects due to mutations in over 504 genes—PIDs exhibit a wide range of clinical manifestations, from asymptomatic cases to severe, life-threatening conditions. Early diagnosis and specialized care are critical for optimal outcomes. Advances in molecular diagnostics, including next-generation sequencing (NGS) and whole exome sequencing (WES), have significantly improved the identification of genetic defects, enabling precise diagnosis and personalized treatment. Laboratory investigations, including immunological and biochemical assays, provide essential clues to the underlying defects. Recent therapeutic advancements, such as gene therapy, targeted therapies, and gene editing technologies such as clustered regularly interspaced short palindromic repeats (CRISPR)-CRISPR-associated protein 9 (Cas9), have revolutionized the management of IEI, offering curative and precision medicine approaches. Despite these advancements, challenges in accessibility, affordability, and diagnostic limitations persist. This chapter provides a comprehensive overview of the clinical features, diagnostic approaches, genetic underpinnings, and recent therapeutic innovations in the management of IEI, highlighting the shift toward precision medicine and the need for continued research and equitable access to care.

INTRODUCTION

Primary immunodeficiency disorders (PIDs) now are diverse inherited conditions affecting the immune system. These patients are at an increased risk to develop infections due to some underlying genetic defects. Some of these patients have immune dysregulation leading to autoimmune manifestation, lymphoproliferation and/or malignancy. To encompass this diverse phenotype

PID is now rechristened as inborn errors of immunity (IEI). Early diagnosis and prompt referral to specialized centers remain crucial for optimal outcomes. The estimated global incidence is 1:10,000, suggesting approximately 140,000 patients may be affected in India alone. With advances in molecular diagnostics, over 555 distinct genetic defects have been identified as causing PIDs. The underlying genetic variant cause disease phenotype by altering the function or expression of the protein function. There are 17 phenocopies due to autoantibodies or somatic mutations. The disease mechanism depends on the type of variant and its mode of inheritance. Monoallelic variants can lead to disease through haploinsufficiency, dominant-negative effects, or gain-of-function (GOF), while biallelic variants (homozygous or compound heterozygous) typically cause autosomal recessive conditions through loss-of-function (LOF), GOF, or neomorphic protein functions. Some X-linked recessive diseases arise from LOF or GOF variants on the X chromosome, affecting males in a hemizygous state or females in a homozygous state. In X-linked carrier females, lyonization can lead to variable expression of the disease depending on the proportion of cells expressing the affected X chromosome.

CLINICAL MANIFESTATIONS SEEN IN PRIMARY IMMUNODEFICIENCY DISORDER

Primary immunodeficiency disorders can manifest with different clinical manifestations with severity ranging from asymptomatic disease to severe and recurrent infections, autoimmunity, and malignancy. The most important clues being:

- Infections with unexpectedly high frequency, unusual presentation, atypical pathogens, and unusual severity.
- Early or atypical onset of autoimmunity, multiorgan involvement.
- Lymphoproliferative disease.

An executive subcommittee of the International Union of Immunological Societies (IUIS) updates a phenotypic classification of PID. The common clinical presentations of the different IUIS categories are listed in **Table 1**.

AGE OF PRESENTATION

The age of presentation depends on the underlying defect. Patients with severe combined immunodeficiency disorder (SCID) usually present in early infancy, though leaky SCID may present later. The patients with X-linked agammaglobulinemia (XLA) present after 6 months of age as the maternal antibodies protect till then. Common variable immunodeficiency disorder is the most common symptomatic PID and can present in adulthood.

INFECTIONS

Recurrent infections are the most common clinical presentation in patients suspected of having PID. Knowing the organism provides important clues to the underlying immune defects **(Table 2)**.

TABLE 1: Common clinical presentation seen different categories of primary immunodeficiency disorder.

IUIS category	Common presentation
Immunodeficiencies affecting cellular and humoral immunity	Recurrent sinopulmonary infections, intractable diarrhea, failure to thrive since infancy, eczematous rash, unusual site or organism
Combined immunodeficiencies with associated or syndromic features	Recurrent infections with characteristic syndromic features like special facial features, cardiac anomalies, etc.
Predominantly antibody deficiencies	Recurrent sinopulmonary infections, chronic diarrhea, septic arthritis, bronchiectasis
Diseases of immune dysregulation	Autoimmune cytopenias, lymphoproliferation
Congenital defects of phagocyte number or function	Recurrent pyogenic infections, poor wound healing, granuloma, delayed cord fall
Defects in intrinsic and innate immunity	Susceptibility to specific organisms such as nontuberculous mycobacteria, herpes simplex, etc.
Autoinflammatory disorders	Periodic fever, sterile arthritis, rashes
Complement deficiencies	Angioedema, systemic lupus erythematous, atypical hemolytic-uremic syndrome

(IUIS: International Union of Immunological Societies)

TABLE 2: Organisms providing clues to the underlying genetic defect.

Infective organism	Probable category of PID/genetic defect
Bacteria	
Staphylococcus aureus	Hyper immunoglobulin (Ig)E syndrome, chronic granulomatous diseases (CGD), leukocyte adhesion deficiency (LAD), XLA, *IRAK4, MYD88*
Pseudomonas	*CD40LG*, congenital neutropenia, CGD
Nontuberculous mycobacteria	Mendelian susceptibility to mycobacterial disease (MSMD), CGD, SCID
Nontyphi salmonella	MSMD
Streptococcus pneumoniae	XLA, complement deficiencies, *IRAK4, MYD88,* congenital asplenia
Nisseria menigitidis	Complement deficiencies
Viruses	
EBV with HLH	*PRF1, RAB27A, SH2D1A, STX11, XIAP, UNC13D*
Chronic EBV viremia	*CD21, CD27, CD70, ITK, MAGT1, PRKCD, PI3KD, SAP, XIAP*
CMV	*SCID, DOCK8, WAS, eNOS*
Fungi	
Candida (Invasive)	*CARD9*, CGD, neutropenia
Chronic mucocutaneous Candidiasis	AIRE, Th17 pathway defect
Aspergillus	CGD, SCID, CIS, Hyper IgE
Parasite	
Giardia	X-linked agammaglobulinemia, common variable immunodeficiency (CVID)

(CMV: cytomegalovirus; EBV: Epstein–Barr virus; HLH: hemophagocytic lymphohistiocytosis; PID: primary immunodeficiency disorder; SCID: severe combined immunodeficiency; XLA: X-linked agammaglobulinemia)

NONINFECTIOUS MANIFESTATIONS

Autoimmune manifestations in monogenic immune disorders often involve multiple organ systems, including hematologic, endocrine, gastrointestinal, and systemic features. Hematologic manifestations primarily consist of autoimmune cytopenias such as autoimmune hemolytic anemia, thrombocytopenia, and neutropenia, as well as lymphoproliferation presenting with hepatomegaly, splenomegaly, and lymphadenopathy. Endocrinopathies are common and include early-onset type 1 diabetes mellitus, hypoparathyroidism, thyroiditis, adrenal insufficiency, growth hormone deficiency, and growth failure. Gastrointestinal symptoms often involve chronic diarrhea, malabsorption, growth failure, and inflammatory bowel disease (IBD)-like inflammation [very early onset IBD (VEOIBD)]. Systemic features may include arthritis, vasculitis, and lupus-like symptoms. These manifestations are often severe, refractory to treatment, and may involve multiple organ systems, and necessitating genetic sequencing for diagnosis **(Table 3)**.

MALIGNANCY

These patients have an increased risk of malignancies, particularly lymphomas, due to defective immune responses and DNA repair mechanisms. Hematopoietic malignancies, such as non-Hodgkin lymphoma (NHL) and Hodgkin lymphoma (HL), are the most common cancers in PID patients, often linked to Epstein-Barr virus (EBV) infections. PIDs like ataxia-telangiectasia (AT), common variable immunodeficiency (CVID), and Wiskott-Aldrich syndrome (WAS) show the highest cancer risks, with NHL being predominant cancer. Solid tumors, including gastric and skin cancers, are also more frequent in PIDs due to chronic inflammation, infections [e.g., *Helicobacter pylori*, human papillomavirus (HPV)], and genetic mutations. Conditions such as severe congenital neutropenia (SCN) and X-linked hyper immunoglobulin M syndrome (XHIGM) further predispose

TABLE 3: Autoimmunity and lymphoproliferation in primary immunodeficiency disorder.

Disease/genes	System/organ involvement
SCID *(RAG1/RAG2, ADA)*	Autoimmune cytopenia
CVID	Autoimmune cytopenia, autoimmune hepatitis, autoimmune manifestations involving skin, lung, brain, and lymphoproliferation
Autoimmune polyendocrinopathy-candidiasis-ectodermal dystrophy (APECED)	Endocrine involvement, hypoparathyroidism, insulin dependent diabetes mellitus (IDDM), Addison disease
STAT3 GOF	Lymphoproliferation, autoimmune cytopenia, endocrine involvement, IDDM, Addison disease
Autoimmune lymphoproliferative syndrome	Lymphoproliferation, autoimmune cytopenia

(GOF: gain-of-function; SCID: severe combined immunodeficiency)

patients to acute myeloid leukemia (AML) and organ-specific carcinomas. Advances in PID management have improved survival, but cancer and immunodeficiency have worse prognosis than in an immunocompetent individual. They need tailored chemotherapy protocols of shorter duration with good infection control and allogeneic blood or marrow transplantation (AlloBMT) to cure the underlying genetic defect. It is important to rule out the same genetic defect in case of a family donor for AlloBMT.

LABORATORY EVALUATION FOR PRIMARY IMMUNODEFICIENCY DISORDER

An aggressive immunological and genetic workup is necessary in patients suspected of having PID. The clinical approach is still relevant in recognizing patterns that would help suspect the type of underlying PIDs **(Table 4)**.

GENETICS OF PRIMARY IMMUNODEFICIENCY DISORDER

The PID being a heterogeneous group of >555 genetic defects WES or targeted panel is the molecular diagnostic method of choice depending on the clinical presentation. Targeted panels can be done when the symptoms match a specific phenotype with supportive immunological investigations. Whereas when the presentation is less specific WES can be employed. It is pragmatic to do WES rather than targeted sequencing. Identifying the underlying genetic defects can help guide the treatment, and provide information on the prognosis and genetic counseling.

SEQUENCING TECHNIQUES

Sanger Sequencing

Sanger sequencing remains the test of choice for parental segregation and sibling screening. It is also useful in patients with a preceding family history with a known genetic defect.

Next-generation Sequencing

With the advent of NGS, massively parallel sequencing is now possible cost-effectively and rapidly. It is now the test of choice for genetic diagnosis for most clinicians. DNA sequencing by NGS is primarily of three types, viz., targeted gene panels, WES, and whole genome sequencing (WGS). In targeted gene panels or clinical exome sequencing, a limited number of genes are covered. Often, commercial vendors perform WES even if targeted panels are requested to optimize runs, however, a focused bioinformatic analysis for a select list of genes is reported. It is useful if there is some evidence to an underlying genetic defect based on the available immunophenotypic work-up. As patients presenting with IEI may sometimes have a broad differential, doing a small panel may not identify the genetic defect. WES covers the entire coding portion of the genome with some

TABLE 4: Laboratory investigations in patients suspected to have primary immunodeficiency disorder.

Category	Basic tests	Supportive tests	Advanced tests
Combined immunodeficiencies	• CBC, differential counts • Lymphocyte subset analysis	• Naïve Th, Naïve Tc cells • T-cell proliferation against phytohemagglutinin (PHA), CD3-CD28 • Phosphorylated *STAT 5* (pSTAT5) expression • CD132, CD127 expression	• T-cell receptor excision circles • Vβ repertoire • ADA/PNP enzyme activity • Radiation sensitivity assay
Antibody deficiencies	• Serum Ig G, A, M, E levels • Lymphocyte subset analysis to look for B-cell numbers	• Class switched B cells • IgG subclass • Specific antibody response against protein and polysaccharide vaccine • Isohemagglutinin titers	• BTK expression • NFKB1/NFKB2 expression
Hemophagocytic lymphohistiocytosis	• Serum ferritin • Serum triglycerides • Serum fibrinogen	Perforin expression, CD107a degranulation assay, sCD25	• K562 cytotoxic assay • NK and CD8 cell exocytic response
Phagocyte disorders	• CBC and differential counts • Peripheral blood smear	• Nitro blue tetrazolium test • Dihydrorhodamine assay • p22, p47, p67 PHOX expression • CD18/11a, 11b, 11c expression • IFNGR1 expression • CD212 expression	• Gene scan for delGT • pSTAT1, pSTAT4 • BCG stimulation assay
Complement deficiencies	C3, C4	CH50/AH50	

(ADA: adenosine deaminase; PNP: purine nucleoside phosphorylase; BCG: Bacillus Calmette Guérin; CBC: complete blood count; BTK: Bruton's tyrosine kinase; Ig: immunoglobulin)

BOX 1: Inborn errors of immunity (IEI) genes with pseudogenes.

ACTB, AK2, CFTR, IGLL1, NCF1, PMS2, RAC2, RNF168, RPSA, SBDS, TRNT1, UNG, XIAP, C19orf40, CD46, CDCA7, CSF2Rb, DCLRE1C, FPR1, HAX1, IKBKG, ITCH, MAGT1, MSN, MTHFD1, NBAS, NCSTN, NHP2, NOP10, PIK3CD, PNP, PTEN, RANBP2, RLTBP2, RLTPR, RNASEH2C, RTEL1, TCF3, TMC6, ZBTB24

flanking regions. It will be able to identify defects in other genes that mimic the phenotype and novel genes. The diagnostic yield of WES for patients suspected to have IEI ranges from 15 to 79%. There are some genes that cannot be covered with WES because of the presence of pseudo-genes **(Box 1)**. Also, some genes have poor coverage around 90% on WES such as *IKBKB, TACI,* and *TBX1* because of regions difficult to sequence.

Copy Number Variants

The copy number variants (CNV) play a significant role in the genetic landscape of IEI, which are disorders caused by genetic defects affecting the immune system. CNVs involve deletions or duplications of chromosomal regions and can disrupt gene function, contributing to the phenotypic heterogeneity observed in IEI. While single nucleotide variants (SNVs) have been extensively studied, CNVs are often underexplored in routine diagnostics despite their potential to increase diagnostic yield. Recent studies, including WES and SNP array analyses, have identified pathogenic CNVs in genes such as *ICOS, TNFAIP3, DOCK8,* and 22q11.2, which are associated with immune dysregulation and susceptibility to infections. Additionally, CNVs can co-occur with SNVs, suggesting potential modifying effects on disease phenotypes. The integration of CNV analysis into diagnostic workflows enhance the understanding of IEI and enables more precise molecular diagnoses, ultimately improving therapeutic management for affected patients.

Somatic Variants

Unlike germline mutations, somatic variants occur in a subset of cells and can lead to mosaicism, where only certain tissues or cell types carry the mutation. These variants can mimic germline IEI, causing similar clinical phenotypes such as autoimmunity, autoinflammation, or immunodeficiency. For example, somatic mutations in genes such as *FAS, NLRP3,* and *UBA1* have been implicated in autoimmune lymphoproliferative syndrome (ALPS), cryopyrin-associated periodic syndromes (CAPS), and VEXAS syndrome, respectively. Detection of somatic variants is challenging due to their low variant allele frequency (VAF) and the need for high-depth sequencing or targeted approaches. These mutations often arise later in life, expanding the scope of IEI diagnoses to include adult-onset diseases. Understanding somatic variants not only improves diagnostic precision but also informs targeted therapies, as seen in conditions like VEXAS syndrome, where somatic mutations drive treatment-refractory inflammation.

Whole Genome Sequencing

The WGS is a comprehensive genetic testing method that analyzes the entire genome, including both exonic intronic regions, as well as mitochondrial DNA. It provides a complete picture of an individual's genetic makeup. This approach is particularly valuable for diagnosing complex or rare genetic disorders, such as IEI, where causative variants may reside in noncoding regions or involve structural variations such as deletions, duplications, or translocations. WGS has the potential to detect a wide range of genetic abnormalities, including SNVs, CNV, and structural variants, making it a powerful tool in clinical diagnostics. However, challenges such as high costs, data storage, and interpretation of vast amounts of genetic data remain significant barriers to its widespread adoption in routine clinical practice.

Recent Modalities

Emerging technologies such as optical genome mapping (OGM) and RNA sequencing (RNA-seq) are enhancing the diagnostic yield by identifying structural variants and transcriptomic changes, respectively. Single-cell sequencing allows for the analysis of genetic variations at the cellular level, improving the detection of mosaicism and rare variants. Additionally, artificial intelligence (AI) and machine learning (ML) are being integrated into genetic diagnostics to streamline variant interpretation, improve risk stratification, and reduce turnaround times. These advancements are paving the way for more precise and personalized approaches to diagnosing and managing genetic disorders.

RECENT UPDATES IN MANAGING INBORN ERRORS OF IMMUNITY

Recent advances in the treatment of IEI have focused on innovative, targeted, and curative approaches **(Table 5)**. BMT is curative in large number of IEI. Gene therapy has seen significant progress, with safer self-inactivating lentiviral vectors enabling successful treatment of conditions such as adenosine deaminase (ADA)-SCID, XR-SCID, and WAS, while reduced-toxicity conditioning regimens have improved immune reconstitution. Gene editing technologies, particularly CRISPR-Cas9, are showing preclinical success in precisely correcting genetic defects, preserving natural gene regulation, and addressing dominant-negative mutations in diseases such as XR-SCID, X-linked hyper-IgM, and IPEX (immune dysregulation, polyendocrinopathy, enteropathy, X-linked). Intravenous immunoglobulin (IVIG)/subcutaneous immunoglobulin (SCIG) remains the mainstay of treatment for antibody deficiencies. Targeted therapies have also expanded **(Table 5)**, with Janus kinase (JAK) inhibitors effectively treating STAT1/STAT3 GOF mutations, Abatacept in cytotoxic T-lymphocyte-associated antigen 4 (CTLA-4) haploinsufficiency and LRBA deficiency, and PI3Kδ inhibitors like leniolisib demonstrating efficacy in activated PI3Kδ syndrome (APDS). Additionally, complement inhibitors such as eculizumab and pozelimab are being tested for CD55 deficiency. Recombinant interferon alpha (r-IFNα) is tried with limited benefit in patients with mendelian susceptibility to mycobacterial disease. These advancements highlight a shift toward precision medicine, offering improved outcomes and quality of life for patients with IEI, though challenges in accessibility and affordability remain.

TABLE 5: Newer therapeutic targets in inborn errors of immunity.

CGD: • Infection • Inflammation	→	Steroids	*STAT3 GOF:* • Autoimmunity • Lymphoproliferation	→	• Steroids • mTOR inhibitors Sirolimus) • JAK inhibitors
ALPS: • Lymphoproliferation • Inflammation	→	mTOR inhibitors (Sirolimus)	*APDS1 GOF:* • Infection • Lymphoproliferation • FTT	→	• P110δ inhibitors (Leniolisib Idelalisib) • mTOR inhibitors (Sirolimus)
STAT1 GOF: • Infection • Inflammation	→	JAK1, 2 inhibitors (Ruxolitinib Baricitinib)	*LRBA/CTLA4:* • Infection • Lymphoproliferation • CVID	→	CTLA4 agonist (Abatacept)
ADA2 deficiency: • Fever • Rash • Inflammation	→	• TNFα • Inhibitors	*Lyn-GOF:* • Liver fibrosis • Autoinflammation • Cytopenias	→	Dasatinib
WHIM: • Infection • Inflammation	→	Plerixafor	*AGS:* • Autoimmunity • Lymphoproliferation	→	• JAK inhibitors • ART
HLH: • Lymphoproliferation • Inflammation	→	• Alemtuzumab • JAK2 inhibitors • Anti-IL18BP	*GvHD:* • Infection • Lymphoproliferation • FTT	→	JAK inhibitors
MSMD: • Infection • Inflammation	→	• INFα • IFNγ	*Autoinflammatory disorders:* Autoinflammation	→	• Anakinra • Adalimumab • Etanercept • Canakinumab • Rilonacept
G6PC3 deficiency: Neutropenia	→	Empagliflozin (Jardiance)	*LAD1:* Autoimmunity	→	• Ustekinumab • Secukinumab

(AGS: Aicardi–Goutières syndrome; APDS1: activated phosphoinositide 1-kinase δ syndrome; ADA2: adenosine deaminase 2; ALPS: autoimmune lymphoproliferative syndrome; CGD: chronic granulomatous diseases; CVID: common variable immunodeficiency; GvHD: graft versus host disease; IFN: interferon; JAK: Janus kinase; LAD1: leukocyte adhesion deficiency 1; LRBA: lipopolysaccharide responsive beige-like anchor; mTOR: mechanistic target of rapamycin; MSMD: Mendelian susceptibility to mycobacterial disease; STAT1 GOF: signal transducer and activator of transcription 1 gain-of-function; TNF: tumor necrosis factor; WHIM: Warts, hypogammaglobulinemia, immunodeficiency, myelokathexis)

CASES

Case 1

A 4-year-old boy presented with bilateral knee joint swelling for past 6 months **(Fig. 1)**.

He had a significant past history of:
- Two admissions with pneumonia and empyema at 2 years and 3 years of age.
- Urinary tract infection at 3 years of age.
- Otitis media and persistent ear discharge between 2 and 3½ years of age.
- Weight 9 kg constant in past 1 year suggesting failure to thrive.

Significant family history: Maternal uncle expired with recurrent pneumonia at 18 years of age.
- *Lab investigation:*
    - IgG, IgM, and IgA were all low.
    - B cells were absent on lymphocyte subset analysis (LSSA).
    - Bruton's tyrosine kinase (BTK) expression by flow cytometry—absent and mother showed carrier pattern **(Figs. 2A and B)**.

Diagnosis: X-linked agammaglobulinemia.

Management: Septran prophylaxis and monthly intravenous immunoglobulin replacement.

Case 2

An 8-month-old male, BK, was admitted with a 1-month history of intermittent fever and progressive abdominal enlargement. His parents are third-degree consanguineous, with a history of adverse pregnancy outcomes: First child (male) died at 3 days of age.

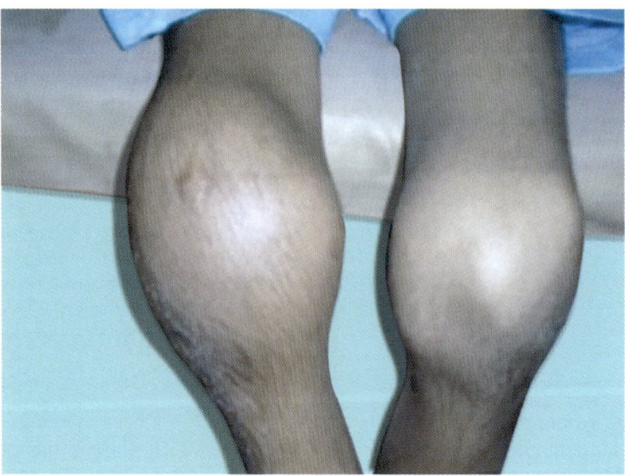

FIG. 1: Bilateral knee joint swelling.

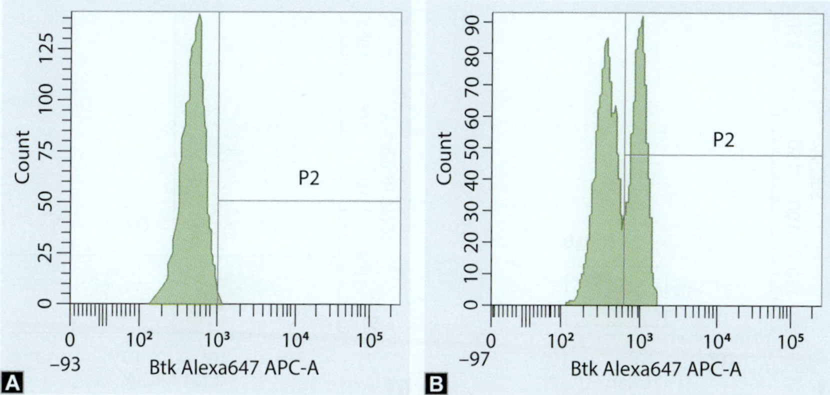

FIGS. 2A AND B: (A) BTK expression by flow cytometry of patient. (B) BTK expression by flow cytometry of mother.

(BTK: Bruton's tyrosine kinase)

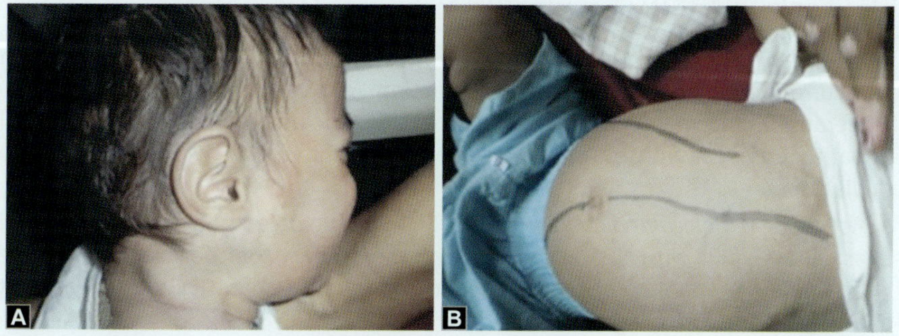

FIGS. 3A AND B: (A) Cervical lymphadenopathy; and (B) Splenomegaly.

Presentation on admission: Afebrile at admission; height, and weight below the 3rd percentile.

Physical examination: Palpable cervical lymph nodes. Hepatomegaly (liver palpable 5 cm below the costal margin). Splenomegaly (spleen palpable 8 cm below the costal margin) **(Figs. 3A and B)**.

Laboratory findings: Hemoglobin—7.7 g/dL, white blood cell count (WBC)—95,700/mm^3, neutrophils 11%, lymphocytes—88%, platelets—196,000/mm^3.

Immunophenotyping: Lymphocyte subset analysis (LSSA) revealed that 87% of lymphocytes were double-negative T-cells (DNT) expressing TCR αβ+, but lacking CD4 and CD8 markers **(Figs. 4A and B)**.

Whole exome sequencing: Homozygous *FAS*:c.110T>A (p.Leu37Ter).

Management: The patient was diagnosed as autoimmune lymphoproliferative syndrome and started on sirolimus with good response.

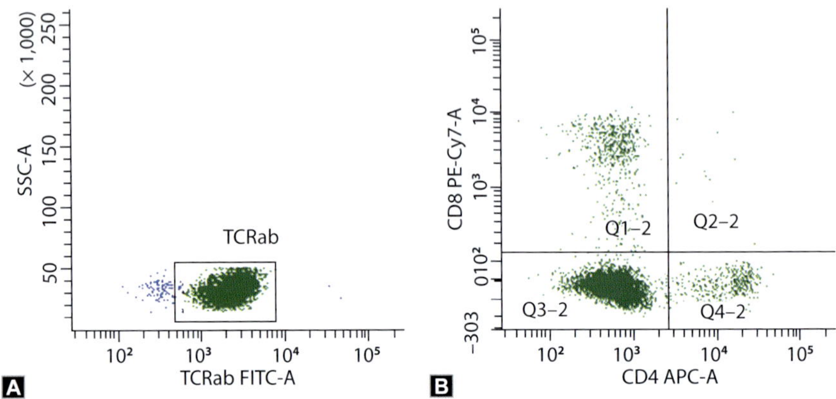

FIGS. 4A AND B: Elevated CD3+ CD4– CD8– TCR αβ T cells.

Take Home Points

- *Diverse clinical manifestations of inborn errors of immunity:* IEI can present with recurrent infections, immune dysregulation (e.g., autoimmunity, lymphoproliferation), and malignancies. Key clinical clues include infections with unusual pathogens, early-onset or atypical autoimmunity, and lymphoproliferative diseases.
- *Advances in molecular diagnostics*: Over 555 genetic defects have been identified as causes of IEI, with NGS and WES being the primary tools for diagnosis. These technologies enable precise identification of genetic variants, guiding treatment and genetic counseling.
- *Emerging therapies and precision medicine:* Recent advancements in targeted therapies (e.g., JAK inhibitors, PI3Kδ inhibitors) and gene therapy are transforming the management of IEI. These approaches offer curative and personalized treatment options, though challenges in accessibility and affordability remain significant barriers to widespread implementation.

SUGGESTED READINGS

1. Tangye SG, Al-Herz W, Bousfiha A, Cunningham-Rundles C, Franco JL, Holland SM, et al. Human inborn errors of immunity: 2022 Update on the Classification from the International Union of Immunological Societies Expert Committee. J Clin Immunol. 2022;42(7):1473-507.
2. Sullivan KE, Stiehm ER. Stiehm's Immune Deficiencies: Inborn Errors of Immunity, 2nd edition. New York: Academic Press; 2020.
3. von Hardenberg S, Klefenz I, Steinemann D, Di Donato N, Baumann U, Auber B, et al. Current genetic diagnostics in inborn errors of immunity. Front Pediatr. 2024;12:1279112.
4. Notarangelo LD, Bacchetta R, Casanova JL, Su HC. Human inborn errors of immunity: An expanding universe. Sci Immunol. 2020;5(49):eabb1662.
5. Aluri J, Cooper MA. Somatic mosaicism in inborn errors of immunity: Current knowledge, challenges, and future perspectives. Semin Immunol. 2023;67:101761.

6. Wan R, Schieck M, Caballero-Oteyza A, Hofmann W, Cochino AV, Shcherbina A, et al. Copy number analysis in a large cohort suggestive of inborn errors of immunity indicates a wide spectrum of relevant chromosomal losses and gains. J Clin Immunol. 2022;42(5): 1083-92.
7. IEI genetics. IUIS IEI data source. [online] Available from https://wp-iuis.s3.eu-west-1.amazonaws.com/app/uploads/2025/01/08170257/IEI-Final-Update-of-2024-Report-Jan-2025.pdf [Last accessed May, 2025].

CHAPTER 31

New Updates in Histiocytic Disorders: Where do We Stand in 2024?

Sarika Singh, Preeti Tripathi, Priyanka Mishra

ABSTRACT

Histiocytic and dendritic cell neoplasms are tumours originating from or showing differentiation toward cells of the mononuclear phagocyte system, which comprise of monocytes, macrophages and dendritic cells. Emerging knowledge on cell of origin and genetic pathophysiology has helped in reclassification and inclusion/exclusion of few entities in this category of disorders. Better diagnostic assays and improved understanding of concepts have led to newer approaches to diagnosing hemophagocytic histiocytic lymphocytic syndrome, confirming suspicion of germline origin in familial Rosai–Dorfman disease and juvenile xanthogranuloma. Targeted therapy has led to emergence of personalized medicine in histiocytic disorders.

INTRODUCTION

Histiocytic neoplasms are rare disorders characterized by the accumulation of myeloid-dendritic cell-derived neoplastic cells with an accompanying inflammatory infiltrate. They are rare disorders with clinical behavior ranging from mild to disseminated, and sometimes, life-threatening forms. Nonspecific and overlapping features often lead to delay in diagnosis and such patients should be referred to centers of expertise for diagnosis and treatment of suspected histiocytic neoplasms.

This category of disorders includes entities originating from mononuclear—macrophage system of the body which include tissue residing macrophages, hematopoietic stem cells (HSC) derived monocytes, and dendritic cells. With origin both from yolk sac/liver and bone marrow, these disorders are difficult to classify. The original classification of histiocytic neoplasms by the Working Group of the Histiocyte Society (1987) initially categorized them as Langerhans cell and non-Langerhans cell predominantly. However, this was not found to be appropriate, as both categories showed many overlapping molecular features.

In 2016, the Histiocyte Society published a revised classification dividing them into five groups of diseases: (1) *L-group*—Langerhans cell related, (2) *C-group*—cutaneous and mucocutaneous (3) *M-group*—malignant histiocytoses, (4) *R-group*—Rosai-Dorfman disease (RDD), and (5) *H group*—hemophagocytic lymphohistiocytic (primary and secondary) syndrome. This classification grouped both neoplastic and reactive disorders into various groups as per their predominant clinical feature. The World Health Organization (WHO) classification of hematolymphoid malignancy, however, follows a slightly different approach and includes only the disorders with neoplastic potential. The recently gained knowledge in the genetic origin of these disorders has led to important changes which are discussed in detail in the following text.

CELL OF ORIGIN AND CHANGE IN CLASSIFICATION AS PER WHO 2022 HEMATOLYMPHOID MALIGNANCY 5TH REVISION

The mononuclear phagocyte system—mononuclear phagocytes are specialized cells of the innate immune system which are the first responder in case of any infection. These include tissue residing macrophages, HSC derived monocytes and dendritic cells as shown in **Figure 1**.

Plasmacytoid dendritic cell (pDC) can be generated from common myeloid progenitors (via common dendritic cell progenitors) as well as from common lymphoid progenitors. In 5th edition of WHO hematolymphoid malignancies, blastic plasmacytoid dendritic cell neoplasm (BPDCN) has been included under category of histiocytic neoplasm rather than myeloid malignancies. Similarly, follicular dendritic cells and fibroblastic reticular cells, which are of mesenchymal

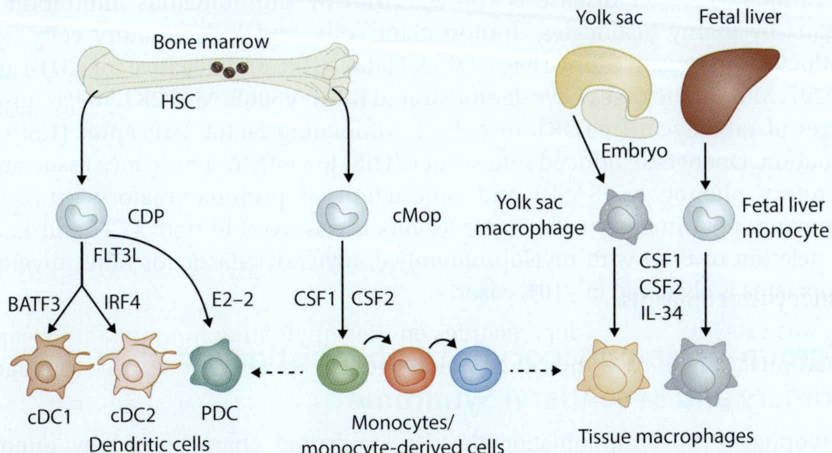

FIG. 1: Display of cell/organ of origin of various components of mononuclear-macrophage system of human body.

(CSF: colony-stimulating factor; HSC: hematopoietic stem cells; IL: interleukin)

origin, are no longer considered part of the mononuclear-phagocyte system. Hence, a separate category of "stromal-derived neoplasms of lymphoid tissues" has been identified for these disorders. Introduction of some new entities such as mature pDC proliferation associated with myeloid neoplasm, Rosai-Dorfman disease, and anaplastic lymphoma kinase (ALK)-positive histiocytosis has been added in the new revised classification.

L-group—Langerhans Cell Histiocytosis-related Group

The L-group comprises Langerhans cell histiocytosis (LCH), Erdheim-Chester disease (ECD) mixed LCH-ECD, and indeterminate cell histiocytosis (ICH). LCH is predominantly seen in children <15 years of age and characterized by infiltration of organs with oval shaped cells with coffee-bean nuclei that are positive for CD207 (langerin), CD1a and S100. Based on the number of sites involved, LCH is classified as single system unifocal, single system multifocal, single system pulmonary, single system central nervous system (CNS), and multisystem with/without risk organ involvement (liver, spleen, or bone marrow). The bone and the skin are the most common sites and multisystem LCH with risk organ involvement have reduced survival rates with risk of relapse.

The most common mutation is BRAF V600E (substitution of valine by glutamate at position 600) seen in approx. 60% of LCH causes constitutive activation of MEK/ERK signaling pathway. Mutations in MAP2K1 encoding for MEK account for 30% of cases. The "activated immature model" proposed initially postulated that aberrant Langerhans cells (LCs) proliferated and migrated to various organs of the body forming the lesions of LCH. This was later replaced by "misguided myeloid DC (dendritic cell) precursor model" arise from different myeloid precursors and severity of disease is determined by the stage of differentiation of the precursor cells.

Erdheim-Chester disease is characterized by xanthomatous infiltration of organs by foamy histiocytes, Touton giant cells, and inflammatory cells. The histiocytes are positive for CD68, CD163, factor XIIIa, and negative for CD1a and CD207. Most of the cases have demonstrated BRAF V600E, MAP2K1, mechanistic target of rapamycin (mTOR), or colony stimulating factor 1 receptor (CSF1R) mutation. Oncogene induced senescence (OIS) leading to senescence associated secretory phenotype (SASP) and production of proinflammatory cytokines attracting inflammatory cells in the lesions is observed in both LCH and ECD. Association of ECD with myeloproliferative, myelodysplastic, or other myeloid neoplasms is observed in ~10% cases.

H-group—Hemophagocytic Lymphohistiocytic (Primary and Secondary) Syndrome

Hemophagocytic lymphohistiocytic is a syndrome characterized by intense immune activation causing fever, cytopenias, hepatosplenomegaly, and hyperferritinemia. It is divided into primary and secondary HLH with both having overlapped clinical features. While primary HLH is a familial disorder, secondary HLH is reactive to underlying infections/malignancy or autoimmune disorders. Symptoms of HLH developing in a patient with an underlying rheumatic condition are historically called macrophage activation syndrome (MAS)—this subset of disorders are called MAS-HLH syndrome. First-line treatment of both primary and secondary HLH is directed to control hyperinflammation but for primary HLH, HSC transplantation (HSCT) is the only available cure, and hence, it is essential to identify this subset of patients.

Primary HLH is associated with impairment or disturbance of the inflammasome formation, however, few still await discovery of exact genetic defect. The HLH 2004 criteria widely used for diagnosis of primary/secondary HLH have certain limitations like nonavailability of certain tests [Natural killer (NK) cell activity] and lack of genetic marker which can lead to fatal delays. Henter et al. has described a three-way approach to diagnosing primary HLH after studying a large cohort of patients with established familial HLH as per the **Table 1**. When and where to use each diagnostic pathway will depend on the clinical situation. The clinical pathway can rapidly help to decide on whether to initiate HLH-directed therapy. The cellular pathway may help at a later stage in giving additional predictions on the likelihood of familial hemophagocytic lymphohistiocytosis (FHL). For decisions on therapeutic options like HSCT, it is advised that primary HLH be confirmed through genetic analysis.

For diagnosing secondary HLH, the most widely used criteria is still the HLH-2004 score proposed by the Histiocyte Society. It was developed in pediatric population with primary HLH. Its use for the diagnosis of secondary HLH has not been validated by any study. In addition, 2 of the 8 criteria (soluble CD25 and NK cell activity) are not commonly available. To address these shortcomings, in 2014, Fardet et al. established a diagnostic probability score entitled the H-score tailored for adult patients with suspected secondary HLH. This serves as a good

TABLE 1: Three-way approach and revised diagnostic criteria to diagnose primary familial hemophagocytic lymphohistiocytic.

Genetic approach	Clinical approach	Clinical approach
Biallelic combination of large deletions, nonsense variants, and other previously well-described disease-causing genetic aberrations in FHL-associated genes	Absent/impaired perforin expression or defective cytotoxic lymphocyte exocytosis	Requires 5 out of 7 criteria: 1. Fever ≥38.5°C 2. Splenomegaly (≥2 cm below the costal margin) 3. Bicytopenia (hemoglobin <90 g/L; platelets $<100 \times 10^9$/L; neutrophils $<1.0 \times 10^9$/L) 4. Hypertriglyceridemia and/or hypofibrinogenemia (fasting triglycerides 23.0 mmol/L and fibrinogen ≤1.5 g/L) 5. Hemophagocytosis in BM/LN/liver/spleen 6. Serum ferritin ≥500 μg/L 7. sCD25 levels (soluble interleukin-2 receptor) ≥2,400 U/mL

clinical indicator to initiate the therapy in cases with high suspicion. The best differentiating cutoff value for the H-score was 169 in her study corresponding to a sensitivity of 93%, specificity of 86%, and accurate classification of 90% of patients, however, authors concluded that the performance of this score should be studied in other larger series.

R-group—Rosai–Dorfman Syndrome

This group includes Rosai–Dorfman disease (also called Rosai-Dorfman-Destombes disease) which is characterized by accumulation of abnormal histiocytes in nodal/extranodal sites showing characteristic emperipolesis. The term sinus histiocytosis with massive lymphadenopathy is no longer acceptable in formal mentions as per WHO 5th edition. Cause is unknown but may be associated with familial, autoimmune, and/or malignant processes and can also co-occur with other hematolymphoid malignancies. Rare inherited disorders predispose to familial RDD including those associated with germline mutations in the nucleoside transporter SCL29A3 (also called H syndrome/Faisalabad histiocytosis), and FAS deficiency with heterozygous germline mutations in *TNFRSF6* gene encoding FAS (autoimmune lymphoproliferative syndrome). These mutations are not known to be associated with sporadic RDD.

The pathogenesis of RDD is incompletely understood but approximately 50% of cases carry gain-of-function mutations in the mitogen-activated protein kinase (MAPK)/ERK pathway, including KRAS, NRAS, MAPK21, ARAF, CSF1R, and BRAF p.V600E, suggesting that at least a proportion of cases of RDD represent a neoplastic disorder. The typical presentation is that of painless, slow-growing massive lymphadenopathy, with B-symptoms. Histopathologic analysis of RDD can be challenging, as RDD tissue tends to contain relatively few lesional cells. Large histiocytic cells with hypochromatic nuclei and an abundant amount of pale cytoplasm showing emperipolesis, specifically intracytoplasmic leukocytes, is a frequently observed feature of RDD. However, emperipolesis may be observed less often in extranodal lesion tissue. Other pathologic hallmarks include the accumulation of CD68-positive, CD163-positive, CD14-positive, and S100-positive histiocytic cells which are negative for CD1a and CD207 (Langerin) but may show positivity for cyclin D1 and OCT2. Molecular testing can be done either in a stepwise fashion or in parallel, depending on clinical indication and institutional protocols. The disease often resolves spontaneously but targeted MEK (encoded by MAP2K1) inhibitors may be helpful in patients with persistent disease or recurrence.

C-group—Cutaneous and Mucocutaneous Histiocytosis

The various diseases included in this family can be defined by the clinical setting, that is, solitary, multiple, or disseminated. Juvenile xanthogranuloma (JXG) is the most common of these. It is a benign disorder which appears during the first years of life and presents with single/multiple nodular lesions. The etiology of JXG is largely unknown but it may occur in patients affected by neurofibromatosis and Wiskott-Aldrich syndrome. MAPK/ERK pathway alterations play a pathogenetic role in JXG. Activating mutations of NRAS, KRAS, ARAF, MAP2K1, and CSF1R,

RNF1::BRAF, and NTRK1 fusions have also been reported. Cases with systemic JXGs with CNS involvement and BRAF p.V600E mutation probably represent ECD instead of JXG.

Histologically, JXG appear as well-circumscribed dermal or dermohypodermal nodules sparing the epidermis. Mature lesions contain foamy cells, foreign-body giant cells, and Touton cells as well as macrophages, lymphocytes, and eosinophils. Older, regressing lesions show proliferation of fibroblasts and fibrosis that replace part of the infiltrate. Immunohistochemistry shows immunophenotype of dermal macrophage (CD68/CD163/Factor XIIIa) with negativity for CD1a/Langerin and ALK. JXG has excellent prognosis, with a self-limiting course and favorable outcome except in uncommon cases with systemic dissemination.

Disseminated JXD affects young men with prominent mucosal and visceral component mainly located on the flexor areas and around the eyes. Diabetes insipidus is encountered in about 40% of cases. The course of the disease is chronic and persistent. Treatment with clofarabine, cladribine, or cytarabine combined with cladribine have been used in these patients with variable response. Treatment with targeted kinase (BRAF) inhibition is also a newer option for those that fail conventional treatment.

M-group—Malignant Histiocytosis

Malignant histiocytosis (MH) is classified as an exceedingly rare subtype of histiocytic neoplasms, with an estimated incidence rate of <1 case per million individuals. This condition can manifest in both children and adults; however, it is more frequently identified within the adult population. MH may occur as a solitary condition (primary MH) or in conjunction with other hematological malignancies, such as leukemia or lymphoma (secondary MH). The classification of MH includes three distinct entities: histiocytic sarcoma (HS), Langerhans cell sarcoma (LCS), and interdigitating dendritic cell sarcoma (IDCS), with HS constituting the majority of MH cases.

The typical age at diagnosis is approximately 60 years; nonetheless, MH has been documented in both pediatric and geriatric patients. MH can impact any organ system, with the lymph nodes, bone, lungs, skin, bone marrow, and CNS being the most frequently affected sites. Approximately one-third of patients with MH present with a single site of disease (unifocal MH), while the remainder exhibit multiple sites of involvement (multifocal MH). The designation "malignant" typically indicates an aggressive disease course; however, there exist several instances of unifocal MH that exhibit indolent behavior and favorable prognoses.

RECENT ADVANCES

Histiocytic/Dendritic Cell Neoplasms

These NEOPLASMS are placed in recent amendments of WHO Classification of Hematolymphoid Neoplasms, after myeloid neoplasms in recognition of the fact that they derive from common myeloid progenitors that give rise to cells of the monocytic/histiocytic/dendritic lineages.

BOX 1: Dendritic cell and histiocytic neoplasms.

Plasmacytoid dendritic cell neoplasms:
- Mature plasmacytoid dendritic cell proliferation associated with myeloid neoplasm
- Blastic plasmacytoid dendritic cell neoplasm

Langerhans cells neoplasms:
- Langerhans cell histiocytosis
- Langerhans cell sarcoma

Other dendritic cell neoplasms:
- Indeterminate dendritic cell tumor
- Interdigitating dendritic cell sarcoma

Histiocytic neoplasms:
- Histiocytic sarcoma
- ALK positive histiocytosis

Key changes in the current edition of the classification include **(Box 1)**:
- Inclusion of clonal pDC diseases in this category.
- Moving follicular dendritic cell sarcoma and fibroblastic reticular cell tumor to a separate category.
- Rosai–Dorfman disease and ALK positive histiocytosis as disease types.

Plasmacytoid Dendritic Cell Neoplasms

Recognition of clonal proliferations detected in association with myeloid neoplasms and refinement/update of the diagnostic criteria for blastic pDC neoplasm.

Mature plasmacytoid dendritic cell proliferation (MPDCP) associated with myeloid neoplasms reflects that these represent clonal proliferation of pDCs with low grade morphology in context of a defined myeloid neoplasm. Clonal MPDCP cells accumulate in the bone marrow of patients with myeloproliferative chronic myelomonocytic leukemia (CMML) harboring activating RAS mutations. Patients with acute myeloid leukemia (AML) can have clonally expanded pDCs (pDC-AML) which share similar mutational aberrations as CD34-positive blasts and frequent association with RUNX1 mutation. Though its relationship with myelodysplastic syndrome (MDS)/MDS-myeloproliferative neoplasms (MPN) and MDS associated AML is yet not well understood, the diagnostic criteria remain the same as earlier and need detailed immunophenotyping.

Dendritic and Histiocytic Neoplasms and Anaplastic Lymphoma Kinase Positive Histiocytosis

These disorders including ECD show mutation in MAPK pathway such as BRAF, ARAF, MAP2K1, NRAS, and KRAS.

The ALK positive histiocytosis shows a broad clinicopathological spectrum with ALK gene mutation (KIF5B: ALK). This is a MAPK signaling pathway derived disease which further mediates ALK activation. These genetic pathways have brought a promising breakthrough in targeted therapy especially using BRAF and MEK inhibitors.

Histiocytic neoplasms in association or following leukemia/lymphoma: A small subset of histiocytic neoplasm occurs in this background especially in association with follicular lymphoma, chronic lymphocytic leukemia, and Tor B-cell acute lymphoblastic leukemia (B-ALL). These lesions can show the same clonal markers and/or genetic changes and at times can show additional genetic aberrations, thus pointing toward transdifferentiation as well as divergent differentiation from a common leukemia/lymphoma progenitor.

Recent advancements in the diagnostic and therapeutic approaches to MH have centered on elucidating its molecular pathophysiology and the formulation of targeted treatment modalities. MH, a rare neoplastic disorder originating from the macrophage-dendritic cell lineage, manifests with diverse clinical presentations and prognoses, frequently impacted by the severity of the disease and the degree of organ involvement. Contemporary research has underscored the importance of genetic alterations, particularly within the MAPK signaling pathway, in the etiology of MH, thereby guiding the innovation of novel therapeutic interventions.

MOLECULAR ABERRATIONS AND DIAGNOSIS

Genetic investigations have uncovered somatic mutations within the MAPK pathway, encompassing genes such as *BRAF* and *MAP2K1*, which imply a clonal neoplastic characteristic of MH. Targeted next-generation sequencing has emerged as an indispensable diagnostic instrument, uncovering pathogenic mutations in 86% of the patient cohort examined, with mutations in the MAPK pathway identified in 73% of the instances.

TREATMENT ADVANCEMENTS

Chemotherapy continues to serve as a prevalent first-line intervention for multifocal MH, while surgical resection is frequently employed for unifocal cases. Targeted therapies, particularly BRAF inhibitors such as vemurafenib and dabrafenib, have demonstrated efficacy in managing high-risk cases. Despite ongoing challenges related to relapse and adverse effects, MEK inhibitors, including cobimetinib, have received approval for use in adult patients, providing an additional pathway for targeted treatment.

PROGNOSIS AND OUTCOMES

- The prognosis for MH is intrinsically linked to the extent of the disease and the involvement of various organs, with multifocal disease correlating with markedly poorer outcomes in comparison to unifocal disease. Patients exhibiting risk organ involvement, including but not limited to the bone marrow, spleen, or liver, experience significantly worse outcomes.
- Despite substantial advancements in the comprehension and management of MH, obstacles persist, particularly regarding the management of therapy interruptions, and the determination of optimal treatment durations. Ongoing research is vital to enhance these treatment strategies and elevate

patient outcomes, underscoring the necessity for continuous investigation into molecular genetics, and targeted therapies within the realm of histiocytic neoplasms.

FUTURE RESEARCH

- Future investigations should concentrate on elucidating the biological disparities among the diverse lineage subtypes of MH to ascertain potential prognostic and therapeutic biomarkers that could ameliorate patient outcomes.
- Additional research with more extensive sample sizes and multivariate analyses is imperative to derive more conclusive insights regarding the influence of phenotypic, clinical, and genotypic characteristics on prognosis.
- Examining the mechanisms that govern the activation of the MAPK signaling pathway and its correlation with cyclin D1 expression may yield valuable understanding of the pathobiology associated with these neoplasms.

Moreover, a thorough investigation of epigenetic mutations in secondary MH cases, particularly those with antecedent B-cell lymphoma, is deemed necessary.

ACKNOWLEDGEMENT

This is to acknowledge Dr Bharani Dharan (Consultant, Apollo Hospital, Chennai) for helping in manuscript preparation with Dr Sarika Singh.

Take Home Points

- *Targeted therapies:* There has been significant progress in the development of targeted therapies for malignant histiocytic disorders, particularly for conditions LCH and histiocytic sarcoma. Drugs targeting specific mutations, such as BRAF and MAPK pathways, have shown promise in clinical trials.
- *Immunotherapy*: Advances in immunotherapy, including checkpoint inhibitors and CAR T-cell therapy, are being explored for treating histiocytic disorders. These approaches aim to enhance the immune response against malignant histiocytes.
- *Genomic profiling*: The use of genomic profiling has become more prevalent, allowing for the identification of specific mutations and alterations in histiocytic disorders. This information can help tailor treatment strategies to individual patients.
- *Combination therapies*: Research is focusing on combination therapies that integrate targeted agents with conventional chemotherapy or immunotherapy to improve outcomes in patients with refractory or relapsed histiocytic disorders.
- *Clinical trials*: There has been an increase in clinical trials dedicated to malignant histiocytic disorders, providing new opportunities for patients to access cutting-edge treatments and contribute to the understanding of these diseases.

- *Improved classification*: Advances in the classification of histiocytic disorders have led to better understanding and differentiation between various subtypes, which is crucial for appropriate management and treatment.
- *Longitudinal studies*: Ongoing longitudinal studies are helping to elucidate the long-term outcomes of patients with malignant histiocytic disorders, aiding in the development of more effective treatment protocols.

SUGGESTED READINGS

1. Emile JF, Abla O, Fraitag S, Horne A, Haroche J, Donadieu J, et al. Revised classification of histiocytoses and neoplasms of the macrophage-dendritic cell lineages. Blood. 2016;127(22):2672-81.
2. Khoury JD, Solary E, Abla O, Akkari Y, Alaggio R, Apperley JF, et al. The 5th edition of the World Health Organization Classification of Haematolymphoid Tumours: Myeloid and histiocytic/dendritic neoplasms. Leukemia. 2022;36(7):1703-19.
3. Go RS, Jacobsen E, Baiocchi R, Buhtoiarov I, Butler EB, Campbell PK, et al. Histiocytic neoplasms, Version 2.2021, NCCN Clinical Practice Guidelines in Oncology. J Natl Compr Canc Netw. 2021;19(11):1277-303.
4. Sconocchia T, Foßelteder J, Sconocchia G, Reinisch A. Langerhans cell histiocytosis: current advances in molecular pathogenesis. Frontiers in Immunology. 2023;14:1275085.
5. Kulkarni AM, Gayam PK, Aranjani JM. Advances in understanding and management of Erdheim-Chester disease. Life Sciences. 2024;348:122692.
6. Henter J-I, Sieni E, Eriksson J, Bergsten E, Myrberg IH, Canna SW, et al. Diagnostic guidelines for familial hemophagocytic lymphohistiocytosis revisited. Blood. 2024;144(22):2308-18.
7. Abla O, Jacobsen E, Picarsic J, Krenova Z, Jaffe R, Emile JF, et al. Consensus recommendations for the diagnosis and clinical management of Rosai Dorfman-Destombes disease. Blood. 2018;131(26):2877-90.
8. Ceppi F, Abla O. Juvenile xanthogranuloma and related Non-LCH disorders. In: Abla O, Janka G (Eds). Histiocytic Disorders. Cham: Springer; 2018.
9. Ruan GJ, Zanwar S, Ravindran A, Schram S, Abeykoon JP, Hazim A, et al. Mayo Clinic-University of Alabama at Birmingham Histiocytosis Working Group. Clinical characteristics, molecular aberrations, treatments, and outcomes of malignant histiocytosis. Am J Hematol. 2024;99(5):871-9.
10. Koh KN, Yoon SH, Kang SH, Kim H, Im HJ. Advancements in the understanding and management of histiocytic neoplasms. Blood Res. 2024;59(1):22.
11. Histiocyte society. [online] Available from https://www.histiocytesociety.org/ [Last accessed May, 2025].
12. WHO. Classification of Tumours. [online] Available from https://tumourclassification.iarc.who.int/[Last accessed May, 2025].

CHAPTER 32

Role of Genomic Techniques in the Management of Acute Leukemia

Prakhar Gupta, Mayur Parihar

ABSTRACT

The genomic landscape of acute leukemia is a complex yet critically informative terrain that shapes modern hematologic oncology. This chapter delves into the transformative role of genomic technologies in decoding the molecular heterogeneity of acute leukemias, thereby guiding diagnosis, risk stratification, minimal residual disease (MRD) monitoring, and targeted therapy. It introduces the full spectrum of diagnostic tools—including karyotyping, FISH, PCR, RT-qPCR, digital PCR, Sanger sequencing, and next-generation sequencing (NGS)—with a comparative analysis of their resolution, sensitivity, advantages, and limitations. With the advent of high-resolution tools clinicians and pathologists now possess unprecedented capabilities to unveil genetic alterations that define distinct leukemic subtypes. Designed for pathology residents, this chapter serves as a foundational framework for understanding the clinical relevance of molecular diagnostics in leukemias. It provides a side-by-side comparison of test modalities, real-world case applications, and guidance on test selection, offering a practical starting point for students aiming to deepen their knowledge and confidently approach hematologic malignancies through a molecular lens.

INTRODUCTION

Genomic profiling of acute leukemias has revolutionized our understanding of tumor biology helping us define the genetic basis of hematological neoplasms, refining the classification of patients into clinically relevant subgroups with identification of new subtypes. The multiple genetic subtypes are characterized by sentinel chromosomal aberrations or mutations that drive the neoplastic process. The abnormalities include chromosomal rearrangements and/or aneuploidies involving genes coding for transcription factors (*RUNX1, TCF3*), epigenetic modifiers *(KMT2A)* cytokine receptors (*CRLF2*), and tyrosine kinases (*ABL1, ABL2*). The founding mutations alter key cellular pathways like those involved in transcription (*CEBPA*), cell cycle regulation (*NPM1*), splicing factor regulation (*SRSF2, SF3B1*), and tumor suppressors (*TP53*).

Identification of these genetic abnormalities is an essential component of modern risk-stratified therapy protocols. The cytogenetic and molecular genetic studies are essential to identify specific genetically defined entities, risk stratification and potential minimal residual disease (MRD) markers to assess clinical progression and response to treatment. The genetic characterization of tumors enables the appropriate intensification of therapy for patients at increased risk for treatment failure as well as the deintensification of therapy (and consequent reduction in treatment-related toxicity) in patients with favorable risk features.

A summary of the primary genetic abnormalities that are diagnostic of defined specific subtypes based on the two recent classification systems [the World Health Organization classification of hematolymphoid tumors (WHO-HAEM) 5th edition and the International Consensus Classification (ICC)] of acute leukemia is elucidated in **Table 1**.

TABLE 1: A comparison of the ICC 2022 and WHO 5th edition, 2022.

ICC 2022 updates	WHO 2022
Acute myeloid leukemia (AML)	
• Acute promyelocytic leukemia (APL) with t(15;17)(q24.1;q21.2)/PML::RARA) (≥10% blasts) • APL with other RARA rearrangements (≥10% blasts)	Acute promyelocytic leukemia with *PML::RARA* fusion*
• AML with t(8;21) (q22;q22.1i)/RUNX1::RUNX1T1) (≥10% blasts)	AML with *RUNX1::RUNX1T1* fusion*
• AML with inv(16)(p13.1;q22) or t(16;16) (p13.1;q22)/iCBFB:MYH11)(≥10% blasts)	AML with *CBFB::MYH11* fusion*
• AML with t(9;11) (p21.3;q23.3)/MLLT3::KTM2A) (≥10% blasts)	• AML with *KMT2A* rearrangement*
• AML with other *KMT2A* rearrangements (≥10% blasts)	• AML with *KMT2A* rearrangement*
• AML with t (6;9) (p22.3;q34.1)/*DEK*::NUP214) (≥10% blasts)	AML with *DEK::NUP214* fusion*
• AML with inv(3)(q21.3q;26.2) or t(3;3)(q21.3;q26.2)/*GATA2::MECOM(EVI1)* (≥10% blasts)	• AML with *MECOM* rearrangements*
• AML with other *MECOM* rearrangements (≥ 10% blasts)	• AML with *MECOM* rearrangements*
• AML with other rare recurring translocations (≥10% blasts), including *NUP98* rearrangement and *RBM15::MRTF1* fusion	AML with other defined genetic alterations (rare fusions)*
AML with t (9;22) (q34.1;q11.2)/BCR:: ABL1) (≥ 20% blasts)	AML with BCR::ABL1 fusion (≥20% blasts)
AML with mutated *NPM1* (≥10% blasts)	AML with *NPM1* mutation*
AML with in-frame bZIP *CEBPA* mutations (≥10% blasts)	AML with *CEBPA* mutation (≥20% blasts)
AML with mutated *TP53* (≥20% blasts)	
AML with myelodysplasia-related gene mutations (*ASXL1, BCOR, EZH2, RUNX1, SF3B1, SRSF2, STAG2, U2AF1, or ZRSR2*) (≥20% blasts)	AML, myelodysplasia-related (≥20% blasts)
AML with myelodysplasia-related cytogenetic abnormalities (≥20% blasts)	AML, myelodysplasia-related (≥20% blasts)
AML not otherwise specified (NOS) (≥20% blasts)	AML, defined by differentiation (≥20% blasts)

Continued

Continued

ICC 2022 updates	WHO 2022
B-cell acute lymphoblastic leukemia (B-ALL) with recurrent genetic abnormalities	
B-ALL with t(9;22)(q34.1;q11.2)/*BCR::ABL1*	B-lymphoblastic leukemia/lymphoma with *BCR::ABL1 fusion*
B-ALL with t(v;11q23.3)/*KMT2A* rearranged	B-lymphoblastic leukemia/lymphoma with *KMT2A* rearrangement
B-ALL with t(12;21)(p13.2;q22.1)/*ETV6::RUNX1*	B-lymphoblastic leukemia/lymphoma with *ETV6*::RUNX1 fusion
B-ALL, hyperdiploid	B-lymphoblastic leukemia/lymphoma with high hyperdiploidy
B-ALL, low hypodiploid	B-lymphoblastic leukemia/lymphoma with hypodiploidy
B-ALL, near haploid	
B-ALL with t(5;14)(q31.1;q32.3)/*IL3::IGH*	B-lymphoblastic leukemia/lymphoma with *IGH::IL3 fusion*
B-ALL with t(1;19)(q23.3;p13.3)/*TCF3::PBX1*	B-lymphoblastic leukemia/lymphoma with *TCF3::PBX1 fusion*
B-ALL, BCR::ABL1-like, *ABL*-1 class rearranged B-ALL, BCR::ABL1-like, JAK-STAT activated	B-lymphoblastic leukemia/lymphoma with *BCR::ABL1*-like features
B-ALL, *BCR::ABL1*-like, NOS	B-lymphoblastic leukemia/lymphoma, NOS
B-ALL with iAMP21	B-lymphoblastic leukemia/lymphoma with iAMP21
B-ALL with HLF rearrangement	B-lymphoblastic leukemia/lymphoma with *TCF3::HLF* fusion
• B-ALL with *MYC* rearrangement • B-ALL with *DUX4* rearrangement • B-ALL with *MEF2D* rearrangement • B-ALL with *ZNF384* rearrangement • B-ALL with *NUTM1* rearrangement • B-ALL with *UBTF::ATXN7L3/PAN3, CDX2* ("CDX2/UBTF") • B-ALL with *IKZF1* N159Y • B-ALL with *PAX5* P80R *Provisional entities*: • B-ALL, *ETV6::RUNX1*-like • B-ALL, with *PAX5* alteration • B-ALL, with mutated *ZEB2* (p.H1038R)/IGH::CEBPE • B-ALL, *ZNF384* rearranged-like • B-ALL, *KMT2A* rearranged-like	B-lymphoblastic leukemia/lymphoma with other defined genetic abnormalities
T-acute lymphoblastic leukemia (T-ALL)	
Early T-cell precursor ALL, *BCL11B*-activated	Early T-precursor lymphoblastic leukemia/lymphoma
Early T-cell precursor ALL, NOS	
T-ALL, NOS	T-lymphoblastic leukemia/lymphoma, NOS
Provisional entity: Natural killer (NK) cell ALL	Entity deleted

*No bone marrow blast number cutoff.

TYPES OF GENETIC ABNORMALITIES–SPECTRUM OF GENETIC ABNORMALITIES

Genetic alterations drive cancer development by disrupting normal cell cycle control, promoting uncontrolled proliferation, and allowing cells to evade apoptosis. A brief description of these genetic abnormalities along with the level of resolution at which they occur and most common cytogenetic and molecular techniques to detect are summarized in **Table 2**. The different genetic abnormalities include the following.

TABLE 2: Genetic alterations with the level of resolution and common techniques in their detection.

Type of abnormality/ genetic alteration	Description	Level of resolution	Common techniques used
Aneuploidy (e.g., whole chromosome gains/losses)	Abnormal number of chromosomes due to mitotic errors, leading to genomic instability	Chromosome level (5–10 Mb)	• *Karyotyping* (detects large chromosomal changes), *FISH* (specific chromosome probes), *array CGH* (high-resolution copy number analysis) • *Whole genome sequencing* • *RNA sequencing*
Chromosomal translocations (e.g., fusion genes)	Exchange of chromosome segments leading to oncogene activation or tumor suppressor inactivation	Chromosome/ subchromosomal (≥3–5 Mb)	*Karyotyping* (large-scale changes), *FISH* (targeted detection), *RT-PCR* (detects fusion transcripts), *NGS* (comprehensive fusion gene analysis)
Chromosomal deletions	Loss of chromosomal regions containing tumor suppressor genes, leading to unchecked cell growth	Subchromosomal (50 kb–5 Mb)	*FISH* (targeted deletions), *Array CGH* (genome-wide deletion detection), *MLPA* (specific region analysis)
Gene amplifications	Multiple copies of oncogenes lead to overexpression and uncontrolled proliferation	Subchromosomal (50 kb–5 Mb)	*FISH* (gene-specific detection), *array CGH* (genome-wide copy number changes), *qPCR* (quantitative amplification analysis)
Single nucleotide variants (SNVs)	Single base-pair changes leading to altered protein function, driving tumor progression	Base-pair level (1 bp)	*PCR* (targeted detection), *Sanger sequencing* (small-scale mutations), *NGS* (high-throughput mutation analysis)

Continued

Continued

Type of abnormality/ genetic alteration	Description	Level of resolution	Common techniques used
Small insertions/ deletions (Indels)	Small base-pair insertions or deletions causing frameshift mutations or altered protein function	Base-pair to few bp level	PCR, Sanger sequencing, NGS
Copy number variations (CNVs)	Large insertions or deletions affecting gene dosage and oncogene activation	Subchromosomal (50 kb–5 Mb)	*Array CGH, MLPA, qPCR, NGS*

(CGH: comparative genomic hybridization; FISH: fluorescence in situ hybridization; MLPA; multiplex ligation-dependent probe amplification; NGS: next-generation sequencing; qPCR: quantitative polymerase chain reaction)

Copy Number Abnormalities

Any gain or loss of genetic material from the genome is defined as a copy number abnormality. Based on the size of the copy number abnormalities can be enumerated as:

- *Aneuploidies:* It is defined as an abnormal gain or loss of chromosomes. It can range from gain or loss of single chromosomes example trisomy 8 and/ or monosomy 7 in acute myeloid leukemia (AMLs) or multiple chromosomes for example high hyperdiploidy (51–65 chromosomes) and hypodiploidy (<40 chromosomes). The pathogenic effect of aneuploidies is gene dosage effect resulting in widespread change in global gene expression.
- *Deletion of a segment or arm of a chromosome:* Deletions involve the loss of a segment or an entire arm of a chromosome, resulting in haploinsufficiency of the genes present on the deleted segment. Example deletion 5q deletion 7q seen in myeloid malignancies, deletion 9p seen in acute lymphoblastic leukemia (ALL).
- *Deletion of an entire gene or deletion of exons/introns within a gene:* Deletion/ loss of an entire gene exons/introns results in haploinsufficiency of the gene product result in either loss of function of the gene or dominant negative isoforms that prevent the normal allele of the gene from functioning optimally. *Example:* Deletion of entire gene—*TP53* in AML; *Intrageneic deletions resulting in dominant negative isoforms*—exons 4–7 deletion in *IKZF1* gene in ALL.
- *Duplication of a segment or an arm of a chromosome:* The pathogenic impact being gene dosage effects. *Example:* Duplication 1q in ALL.
- *Amplification of a gene:* Amplification of genes results in multiple copies of a gene arising from breakage-fusion-bridge cycles, a mechanism driven by chromosomal instability. *Examples:* Intrachromosomal amplification of the *MLL/KMT2A* gene in AML and iAMP21 in ALL.

- *Insertion/deletion of nucleotides:* These insertions or deletions of nucleotides disrupt the reading frame/coding sequence resulting in abnormal transcription and translation. *Example: FLT3 ITD, NPM1* indel mutations.

Translocations

Chromosomal translocations are a result of exchange of segments or regions of chromosomes that may or may not result in formation of fusion genes. The translocations may further be classified as balanced or unbalanced translocation. Balanced translocations do not result in loss or gain of genetic material whereas, unbalanced translocations result in loss or gain of genetic material. Some of the translocations are cryptic and cannot be identified on karyotype, example, t(12;21)(p13;q22)/*ETV6::RUNX1* fusion and can only be identified by fluorescence in situ hybridization (FISH) or molecular techniques. Certain translocations like t(8;14)(q24;34) result in juxtaposition of genes to enhancer elements resulting in overexpression of the gene without the formation of a chimeric transcript. These translocations are identified by DNA-based tests rather than RNA-based tests.

Single Nucleotide Variants/Mutations

In acute leukemia single nucleotide variants (SNVs) can impact transcription factors, oncogenes, tumor suppressor genes, genes involved in cell cycle, and signaling pathways. Mutations in some genes also increase germline predisposition to develop leukemias (e.g., *RUNX1*).

These mutations can be identified either by specific polymerase chain reaction (PCRs), Sanger sequencing, or next-generation sequencing (NGS) either targeted or exome or whole genome.

SAMPLE SELECTION FOR MOLECULAR TESTING

Sample selection and optimal anticoagulant are crucial to produce reliable results in a clinical laboratory. Blood and bone marrow samples for cytogenetic analysis are best preserved using heparin, an anticoagulant that binds to antithrombin III, effectively inhibiting thrombin activation and preventing clot formation. However, heparin interferes with the PCR-based assays because of its inhibitory effect on the polymerase enzyme, hence, is not suitable for molecular studies.

The results of a molecular test depend largely on the quantity and quality of nucleic acid isolated from a sample, which are highly dependent on the source and quality of the starting material. Inhibitory substances such as hemoglobin, heparin, triglycerides, and endogenous proteins are significant factors that may impair molecular analysis or cause false-negative results. Blood and bone marrow samples for molecular tests are best preserved using ethylenediaminetetraacetic acid (EDTA) which acts by chelating the calcium and prevents clot formation.

The choice of the test depends on the clinical context and type of genetic abnormality. A summary of genetic tests, their resolution, and advantages and disadvantages are summarized in **Table 3**.

TABLE 3: List of the genetic tests with advantages and limitations.

Method	Resolution	Sensitivity	Advantages	Limitations
Conventional karyotyping (G-banding)	5–10 Mb	5–10% of abnormal cells	Gold standard for chromosomal abnormalities; provides an overview of genome-wide changes	Low resolution; requires dividing cells; misses submicroscopic changes
Fluorescence in situ hybridization (FISH)	50–100 kb	1–5% of abnormal cells in dual color dual fusion probes. 10% in deletion probes	Higher resolution than karyotyping; detects cryptic translocations and deletions	Limited to targeted abnormalities; does not detect unknown alterations
Array comparative genomic hybridization (array CGH)	50–100 kb	20–25% abnormal cells	Higher resolution than karyotyping; detects submicroscopic CNVs	Cannot detect balanced translocations or low-level mosaicism
Single nucleotide polymorphism (SNP) array	10–50 kb	20–25% abnormal cells	Higher sensitivity for small alterations	Does not detect balanced translocations or mutations
Polymerase chain reaction (PCR)	1 bp	0.01–1% mutant allele frequency (MAF)	Highly specific and rapid; applicable to small samples	Only detects known mutations or rearrangements
Quantitative PCR (qPCR/RT-qPCR)	1 bp	0.001–1% MAF	High sensitivity; allows minimal residual disease (MRD) monitoring	Limited to known targets; cannot detect new mutations
Digital PCR	1 bp	0.001–0.0001% MAF	High sensitivity; allows MRD monitoring	Limited to known targets; cannot detect new mutations
Multiplex ligation-dependent probe amplification (MLPA)	50–100 bp	20–25% abnormal cells	Detects small copy number changes; more sensitive than FISH	Cannot detect point mutations or balanced rearrangements
Sanger sequencing	1 bp	10–20% MAF	Gold standard for single-gene mutations; useful for confirming NGS results	Low sensitivity; not ideal for low-frequency mutations
Next-generation sequencing (NGS, targeted panel/whole exome/genome)	1 bp	0.1–1% MAF	High resolution; allows personalized treatment decisions; detects clonal evolution	Expensive; requires bioinformatics expertise; may generate variants of unknown significance (VUS)

DETECTION OF ANEUPLOIDY AND CHROMOSOMAL DELETIONS

Aneuploidy refers to an abnormal gain or loss of entire chromosomes. In acute leukemias, specific aneuploidy patterns are associated with distinct prognostic implications. For example, pediatric ALL, with high-hyperdiploidy (51–65 chromosomes) is associated with a favorable prognosis. Conversely, hypodiploidy (<40 chromosomes) is linked to poor outcomes. In AML, aneuploidy is less frequent and usually occurs in complex karyotypes signifying poor prognosis as per the European Leukemia Network (ELN) 2022 guideline. Monosomy 7 and monosomy 5 are recurrent abnormalities associated with poor prognosis in AMLs. Deletions result in haploinsufficiency of genes and intrageneic deletions result in alternative transcripts and isoforms that may result in dominant negative effect.

To detect the aneuploidies various techniques are used.

Conventional Cytogenetics (Karyotyping)

Karyotyping is a traditional cytogenetic technique used to analyze the number and structure of chromosomes. It involves cell culture followed by arresting them in metaphase using mitotic inhibitors (e.g., colchicine), staining the chromosomes (commonly with Giemsa for G-banding), and then analyzing their banding patterns using a microscope. This method allows the detection of large structural abnormalities, including translocations, deletions, duplications, and aneuploidy.

Advantages

- *Global chromosomal overview:* Provides a comprehensive analysis of all chromosomes in a single assay.
- *Detection of balanced and unbalanced rearrangements:* Identifies large-scale structural changes, including translocations and numerical abnormalities.

Limitations

- *Requires actively dividing cells:* Only fresh samples can be used for karyotyping. Not applicable to nondividing cells and archival samples.
- *Low resolution (~5–10 Mb):* Cannot detect cryptic or small-scale translocations and submicroscopic alterations.
- Labor intensive and subjective.

Fluorescence In Situ Hybridization

The FISH is a molecular cytogenetic technique used to detect specific DNA sequences on chromosomes using fluorescently labeled DNA probes. This process involves denaturing both the probe and the target DNA followed by hybridization of complementary sequences and postwashing of unbound probes the samples are examined under a fluorescence microscope. FISH can not only detect aneuploidies but also detect chromosomal abnormalities such as translocations, deletions, and duplications. The fluorescent probes used in FISH can be fusion or break apart probes.

Advantages

- *High sensitivity and specificity:* FISH can detect chromosomal abnormalities with high precision, up to a single-cell level.
- *Works on nondividing cells:* Since FISH can be performed on interphase nuclei, it can also be performed on archival samples.
- *Rapid results:* The turnaround time is quicker compared to conventional karyotyping.
- *Detects cryptic rearrangements:* The power of resolution of FISH (up to 50–100 kb).

Limitations

- Target-specific and cannot provide genome-wide analysis.
- *Limited resolution:* Small mutations or unknown genomic alterations are not detected by FISH.
- *Expensive compared to karyotyping:* Requires specialized probes and fluorescence imaging equipment.

Comparative Genomic Hybridization and Array–Comparative Genomic Hybridization

Comparative genomic hybridization (CGH) is a molecular cytogenetic technique used to detect DNA copy number variations (CNVs) such as deletions, duplications, and amplifications across the genome. Traditional CGH involves co-hybridizing differentially labeled test (patient) and reference (normal) DNA to metaphase chromosomes. Differences in fluorescence intensity indicate gains or losses of genetic material. The resolution of CGH is limited to about 3–10 Mb.

Array-CGH (aCGH) is an advanced version of CGH that replaces metaphase chromosomes with a microarray containing thousands to millions of DNA probes, providing higher resolution and genome-wide coverage. This allows for the detection of smaller CNVs that would be missed by conventional CGH.

Advantages

- *High-resolution CNV detection:* aCGH provides much higher resolution than conventional CGH and karyotyping. In theory, resolution of array CGH is only limited by the number and quality of DNA targets arrayed on the slide.
- Genome-wide analysis.
- *Does not require dividing cells:* Can be performed on DNA extracted from any tissue, including archived samples.

Limitations

- Cannot detect balanced rearrangements.
- No information on gene mutations.
- *Relatively expensive:* Higher cost compared to conventional cytogenetic techniques.

DETECTION OF CHROMOSOMAL TRANSLOCATIONS (FOR EXAMPLE, FUSION GENES)

Chromosomal translocations are a major class of genetic alterations in acute leukemias. These genetic alterations result from the rearrangement of chromosome segments, often resulting in oncogene activation or fusion genes that drive leukemogenesis. Various cytogenetic and molecular techniques are used to identify chromosomal translocations, each method has its merits and limitations.

Techniques for Detecting Chromosomal Translocations

Conventional Cytogenetics (Karyotyping)

Karyotyping can detect large structural chromosomal abnormalities, including translocations, by staining and visualizing metaphase chromosomes under a microscope.

Fluorescence in Situ Hybridization

The FISH technique can detect chromosomal translocations using either fluorescently labeled DNA probes which hybridize to the specific chromosomal regions (fusion probes) or probes which target sequences on either side of a known chromosomal breakpoint (break-apart). The difference between break-apart probe and fusion probes is summarized in **Table 4**.

RNA Sequencing

RNA-Sequencing is an indispensable tool for transcriptome-wide analysis of differential gene expression and differential splicing of mRNAs. It provides an unbiased analysis of gene expression, alternative splicing, and fusion transcripts. The standard workflow of RNA sequencing begins with RNA extraction, followed by mRNA enrichment or ribosomal RNA depletion, complementary DNA (cDNA) synthesis, and preparation of an adaptor-ligated sequencing library. The library is then sequenced to a read depth of 10–30 million reads per sample on a high-throughput platform (usually Illumina). The final steps are computational: aligning and/or assembling the sequencing reads to a transcriptome, quantifying reads that overlap transcripts, filtering and normalizing between samples, and statistical modeling of significant changes in the expression levels of individual genes and/or transcripts between sample groups.

Advantages

- *Unbiased detection:* RNA-Sequencing does not require prior knowledge of translocations, allowing for novel fusion discovery.
- *High sensitivity and resolution:* RNA-Sequencing can detect low-abundance fusion transcripts with high accuracy.
- *Comprehensive transcriptome profiling:* It provides insights into gene expression changes, alternative splicing, and allele-specific expression.

TABLE 4: Break-apart versus fusion probes.

	Break-apart probes	Fusion probes
Design	• Consists of two differently colored fluorescent probes that hybridize to opposite sides of a specific gene or chromosomal region • For example, in APL, break-apart probes target the *RARA gene locus*, with one probe binding upstream and the other downstream of the typical breakpoint site	• Consists of two differently colored fluorescent probes designed to hybridize to two specific genes or chromosomal regions known to form a fusion • For example, in APL, fusion probes are designed for *PML* (on chromosome 15) and *RARA* (on chromosome 17)
Signals	Split signals when a rearrangement is present	Fused signals when a fusion is present
Purpose	• Detects *rearrangements* or structural abnormalities, such as translocations, without requiring knowledge of the partner gene • If the gene is intact, the probes will emit a single fused signal • When the gene is rearranged (e.g., in a translocation), the probes separate, showing two distinct signals (e.g., red and green)	• Specifically identify known *fusion genes* or translocations • When the two target regions fuse due to a translocation, the probes come into close proximity, creating a single fused signal (e.g., yellow from overlapping red and green signals)
Use in APL	• Detects abnormalities involving the *RARA gene*, even if the translocation partner is unknown or uncommon • Useful for identifying variant APL cases that involve rearrangements with partners other than PML	• Confirms the presence of the *PML-RARA fusion*, characteristic of classical APL • Helps differentiate classical APL from variant APL cases that do not involve PML

(APL: acute promyelocytic leukemia)

Limitations

- High cost and turnaround times.
- *Computational complexity:* Analysis requires sophisticated bioinformatics pipelines and significant computational resources.
- *Sequence biases:* GC-content and PCR amplification biases may affect transcript quantification.
- *RNA degradation issues:* Poor RNA quality from clinical samples can impact sequencing efficiency.

Reverse Transcription Polymerase Chain Reaction

To study the specific genes expression in a cell the most practical way is by analyzing the mRNA sequence. Since the RNA is more unstable, it is difficult to work with in the laboratory, so it is converted into the cDNA by a process known as reverse transcription. The resultant cDNA is much more stable than the mRNA. Reverse transcription is so named because RNA is used as the template to direct the production of cDNA, the reverse of normal cellular transcription, where DNA is used by RNA polymerase to direct the production of mRNA.

Reverse transcriptase enzyme is made by some RNA viruses and similar to the DNA polymerase, it requires a DNA primer to initiate its function. As mRNA has a poly(A) tail at its 3'-end, an ideal primer for reverse transcription of mRNA species would be a poly(T) oligonucleotide (oligo dT). The enzyme starts transcription at the 3'-end of template RNA [the 5'-end of the nascent (new) cDNA strand] and proceeds in a 5'- → 3'-direction on the nascent strand ("first strand synthesis"). In this fashion, all the mRNA (or total RNA) present in a cell is transcribed into complementary DNA. The mRNA sequences that are present at a high copy number in the cell will be reverse transcribed to a high cDNA copy number compared with those mRNA sequences which are rare in a cell. Then in the following PCR cycle [in the second cycle of a one-step reverse transcription polymerase chain reaction (RT-PCR)] and in second PCR of two-step RT-PCR) and sequence specific primer pairs hybridize to the cDNA and generate millions of copies of the target region of interest over next 30–40 cycles. The amplified products are then visualized by a variety of techniques most commonly by an Agarose gel electrophoresis using appropriate positive, negative controls, and ladder sequence. The captured image of the gel electrophoresis is interpreted to obtain the result. The differences in one-step and two-step RT/RQ-PCR are summarized in **Table 5**.

Advantages of Reverse Transcription Polymerase Chain Reaction

- High sensitivity and specificity.
- *Rapid and efficient:* Provides results within hours.
- *High sensitivity:* The sensitivity of RT-PCR assay is high and can be further increased by utilizing nested assays (~0.01–0.001%).

Disadvantages of Reverse Transcription Polymerase Chain Reaction

- *RNA degradation:* RNA is highly unstable and prone to degradation, requiring careful handling. Poorly preserved or degraded RNA can lead to false-negative reporting **(Fig. 1)**.

TABLE 5: Comparison of one-step and two-step RT-qPCR.

Parameter	One-step RT-qPCR	Two-step RT-qPCR
Workflow	Single tube, combined RT and qPCR	Separate RT and qPCR steps
Time	Faster	Slower
Handling	Minimal handling, lower contamination risk	More handling, higher contamination risk
Flexibility	Less flexible	More flexible
Sensitivity	May be lower for low-abundance targets	Higher sensitivity
Sample throughput	Suitable for high-throughput analysis	Suitable for multiple targets from one sample
Cost	Lower cost per reaction	Higher cost due to additional reagents

(RT-qPCR: real-time quantitative polymerase chain reaction)

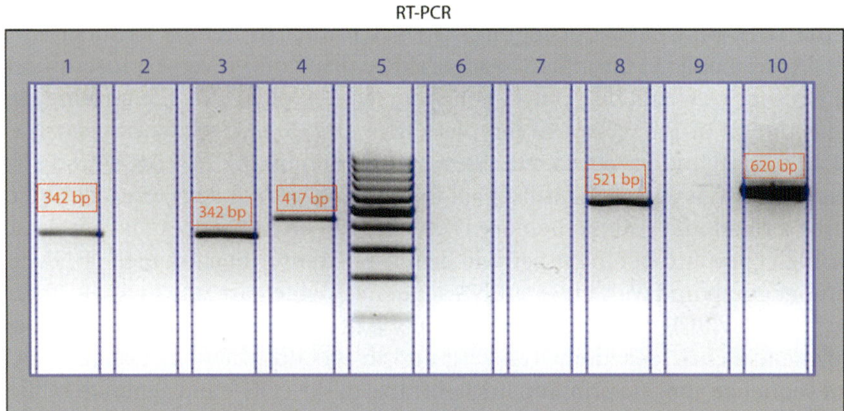

FIG. 1: Qualitative *RT-PCR* to detect BCR-ABL1 fusion transcript in a case of Ph+ve B-ALL. Lane 1 and 6: Patient's sample to detect p210 and p190 transcripts respectively. Lane 3: Positive control for p210 (e13a2) transcript showing band at 342 bp. Lane 4: Positive control for p210 (e14a2) transcript showing band at 417 bp. Lane 8: Positive control for p190 transcript showing band at 521 bp. Lane 5: 100 bp DNA ladder. Lane 2, 7 and 9: No template control (NTC) for detecting contamination or non-specific amplification. Lane 10: Housekeeping gene (*GUS* gene) as endogenous control for sample integrity showing band at 620 bp.

- *Risk of contamination:* PCR is highly sensitive, making it susceptible to false positives due to sample contamination.
- *Limited to known sequences:* RT-PCR requires prior knowledge of target sequences, making it unsuitable for detecting unknown mutations.

DETECTION OF MOLECULAR ALTERATIONS–SINGLE NUCLEOTIDE VARIANTS, INDELS (e.g., FUSION GENES): POLYMERASE CHAIN REACTION AND MODIFICATIONS

Nucleic acid amplification by PCR since its Nobel award winning discovery by Mullis and colleagues in the mid-1980s has revolutionized the field of molecular biology as it is used to amplify a specific DNA region of interest.

The principle of PCR has been extensively described in the literature. At its simplest, the "six key ingredients" of a PCR reaction include (1) DNA template, (2) a reaction buffer, (3) cocktail of deoxy nucleotide triphosphates (dNTPs), (4) a heat-table DNA polymerase enzyme, magnesium ions (Mg^{2+}), (5) specific DNA primer pairs that flank the region of interest, and (6) the template (containing the target region of interest). A PCR cycle is divided into three steps, (1) *Denaturation step*—thermal-induced separation of the double-stranded target DNA, (2) *Annealing step*—oligonucleotide primers anneal to the target sequence, and (3) *Extension step*—the DNA polymerase synthesis new strand on the annealed primer-target sequence. This cycle is repeated 25–40 times to generate millions of copies of the region of interest. The amplified PCR products are then analyzed and/or quantified by a variety of methods. Modifications of PCR reagents, steps, and detection methods are central to the detection of the many genetic alterations in hematological neoplasms and acute leukemia **(Figs. 2 and 3)**.

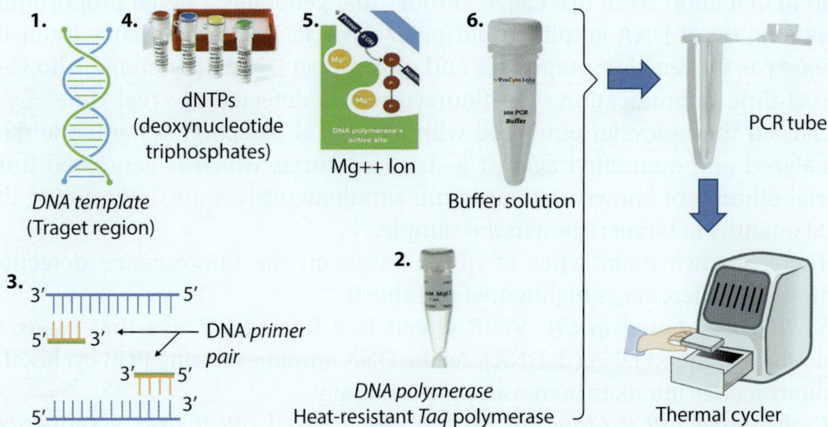

FIG. 2: PCR reaction components—six critical agents of a PCR reaction: 1. Template DNA: Contains the Region of interest; 2. DNA Polymerase (Taq Polymerase): a thermostable polymerase enzyme; 3. Primers: Oligonucleotide pairs designed to flank the region of interest on both the sense and antisense strands; 4. dNTPs; 5. Mg2; 6. Buffer.

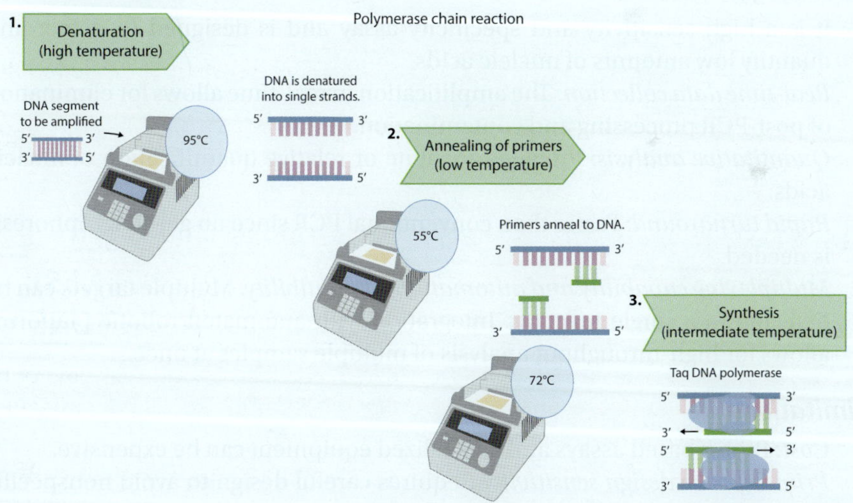

FIG. 3: The steps of polymerase chain reaction. 1. Denaturation; 2. Annealing; and 3. Exetension.

Reverse Transcription Polymerase Chain Reaction and Real-time Quantitative Polymerase Chain Reaction

Real-time quantitative polymerase chain reaction (RT-qPCR) is a modification of the conventional PCR that allows for the amplification and quantification of DNA or RNA in real-time. Unlike conventional PCR, which only provides end-point analysis, qPCR monitors the amplification process in real-time using fluorescent dyes or probes.

In qPCR, DNA is amplified using a thermostable DNA polymerase, primers, and a template. The key difference compared to the conventional PCR is the addition of a fluorescent dye called "Probe" that generates a signal proportional to the amount of DNA amplified during each cycle. The fluorescence intensity increases as the reaction progresses and more target DNA is generated, allowing for real-time quantification. The fluorescence is detected in "real time" by a specialized thermocycler equipped with an optical detection system. The data is analyzed and quantified against a standard curve, which is generated from a serial dilution of known standards run simultaneously, thus determining the initial quantity of target region in the sample.

There are two main types of qPCR based on the fluorescence detection method, the difference is highlighted in **Table 6**.

1. *SYBR Green-based qPCR:* SYBR Green is a fluorescent dye that binds to double-stranded DNA (dsDNA). As the DNA amplifies during PCR cycles, the fluorescence intensity increases proportionally.
2. *Probe-based qPCR (TaqMan assay):* Probe-based qPCR uses a sequence-specific fluorescent probe (e.g., TaqMan probe, molecular beacons) that hybridizes to the target DNA. These probes contain a reporter dye and a quencher dye. During amplification, the DNA polymerase cleaves the probe, separating the reporter from the quencher, generating a fluorescence signal.

Advantages

- It is a high sensitivity and specificity assay and is designed to detect and quantify low amounts of nucleic acids.
- *Real-time data collection:* The amplification in real-time allows for elimination of post-PCR processing and contamination.
- *Quantitative analysis*: Provides absolute or relative quantification of nucleic acids.
- *Rapid turnaround:* Faster than conventional PCR since no gel electrophoresis is needed.
- *Multiplexing capability and automation compatibility:* Multiple targets can be detected in a single reaction. Integration with automated robotic platforms allows for high-throughput analysis of multiple samples at once.

Limitations

- *Cost:* Probe-based assays and specialized equipment can be expensive.
- *Primer/probe design sensitivity:* Requires careful design to avoid nonspecific amplification.

TABLE 6: SYBR Green qPCR versus probe-based qPCR (TaqMan).

Feature	SYBR Green qPCR	Probe-based qPCR (TaqMan)
Cost	Lower	Higher
Specificity	Lower (binds to any dsDNA)	Higher (sequence-specific probe)
Multiplexing	Difficult	Easier (multiple probes with different fluorophores)
Sensitivity	Moderate	High
Ease of design	Simple (only primers needed)	Complex (requires probe design)

(dsDNA: double-stranded DNA; qPCR: quantitative polymerase chain reaction)

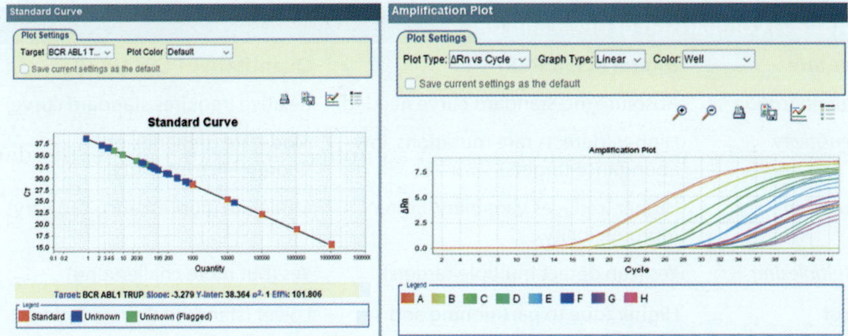

FIG. 4: BCR-ABL1 and ABL1 qPCR Standard Curve and amplification plot: The standard curve plot show standards (Red) which help in generating the reference plot against which unknown samples (Blue) are compared. The amplification plot shows relative fluorescence with a normalized reporter value on the y-axis and x-axis is the cycle number of the PCR. The amplification is proportional to the amount of target DNA in the sample.

- *Inhibition by contaminants:* PCR inhibitors from samples (e.g., blood, plant extracts) can affect results.
- *Limited dynamic range:* Although sensitive, it may not be as effective for very high target concentrations without dilution.
- *RNA degradation (for RT-qPCR):* In RNA-based assays, RNA degradation can affect accuracy **(Fig. 4)**.

Digital Polymerase Chain Reaction

Digital PCR (dPCR) is the third generation of qPCR that allows for absolute quantification of nucleic acids without the need for standard curves. dPCR physically partitions the sample into thousands or millions of individual reactions, where each partition acts as an independent PCR reaction. The partitions follow a Poisson distribution; thus the absolute number of target molecules is calculated based on the proportion of positive reactions, without needing a standard curve. This enables for a precise and highly sensitive detection of target DNA or RNA, making it useful for applications requiring ultra-sensitive quantification, rare mutation detection, and low-abundance nucleic acid analysis. This makes it a lucrative technique to be utilized in MRD monitoring. The differences between dPCR and qPCR are summarized in **Table 7**. There are three main types of dPCR based on the method of sample partitioning:

1. *Droplet digital PCR (ddPCR)*: An oil-water emulsion is used to divide the sample into thousands to millions of tiny droplets. Each droplet acts as an independent PCR reaction chamber. After amplification, droplets are analyzed for fluorescence, with positive droplets containing the target DNA. *Example platform:* Bio-Rad QX200 ddPCR system.
2. *Microfluidic chamber-based dPCR*: A microfluidic chip with predefined small wells is used to physically partition the sample into thousands of reactions. Amplification occurs within the chip, and fluorescence is detected per chamber. *Example platform:* Fluidigm Biomark system.

TABLE 7: Comparison of dPCR and qPCR.

Feature	Digital PCR (dPCR)	Quantitative PCR (qPCR)
Quantification	Absolute (no standard curve needed)	Relative (requires standard curve)
Sensitivity	Higher (detects rare mutations, low-abundance targets)	Moderate (depends on fluorescence intensity)
Precision	Higher (reduces variability, better reproducibility)	Moderate (fluorescence can vary)
Multiplexing	Yes (can detect multiple targets)	Yes (but more challenging)
Cost	Higher (due to partitioning and specialized equipment)	Lower (standard thermocyclers can be used)
Dynamic range	Moderate	Wider dynamic range
Ease of use	More complex (partitioning, specialized equipment)	Simpler (no partitioning needed)
Detection of rare variants	Excellent (as low as 0.01%)	Less sensitive for rare mutations

3. *Plate-based or array-based dPCR:* A 96-well or 384-well plates with each well acting as an individual reaction chamber is used for physical partitioning. *Example platform:* QuantStudio absolute Q dPCR system.

Advantages

- *Absolute quantification:* Unlike qPCR, dPCR provides direct quantification of nucleic acids without requiring standard curves.
- *High sensitivity:* Can detect rare mutations, low-abundance DNA/RNA, and single-copy variations with high accuracy.
- *Better reproducibility:* Reduces variability due to sample partitioning, making it more consistent than qPCR.
- *Resistant to PCR inhibitors:* More robust in challenging samples (e.g., blood, environmental samples) where inhibitors can affect qPCR performance.
- *Multiplexing capability:* Can detect multiple targets simultaneously in different partitions.

Limitations

- *High cost:* Requires specialized equipment and consumables, making it more expensive than qPCR.
- *Lower throughput compared to qPCR:* Since dPCR partitions samples into individual reactions, it may not process as many samples at once.
- *Complex workflow:* Droplet or chip-based methods require careful handling and optimization.
- *Limited dynamic range:* dPCR is excellent for low-copy-number detection but has a narrower range for high concentrations compared to qPCR.
- *Longer run time:* Takes more time than qPCR due to partitioning, amplification, and fluorescence analysis.

Fragment Analysis

Fragment analysis is a simple technique which determines the DNA fragments based on the differences in their length and size variations. Fragment analysis is performed using a capillary electrophoresis (CE), where fluorescently labeled DNA fragments migrate through a polymer matrix and are separated according to their size. The electropherogram provides a visual representation of DNA fragment sizes in the sample and their relative abundance. The key steps include:

- *DNA extraction and PCR amplification:* One primer in the PCR reaction is labeled with a fluorescent dye (e.g., FAM, HEX, VIC) for detection.
- *Capillary electrophoresis:* Allows for fragment separation according to their size.
- *Data analysis:* Electropherogram interpretation—the size of each fragment is determined by comparing it to a size standard (ladder).

Advantages

- *High sensitivity and accuracy:* Can detect small insertions, deletions, and repeat expansions with precision.
- *Multiplexing capability:* Allows analysis of multiple DNA markers in a single run, increasing efficiency.
- *High throughput and cost-effective:* Faster and cheaper than whole-genome sequencing, making it ideal for genotyping and forensic analysis.
- *Automated and reproducible:* Capillary electrophoresis-based systems provide highly reproducible results with minimal human error.
- *Applicable to a wide range of genetic studies:* Used in genetic disease screening, forensic DNA analysis, chimerism, and clonality assays.

Limitations

- *Limited to known genetic markers:* Requires prior knowledge of the target DNA sequence for primer design and cannot detect novel mutations.
- *Does not provide sequence information:* Only determines fragment sizes, not the actual nucleotide sequence. Moreover, mutations within the same fragment size cannot be distinguished.
- *Potential for artifacts:* Stutter peaks, preferential amplification, or PCR artifacts can interfere with interpretation.

The comparison of fragment analysis with sequencing is tabulated in **Table 8**.

Sanger Sequencing

Sanger sequencing, also known as the chain termination method, is a DNA sequencing technique developed by Frederick Sanger in 1977. It is based on the selective incorporation of chain-terminating dideoxynucleotides (ddNTPs) during DNA replication. These ddNTPs lack a 3′-OH group, which prevents further extension of the DNA strand when incorporated. This results in the generation of DNA fragments of varying lengths, which can then be separated and analyzed to determine the DNA sequence by CE.

TABLE 8: Comparison of fragment analysis and sequencing.

Feature	Fragment analysis	DNA sequencing (Sanger/NGS)
Purpose	Measures fragment size differences	Determines nucleotide sequence
Throughput	High (can analyze multiple fragments at once)	Lower for Sanger, very high for NGS
Sensitivity	High (detects minor genetic variations)	Higher for sequence-level changes
Data output	Electropherogram (size and intensity)	Sequence chromatogram or FASTQ files
Mutation detection	Good for indels and repeats	Best for all mutation types
Cost	Lower than sequencing	Higher for whole-genome sequencing
Speed	Faster (hours)	Slower for sequencing (days)

(NGS: next-generation sequencing)

Steps in Sanger Sequencing

- *DNA template preparation:* A short primer complementary to the target sequence is annealed to the single-stranded DNA (obtained by denaturation of DNA).
- PCR amplification with chain-terminating nucleotides (incorporation of ddNTPs).
- Capillary electrophoresis (fragment separation).
- Data analysis (sequence determination).

Advantages

- *High accuracy:* Considered as the gold standard for sequencing, with an accuracy of > 99.9%.
- *Long read lengths:* Generates reads up to 1,000 base pairs (bp), making it ideal for sequencing single genes or long DNA fragments.
- *Reliable for small-scale sequencing:* Well-suited for sequencing small genes or PCR products.
- *Low error rate:* Unlike NGS, which requires high coverage to reduce sequencing errors, Sanger sequencing provides clean and reliable data.
- *Ease of use:* Automated sequencing instruments and standardized protocols make it simple to perform in most labs.

Limitations

- *Low throughput:* Can only sequence one DNA fragment at a time, making it inefficient for large-scale sequencing (e.g., whole-genome sequencing).
- *High cost per sample:* More expensive than NGS for high-throughput applications but cost-effective for small projects.
- *Limited sensitivity for low-frequency variants:* Cannot detect rare mutations in mixed populations as effectively as dPCR or NGS.
- *Requires high-quality DNA:* DNA samples with degradation or impurities may result in poor-quality reads.
- *Limited to known targets:* Requires prior knowledge of the target sequence for primer design, making it unsuitable for de novo sequencing of unknown genomes.
- *Time-consuming:* Requires multiple steps, including PCR, electrophoresis, and data analysis, making it slower than NGS.

The comparison of Sanger sequencing and NGS is summarized in **Fig. 5** and **Table 9**.

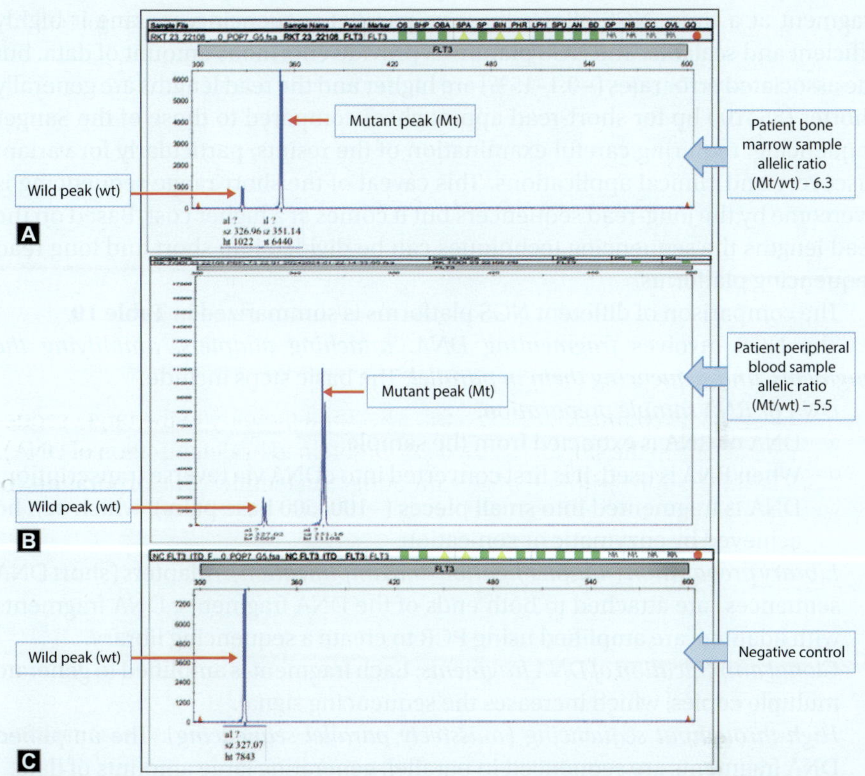

FIGS. 5A TO C: Fragment analysis to detect FLT3-ITD mutation: (A) Orthogonal technique—GeneMapper Software Fragment Analysis image of bone marrow sample: The image shows the insertion of 24 base pairs in the patient sample (Allelic Ratio - 6.3). (B) Orthogonal technique-GeneMapper Software Fragment Analysis image of Peripheral Blood sample: The image shows the insertion of 24 base pairs in the patient sample (Allelic Ratio - 5.5). (C) No template Control for FLT3-ITD.

TABLE 9: Comparison of Sanger sequencing and next-generation sequencing.

Feature	Sanger sequencing	Next-generation sequencing (NGS)
Throughput	Low (one sequence at a time)	High (millions of sequences in parallel)
Read length	Long (500–1,000 bp)	Short (50–300 bp per read)
Accuracy	Very high (99.9%)	High (lower for single reads, but improved with depth)
Cost	Expensive per sample but cheaper for small projects	High upfront cost but cheaper for large-scale sequencing
Speed	Slower (hours to days)	Faster (hours)
Best use case	Small DNA fragments, mutation validation	Whole genome, transcriptomics, high-throughput analysis

Next-generation Sequencing

The NGS works by sequencing millions to billions of DNA fragments simultaneously. Unlike traditional Sanger sequencing, which sequences a single DNA fragment at a time, NGS allows massive parallel sequencing, making it highly efficient and scalable. The NGS platforms provide enormous amount of data, but the associated error rates (~0.1–15%) are higher and the read lengths are generally shorter (35–700 bp for short-read approaches) compared to those of the Sanger sequencing, requiring careful examination of the results, particularly for variant discovery and clinical applications. This caveat of the short-range sequencing is overcome by the long-read sequencers but it comes at a higher cost. Based on the read lengths the sequencing techniques can be divided into short and long read sequencing platforms.

The comparison of different NGS platforms is summarized in **Table 10**.

The NGS involves *fragmenting DNA, attaching adapters, amplifying the fragments, and sequencing them in parallel*. The basic steps include:

- *DNA or RNA sample preparation*:
    - DNA or RNA is extracted from the sample.
    - When RNA is used, it is first converted into cDNA via reverse transcription.
    - DNA is fragmented into small pieces (~100–500 base pairs), which can be achieved by enzymatic or sonication.
- *Library preparation (adapter ligation and amplification)*: Adapters (short DNA sequences) are attached to both ends of the DNA fragments. DNA fragments with adapters are amplified using PCR to create a sequencing library.
- *Clonal amplification of DNA fragments*: Each fragment is amplified to generate multiple copies, which increases the sequencing signal.
- *High-throughput sequencing (massively parallel sequencing)*: The amplified DNA fragments are sequenced in parallel, generating large amounts of data.
- *Data analysis and interpretation*:
    - The generated raw sequence reads are processed using bioinformatics tools. Reads are aligned to a reference genome or assembled de novo.
    - Variant calling detects mutations such as single nucleotide polymorphisms (SNPs), insertions/deletions (indels), and structural variations.

TABLE 10: Comparison of next-generation sequencing (NGS) platforms.

Feature	Illumina	Ion Torrent	PacBio	Oxford Nanopore
Read length	Short (50–300 bp)	Short (~200–400 bp)	Long (10–60 kb)	Ultra-long (>100 kb)
Accuracy	High (>99%)	Moderate	High (~99%)	Moderate (~90–95%)
Throughput	Very high	Moderate	Moderate	Low
Speed	Slow (~1–2 days)	Fast (~hours)	Slow (~1–2 days)	Real-time
Cost per base	Low	Low	High	High
Best used for	WGS, RNA-seq	Targeted sequencing	De novo assembly	Portable sequencing

(WGS: whole genome sequencing)

- *Variant interpretation*: Variant interpretation involves multiple steps:
  - *Quality control:* Filtering out sequencing errors.
  - *Comparison to databases:* Identifying known variants [ClinVar, single nucleotide polymorphism database (dbSNP), genome aggregation database (gnomAD)].
  - *Pathogenicity prediction:* Tools such as sorting intolerant from tolerant (SIFT) and polymorphism phenotyping (PolyPhen) predict functional impact.
  - *Clinical correlation and variant annotation:* Finally, the variants are annotated according to the standards and guidelines for the interpretation of sequence variants proposed by Joint Consensus Recommendation of the American College of Medical Genetics and Genomics and the Association for Molecular Pathology and are classified using specific standard terminology: "pathogenic," "likely pathogenic," "uncertain significance," "likely benign," and "benign" as per the phenotypic data.

Advantages

- *High throughput:* Multiple samples are processed together which enables simultaneous sequencing of millions of RNA/DNA fragments at once allowing for a rapid processing compared to traditional Sanger sequencing.
- *Cost-effective:* The multiplexing of many samples in a single run reduces the overall cost of sequencing per base compared to Sanger sequencing.
- *Scalability:* The flexibility of the NGS panels allows for the sequencing of entire genomes, exomes, or specific targeted regions, depending on research or clinical needs.

Whole Genome Sequencing

- This technique helps in capturing the complete DNA sequence of an organism.
- It provides comprehensive genomic information, including exonic as well as intronic regions. This requires high sequencing depth and computational power, making it expensive and data intensive.
- It is seldom used in routine practice. The technique can identify variants in undiagnosed genetic disorders.

Whole Exome Sequencing

- This technique focuses on sequencing only the exonic (protein-coding) regions, which constitute about 1–2% of the genome.
- It is more cost-effective than whole genome sequencing (WGS) while still identifying most disease-associated variants. However, it can miss the variants in the regulatory, noncoding and deep intronic regions which might influence gene expression.
- It is seldom used in routine practice and is utilized in specific clinical queries like in diagnostic workup of rare genetic disorders, inherited conditions, and monogenic diseases.

Targeted Gene Panels

A targeted panel is designed to look at specific genes or regions of interest that are typically associated with a known disease.

- It provides high-depth sequencing at a lower cost with reduced data complexity and is the most frequently used NGS methodology in routine clinical practice.
- However, the limited scope and panel design make it unsuitable for discovering novel mutations.

Disadvantages

- *High initial cost:* The initial investment cost is substantial due to the high price of sequencing instruments and the significant computational infrastructure required for data processing and analysis.
- *Complex bioinformatics:* Processing vast amounts of raw sequencing data requires a skilled bioinformatician.
- *Error rates:* The short-read platforms struggle with repetitive or complex genomic regions, while the long-read sequencers have higher error rates. However, newer techniques are being developed to overcome this caveat **(Fig. 6 and 7, Flowchart 1)**.

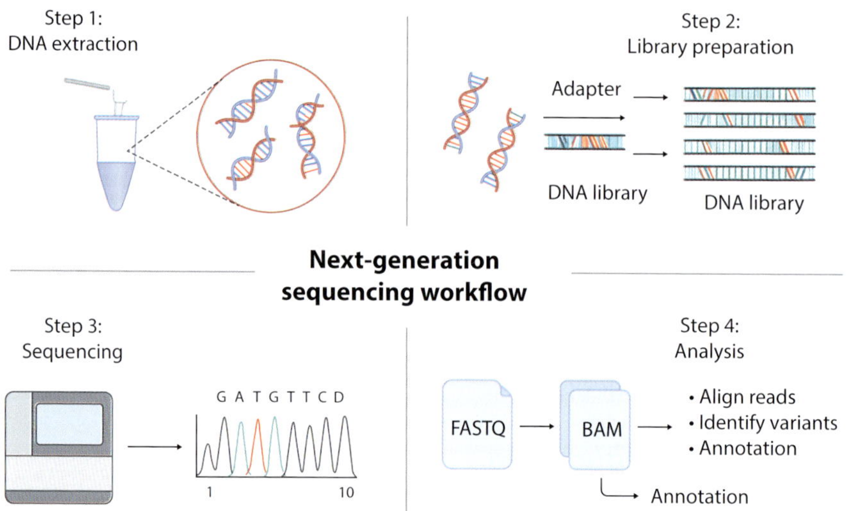

FIG. 6: The workflow of next-generation sequencing.

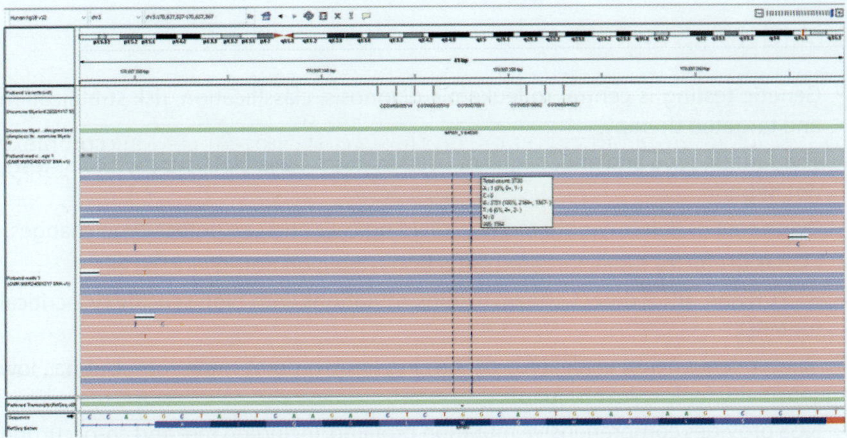

FIG. 7: Integrated genome viewer NM_002520.7:c. c.860_863dup p.Trp288Cysfs*12 (VAF-56%) showing insertion of the bases.

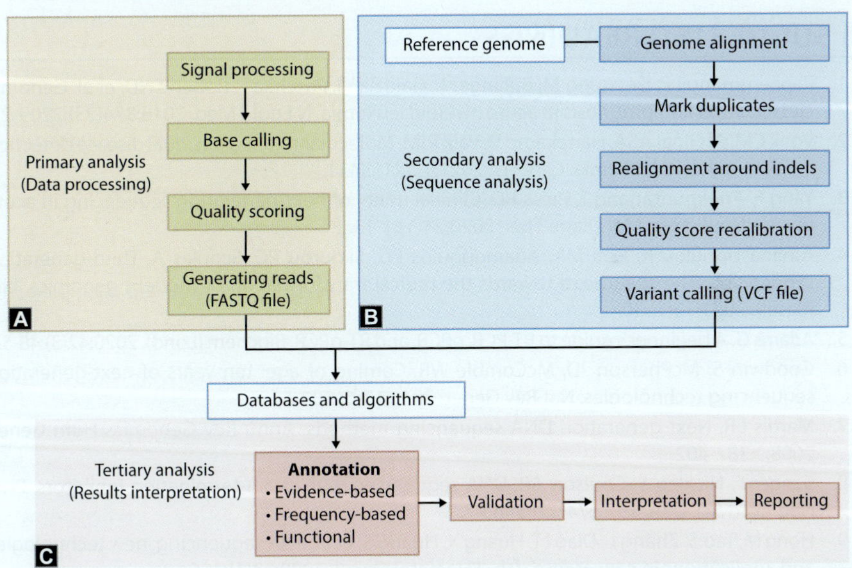

FLOWCHART 1: Workflow of data analysis in next-generation sequencing (NGS) - (A) Primary Analysis (Data Processing): This initial phase involves processing raw signals generated by sequencing instruments. (B) Secondary Analysis (Sequence Analysis): The FASTQ files are aligned to a reference genome. The outcome of this analysis is a Variant Call Format (VCF) file containing the identified genetic variants. (C) Tertiary Analysis (Results Interpretation): The identified variants are further annotated using various databases and algorithms. Annotation is based on evidence, population frequency, and predicted functional impact. This is followed by validation, biological and clinical interpretation, and generation of a final report.

Take Home Points

- Genetic testing is central to leukemia diagnosis, classification, risk stratification and targeted therapy.
- The sample type and anticoagulant used matters—use EDTA for molecular tests, not heparin.
- Cytogenetics (karyotyping) requires dividing cells and can detect large changes.
- FISH is useful for rapid, targeted detection—even on non-dividing cells.
- RT-PCR and qPCR detect known fusions/mutations with high sensitivity—critical for MRD.
- Sanger sequencing is ideal for confirming known point mutations, but has low sensitivity for low-level variants.
- NGS provides comprehensive mutation profiling, including rare and co-occurring variants.
- Always correlate molecular findings with morphology, immunophenotype, and clinical data.

SUGGESTED READINGS

1. Papaemmanuil E, Gerstung M, Bullinger L, Gaidzik VI, Paschka P, Roberts ND, et al. Genomic classification and prognosis in acute myeloid leukemia. N Engl J Med. 2016;374(23):2209-21.
2. Vonk CM, Al Hinai ASA, Hanekamp D, Valk PJM. Molecular minimal residual disease detection in acute myeloid leukemia. Cancers. 2021;13(21):5431.
3. Yang F, Anekpuritanang T, Press RD. Clinical utility of next-generation sequencing in acute myeloid leukemia. Mol Diagn Ther. 2020;24(1):1-13.
4. Athanasopoulou K, Boti MA, Adamopoulos PG, Skourou PC, Scorilas A. Third-generation sequencing: The spearhead towards the radical transformation of modern genomics. Life (Basel). 2021;12(1):30.
5. Adams G. A beginner's guide to RT-PCR, qPCR, and RT-qPCR. Biochem (Lond). 2020;42(3):48-53.
6. Goodwin S, McPherson JD, McCombie WR. Coming of age: ten years of next-generation sequencing technologies. Nat Rev Genet. 2016;17(6):333-51.
7. Mardis ER. Next-generation DNA sequencing methods. Annu Rev Genomics Hum Genet. 2008;9:387-402.
8. Sanger F, Nicklen S, Coulson AR. DNA sequencing with chain-terminating inhibitors. Proc Natl Acad Sci. USA. 1977;74(12):5463-7.
9. Hong M, Tao S, Zhang L, Diao LT, Huang X, Huang S, et al. RNA sequencing: new technologies and applications in cancer research. J Hematol Oncol. 2020;13(1):166.
10. Stark R, Grzelak M, Hadfield J. RNA sequencing: the teenage years. Nat Rev Genet. 2019;20(11):631-56.
11. Marguerat S, Bähler J. RNA-seq: from technology to biology. Cell Mol Life Sci. 2010;67(4):569-79.
12. Jovic D, Liang X, Zeng H, Lin L, Xu F, Luo Y. Single-cell RNA sequencing technologies and applications: A brief overview. Clin Transl Med. 2022;12(3):e694.
13. Taylor SC, Laperriere G, Germain H. Droplet digital PCR versus qPCR for expression analysis with low abundant targets: from variable nonsense to publication quality data. Sci Rep. 2017;7:2409.
14. Gabert J, Beillard E, van der Velden V, Grimwade D, Pallisgaard N, Barbany G, et al. Standardization and quality control studies of 'real-time' quantitative reverse transcriptase polymerase chain reaction of fusion gene transcripts for residual disease detection in leukemia—a Europe against cancer program. Leukemia. 2003;17:2318-57.

15. Patnaik MM. The importance of FLT3 mutational analysis in acute myeloid leukemia. Leuk Lymphoma. 2018;59(10):2273-86.
16. Li MM, Datto M, Duncavage EJ, Kulkarni S, Lindeman NI, Roy S, et al. Standards and guidelines for the interpretation and reporting of sequence variants in cancer: A Joint Consensus Recommendation of the Association for Molecular Pathology, American Society of Clinical Oncology, and College of American Pathologists. J Mol Diagn. 2017;19(1):4-23.
17. He R, Wiktor AE, Hanson CA, Ketterling RP, Kurtin PJ, Van Dyke DL, et al. Conventional karyotyping and fluorescence in situ hybridization: an effective utilization strategy in diagnostic adult acute myeloid leukemia. Am J Clin Pathol. 2015;143(6):873-8.
18. Khehra N, Padda IS, Swift CJ. Polymerase chain reaction (PCR). In: StatPearls. Treasure Island (FL): StatPearls Publishing; 2025.
19. Life Technologies. Real-time PCR handbook. Carlsbad: Thermo Fisher Scientific; 2010.

CHAPTER 33

Thrombophilia Workup: When, Whom, and What to Test?

Prerna Arora, Vijay Kumar

ABSTRACT

Thrombophilias are defined as either hereditary or acquired conditions which increase the predisposition to develop arterial or venous thrombosis. It is a known fact that the risk of thrombosis increases with a number of risk factors; however, the different risk factors are known to have variable predictive values. Guidelines on testing for thrombophilia are controversial. This chapter provides an overview of performing thrombophilia workup, including when, when not, and whom to test for thrombophilia, along with a brief summary of the tests to be performed.

INTRODUCTION

Thrombophilias are a group of acquired and hereditary conditions that increase the risk of either arterial or venous thrombi (**Table 1**). Deep venous thrombosis (DVT) and/or venous thromboembolism (VTE) have a higher association with thrombophilia in comparison to arterial thrombosis. Increasing age also increases the risk of thrombosis. As per Brækkan SK et al., the incidence of thrombosis increases from 1 per 10,000 persons per year in young adults to 1 per 100 persons per year in the elderly. The incidence of VTE in children is 0.07–0.14 per 10,000 children per year, with increased incidence in hospitalized children. However, the data to determine the incidence of VTE among Asian Indians is extremely sparse. Recent reports of the NAMS task force have determined the incidence of 1.79 per thousand DVT in Indians, among the general population.

PATHOGENESIS AND RISK OF THROMBOSIS

Virchow's triad, comprising stasis, endothelial injury, and hypercoagulability, is considered to be the cornerstone for the pathogenesis of VTE. At least one of the elements of Virchow's triad can be identified for the development of

TABLE 1: List of factors predisposing to thrombosis.

Inherited thrombophilia	Acquired thrombophilia
Protein C, protein S deficiency	Antiphospholipid syndrome (APS)
Antithrombin deficiency	Myeloproliferative neoplasms (MPNs) and JAK2 mutation positivity
Factor V Leiden mutation (FVL)	Paroxysmal nocturnal hemoglobinuria (PNH)
Prothrombin G20210A mutation	Immobilization, fractures, and prolonged surgery
Elevated factor VIII levels	Estrogen therapy (contraceptive pills), pregnancy
Plasminogen deficiency	Nephrotic syndrome and heparin-induced thrombocytopenia (HIT)
Tissue plasminogen activator deficiency and tissue factor pathway inhibitor	Malignancies, SARS-CoV-2 disease (COVID-19)

TABLE 2: Relative risk of thrombosis due to various etiologies.

Thrombophilia	Relative risk of initial venous thromboembolism (VTE)	Relative risk of recurrent VTE
FVL heterozygous	4–6	1–2
FVL homozygous	7–19	2
Prothrombin mutation heterozygous	2–4	1–2
Prothrombin mutation homozygous	2–21	Uncertain
Protein C deficiency	10	2
Protein S deficiency	10	1
Antithrombin deficiency	10–30	3
Antiphospholipid antibodies (aPL)	7	2–7

VTE. However, the predictive value of the risk factors for the development of thrombosis is highly variable. For example, factor V Leiden (FVL) mutation carries a low thrombosis risk, while protein C or S deficiency is much rarer in occurrence but carries a significant thrombosis risk **(Table 2)**.

Antiphospholipid antibodies (aPL) are the most common acquired cause of arterial thrombosis, microvascular events as well as VTE. Thrombosis at unusual sites such as the portal vein, mesenteric vein, splenic vein, Budd–Chiari syndrome, and cerebral venous sinus thrombosis can be caused by acquired causes such as paroxysmal nocturnal hemoglobinuria (PNH) and myeloproliferative neoplasms (MPN), along with aPL.

WHEN, WHEN NOT, AND WHOM SHOULD I TEST FOR THROMBOPHILIA?

When to initiate a laboratory workup for thrombophilia is a complex decision. When and what not to order for thrombophilia testing is as important and pertinent to know as what tests to order for thrombophilia. Testing for thrombophilia should only be undertaken when the results will significantly alter the management, like in determining the duration of anticoagulation or in aiding the primary prevention of thrombosis in relatives of affected patients. For example, anticoagulation is usually not necessary in a patient with the presence of thrombophilia with no history of thromboembolism. On the other hand, if there is recurrent thromboembolism, anticoagulation should be given irrespective of the results of thrombosis testing. Tests for thrombophilia hence are only informative if done in the right patient at the right time. As per Darlow et al., the following are the indications for the thrombophilia workup:

- Thrombosis at a young age (<40 years), especially in association with weak provoking factors (minor surgery, combined oral contraceptives, or immobility) or unprovoked VTE
- Strong family history of VTE (first-degree family members affected at a young age)
- Recurrent VTE events, especially at a young age
- VTE in unusual sites

In addition, recent American Society of Hematology 2023 (ASH) guidelines on thrombophilia conditionally recommend testing in the following scenarios:

- Patients with VTE associated with nonsurgical major transient or hormonal risk factors
- Patients with cerebral or splanchnic venous thrombosis, in settings where anticoagulation would otherwise be discontinued
- Individuals with a family history of antithrombin, protein C, or protein S deficiency, when considering thromboprophylaxis for minor provoking risk factors, and for guidance to avoid combined oral contraceptives or hormone replacement therapy
- Pregnant women with a family history of high-risk thrombophilia types
- Patients with cancer who are at low or intermediate risk of thrombosis and have a family history of VTE

Testing in neonates and children constitutes a special subcategory. The prevalence of heritable thrombophilia in neonates with VTE has been found to be the same as that in the healthy population; hence, screening neonates with VTE for heritable thrombophilia is not necessary and does not influence the treatment. However, thrombophilia testing should be considered in neonates and children if there is a strong family history of VTE. Also, protein C and S levels should be undertaken in neonates and children presenting with purpura fulminans. **Flowchart 1** highlights the approach to thrombophilia testing.

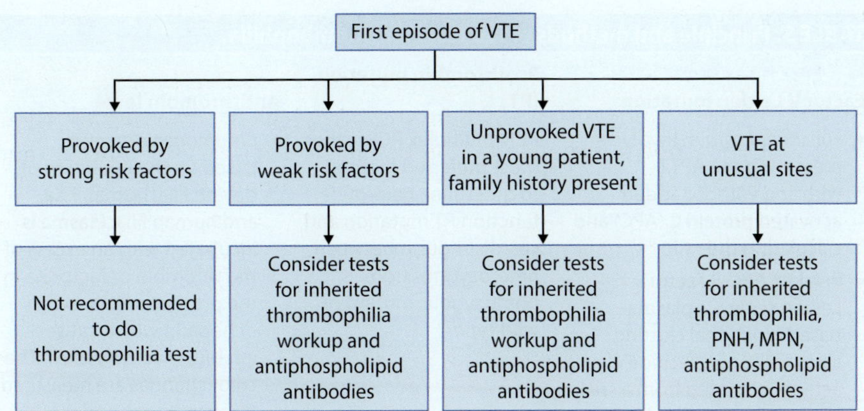

FLOWCHART 1: Algorithm depicting the selection of patients for thrombophilia testing.
(MPN: myeloproliferative neoplasm; PNH: paroxysmal nocturnal hemoglobinuria; VTE: venous thromboembolism)

When Not to Test for Thrombophilia?

- Thrombophilia testing is not recommended following an episode of provoked VTE, as it is not sufficient to give extended anticoagulation.
- There is a limited role of thrombophilia screening tests in asymptomatic relatives of patients with known thrombophilia; however, relatives can be counseled regarding the use of prophylaxis in high-risk situations.
- Association of heritable causes of thrombophilia with arterial events such as ischemic stroke or myocardial infarction is weak and does not alter the management; however, aPL should be considered in the absence of significant causes of vascular risk factors.
- Testing for heritable thrombophilia in neonatal VTE is debatable and not clear, thus, screening is not routinely recommended for neonatal stroke.

What to Test for Thrombophilia?

Judicious testing for thrombophilia, keeping in mind the diagnostic pitfalls, can ensure meaningful results of the thrombophilia workup. This is particularly important as treatment may not change even on identification of an underlying thrombophilia, particularly for heritable diseases.

A full thrombophilia panel includes the following tests:

- Factor V Leiden mutation
- Prothrombin G20210A gene mutation
- Antithrombin deficiency
- Protein C deficiency
- Protein S deficiency
- aPL and lupus anticoagulant

A brief outline of various tests is described in **Tables 3 and 4**.

TABLE 3: Principle and methods of lab tests for thrombophilia.

Factor V Leiden mutation	Prothrombin mutation (PT)	Antithrombin level
• *Functional assays*: Involves measuring the APTT with and without added activated protein C (APC) and calculating the ratio • Pefakit® APC-R Factor V Leiden screen is plasma-based functional clotting assay utilizing specific FV activator isolated from a snake venom (*Daboia russelli*). The test is performed with and without the addition of APC and involves a predilution of patient plasma with factor V-deficient plasma • *Mutation testing*: Different amplification products/ amplicons are produced as a result of the mutation which are analyzed by PCR/RFLP	PCR/multiplex PCR is the most preferred method to determine gain-of-function PT mutation and can distinguish between heterozygous from homozygous mutant or wild type	• *Chromogenic assay* is based on the inhibition of bovine FIIa, human FXa, and human FIIa. Plasma is incubated with an excess of the thrombin or factor Xa in the presence of an excess of heparin which causes inhibitory activity of AT. The color changes are measured by absorbance and are inversely proportional to the AT levels in the sample • *Immunogenic assay*: Various modalities can be used like ELISA assay, Laurell electroimmunoassay • *Clotting-based assay*: Exogenously added thrombin is neutralized by AT, leading to prolongation of the clotting time

(APC: activated protein C; APTT: activated partial thromboplastin time; ELISA: enzyme-linked immunosorbent assay; PCR: polymerase chain reaction; RFLP: restriction fragment length polymorphism)

TABLE 4: Principle and methods of lab tests for thrombophilia.

Protein C	Protein S (free protein S)	Antiphospholipid syndrome
• *Chromogenic method*: Plasma is incubated with the protein C activator, e.g., Protac, and a chromogenic substrate for activated protein C is added. The change in optical density is measured, and the protein C level can be determined • *Immunological assay*: ELISA-method, which measures protein C level but not its functional activity • *Clotting-based functional assay* can be APTT based, which uses protein C activator	• *Immunological assay*: Can be based on ELISA or Latex particle-based agglutination assay. ELISA can determine free as well as total protein S • *Functional assay*: Can be based on PT or APTT assays and measures only free protein S levels as it is the functional form	• LA testing uses screening and a confirmatory test • *Screening test*: Phospholipid-dependent test such as aPTT or dilute Russel viper venom test (dRVVT) • *Confirm test*: Addition of excess phospholipid to demonstrate phospholipid dependence • *Immunological assay*: aCL and anti-B2GP1 (IgG and IgM antibody) titers

(aCL: anticardiolipin antibodies; aPTT: activated partial thromboplastin time; ELISA: enzyme-linked immunosorbent assay)

TABLE 5: Various factors affecting levels of inherited thrombophilia causes.

Protein C levels	Free protein S levels	Antithrombin level
• *Reduced levels*: Neonates and children, liver diseases, DIC, acute inflammation/ infections, trauma/surgery or uremia, cancer, and vitamin K deficiency/ warfarin therapy • *Artefactual decrease*: Factor V Leiden if using clot-based assays	• *Reduced levels*: Neonates pregnancy, oral anticoagulation/warfarin therapy, nephrotic syndrome, OCPs, DIC, SLE, HIV infection, and liver disease • *False decrease*: Factor V Leiden if using clot-based assays	*Reduced levels*: Neonates, proteinuria, surgery, heparin renal disorders, liver dysfunction, DIC, L-asparaginase therapy

(DIC: disseminated intravascular coagulation; HIV: human immunodeficiency virus; OCP: oral contraceptive pill; SLE: systemic lupus erythematosus)

POTENTIAL PITFALLS IN TESTING FOR THROMBOPHILIA

- The clotting-based tests for thrombophilia should be avoided while patients are on anticoagulants or during active thrombosis within the last 3 months. This is because the consumption of coagulation factors or an increase in acute phase reactants (factor VIII, fibrinogen, or C-reactive protein) in such cases may give erroneous results. Underlying medical conditions such as nephrotic syndrome, infection, disseminated intravascular coagulation (DIC), or liver impairment can also cause interferences **(Table 5)**.
- If the patient is on heparin, functional activity of AT should not be determined.
- Warfarin should be stopped 2 weeks before testing as warfarin can invalidate protein C and S and lupus anticoagulant assays.
- Patients on low molecular weight heparin (LMWH) can be tested for thrombophilia, but samples should be drawn at least 12 hours after the last dose, as heparin use produces a false-positive lupus anticoagulant test.
- Direct oral anticoagulants (DOACs) should be stopped 48 hours before testing and earlier in patients with renal impairment.
- Diagnostic accuracy of molecular mutation testing or immunoassays is not affected and can be performed even during an acute episode or on anticoagulant therapy.

THROMBOPHILIA TESTS IN SPECIAL CIRCUMSTANCES

Patients with thrombosis at unusual sites can be tested to rule out PNH clone and myeloproliferative neoplasms in the presence of abnormal hematological parameters (i.e., cytopenia or evidence of hemolysis) or blood count or morphological abnormalities in cases of MPN, respectively.

An extended "thrombophilia panel" may include homocysteine, factor VIII, lipoprotein(a) levels, plasminogen activator inhibitor-1 (PAI-1) levels, and methylenetetrahydrofolate reductase (MTHFR) polymorphisms. However, guidance is lacking on how these results might influence patient management, hence, these are not routinely recommended.

CASE-BASED APPROACH

Case 1: A 60-year-old female with a medical history of hypertension undergoes hysterectomy. On postoperative day 20, she presents with pulmonary embolism. What should be the patient care approach in this case?

Recommendation: No thrombophilia testing. Treatment with anticoagulation for 3 months and stop anticoagulation.

Category: Provoked, strong trigger

Case 2: A 22-year-old female presents with ankle sprain and is advised 10 days of bed rest. Mother and sister: History of DVT is present. The patient wants to start oral contraceptive pills (OCPs) for pregnancy prevention. What should be the patient care approach in this case?

Recommendation: Thrombophilia testing with suggestion to prevent OCP if the thrombophilia screen is positive.

Category: Family history and minor risk factor, contemplating to start OCP.

Take Home Points

- Thrombophilia (inherited or acquired) increases the risk for venous thrombosis and VTE.
- Thrombophilia testing should be used in a highly selective manner, and only in circumstances where the information obtained will influence a decision important to the patient and outweigh the potential risks of testing.
- Thrombophilia testing includes a battery of investigations using molecular mutation studies as well as immunological, functional, and clot-based assays.
- Testing for thrombophilia should not be performed during acute thrombosis or during the initial (3-month) period of anticoagulation.
- Guidance is not clear for thrombophilia testing in conditions of stroke, myocardial infarction, or peripheral arterial thrombosis.

SUGGESTED READINGS

1. Stevens SM, Woller SC, Bauer KA, Kasthuri R, Cushman M, Streiff M, et al. Guidance for the evaluation and treatment of hereditary and acquired thrombophilia. Journal of thrombosis and thrombolysis. 2016;41:154-64.
2. Brækkan SK, Hansen JB. VTE epidemiology and challenges for VTE prevention at the population level. Thrombosis Update. 2023;10:100132.
3. Lassandro G, Palmieri VV, Palladino V, Amoruso A, Faienza MF, Giordano P. Venous Thromboembolism in Children: From Diagnosis to Management. Int J Environ Res Public Health. 2020;17(14):4993.
4. NAMS task force report on Venous thromboembolism. Annals of the National Academy of Medical Sciences, India. 2024;60(1).
5. Connors JM. Thrombophilia testing and venous thrombosis. N Engl J Med. 2017;377:1177-87.
6. Darlow J, Mould H. Thrombophilia testing in the era of direct oral anticoagulants. Clin Med. 2021;21(5):e487-91.

7. Nicolaides AN, Fareed J, Kakkar AK, Comerota AJ, Goldhaber SZ, Hull R, et al. Prevention and treatment of venous thromboembolism- International Consensus Statement. Int Angiol. 2013;32(2):111-260.
8. Middeldorp S, Nieuwlaat R, Baumann Kreuziger L, Coppens M, Houghton D, James AH, et al. American Society of Hematology 2023 guidelines for management of venous thromboembolism: thrombophilia testing. Blood Adv. 2023;7(22):7101-38.
9. Klaassen IL, van Ommen CH, Middeldorp S. Manifestations and clinical impact of pediatric inherited thrombophilia. Blood. 2015;125(7):1073-7.
10. Arachchillage DJ, Mackillop L, Chandratheva A, Motawani J, MacCallum P, Laffan M. Thrombophilia testing: a British Society for Haematology guideline. Br J Haematol. 2022;198(3):443.

CHAPTER 34

Amyloidosis: Newer Insights in Diagnosis

Vikram Singh, Kanwaljeet Singh

ABSTRACT

This chapter is intended to highlight the newer insights and molecular techniques in amyloid diagnostics, which in conjunction with traditional diagnostic modalities, can be extremely beneficial in the timely diagnosis and prognostication of the affected patients so that proper management protocol can be established in the affected patients with an ultimate aim to reduce morbidity and mortality.

INTRODUCTION

Amyloidosis refers to a heterogeneous group of rare disorders characterized by the extracellular deposition of abnormally folded insoluble fibrillar proteins, known as amyloid, within various tissues and organs. These amyloid fibrils are formed from normally soluble globular proteins that undergo misfolding and aggregation, ultimately leading to progressive organ dysfunction and damage. These amyloid fibrils are nonbranching rigid structures, characteristically measuring 8–12 nm in diameter on electron microscopy and are formed by the process of fibrillogenesis, which leads to the formation of predominantly β-pleated sheet secondary structural conformation. This β-pleated sheet structure is insoluble, nonfunctional, and resistant to degradation, leading to its pathological accumulation. Amyloid genesis is affected multifactorial causes ranging from hereditary mutations to acquired genetic alterations.

CLASSIFICATION

The classification of amyloidosis is primarily based on the biochemical nature of the precursor protein forming the amyloid fibrils. To date, over 30 different amyloidogenic proteins have been identified in humans.

- *Immunoglobulin-derived amyloidosis*:
    - Light chain (AL) amyloidosis: Results from the deposition of monoclonal immunoglobulin light chains, typically associated with plasma cell dyscrasias. It is the most common form of systemic amyloidosis.

  - Heavy chain (AH) amyloidosis: Involves deposition of immunoglobulin heavy chains
- *Serum amyloid A protein-derived amyloidosis*:
  - AA amyloidosis: Occurs secondary to chronic inflammatory conditions, leading to elevated serum amyloid A protein levels and subsequent deposition
- *Transthyretin-derived amyloidosis*:
  - *Transthyretin amyloidosis (ATTR)*: Involves deposition of transthyretin (TTR) protein. It has two subtypes:
    i. Hereditary (hATTR): Caused by mutations in the *TTR* gene
    ii. Wild-type (wtATTR): Formerly known as senile systemic amyloidosis, occurs without TTR mutations
- *β2-microglobulin-derived amyloidosis*:
  - Aβ2M amyloidosis: Associated with long-term hemodialysis, leading to β2-microglobulin deposition, primarily affecting musculoskeletal tissues.
- *Apolipoprotein-derived amyloidosis*:
  - AApoAI, AApoAII, AApoAIV, AApoCII, AApoCIII amyloidosis: Result from mutations in apolipoprotein genes, leading to amyloid deposits in various organs, often with renal involvement
- *Fibrinogen A alpha-chain amyloidosis*:
  - AFib amyloidosis: Caused by mutations in the fibrinogen alpha-chain gene, leading to predominant renal amyloid deposits
- *Gelsolin-derived amyloidosis*:
  - AGel amyloidosis: Results from mutations in the gelsolin gene, leading to amyloid deposits affecting the eyes, nerves, and skin
- *Lysozyme-derived amyloidosis*:
  - ALys amyloidosis: Due to mutations in the lysozyme gene, leading to systemic amyloidosis with renal and hepatic involvement
- *Cystatin C-derived amyloidosis*:
  - ACys amyloidosis: Known as hereditary cerebral hemorrhage with amyloidosis, Icelandic type (HCHWA-I), caused by mutations in the cystatin C gene, leading to amyloid deposits in cerebral vessels
- *Amyloid beta protein-derived amyloidosis*:
  - *Aβ amyloidosis*: Associated with Alzheimer's disease, involving deposition of amyloid beta peptides in the central nervous system
- *Prion protein-derived amyloidosis*:
  - APrP amyloidosis: Involves deposition of prion proteins, associated with transmissible spongiform encephalopathies like Creutzfeldt–Jakob disease.
- *Islet amyloid polypeptide-derived amyloidosis*:
  - AIAPP amyloidosis: Occurs in the pancreatic islets, associated with type 2 diabetes mellitus
- *Atrial natriuretic factor-derived amyloidosis*:
  - AANF amyloidosis: Involves deposition of atrial natriuretic peptides, primarily affecting the cardiac atria

TABLE 1: Amyloid proteins and common location of accumulation.

Type of amyloid	Protein	Common location
AA amyloid	Serum amyloid A	Kidney, liver, and spleen
AL amyloid	Immunoglobulin light chain	Heart, kidneys, and nerves
ATTR amyloid	Transthyretin	Heart and peripheral nervous system
Aβ amyloid	Amyloid beta	Brain (Alzheimer's Disease)
AE amyloid	Endocrine amyloid proteins	Pancreatic islets (type 2 diabetes)
APrP amyloid	Prion protein	Brain (prion diseases)
A β2M amyloid	Beta-2 microglobulin	Joints (dialysis-related)

- *Prolactin-derived amyloidosis*:
    - APro amyloidosis: Associated with prolactinomas, involving deposition of prolactin-derived amyloid
- *Calcitonin-derived amyloidosis*:
    - ACal amyloidosis: Occurs in medullary carcinoma of the thyroid, involving deposition of calcitonin-derived amyloid

Table 1 shows the locations involved related to the type of amyloid and the protein involved.

CLINICAL PRESENTATION AND COMPLICATIONS

Amyloidosis leads to a range of complications depending on the organs involved. Cardiac involvement is common, with amyloid deposits reducing the heart's ability to fill with blood between beats, leading to restrictive cardiomyopathy, heart failure, and arrhythmias. Cardiac amyloidosis leads to symptoms such as dyspnea, orthopnea, fatigue, and edema.

Renal complications often manifest as proteinuria, progressing to nephrotic syndrome, hypoalbuminemia, edema, chronic renal disease, and potentially culminating in end-stage kidney disease requiring dialysis.

Neurological manifestations include peripheral neuropathy, presenting as tingling and pain typically in "stocking and glove distribution" weakness, or loss of sensation, and autonomic dysfunction, which can cause orthostatic hypotension, gastroparesis, diarrhea, and erectile dysfunctions.

Gastrointestinal involvement includes macroglossia, dysphagia, malabsorption, and diarrhea.

Hepatic involvement may lead to hepatomegaly and impaired liver function.

Musculoskeletal involvement includes bilateral swelling over the shoulders due to amyloid deposition (shoulder pad sign) and arthropathy.

Hematological manifestations of amyloidosis include a bleeding tendency due to infiltration of blood vessels and coagulation factor X deficiency.

Pulmonary involvement includes pulmonary nodules or infiltrates, which are rare, along with pleural effusion.

Skin involvement includes purpura/ecchymosis, around the eyes (raccoon eyes) due to vascular fragility.

Additionally, amyloidosis can affect the spleen and adrenal glands, leading to diminished function. It is important to note that amyloidosis can also lead to thrombotic and bleeding complications, with patients experiencing significant risks of both thrombotic events and bleeding.

Early recognition and management of these complications are crucial to improving patient outcomes.

DIAGNOSIS

Accurate and early diagnosis is crucial for effective management. Recent advancements have enhanced the diagnostic capabilities available to pathologists.

Tissue Biopsy and Histological Analysis

- *Biopsy*: Obtaining a tissue sample from an affected organ remains the gold standard for diagnosing amyloidosis. Organ biopsies, such as those from the kidney or heart, offer high sensitivity (kidney: 99%; heart: 100%) and are preferred in cases of localized amyloidosis or when differential diagnoses are considered. Less invasive sites, such as bone marrow, abdominal fat, or minor salivary glands, can be utilized, achieving diagnostic success in up to 85% of cases. On hematoxylin and eosin (H&E), amyloid deposits appear as pale pink, amorphous, extracellular, glassy, hyaline material, predominantly in vascular or perivascular locations. Characteristic cracking artifacts may be observed, and macrophages or foreign body giant cells can be present around deposits. Apart from tissue biopsy/histopathology, fine needle aspiration from the abdominal fat pad is minimally invasive and can be a widely used method for diagnosing systemic amyloidosis, with sensitivity ranging from 70 to 90% and specificity approaching almost 95–100% when combined with Congo red stain and polarized microscopy. **Figures 1A to D** show an example of gastric amyloidosis.
- *Histochemical staining*: Congo red staining is a cornerstone in the histopathological diagnosis of amyloidosis, enabling the visualization of amyloid deposits within tissue sections. When applied to adequately prepared tissue samples, Congo red binds specifically to amyloid fibrils. Under standard light microscopy, these deposits exhibit a characteristic red or salmon-pink coloration. However, the definitive diagnostic feature of amyloid is observed under polarized light, where the stained deposits display apple-green birefringence. This birefringence results from the unique alignment of Congo red molecules within the beta-pleated sheet structure of amyloid fibrils, causing differential refraction of polarized light.
- *Other stains which are useful in staining amyloid deposits include*:
    - Thioflavin T, which is a fluorescent dye binding to amyloid fibrils and green fluorescence, is obtained in amyloid deposits under ultraviolet light.
    - Periodic acid-Schiff (PAS) stain highlights amyloid deposits as pink material and is often used in conjunction with other stains for specificity.
    - Crystal violet stain displays metachromatic staining of amyloid fibrils in light microscopy.

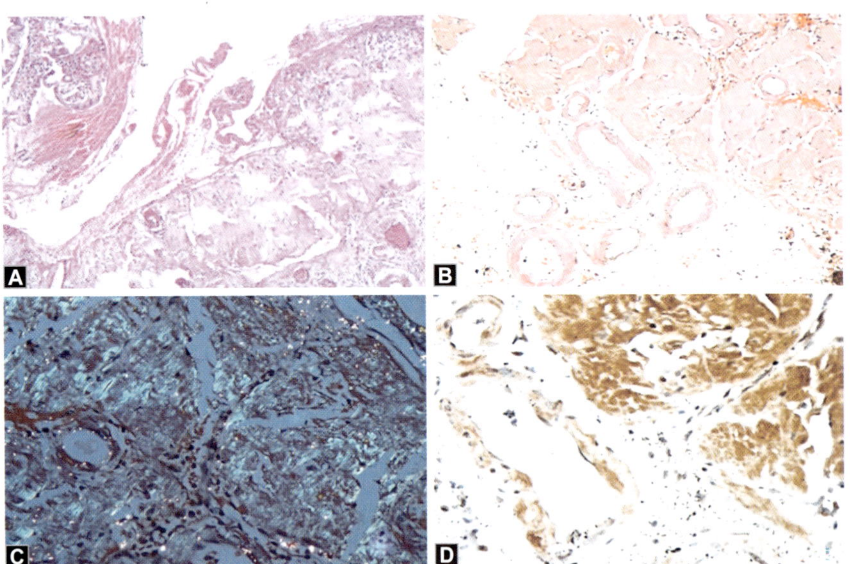

FIGS. 1A TO D. Photomicrograph of the stomach. (A) Ulcerated surface epithelium of gastric mucosa with presence of pale, acellular, homogenous, eosinophilic material (H&E, 20×); (B) Congo red stain—both vascular and extracellular areas show presence of congophilic material (20×); (C) Polarizing microscopy—showing characteristic apple-green birefringence on polarizing microscopy (40×); (D) Serum amyloid A (SAA) protein positivity was noted, both in the vascular and extracellular area (40×).

Amyloid Typing

- *Immunohistochemistry (IHC)*: IHC utilizes antibodies specific to amyloidogenic proteins to determine the amyloid type. There are certain disadvantages for IHC:
  - Detects limited types of amyloid (e.g., AA, ATTR, and AL)
  - Requirement of frozen tissue for immunofluorescence and special fixation and electron microscopy for immunogold labeling, which involves using antibodies tagged with gold particles that specifically bind to amyloid proteins, allowing for precise identification of amyloid deposits under transmission electron microscope (TEM)
  - Antibodies are not optimized for recognizing the mutant and truncated forms of the amyloidogenic protein.
  - The antibodies and fibrils interact in a nonspecific way due to the β-pleated sheet conformation.
- *Proteomics*: Proteomics is rapidly emerging as a pivotal tool in diagnosing amyloidosis, a condition where the implicated protein plays a central molecular role. Shotgun proteomics, which directly identifies proteins in deposits, aligns perfectly with this diagnostic need. This approach involves digesting amyloid proteins into peptides and analyzing them through liquid chromatography-tandem mass spectrometry (LC-MS/MS). Laser-capture microdissection (LID) is applied for clinical amyloid subtyping by isolating

specific areas from formalin-fixed paraffin-embedded (FFPE) tissues, followed by LC-MS/MS analysis. First successfully implemented in 2009 by Vrana and colleagues at the Mayo Clinic, this technique was validated in a cohort of 91 cases. An independent study at Kumamoto University, Japan, highlighted LMD-LC-MS/MS's superiority over IHC for quantifying genetic variants. Thirteen subsequent studies have confirmed its accuracy in amyloid typing. LMD is an advanced technology used in molecular pathology to isolate specific cells or tissues from a heterogenous sample with high precision. It involves the use of a focused laser beam to cut and capture target areas of interest, while maintaining the integrity of surrounding material. This process enables researchers to analyze DNA, RNA, and proteins, including the different amyloid proteins from specific cell population, making it particularly valuable in diagnostic applications and gene expression studies or proteomics.

This method's key advantage lies in selectively excising Congo Red-positive (CR) deposits, enhancing specificity by minimizing interference from normal tissue, and requiring only minimal CR-positive material for analysis. LC-MS/MS has been instrumental in amyloidosis research, identifying and characterizing novel amyloid types, including AApoCII, AApoCIII, AApoAIV, AEnf, and ALECT2. It also detects amino acid sequence variants in amyloid proteins via sequence tagging or custom protein sequence databases. Additionally, LC-MS/MS enables the identification of novel mutant peptides and multiple amyloidogenic amino acid substitutions in various amyloid types such as ATTR, AApoA1, AApoCII, AFib, AGel, and Alys. Proteomics achieves high sensitivity (92% for known substitutions; 82% for novel) and specificity (100% for known; 99% for novel) in detecting amino acid substitutions, though its clinical validation for mutation detection remains pending.

Although targeted mass spectrometry is widely utilized in clinical research for small molecule analysis, the LC-MS/MS amyloid typing assay is the first semi-quantitative shotgun proteomics platform transitioned from research to clinical application. However, its complexity poses challenges, including limited sample material due to microdissection, processing difficulties, and the need for expertise in interpreting proteomic profiles. To facilitate broader clinical use, robust sample processing platforms, standardized quality controls, and a quality management system are essential for consistent results over time despite changes in equipment or consumables. Adequate training and qualification of clinical laboratory personnel are also crucial. Dissemination of the assay's performance to regulatory agencies is necessary for approval, and educating clinicians is key to increasing referrals and usage. Importantly, the shotgun proteomics amyloid typing assay should complement, not replace, conventional diagnostics. Final diagnoses should be rendered by experienced surgical or hematopathologists specializing in amyloidosis.

The diagnostic algorithm of amyloidosis is shown in **Flowchart 1**.

Imaging Techniques

- *Nuclear medicine scans*: Nuclear medicine imaging plays a pivotal role in diagnosing and differentiating types of cardiac amyloidosis, particularly

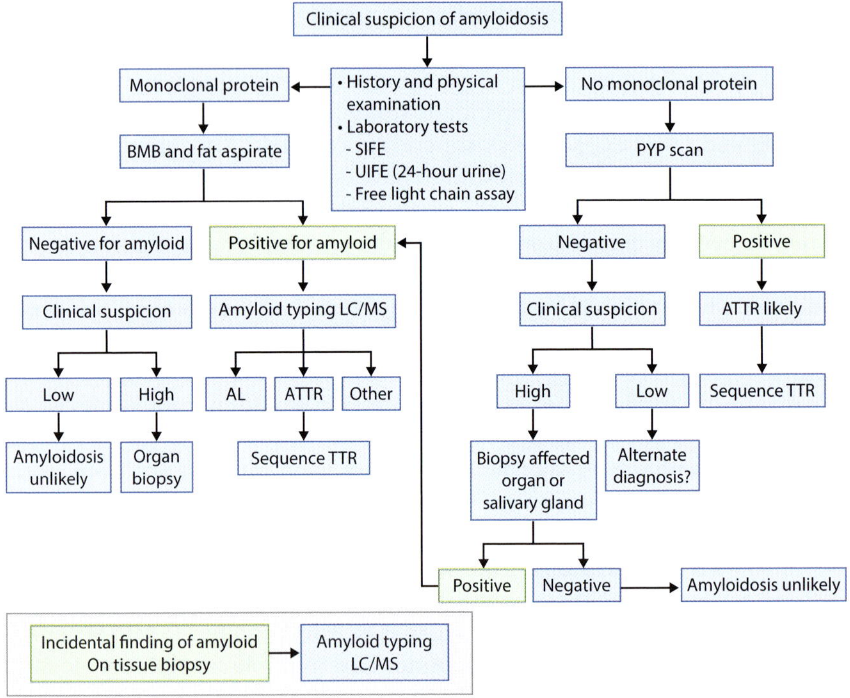

FLOWCHART 1: Diagnostic algorithm for patients that are being evaluated for a syndrome compatible with systemic amyloidosis.

[AL: immunoglobulin light chain amyloidosis; ATTR: transthyretin amyloidosis; BMB: bone marrow biopsy; PYP: (99 m)Tc-pyrophosphate scintigraphy; SIFE: serum immunofixation electrophoresis; TTR: transthyretin; UIFE: urine immunofixation electrophoresis; LC/MS: liquid chromatography-coupled tandem mass spectrometry]

ATTR and light-chain amyloidosis (AL). The primary imaging modalities include bone-seeking radiotracers and amyloid-specific agents. Technetium-99m-labeled compounds, such as pyrophosphate (Tc-99m PYP), 3,3-diphosphono-1,2-propanodicarboxylic acid (Tc-99m DPD), and hydroxy methylene diphosphonate (Tc-99m HDP), are commonly used. These tracers exhibit affinity for myocardial amyloid deposits, particularly in ATTR amyloidosis. The imaging procedure involves intravenous administration of the tracer, followed by planar and single-photon emission computed tomography

- Echocardiography (ECHO) patterns of cardiac involvement in amyloidosis include structural findings (increased ventricular wall thickness, small left ventricular cavity size, atrial enlargement, and valvular thickening) and functional findings (diastolic dysfunction, reduced longitudinal strain, and pericardial effusion). The interventricular spectrum exhibits a speckled pattern.
- Magnetic resonance imaging (MRI) findings in amyloidosis include increased myocardial thickness and small left ventricular size.

Genetic and Molecular Analysis

Genetic testing: Genetic testing plays a pivotal role in diagnosing and managing hereditary forms of amyloidosis, particularly ATTR. This condition arises from mutations in the *TTR* gene, leading to the production of unstable transthyretin proteins that misfold and aggregate into amyloid fibrils. Genetic testing involves sequencing the *TTR* gene to detect pathogenic variants.

Over 120 mutations have been identified, each associated with varying clinical manifestations and disease progression rates. For instance, the V30M mutation is commonly linked to neuropathic symptoms, while the V122I mutation predominantly leads to cardiac involvement.

Certain TTR mutations may influence therapeutic decisions. For example, the efficacy of transthyretin stabilizers, such as tafamidis, may vary depending on the specific mutation present. Additionally, some mutations are associated with a more aggressive disease course, prompting consideration of early intervention with gene-silencing therapies such as patisiran or inotersen.

Emerging Diagnostic Modalities

- *Artificial intelligence (AI) and deep learning (DL)*: AI and DL are revolutionizing the diagnostic landscape of amyloidosis by enhancing accuracy and expediting detection. Deep learning algorithms applied to autofluorescence microscopy images can virtually replicate Congo red staining and birefringence patterns, potentially streamlining the diagnostic workflow.

  Deep learning, a subset of AI, employs neural networks to process large datasets, enabling the identification of subtle features in medical images that may elude human observers. In cardiac amyloidosis, DL models have been trained to analyze cardiovascular magnetic resonance (CMR) images, echocardiograms, and other imaging modalities. For instance, a study demonstrated that a deep learning model could accurately detect CA from CMR images, potentially distinguishing it from other cardiomyopathies.
- *Multimodal data integration*: Combining echocardiographic data with electronic health records through machine learning models has shown promise in detecting cardiac amyloidosis, potentially facilitating earlier diagnosis and treatment. AI models integrate data from electronic health records to enhance diagnostic precision. By combining echocardiographic data with patient demographics and laboratory results, AI can improve the detection of cardiac amyloidosis.

  A case study highlighting the importance of amyloid, which masqueraded as malignancy in a patient is as follows: A 47 years old patient presented with massive hematemesis from a large ulcer in stomach due to which patient underwent total gastrectomy as an emergency lifesaving procedure, and specimen was sent to laboratory for histopathological evaluation (HPE). Gross evaluation of the gastrectomy specimen showed a hemorrhagic gastric ulcer involving the body, fundus, and sparing the antral part. HPE of relevant sections showed ulcerated mucosa along with presence of extensive deposits of extracellular, homogeneous, eosinophilic material on H&E stain.

Congo red stain showed the congophilic nature of this material, and apple green birefringence was noted on polarized microscopy. Further IHC for serum amyloid A (SAA) was positive, suggesting the diagnosis of secondary amyloidosis

CONCLUSION

For systemic amyloidosis patients, unequivocal identification of the amyloid type is mandatory for optimal treatment. Through close collaborations between clinicians, pathologists, and proteomics researchers, mass spectrometry-based proteomics has become the new gold standard for amyloid typing, used in conjunction with current clinical and antibody-based tests at multiple centers internationally. However, as the establishment of this platform by a clinical laboratory is challenging and requires meticulous attention to standardization and quality control as well as advanced bioinformatics, it should be undertaken only by institutions with sufficient resources and expertise to invest in this endeavor.

Take Home Points

- *Early recognition is key*: Amyloidosis is a rare but serious condition caused by abnormal protein deposits (amyloid) in tissues and organs. Early diagnosis improves outcomes significantly.
- *Multisystem involvement*: Look for unexplained symptoms in multiple organs, such as kidney dysfunction, cardiomyopathy, neuropathy, or hepatomegaly.
- *Confirmatory testing*: Diagnosis requires histological confirmation (biopsy) with Congo red staining and identification of amyloid type via IHC or mass spectrometry.
- *Comprehensive management*: It involves treating the underlying cause and addressing organ damage.

SUGGESTED READINGS

1. Fogo AB, Lusco MA, Najafian B, Alpers CE. AJKD Atlas of Renal Pathology: AL Amyloidosis. Am J Kidney Dis. 2015;66(6):43-55.
2. Kebbel A, Röcken C. Immunohistochemical classification of amyloid in surgical pathology revisited. Am J Surg Pathol. 2006;30(6):673-83.
3. Fotiou D, Theodorakakou F, Spiliopoulou S, Gavriatopoulou M, Migkou M, Kanellias N, et al. Thrombotic and bleeding complications in patients with AL amyloidosis. Br J Haematol. 2024;204(5):1816-24.
4. Singh V, Singla S, Singh H, Sharma V, Das A. Massive hematemesis in a case of gastric amyloidosis masquerading as gastric carcinoma. Autops Case Rep. 2019;9(1):e2018074.
5. Brambilla F, Lavatelli F, Merlini G, Mauri P. Clinical proteomics for diagnosis and typing of systemic amyloidosis. Proteom Clin Appl. 2013;7:136-43.
6. Vrana JA, Gamez JD, Madden BJ, Theis JD, Bergen HR, 3rd; Dogan A. Classification of amyloidosis by laser microdissection and mass spectrometry-based proteomic analysis in clinical biopsy specimens. Blood. 2009;114:4957-9.
7. Hasib Sidiqi M, Gertz MA. Immunoglobulin light chain amyloidosis diagnosis and treatment algorithm 2021. Blood Cancer J. 2021;11:90.

8. Ando Y, Nakamura M, Araki S. Transthyretin-related familial amyloidotic polyneuropathy. Arch Neurol. 2005;62:1057-62.
9. Yang X, Bai B, Zhang Y, Aydin M, Li Y, Selcuk SY, et al. Virtual birefringence imaging and histological staining of amyloid deposits in label-free tissue using autofluorescence microscopy and deep learning. Nat Commun. 2024;15(1):7978.
10. Martini N, Aimo A, Barison A, Della Latta D, Vergaro G, Aquaro GD, et al. Deep learning to diagnose cardiac amyloidosis from cardiovascular magnetic resonance. J Cardiovasc Magn Reson. 2020;22(1):84.

CHAPTER 35

Minimal/Measurable Residual Disease in Myeloma

Asish Rath

ABSTRACT

Over the past decade, treatment responses and survival outcomes for multiple myeloma (MM) patients have significantly improved, thanks to the development of novel therapies. Minimal/measurable residual disease has emerged as a powerful prognostic marker and a key tool for assessing deeper treatment responses following therapy with new drug regimens and targeted treatments. Achieving MRD negativity is an independent predictor of better outcomes across all disease stages and risk categories.

Traditional MRD evaluation methods, such as multiparameter flow cytometry (MFC) and allele-specific oligonucleotide polymerase chain reaction (ASO-PCR), have been largely replaced by more sensitive techniques. Next-generation flow cytometry (NGF) and next-generation sequencing (NGS) are now the preferred and guideline-recommended methods for MRD assessment. Additionally, less invasive blood-based techniques are under investigation and show promise for serial disease monitoring at various time points. This chapter provides an overview of the technological advancements in MM MRD evaluation.

INTRODUCTION

Multiple myeloma (MM) is defined by clonal proliferation of plasma cells, the production of monoclonal immunoglobulin (M-protein), and associated end-organ damage. Over the past decade, the treatment landscape for MM has undergone a significant transformation with the introduction of novel therapeutic regimens, targeted therapies, and chimeric antigen receptor (CAR)-T cell therapies. Despite these advancements, achieving a complete cure for MM remains elusive, even though a majority of patients attain a complete response (CR) or better.

In 2016, the International Myeloma Working Group (IMWG) updated the response assessment criteria to include minimal/measurable residual disease (MRD) as an additional level of response. MRD refers to the ability to detect a very small number of residual clonal plasma cells during or after treatment. The evaluation of MRD has proven to significantly enhance response assessment and prognostic stratification across all patient subgroups, including those eligible or ineligible for stem cell transplant and those with relapsed/refractory disease. Numerous clinical trials have demonstrated that MRD negativity is associated with superior progression-free survival (PFS) and overall survival (OS). Additionally, MRD serves as a surrogate marker for clinically relevant endpoints in drug development trials. The IMWG recommends the use of positron emission tomography with computed tomography (PET-CT), standardized next-generation flow cytometry (NGF), and next-generation sequencing (NGS)-based methods for MRD evaluation. Recent years have seen advancements in existing techniques as well as the development of newer, more sensitive methods for MRD detection, further refining the ability to monitor and predict treatment outcomes in MM.

CONVENTIONAL TECHNIQUES IN MINIMAL/MEASURABLE RESIDUAL DISEASE EVALUATION

Various techniques have been employed for MRD evaluation in MM, including multiparameter flow cytometry (MFC), allele-specific oligonucleotide-polymerase chain reaction (ASO-PCR), NGS, and whole-body imaging techniques such as ^{18}F-fluorodeoxyglucose (FDG) PET-CT. Traditionally, MFC and molecular methods have relied on bone marrow (BM) aspirate samples for MRD analysis. Each of these techniques comes with its own set of advantages and limitations.

Conventional MFC is widely used for detecting clonal plasma cells but has restricted utility due to its relatively low sensitivity (approximately 10^{-4}), lack of standardization, and issues with reproducibility. On the other hand, ASO-PCR-based MRD testing leverages the unique monoclonal rearrangements in immunoglobulin heavy (IgH) and light chains (IgK/IgL). However, its applicability is limited to 80–90% of cases due to challenges such as the patchy distribution of MM cells in the bone marrow, a high rate of somatic hypermutation, and the presence of a polyclonal background following therapy. These factors highlight the need for more advanced and standardized methods to improve MRD detection and monitoring in MM.

ADVANCEMENTS IN FLOW CYTOMETRY FOR MINIMAL/MEASURABLE RESIDUAL DISEASE EVALUATION IN MULTIPLE MYELOMA

In 2017, the EuroFlow group introduced a significant advancement in flow cytometry for MRD detection in MM. They developed a validated antibody panel and a new sample processing protocol, termed NGF, which allows for the acquisition of a higher number of cells, significantly improving sensitivity and reliability.

The EuroFlow NGF approach uses a two-tube, 8-color antibody panel with a total of 10 antibodies **(Table 1)**. This design enables the detection of clonal plasma cells with a sensitivity of 2×10^{-6} when at least 10 million cells are

TABLE 1: EuroFlow MM MRD panel.

	BV421	BV510	FITC	PE	PERCP CY5.5	PECY7	APC	APCC750
Tube 1	CD138	CD27	CD38	CD56	CD45	CD19	CD117	CD81
Tube 2	CD138	CD27	CD38	CD56	CD45	CD19	Kappa	Lambda

TABLE 2: MM MRD antibody panel at Tata Medical Center, Kolkata.

V450	BV510	BV605	BV711	BV786	FITC	PE	PERCP CY5.5	PECY7	APC	APCH7	APCR700
CD38	CD56	CD81	CD117	CD229	Lambda	Kappa	CD20	CD19	CD138	CD45	CD27

acquired. The IMWG recommends using validated NGF for MRD analysis, with a minimum sensitivity of 10^{-5} and a requirement to acquire at least 5 million cells. The use of lyophilized antibodies in the two-tube panel reduces sample processing time and enhances the reliability of MRD results. Automated Gating Software like Infinicyt™ (Cytognos, SL) minimizes intraobserver variability and ensures consistent and uniform MRD detection. Other advancements include the development of single-tube panels incorporating 10 or more antibodies. These panels allow simultaneous evaluation of multiple antigen expressions, further reducing processing time and improving efficiency. The use of ≥8-color antibody panels also facilitates the incorporation of newer antibodies, which is particularly useful for detecting plasma cells after targeted therapies. We, at our institute, use a 12-color MM MRD panel **(Table 2)**.

The widespread use of anti-CD38 therapies, such as daratumumab and isatuximab, has introduced challenges in MRD detection. These therapies can lead to the masking or absence of CD38 on plasma cells, which may persist for 4–6 months post-treatment. Traditional gating strategies relying on CD38 and CD138 may underestimate the number of abnormal plasma cells in such cases. To address these challenges, newer strategies and antibodies are being incorporated into MRD panels. Antibodies targeting CD229 (SLAMF3) and CD319 (SLAMF7) are being used to detect plasma cells post-anti-CD38 therapy. Conventional gating strategy and post-daratumumab gating strategy are shown in **Figures 1 and 2**, respectively. Intracytoplasmic markers like VS38c, which target the cytoskeletal protein P63 localized in the rough endoplasmic reticulum of plasma cells, are promising alternatives. Multiepitope anti-CD38 antibodies are used in the EuroFlow MRD panel. These antibodies can identify multiple epitopes on plasma cells, overcoming the issue of antigen masking. New gating approaches are being developed to improve the accuracy of plasma cell detection in the presence of anti-CD38 therapies.

These advancements in flow cytometry, particularly the development of NGF and innovative antibody panels, have significantly enhanced the sensitivity, reliability, and applicability of MRD evaluation in MM, even in the context of modern targeted therapies.

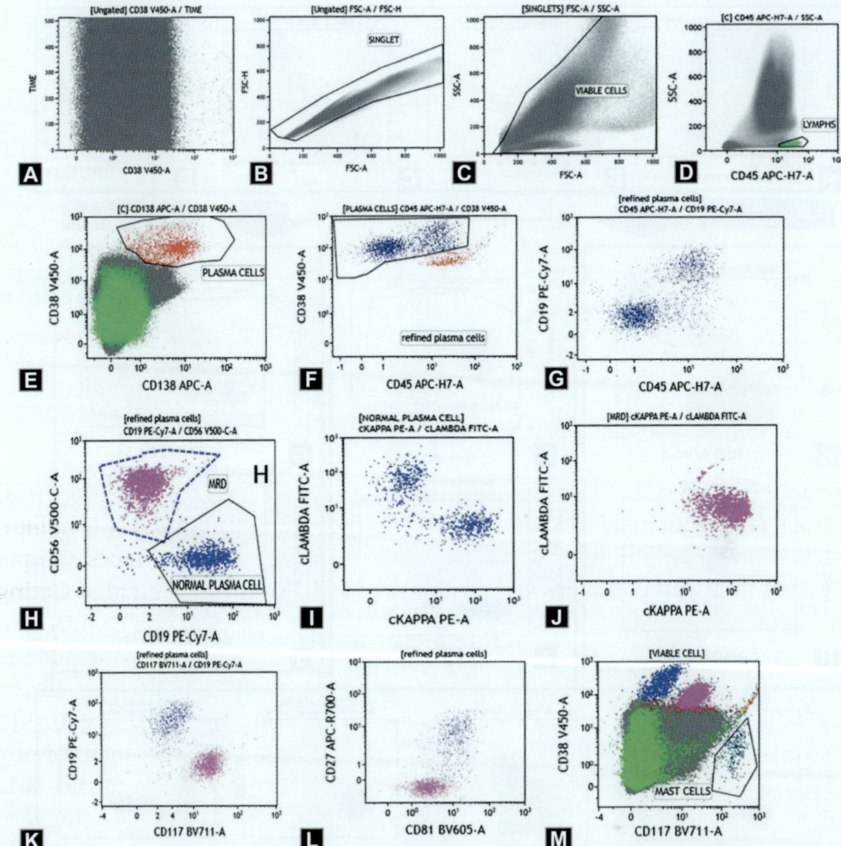

FIGS. 1A TO M: Conventional gating strategy for MM MRD. (A) Time gate for acquisition smoothness; (B) FSC-A versus FSC-H to include only singlet events; (C) FSC-A versus SSC-A to gate viable events; (D) CD45 versus SSC-A to visualize major populations; (E) CD38 versus CD138 to broadly gate all plasma cells; (F) CD38 versus CD45 to refine the plasma cell gating and to include all CD38 bright population only; (G) CD19 versus CD45 shows two clusters of plasma cells CD19+/CD45+ and CD19−/CD45−; (H) CD56 versus CD19 shows CD56 bright/CD19− (pink) abnormal plasma cells/MRD and CD19+/CD56− (blue) normal plasma cells; (I) normal polyclonal plasma cells; (J) MRD/abnormal plasma cells show kappa light chain restriction; (K) normal plasma cells CD19+/CD117− and MRD events CD19−/CD117+; (L) Normal plasma cells CD27+/CD81+, MRD events CD27−/CD81−; (M) CD117 bright mast cells (cyan).

(MM: multiple myeloma; MRD: minimal/measurable residual disease)

CIRCULATING TUMOR CELL DETECTION BY MULTIPARAMETER FLOW CYTOMETRY IN MULTIPLE MYELOMA

Current methods for MRD evaluation in MM rely on BM aspirate samples. However, serial monitoring of MRD using invasive procedures such as BM aspiration is often impractical. BM-based MRD assessment in MM is further complicated by the spatial heterogeneity of the disease and frequent sample

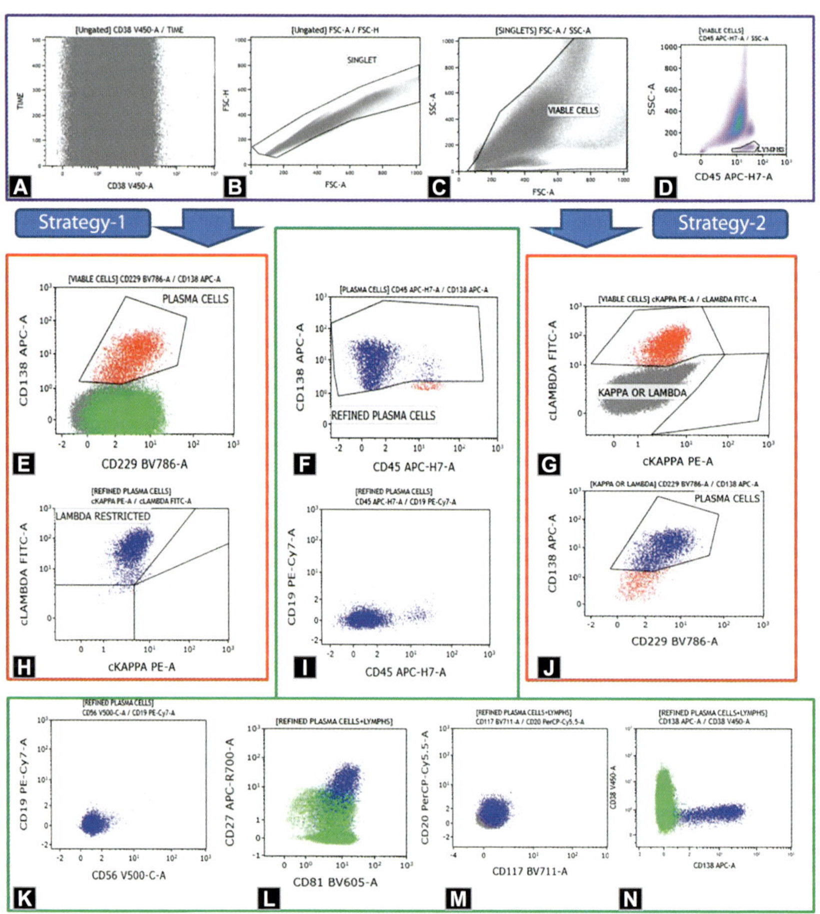

FIGS. 2A TO N: Gating strategy post-daratumumab (anti-CD38) therapy. (A) Time gate for acquisition smoothness; (B) FSC-A versus FSC-H to include only singlet events; (C) FSC-A versus SSC-A to gate viable events; (D) CD45 versus SSC-A to visualize major populations. Plasma cells gating strategy-1; (E) CD229 versus CD138 to broadly gate all plasma cells; (F) Lambda restricted abnormal plasma cells/MRD (blue). Plasma cells gating strategy-2; (G) Kappa versus lambda to identify all cells bound to kappa and lambda stain; (H) Identifying plasma cells of all kappa and lambda stained cells; (I) Refining plasma cells on CD138 versus CD45; (J) CD19 versus CD45 shows majority MRD CD19–/CD45–; (K) CD56 versus CD19 shows CD56–/CD19– MRD; (L) MRD events CD27+/CD81+; (M) CD117 negative in MRD; (N) CD38 negative in MRD post-daratumumab (anti-CD38).

hemodilution. In contrast, the detection of circulating tumor cells (CTCs) in peripheral blood (PB) using NGF has emerged as a prognostically significant tool for newly diagnosed MM patients. It also enhances risk stratification in this population. The presence of CTCs is linked to an elevated risk of malignant progression to symptomatic MM in both monoclonal gammopathy of undetermined significance (MGUS) and smoldering MM, as well as poorer survival outcomes in symptomatic newly diagnosed and relapsed/refractory MM cases. CTCs share similarities with CD34+ stem cells, exhibit a distinct genetic profile, and play a role in disease dissemination and progression.

Published studies have demonstrated that detectable MRD in PB correlates with worse PFS and OS in MM. Additionally, PB-based MRD assessment offers several advantages, including the ability to monitor MM patients more frequently, detect MRD in extramedullary and multifocal disease, and identify impending disease progression. PB MRD is noninvasive and reproducible and avoids the issue of hemodilution. However, it requires the acquisition of a large number of cells (10–50 million), necessitating a larger volume of peripheral blood. Techniques such as immunomagnetic selection of plasma cells and flow cytometry from PB have also been explored. A promising and highly sensitive method (with a sensitivity of ~10^{-7}) combining immunomagnetic enrichment of plasma cells and NGF is now being utilized for PB MRD detection.

DNA PLOIDY GUIDING MINIMAL/MEASURABLE RESIDUAL DISEASE TESTING

In most cases of MM, clinical response evaluation is often incomplete prior to BM testing. As a result, MRD testing is frequently performed even when the BM plasma cell clone is significantly large and often morphologically detectable. To address the need for MRD testing, a method using DNA ploidy was developed at the Mayo Clinic as a screening tool, termed the Plasma Cell Proliferation Index (PCPRO). This approach utilizes a simple panel of markers, including CD19, CD38, CD138, CD45, kappa, lambda, and 4′,6-diamidino-2-phenylindole (DAPI), a DNA-binding dye. The ploidy status is determined by calculating the DNA index (DI), which is the ratio of the mean fluorescence intensity between the G0–G1 peaks of abnormal and normal plasma cells. Additionally, this method allows for the simultaneous evaluation of the S-phase fraction, a known prognostic factor in MM. PCPRO was able to detect MRD in 75% of cases, while the remaining 25% required NGF for further analysis in a study conducted at the Mayo Clinic. DNA ploidy testing serves as an effective screening tool, helping to avoid unnecessary MRD testing while providing valuable additional information.

MM MRD BY NGS AND DROPLET DIGITAL PCR

The biggest limitation of ASO-PCR for MRD detection is its restricted applicability due to the reasons mentioned earlier. NGS-based MRD has emerged as a viable alternative, overcoming many of the disadvantages associated with PCR-based MRD. Amplicon-based sequencing technology is particularly favored due to its cost-effectiveness and superior sensitivity. The primary principle of NGS-based MRD in MM involves sequencing the immunoglobulin (Ig) receptor to identify clonal sequences. Consensus multiplex PCR using IGHV and IGHJ primers enables the sequencing of nearly all rearrangements (VDJ rearrangements) in the immunoglobulin receptor gene. The introduction of adapters and index sequences further enhances sensitivity. A threshold of >5% identical sequences among all identified sequences is used to define clonality at baseline. Post-therapy, patient-specific clonotypes are utilized for MRD evaluation.

The clonoSEQ assay (Adaptive Biotechnologies, Seattle, WA) is currently the only FDA-approved assay for MM MRD. This assay is highly sensitive, capable of detecting 1 clonal plasma cell in a million cells (sensitivity ~10^{-6}). NGS-based MRD is applicable to over 90% of MM patients. At a sensitivity level of 10^{-5}, the results of NGS and NGF MRD are highly concordant. While NGF allows for the simultaneous evaluation of the immune microenvironment and detection of hemodilution by assessing the mast cell compartment, it always requires fresh first-pull samples and is user-dependent. In contrast, NGS-based MRD requires fewer cells to achieve the desired sensitivity and does not necessitate fresh samples. However, somatic hypermutation can render the initial clone unidentifiable in approximately 10% of cases.

Droplet digital PCR (ddPCR) is another precise and highly sensitive method for MRD detection in lymphoid malignancies. Unlike traditional real-time PCR, ddPCR does not require a standard curve and provides absolute quantification of rare events. It can accurately track clonal immunoglobulin gene rearrangements, fusion transcripts, and known mutations.

CIRCULATING TUMOR DNA

Cell-free DNA (cfDNA) assessment, often referred to as liquid biopsy, is an emerging diagnostic tool for evaluating disease burden and MRD. Circulating tumor DNA (ctDNA), a fraction of the total cfDNA, is released by neoplastic cells into the blood and other body fluids. ctDNA carries cancer-specific genomic abnormalities, making it a valuable biomarker. In MM, spatial and genomic heterogeneity can lead to false-negative results from single-site BM evaluations, despite the invasive nature of the procedure. ctDNA monitoring is particularly beneficial in oligosecretory or nonsecretory MM cases and in extramedullary disease. However, detecting ctDNA is challenging due to its low concentration in peripheral blood.

The primary molecular approaches for cfDNA quantification include digital PCR and ultradeep NGS. Recent studies have demonstrated that ultra-low-pass whole genome sequencing (ULP-WGS) is a rapid and effective tool for detecting tumor burden and copy number variations (CNVs) in MM ctDNA. Various recurrently mutated genes have been identified in MM, such as *KRAS*, *NRAS*, and *BRAF* in the MAPK pathway, genes involved in NF-κB signaling, and others such as FGFR3, TRAF3, and TP53. Additionally, novel mutations in genes related to RNA processing, protein homeostasis, MYC transcription regulation, and linker histones have been reported. Ultra-deep targeted sequencing, combined with error-correcting unique molecular identifiers (UMIs), can detect and track single-nucleotide variations (SNVs) and insertions/deletions (indels). The combination of ULP-WGS and ultra-deep targeted sequencing is shown to effectively monitor tumor dynamics and predict disease progression in MM patients.

MASS SPECTROMETRY MINIMAL/MEASURABLE RESIDUAL DISEASE

Mass spectrometry (MS) has emerged as an ultra-sensitive tool over the past decade for detecting serum M-protein after therapy. Two primary methodologies are used in MS: The bottom-up technique (clonotypic peptide approach) and the intact protein approach. Both methods operate on the principle of detecting M-proteins, as each plasma cell produces a unique immunoglobulin (Ig) protein with a specific mass that can be identified by MS.

The intact protein approach is easier to standardize and is more time-efficient for measuring M-protein concentration in serum. Its result interpretation is similar to serum protein electrophoresis (SPEP) or immunofixation electrophoresis (IFE), as it appears as a peak in the mass-to-charge ratio distribution. This method is widely used in routine diagnostics due to its high specificity and faster turnaround time, though it lacks the sensitivity required for MRD evaluation. The intact protein MS assay typically employs matrix-assisted laser desorption/ionization-time of flight (MALDI-TOF) technology. The MASS-FIX technology, which combines MALDI-TOF-MS with immunoglobulin enrichment, offers improved sensitivity compared to SPEP and IFE but still falls short of the sensitivity needed for MRD assessment.

The clonotypic MS assay, on the other hand, is ultra-sensitive and both disease- and patient-specific. In this technique, clonotypic peptides are first identified, either by sequencing myeloma cells or through a blood-based method. Immunoglobulin peptides are obtained by enzymatically digesting the immunoglobulin variable region, followed by analysis using liquid chromatography tandem MS (LC-MS). Clonotypic MS MRD is 1,000 times more sensitive than SPEP. Additional techniques for immunoglobulin purification further enhance the sensitivity of MS-based MRD detection.

However, MS-based MRD faces several technical and disease-related challenges. It is labor-intensive and time-consuming and requires patient-specific calibrators, which can be costly. Additionally, even when BM MRD is negative by NGF or NGS, serum MS MRD may still detect residual M-protein due to the prolonged half-life of M-protein clearance rather than active disease.

WHOLE BODY IMAGING AND MINIMAL/MEASURABLE RESIDUAL DISEASE

Positron emission tomography with computed tomography and whole-body magnetic resonance imaging (WB-MRI) are essential for characterizing bone lesions and detecting extramedullary disease. FDG-PET-CT is a highly sensitive technique for identifying active disease, and PET positivity post-therapy has been established as a poor prognostic factor. New PET-CT radiotracers, such as CD38 radiolabeled antibodies and VLA-4, are under investigation and show promise for improved sensitivity. For example, zirconium-89 (Zr) conjugated with daratumumab has demonstrated greater sensitivity in detecting active lesions compared to traditional FDG-PET. Additionally, diffusion-weighted imaging (DWI) MRI provides accurate detection of both bony and extramedullary lesions. The IMWG guidelines recommend PET/CT to define imaging-based MRD negativity when combined with NGS or NGF.

MINIMAL/MEASURABLE RESIDUAL DISEASE TECHNIQUES—WHICH, WHEN, WHOM, HOW?

Despite advancements in MRD detection methods, NGS and NGF remain the gold standard for BM MRD evaluation. Complementary imaging techniques, such as PET/CT or WB-MRI, are particularly valuable for patients with high-risk cytogenetics and extramedullary disease. Due to the dynamic nature of MRD, multiple evaluations over time provide more comprehensive insights. Pre- and post-transplant MRD assessments have been consistently shown to carry significant prognostic value across clinical trials.

The IMWG guidelines have introduced the concept of *sustained MRD negativity*, defined as BM and imaging-based MRD negativity confirmed at least 1 year apart. The guidelines also recommend follow-up MRD evaluations at different timepoints to confirm MRD negativity. MRD assessment is advised for patients who achieve at least a very good partial response (VGPR) or better.

While MRD negativity is a robust prognostic marker, its role in guiding therapeutic decisions remains under investigation. Further research is needed to determine how MRD status can be integrated into treatment strategies to optimize patient outcomes.

Take Home Points

- MRD negativity is a strong, independent prognostic factor across all disease stages and risk categories in MM.
- Traditional methods such as MFC and ASO-PCR have been replaced by more sensitive techniques. NGF and NGS are now the gold standard for MRD evaluation.
- NGF and NGS offer higher sensitivity (up to 10^{-6}), enabling the detection of very low levels of residual disease.
- NGS-based methods, such as the clonoSEQ assay, are FDA-approved and widely applicable.
- Blood-based MRD techniques, such as circulating tumor DNA (ctDNA) and mass spectrometry (MS), are emerging as promising, less invasive tools for serial monitoring. These methods are particularly useful for oligosecretory/nonsecretory MM and extramedullary disease.
- PET-CT and whole-body MRI (WB-MRI) are critical for detecting extramedullary disease and active lesions.
- The concept of *sustained MRD negativity* (confirmed at two timepoints, 1 year apart) is a key goal in MM treatment. Serial MRD evaluations provide valuable insights into disease dynamics and progression.
- MRD negativity is a robust prognostic marker, but its role in guiding therapeutic decisions is still under investigation. Ongoing research aims to integrate MRD status into treatment strategies for personalized MM management.

SUGGESTED READINGS

1. Medina-Herrera A, Sarasquete ME, Jiménez C, Puig N, García-Sanz R. Minimal residual disease in multiple myeloma: past, present, and future. Cancers. 2023;15(14):3687.
2. Szalat RE, Anderson KC, Munshi NC. Role of minimal residual disease assessment in multiple myeloma. Haematologica. 2024;109(7):2049.
3. Wijnands C, Noori S, Donk NW, VanDuijn MM, Jacobs JF. Advances in minimal residual disease monitoring in multiple myeloma. Crit Rev Clin Lab Sci. 2023;60(7):518-34.
4. Pugh TJ. Circulating tumour DNA for detecting minimal residual disease in multiple myeloma. Semin Hematol. 2018;55(1):38-40.
5. Flores-Montero J, Sanoja-Flores L, Paiva B, Puig N, García-Sánchez O, Böttcher S, et al. Next Generation Flow for highly sensitive and standardized detection of minimal residual disease in multiple myeloma. Leukemia. 2017;31(10):2094-103.
6. Ferla V, Antonini E, Perini T, Farina F, Masottini S, Malato S, et al. Minimal residual disease detection by next-generation sequencing in multiple myeloma: Promise and challenges for response-adapted therapy. Front Oncol. 2022;12:932852.

CHAPTER 36

Quality Control in Hematology Cell Counters and Coagulation Laboratory: Good Laboratory Practices

Prabhu Manivannan, Gaurav Chhabra, Harish Chandra

ABSTRACT

The reports generated from the hematology laboratory play a central role in healthcare delivery; therefore, the results issued to the patients must be both accurate and precise. The robust quality control (QC) implemented in the laboratory through good clinical laboratory practices (GCLP) is therefore essential to maintain the trust and reliability of these reports, especially those which are generated by an automated analyzer from the hemogram and coagulation laboratory. The QC program encompasses various internal and external QC measures in order to maintain compliance with accreditation bodies. The internal quality control (IQC) involves regular monitoring by in-house testing of control material with preassigned values and other strategies such as delta check, duplicate sample testing, retained sample analysis, and employing various statistical procedures and graphical displays to detect errors and maintain the reproducibility of the data generated by the automated analyzer. The external quality assessment program compares the laboratory's test performance with the peer group using the same methodology, reagents, and instruments. It complements the IQC processes by providing interlaboratory comparison, ensuring the accuracy of the reports generated, and improving the overall outcome.

INTRODUCTION

The hematology laboratory plays a central role in healthcare delivery, and most commonly ordered investigations include hemogram and baseline coagulation tests. These basic investigations provide the initial framework and help in establishing the diagnosis, monitoring, and prognosis of various disease states. Therefore, these tests should be both accurate and precise; every step should be taken to avoid errors, and the same is applicable to all other investigations as well. We should have a better understanding of the various definitions used related to the quality. In simple terms, "quality is doing the right things and doing those things right".

"Quality management system (QMS)" refers to the overall activities related to the management function, such as determining the objectives related to quality policies and their implementation. It includes quality planning, quality assurance, quality control, and quality improvement within the system. "Quality assurance (QA)" is defined as a proactive systematic process where all the planned actions which are deemed necessary are taken to provide the adequate confidence that the service or the product satisfies all the given quality requirements. It is the comprehensive terminology covering all the aspects of operation beginning from preparing the patient for sample collection till the dispatch of results. "Quality control (QC)" refers to the set of protocols and procedures designed to monitor and maintain reliability that the results generated by the laboratory meet the established regulatory standards.

The effective QA program should dictate a set of principles called "good clinical laboratory practices (GCLP)" that defines the quality system within the concerned organization and the conditions where the entire laboratory studies will be carried out. This will help laboratories to minimize errors, maintain compliance with accreditation bodies such as the National Accreditation Board for Testing and Calibration Laboratories (NABL), the International Organization for Standardization (ISO), and thereby ensuring safety. The following section is divided to understand the general concepts related to QC and the specific measures taken in the hemogram and the coagulation laboratory.

GENERAL CONCEPTS RELATED TO QUALITY CONTROL

The "laboratory director" has the major responsibility in setting up the organization, and "quality manager" assists in developing the various policies related to QMS and its effective implementation. QC encompasses various internal and external QC measures implemented to verify that its performance is within predefined acceptable limits and meets the expected standards. It is essential that the reliable results are both accurate and precise and genuinely represent the underlying clinical condition. "Accuracy" is defined as closeness of the measured value to the true value, and "precision (reproducibility)" is defined as closeness of the measured value on repeated measurements under specified conditions **(Figs. 1A to D)**.

The definition of "bias" refers to the difference between the expected test results or measured value and a true value. It should also be kept in mind that

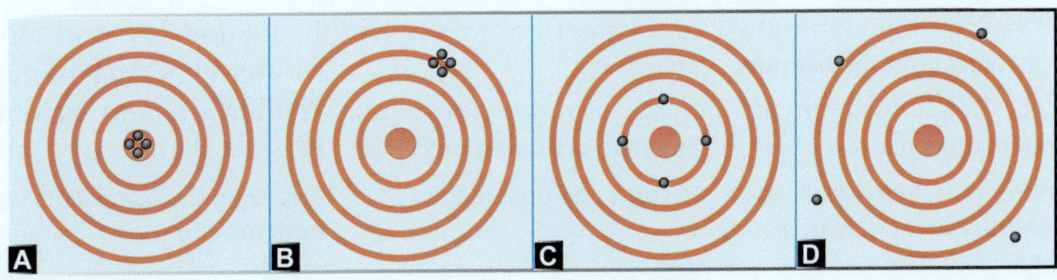

FIGS. 1A TO D: (A) Accurate and precise; (B) Not accurate but precise; (C) Accurate but not precise; (D) Neither accurate nor precise.

due to various factors, there is always a chance that deviation from the expected standards exists, which are called "nonconformities". The "risk management" is an effective approach that should be implemented in each laboratory which involves various steps in identifying the errors from occurring, so that preventing the harm to the person. Each procedure performed should follow the step-by-step instructions as written in the standard operating procedure (SOP) manual adopted in the individual laboratory.

In India, getting the laboratory accreditation by NABL is still voluntary and should follow the specific document 112 and ISO 15189:2022 for ensuring the quality in the laboratory. Similarly, there are other guidelines such as International Council for Standardization in Hematology (ICSH), British Committee for Standards in Hematology (BCSH), and College of American Pathologists (CAP), which are beyond the scope of this discussion. The laboratory testing is highly complex, which comprises testing cycle divided into pre-examination, examination, and postexamination phases. **Table 1** highlights the major determinants in each of these phases affecting the entire testing process.

Pre-examination Phase

The majority of the laboratory errors happen before the actual analysis takes place. **Table 2** highlights the different pre-examination variables affecting the laboratory testing. Most of the healthcare facilities use hospital integrated systems (HISs) and laboratory information systems (LISs) for ordering the tests. It provides necessary patient information, such as medical history/records, and different guidelines recommend its use to enter the test results. It is good practice to label the vacutainer tubes immediately before sample collection, preferably using a bar code system. If not possible, manual labeling should include their first and last name, age, hospital number, date, and time of collection. The two-point identification system should be followed, which includes the phlebotomist

TABLE 1: Major determinants affecting the entire laboratory testing.

Pre-examination phase	Examination phase	Postexamination phase
Ordering appropriate tests	Laboratory environment	Interpretation of reports
Patient preparation	Laboratory personnel	Turnaround time
Correct identification of the patient and the right sample collected	Reagents and consumables	Critical values
Right labeling at the bedside/ collection room	Equipment	Ensuring the correctness of the report
Correct order of draw	Standard operating procedure	Releasing the reports
Appropriate anticoagulants with the correct ratio of blood to anticoagulant	Records and documents	Analyzing the complaints from the end-users
The right method of sample collection, transport, and storage before testing	Safe handling of samples	Rectifying nonconformities, corrective and preventive actions

TABLE 2: Variables affecting the pre-examination phase of laboratory testing.

Patient related	Sample collection related	Sample in-transit related and others
Fasting/Random sample	Posture of the patient	Pneumatic chute/manual transportation
Exercise	Collection timing—diurnal variation	Temperature
Smoking and alcoholism	Fresh venipuncture/ indwelling catheter	Humidity
Drug exposure	Order of draw	Exposure to light
Antisera/Vaccine exposure	Correct anticoagulant	Centrifugation
Hydration status	Vacutainer/syringe and needle	Storage
Icterus	Hemolysis during collection	Accepted sample processing time
Lipemia	Correct volume	Quality check for reagents, consumables, and instruments

asking the name of the patient and matching it with the requisition forms as well as second question regarding his address or father's name.

It is recommended that the tourniquet should not be applied for more than 2 minutes at the time of blood collection. The correct order of blood draw should be followed when taking multiple samples from the same person. Generally, closed systems such as vacutainers with 19-21 G needles in adults and 22-23 G needles in children are preferred. However, in infants, small-bore needles (25-27 G) can be used. The sample must be mixed gently by doing 8–10 inversions after collection in a vial. Dipotassium salts of ethylene diamine tetra-acetic acid anticoagulant are recommended for hemogram because of better morphologic preservation of cells, and 3.2% (109 mmol/L) trisodium citrate should be used for coagulation testing.

Examination Phase

The proficiency of the laboratory personnel is of utmost importance as their basic qualification, adequate training, and motivation to continually learn about the quality are essential to provide reliable results. The basic knowledge about the equipment, reagents, and consumables, and the other factors influencing the examination phase is depicted in **Table 3**.

It is essential to have proper calibration of the instrument, and this involves adjusting the instrument to ensure the results generated are consistent and accurate. This is done by using "calibrators" which are standardized materials or devices with known values that are used to compare the other materials or devices. This is generally performed at the time of installation or after a major breakdown, or according to the local quality policies. This needs to be differentiated from the "control samples" which should be treated exactly similarly to the patient samples. These are generally provided by the manufacturer or third parties, or

TABLE 3: Variables affecting the examination phase of laboratory testing.

Variables	Influencing factors
Personnel proficiency	Educational qualification, adequate training, continual improvement by attending conferences, and workshops
Equipment reliability	Technical specification, comprehensive annual maintenance, user-friendly, and cost-effectiveness
Reagents and consumables	Technical specification meeting the necessary demands, lot number, continuous availability, and stability
Sensitivity and specificity of the test	Validation of the newer test against the reference method, acceptable standards, cost-effective, and easily reproducible method
Procedural reliability	Standard operating procedure
Documents and records	Confidentiality, accessibility, and updated maintenance
Using appropriate controls	Internal and external quality control/interlaboratory comparative program, expected to meet the national and international standards

"in-house" controls can also be used, provided that they are properly validated before their use. These control samples have preassigned values which are used to monitor the analytical performance within the desired limits.

The reliability of the test results depends on internal QC (IQC) and the External Quality Assessment Scheme (EQAS). The IQC monitors and verifies the precision of results by running the control samples daily, whereas the EQAS assesses the accuracy of the analytical process and the overall performance of the instrument.

Postexamination Phase

The personnel in the laboratory should have a thorough knowledge related to assay interpretation and troubleshooting. There should be scope for quality improvement practices such as Six Sigma methods. These ensure that the correct report would reach the correct person at the correct time, and **Table 4** highlights different variables affecting this phase of laboratory testing. The data privacy and handling policies should be strict to provide the confidentiality to the end-users, and safe disposal of processed samples should meet the locoregional and national standards.

Appropriate key performance indicators or quality indicators should be used for monitoring and achieving the goals related to quality policies. It is a good practice to conduct the audit, which means an "independent, systematic, and recording process for acquiring evidence and estimating it impartially to conclude the range to which necessary criteria are satisfied". It is encouraged to get the feedback/complaint and necessary corrective and preventive actions to be taken to address the nonconformities.

TABLE 4: Variables affecting the postexamination phase of laboratory testing.

Variables	Influencing factors
Reporting of results	Thorough knowledge about the interpretation of the test and also about the troubleshooting
Releasing of reports	Completely error free and should be screened by one and preferably validated by other qualified persons
Turnaround time	Reasonable time would be 4–8 hours and within 1–2 hours for emergency samples in hemogram and coagulation laboratory
Critical alert values	Should be clearly defined in the SOP, must be known to all the technical persons working in the laboratory who assist in the emergency/necessary management
Retention of samples/reports	Should meet the national standards
Disposal of samples	Locoregional and national guidelines for safe disposal of biological agents
Confidentiality	Restricted accessibility to vital documents and informed consent and data privacy policies
Feedback/Complaints	Both positive and negative suggestions from end-users/ clients (patients and clinical colleagues)
Measures to avoid nonconformities	Root cause analysis, corrective and preventive actions
Quality indicators	Number of error reports, performance in EQAS (Z-score), accident/incident report, number of blood spills/exposure to toxins/pathogens, major breakdown, and others

SPECIFIC MEASURES RELATED TO HEMATOLOGY CELL COUNTERS

The hemogram is one of the most frequently ordered medical tests, and the assessment of blood cell counts has transitioned from manual microscopy-based methods to fully automated hematology cell counters offering higher throughput, better accuracy, improved precision, and minimized human errors and subjectivity.

The robustness of the QC procedures should be clearly outlined in the SOP manual and more than 20 specific points to be highlighted according to NABL. Some of them include purpose and principle of examination, patient preparation, sample rejection/acceptance criteria, proper calibration, linearity assessment, measurement of uncertainty, establishing the biological reference intervals, testing methodology, interfering substances, critical alert values, clinical interpretation, and environmental and safety measures adopted in the laboratory. The following section is mainly focused on different methods used for assessing IQC in hematology cell counters.

Selection of Internal Quality Control Material

The commercial IQC materials are specially prepared and stabilized whole blood samples from a human or a mammalian source which are available in three levels, representing "high, normal, and low" levels to assess the complete measurement range of the analytical system. It should be compatible and specific to the model of the cell counter being used in the laboratory.

Establishing the Control Sample Ranges

The control means, standard deviation (SD), and coefficient of variation (CV) are established by repeatedly testing control samples with a minimum of 20 runs, and this will be valid till the lot number changes. The commercial IQC material comes with a preassigned target value or the mean with ±2 or 3 SD. However, it is recommended that every laboratory should verify and establish its own mean and SD.

Monitoring Quality Control

The ICSH recommends using Levey-Jennings (LJ) charts at least for the clinically important parameters such as "white and red blood cells count (WBC and RBC), hemoglobin (Hb), mean corpuscular volume (MCV), and platelets." It is a graphical plot of control results versus the time to plot successive (run-to-run or day-to-day) results of the QC. The software plots the QC results, and if the runs are "in-control", the values will be hovering around the mean and ±2 SD. Likewise, a chart is generated for each test parameter and for each level of control material ("high, normal, and low"), providing a visual representation of trends (gradual deviations), shifts (sudden changes), or outliers (values falling outside the acceptable ±2 or 3 SD limits) and should trigger immediate troubleshooting. The "Westgard rules" **(Box 1 and Fig. 2)** are applied to decide whether an analytical

BOX 1: Westgard's rules for interpreting the Levy–Jennings' chart.

- 1_{2s} *Rule*: One observation exceeding ±2 SD limit from the mean, suggesting a random error*, and is used as a warning rule to closely evaluate the procedures along with the other set of rules
- 1_{3s} *Rule*: One observation exceeding ±3 SD from the mean suggests a random error. If this rule is violated, the run is rejected, and troubleshooting for the underlying cause is warranted
- 2_{2s} *Rule*: Two consecutive observations exceeding ±2 SD on the same side of the mean, suggesting systematic error* and detecting bias, the run is rejected following the violation
- R_{4s} *Rule*: Two consecutive observations within the same level run show a difference greater than 4 SD, i.e., one observation exceeds the mean +2 SD, and the other exceeds the mean—2 SD, indicating a random error, leading to rejection of the run
- 4_{1s} *Rule*: This rule is violated when four consecutive observations exceed ±1 SD on the same side of the mean, depicting systematic error and leading to rejection of the run
- 10_{x} *Rule*: Ten consecutive observations falling on the same side of the mean if using the same level control or five consecutive observations when analyzing two different level controls indicating a bias or systematic error

*Random error means the error is occurring by chance, leading to imprecision, whereas systematic error means there is a potential error in the environment, reagents, consumables, equipment or instruments, and continues to occur till it is rectified, resulting in inaccurate results.

run is "in-control" or "out-of-control". These rules provide a systematic approach in identifying errors and should be stressed that no single rule can identify the errors perfectly, and the overall efficiency is improved by using multiple rules together. **Figure 3** shows the IQC "level 1" sample run for the common reportable parameters in the hemogram laboratory and its Levy-Jennings chart in our laboratory.

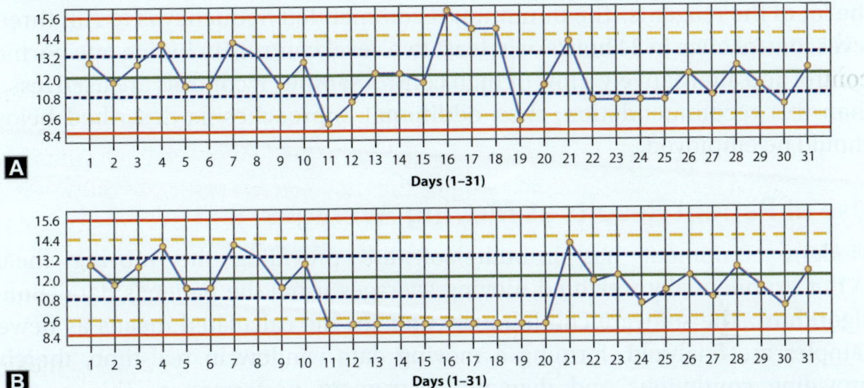

FIGS. 2A AND B: Levy–Jennings chart for hemoglobin. The green line represents the mean value with corresponding ±1 SD (dotted blue), ±2 SD (dashed yellow), and ±3 SD (red) lines, and the orange dot represents individual run results. (A) The results on day 11, day 16, days 17 and 18; days 18 and 19, days 22–25 violating 1_{2s}, 1_{3s}, 2_{2s}, R_{4s} and 4_{1s}, respectively (B) violating the 10_x Westgard rule from day 11 to 20.

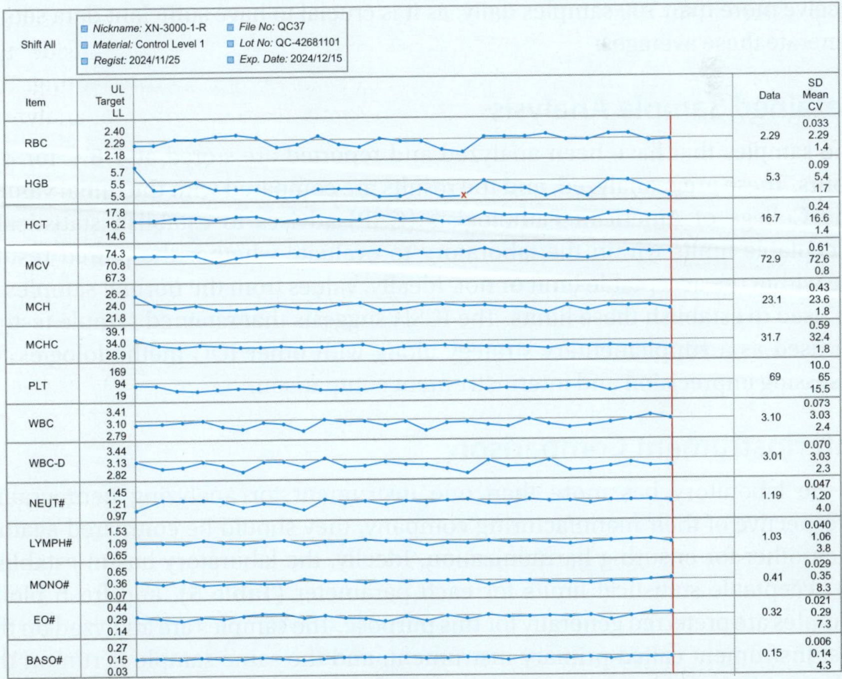

FIG. 3: Internal quality control "level 1" sample run for the common reportable parameters in the hemogram laboratory and its Levy–Jennings chart.

Frequency of Control Sample Measurements

This is based on the workload of the laboratory, analytical stability of the test method, risk appetite of the laboratory, any specific requirements of their quality policy, and any advisory or guidelines issued by a regulatory and statutory agency. Additionally, it is advisable to run controls following any major maintenance of the instrument or calibration or following the change in the lot of the reagents. The minimum recommended frequency is to run three-level control once in 24 hours or at least two-level control, including one normal control and alternatively a low or high control sample. If controls are used lesser than this recommendation, then additional approaches as described below should be employed.

Use of Patient Results as Moving Averages

Modern equipment has in-built software providing the moving mean ($\bar{X}$) or exponentially weighted moving averages using the patient's data (Bull's algorithm). The software continuously updates the calculated means as newer samples are analyzed, forming a moving data window in real-time, thereby providing continuous and dynamic instrument performance. This method involves calculating the mean value of specific parameters (e.g., Hb, MCV, WBC count) from a group of 20 consecutive samples. These averages are then compared to established baseline values or expected target ranges. This ensures QC by identifying the gradual shifts or any trends indicating analytical errors or the accuracy of the analyzer. The major limitation is that the laboratory should receive more than 100 samples daily, as it is crucial to have sufficient data sets to generate these averages.

Retained Sample Analysis

The samples that have been analyzed and reported are stored at 4–8°C for <12 hours. These are reanalyzed, and the results are compared with the initial values. The College of American Pathologists (CAP) advises to establish statistically acceptable limits within the laboratory to evaluate whether the paired results are within the acceptable limit or not. Ideally, values from the normal samples to be used to establish these limits. The ICSH suggests that retained sample testing be used as a supplementary strategy along with other IQC methodologies for assessing imprecision and interinstrument comparison.

Interinstrument Comparison

If the laboratory has more than one instrument for analyzing hemograms, irrespective of their manufacturing company, they should be compared against each other for ensuring harmonization. Ideally, the laboratory has to establish its acceptable statistical limits for each parameter **(Table 5)**, and fresh blood samples are preferred generally for this purpose. The samples are analyzed on the first instrument called primary instrument, and the same sample is run on the other secondary instruments for daily QC of those instruments.

TABLE 5: Interinstrument comparison in the hematology cell counters for WBC count.

Instrument's number		Run	WBC	Average	Deviation	Z-score	Report
C.LAB-WS-I (1062)	Right	I	8.37	8.41	0.00	0.08	Satisfactory
		II	8.44				
	Left	I	8.41	8.47	0.07	1.37	Satisfactory
		II	8.53				
C.LAB-WS-II (1065)	Right	I	8.21	8.34	–0.06	–1.21	Satisfactory
		II	8.47				
	Left	I	8.37	8.42	0.01	0.28	Satisfactory
		II	8.46				
24x7-WS-II (1066)	Right	I	8.42	8.43	0.03	0.58	Satisfactory
		II	8.44				
	Left	I	8.36	8.35	–0.06	–1.11	Satisfactory
		II	8.33				
Mean			8.4			Similarly, establish for the other reportable parameters	
SD			0.05				
2SD			0.10				
95% confidence interval			8.36–8.44				
2 SD interval			8.30–8.50				

Running Samples in Duplicate or Split Sample Testing

Duplicate samples can be obtained by splitting a whole blood sample (split sample testing) into two parts or collected independently in the same phlebotomy in two vials. This approach helps in checking the precision and detecting random errors or other preanalytical issues by reanalyzing and comparing the results.

Delta Check

This is used to monitor for significant changes or differences in consecutive test results for the same patient within a defined time frame to rule out errors in sample handling or analysis. These checks are helpful for parameters that do not fluctuate significantly under normal physiological conditions, such as Hb, hematocrit (Hct), RBC indices, or platelet count. These checks help to detect potential preanalytical, analytical, or postanalytical errors that might go unnoticed otherwise.

Correlation Check

The comparison between the morphological examination of peripheral smear or complete clinical details and the cell counter results represents a vital postexamination QC check. This helps in identifying any discrepancies, assess the accuracy of the analyzer, and the laboratory should specify the indications for peripheral smear review for flagged results.

External Quality Assessment Scheme

In EQAS program, the proficiency testing (PT) provider circulates the standardized samples with known or consensus values to the participating laboratories for analysis, which in turn submit their results back to them. The PT provider in our country for the hemogram, reticulocyte, and peripheral smear is the All India Institute of Medical Sciences, New Delhi, and the performance of our laboratory is shown in **Figure 4**. They compare the results received from

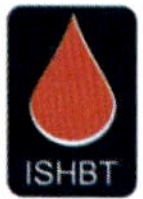

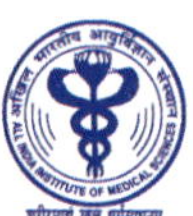

PROFICIENCY TESTING REPORT
ISHTM-ALIMS EXTERNAL QUALITY ASSURANCE PROGRAMME
NABL accredited program as per ISO/IEC 17043:2010 standard
Organized By Department of Hematology, AIIMS, New Delhi-110029

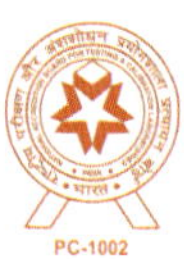

Duration of stability testing-minimum upto 8 days at ambient temp. after dispatch of specimens

EQAP CODE No.: 1065 | Distribution No.: 164-C | Month/Year: June/2024
Instrument ID: SYSMEX | Model Name.: XN-3000 | Serial No.: 48081

Name & Contact No. of PT Co-ordinator: Dr. Manoranjan Mahapatra (Prof. & Head), Hematology, AIIMS, Delhi,
Tel: 9013085730, E-Mail: info@ishtmaiimseqap.com
Date of issue & status of the report: 23-07-2024 [Final]

CBC and Retic Assessment

Test Parameters	S.No.			Among Lab (Accuracy Testing)				Within Lab (Precision Testing)			
		Your Result 1	Your Result 2	Your Results Sum of 2 Value	Consensus result sum of 2 values (Assigned Value)	Uncertainty of Assigned Values	Z Score	Yours Results Diff. of 2 Values	Consensus Result Diff. of 2 values (Assigned Value)	Uncertainty of Assigned Values	Z Score
WBC x10^3/µl	1	5.4	5.33	10.73	16.14	0.281	-0.32	0.07	0.07	0.013	0.47
RBC x10^5/µl	1	3.62	3.6	7.22	7.43	0.016	-0.46	0.02	0.02	0.002	-0.54
Hb g/dl	1	11.7	11.6	23.3	24.4	0.056	-0.69	0.1	0.1	0.007	0.00
HCT%	1	36	36	72	76.9	0.269	-0.60	0	0	0.023	-0.08
MCV-fl	1	100	99.4	199.4	205.1	0.470	-0.42	0.6	0.6	0.022	0.81
MCH-Pg	1	32.3	32.2	64.5	65.8	0.090	-0.57	0.1	0.1	0.017	-0.67
MCHC-g/dl	1	32.5	32.2	64.7	63.8	0.182	0.18	0.3	0.3	0.013	0.00
Plt.x10^3/µl	1	100	93	193	209	2.172	-0.25	7	7	0.290	0.39
Retic %	2	2.5	2	4.5	12.6	0.181	-1.63	0.5	0.5	0.023	0.00

P.S. Assesment

		YOUR REPORT	CONSENSUS REPORT
DLC%	3	Nrbcs=0, Poly-07 L-11, E-01, Mono/Promono-18, 81-60 P.M.-0, Mye 02, Meta-01, Other-0	Blast: 45-64, Poly: 10-16, Lympho: 9-18,, Mono: 3-13.75, Myelo/Meta/Bos/Mono/Promyelo/Baso: 0-5
RBC Morphology	3	Normocytic normochromic	Predominantly: Normocytic/ Normochromic, Moderate: Anisocytosis, Macrocytic
Diagnosis	3	Acute Myeloid Leukemia	Acute Leukemia-(AML)

FIG. 4: Proficiency testing report for hemogram, reticulocyte, and peripheral smear showing acceptable accuracy among the laboratories and with acceptable precision within the laboratory.

each participant with a consensus value derived from the peer group's results using the same testing methodology and instrument. The performance of the participating laboratories is based on their "Standard Deviation Index" or the "Z-score" and according to the ISO13528:2022 standard, the value of "Z-score" of 0 ± 2 is acceptable, ±2 to ±3 indicates warning signal and beyond ±3 is considered unacceptable.

SPECIFIC MEASURES RELATED TO COAGULATION LABORATORY

In hemostasis and thrombosis testing, thorough history taking would give a solution in 80–90% of cases and recommended to use a bleeding assessment tool for an objective evaluation. The commonly performed tests are broadly divided to basic screening and specific assays to identify the factor deficiency, anticoagulant/drug monitoring, lupus anticoagulant, platelet testing, and thrombosis work-up.

Pre-examination Issues in Coagulation Laboratory

The majority of errors (33–75%) occur in the pre-examination phase, and most of them stem from incorrect ordering of tests, issues in blood sample collection, handling, storage, or transport. Recently, ICSH gave their recommendations, especially to avoid these pre-examination errors, processing of samples for coagulation testing, and a few of the salient features are briefed in the following section.

The patient should be given proper instructions to avoid strenuous exercise, abstain from smoking, alcohol, certain foods, and drugs before sampling, which might affect the test results. Whenever possible, samples should be collected within or in a place close to the laboratory and preferable to use fresh venipuncture with tourniquet applied for <1 minute. If this is not possible, the alternate option is to discard the first 5–10 mL of blood if collected from an indwelling catheter or using a butterfly needle.

The trisodium citrate anticoagulant to blood ratio should be maintained strictly as 1:9, and ICSH recommends sample rejection when the amount of blood is <80% of the recommended volume. After collection, the sample should reach the laboratory as early as possible at the room temperature. It is recommended that for performing the platelet function test (PFT), the sample should not be transported via a pneumatic tube system. Earlier transportation is recommended for factor assays, and the sample should reach within 15–30 minutes after receiving the plasma products/recombinant factors.

Most commonly, single centrifugation at room temperatures (18–24°C) is used to prepare platelet poor plasma (PPP), ensuring the platelet count is <10 × 10^9/L; refrigerated centrifuge is not useful for PFT, lupus anticoagulant (LAC), and activated protein C resistance. Double centrifugation is intended for LAC or those with unfractionated heparin for activated partial thromboplastin time (APTT) or anti-Xa testing and before sample freezing.

After centrifugation, one should look for the evidence of in vitro hemolysis and lipemia, because of its interference with plasma-based testing. The Clinical and Laboratory Standard Institute (CLSI) recommends to adjust the citrate-to-blood ratio if the Hct exceeds 55%. The formula used is "volume of citrate (C) in (mL) = (1.85×10^{-3}) (100 – Hct) (volume of blood in mL)".

Every measure should be taken to complete the sample processing within 4 hours of its collection. If delay is expected, sample should be kept at 4°C unless tested and 18–24°C for prothrombin time, LAC, and factor VII assays. Secondary aliquots of the sample should be kept frozen in polypropylene vials with a frequent freeze-thaw cycle of >2 cycles to be avoided until validated in the laboratory. A frost-free freezer should be avoided because the temperature will not be maintained during the warming cycles. Some tests, such as LAC and for thrombophilia, will be done in batches for which PPPs are usually kept frozen at –20°C for 2 weeks and –70°C for up to 6 weeks.

Examination Phase Quality Control

The stringent mandatory requirements to be used for selecting an automated coagulation analyzer because most of the tests are performed in batches. The majority of them work on endpoint detection by mechanical, electromagnetic, or optical methods; and whenever possible, chromogenic assay is preferred over one-stage clot-based detection methods. The instrument calibration is performed at the time of installation, along with process validation performed through installation, operational, and performance qualification.

The utmost care should be taken in selecting the reagents, which should be compatible for use in the coagulation analyzer available in the laboratory. It is good practice to select the APTT reagents sensitive to heparin and LAC, and similarly for prothrombin time, reagents should have an international sensitivity index value close to one. The stability of reagents should be ensured under appropriate storage conditions, and newer lot verification must be performed by comparing the sample results with older lots of reagents. If these reagents are reconstituted before use, proper labeling should be used comprising their concentration, reconstituted date with expiry date with appropriate storage conditions.

In most of the assays, a commercial calibrator is preferred, which is already calibrated against the reference standard because of its traceability. The standard curve is used along with either the commercially available or already validated "in-house" controls at two/three different levels as a part of quality measures. However, in order to monitor certain drugs such as direct oral anticoagulants, a separate calibration curve should be obtained using the specific drug to be studied.

It is generally recommended to pool the plasma from at least 20 healthy volunteers, involving both genders and a broader age distribution, which serves as a normal control and is mandatory to establish the biological reference range for hemostasis and thrombosis testing. In the cost-constrained scenario, aged serum and adsorbed plasma need to be used for mixing studies instead of commercial factor-deficient plasma.

Generally, plastic tubes should be used for sample dilutions, reagent preparation, and storage, whereas actual tests are performed using glass tubes. Centrifuge and pipettes should be periodically calibrated, and a water bath with plastic or glass sides and an in-built monitor/thermometer is preferable to maintain the temperature within a very tight range of 37 ± 0.5°C. Geometric mean is preferred over the arithmetic mean in prothrombin time because the skewed data is covered in the former for calculating international normalized ratio.

Postexamination Quality Measures

The correlation check with the provided clinical details should be ascertained before releasing the test results. It is also good practice to look at the data capturing mechanism in HIS/LIS or follow-up cards or delta check, especially for factor deficiency/inhibitors/thrombotic testing.

The proficiency test provider for coagulation is Christian Medical College, Vellore, and EQAS performance of the laboratory is depicted using histograms and a Youden plot. It is a graphical plot used to identify the variability within the laboratory as well as between the laboratory, provided all of them have analyzed two samples. **Figure 5** shows our performance for APTT with acceptable performance limits, CV (%), and our performance (within consensus) for both the samples.

CONCLUSION

The major role of a hematology laboratory is to deliver the consistent, reliable, and reproducible results for the basic investigations such as hemogram and screening and confirmatory work-up for bleeding/thrombotic disorders. Every laboratory should have documented quality policies and objectives to meet the national and international standards using the GCLP. This policy should be developed collaboratively by all the stakeholders, including the executive from the management, laboratory director, quality manager, other laboratory professionals, and clinical colleagues, and should ultimately benefit the patients/end-users. The QA program should encourage audit-guided intervention, necessary corrective and preventive action, and continual improvement to meet the quality objectives. Integrating the conventional and advancing technology including the QC adds to the complexity of laboratory management. Overall, wider visibility of quality ensures profitability for management, ethical and GCLP for laboratory professionals, satisfaction for the clinical colleagues, and safety/confidentiality for the end-users.

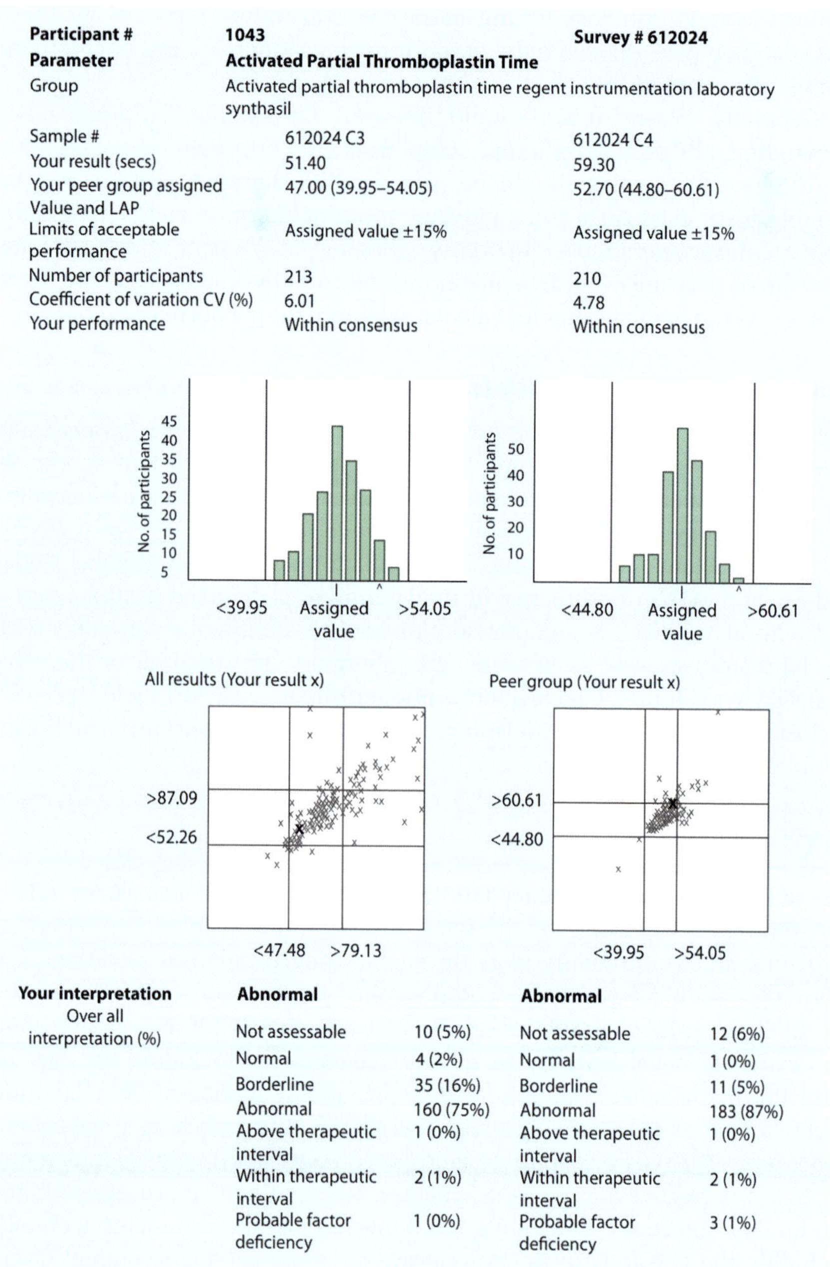

Participant #	**1043**	**Survey # 612024**
Parameter	**Activated Partial Thromboplastin Time**	
Group	Activated partial thromboplastin time regent instrumentation laboratory synthasil	
Sample #	612024 C3	612024 C4
Your result (secs)	51.40	59.30
Your peer group assigned Value and LAP	47.00 (39.95–54.05)	52.70 (44.80–60.61)
Limits of acceptable performance	Assigned value ±15%	Assigned value ±15%
Number of participants	213	210
Coefficient of variation CV (%)	6.01	4.78
Your performance	Within consensus	Within consensus

Your interpretation Over all interpretation (%)	**Abnormal**		**Abnormal**	
	Not assessable	10 (5%)	Not assessable	12 (6%)
	Normal	4 (2%)	Normal	1 (0%)
	Borderline	35 (16%)	Borderline	11 (5%)
	Abnormal	160 (75%)	Abnormal	183 (87%)
	Above therapeutic interval	1 (0%)	Above therapeutic interval	1 (0%)
	Within therapeutic interval	2 (1%)	Within therapeutic interval	2 (1%)
	Probable factor deficiency	1 (0%)	Probable factor deficiency	3 (1%)

FIG. 5: Performance of our laboratory in coagulation EQAS is "within consensus" as demonstrated in the Youden's plot as (x).

Take Home Points

- Robust QC practices form the foundation of reliable hematological testing and contribute to improved patient outcomes.
- Effective IQC practices involve selecting appropriate control materials, establishing QC ranges, monitoring QC data using tools such as Levey-Jennings charts and Westgard rules, and employing supplementary strategies such as delta checks and retained sample analysis
- Participation in EQA programs ensures accuracy by enabling interlaboratory comparisons and benchmarking against national and international standards.
- Integrating IQC, EQA, and error detection strategies ensures the reliability of hematological testing, supporting accurate diagnosis, regulatory compliance, and improved outcomes.
- Accept any feedback/complaints, root cause analysis, and the necessary corrective and preventive action must be taken for the continual improvement. These GCLPs will definitely improve the overall quality of the laboratory, and we can gain the trust of our clients (patients as well as our clinicians).

Review Exercises

CASE 1

A 45-year-old male patient from the general ward is being evaluated for unexplained bleeding. A blood sample is collected for PT and APTT testing. However, the sample is transported without using a pneumatic system, and it takes 2 hours to reach the coagulation laboratory. Upon examination, the sample shows evidence of hemolysis. Which preanalytical issue is most likely to affect the validity of the results in this case?

A. Delayed sample transport
B. Hemolysis during transport
C. Collection in the wrong anticoagulant
D. Insufficient blood volume in the tube

Correct answer: B

CASE 2

A sample for APTT testing is collected from a 60-year-old patient receiving unfractionated heparin therapy. The sample reaches the coagulation laboratory after 90 minutes. The laboratory policy states that analysis must be completed within 4 hours of sample collection. What should the laboratory staff do to ensure reliable results for this sample?

A. Reject the sample and request a new one
B. Inappropriate test ordered
C. Perform a centrifugation before analysis for platelet-poor plasma
D. Store the sample at room temperature for later testing

Correct answers C

SUGGESTED READINGS

1. McCafferty R, Cembrowski G, De La Salle B, Peng M, Urrechaga E. ICSH guidance for internal quality control policy for blood cell counters. Int J Lab Hematol. 2024;46:227-33.
2. McCafferty R, Cembrowski G, De La Salle B, Peng M, Urrechaga E. ICSH review of internal quality control policy for blood cell counters. Int J Lab Hematol. 2024;46:216-26.
3. Miller WG. Quality Control. In: McPherson Richard A, Pincus Matthew R (Eds). Henry's Clinical Diagnosis and Management by Laboratory Methods, 24th edition. Philadelphia: Elsevier; 2022. pp. 130-49.
4. Salle BD La, Perry DJ. Quality Assurance. In: Bain BJ, Bates I, Laffan MA, Lewis Mitchell S (Eds). Dacie and Lewis Practical Haematology. 12th edition. Elsevier; 2017. pp. 533-45.
5. Tambwekar S. In: Handbook of Quality Assurance in Laboratory Medicine, 1st edition. New Delhi: BI Publications Pvt Ltd.; 2009.
6. Westgard JO, Barry PL, Hunt MR, Groth T. A multi-rule Shewhart chart for quality control in clinical chemistry. Clin Chem. 1981;27:493-509.
7. DeVries H, Fritsma GA. Quality Assurance in Hematology and Hemostasis Testing. In: Keohane Elaine M, Otto Catherine N, Walenga Jeanine M (Eds). Rodak's Hematology: Clinical Principles and Applications, 6th edition. St. Louis, Missouri: Elsevier; 2020. pp. 8-30.
8. Green SF. The cost of poor blood specimen quality and errors in preanalytical processes. Clin Biochem. 2013;46:1175-9.
9. Salvagno GL, Lippi G, Bassi A, Poli G, Guidi GC. Prevalence and type of pre-analytical problems for inpatients samples in coagulation laboratory. J Eval Clin Pract. 2008;14:351-3.
10. Kitchen S, Adcock DM, Dauer R, Kristoffersen AH, Lippi G, Mackie I, et al. International Council for Standardisation in Haematology (ICSH) recommendations for collection of blood samples for coagulation testing. Int J Lab Hematol. 2021;43:571-80.
11. Kitchen S, Adcock DM, Dauer R, Kristoffersen AH, Lippi G, Mackie I, et al. International Council for Standardization in Haematology (ICSH) recommendations for processing of blood samples for coagulation testing. Int J Lab Hematol. 2021;43:1272-83.
12. Ray MJ. An artefact related to the ratio of sample volume to the blood collection vial size which effects the APTTs of specimens taken to monitor heparin therapy. Thromb Haemost. 1991;66:387-8.
13. Kitchen S, McGraw A, Enchenagucia M. Diagnosis of Hemophilia and Other Bleeding Disorders: A Laboratory Manual, 2nd edition; 2010.
14. Clinical Laboratory Standards Institute. Collection, Transport and Processing of Blood Specimens for Testing Plasma–Based Coagulation Assays and Molecular Homeostasis Assays: Approval Guidelines, 5th edition. CLSI H21–A5 10; 2008.
15. Schouwers SM, Delanghe JR, Devreese KM. Lupus Anticoagulant (LAC) testing in patients with inflammatory status: does C-reactive protein interfere with LAC test results? Thromb Res. 2010;125:102-4.
16. Monika P, Puneet KN, Vijay K. In: ICMR Guidelines for Good Clinical Laboratory Practices (GCLP) 2021, 2nd edition. New Delhi (India): ICMR, Department of Health Research, Government of India; 2021.

CHAPTER 37

Immunohematology in Solving Cases of Autoimmune Hemolytic Anemia

Sangeeta Pahuja, Satyam Arora, Shamee Shastry

ABSTRACT

Autoimmune hemolytic anemia (AIHA) is group of heterogeneous disorders, characterized by decompensated acquired hemolysis caused by the host's immune system acting against its own red cell antigens. It can occur at any age but incidence rises with increasing age. AIHA is broadly classified as Warm, Cold (CAD and PCH), Mixed and Drug induced AIHA; depending on type, thermal reactivity and specificity of antibodies. Diagnosis is established by clinical, hematological, biochemical and serological workup to ascertain immune nature of hemolysis. Complete evaluation is imperative to ascertain proper diagnosis and to ensure adequate management of patients.

INTRODUCTION

Autoimmune hemolytic anemia (AIHA) is a decompensated acquired hemolysis mediated through the host's immune response, specifically humoral antibodies acting against its own red cells. AIHA is a heterogeneous group of disorders, and thorough clinical and serological workup is required for proper characterization and management.

The incidence is approximately 1 per 100,000/year. It can occur at any age, but the incidence rises with increasing age. The age-wise incidence of individual types of AIHA is also associated with underlying etiopathogenesis.

Diagnosis of AIHA requires serologic evidence of antibodies and evidence of hemolysis caused by autoantibody. Hemolysis is evidenced by:

- *Fall in hemoglobin (and hematocrit):* Bone marrow compensates by increasing production, which is reflected as anisocytosis, polychromasia, and nucleated red blood cells (RBCs) on peripheral smear (PS).
- Reticulocytosis is seen in most cases. However, some patients may show reticulocytopenia, which may be due to inadequate bone marrow capacity (e.g., after chemotherapy, myelophthisis), aplastic anemia, infections (e.g., parvovirus B19 infection), hematinic deficiency, etc. Some anti-RBC antibodies may bind to erythroid precursors, leading to reticulocytopenia

- Increased bilirubin (mainly unconjugated), increased serum lactate dehydrogenase (especially isoenzyme 1)
- In patients with intravascular hemolysis, laboratory studies reveal hemoglobinemia, hemoglobinuria, methemoglobinemia, reduced haptoglobin, and hemosiderinuria.
- Complement levels are reduced in cold agglutinin disease (CAD) due to consumption.
- PS may show microspherocytes (in extravascular hemolysis) or RBC agglutinates (in cold AIHA).

Depending on the type of autoantibody and nature of disease, AIHA has been classified as WAIHA, cold AIHA [includes CAD/secondary cold agglutinin syndrome (CAS) and paroxysmal cold hemoglobinuria (PCH), mixed AIHA, or drug-induced AIHA (DI-AIHA)] **(Table 1)**.

SEROLOGIC EVIDENCE OF AUTOANTIBODY

There are several armamentaria in an immunohematologist's cache to resolve the diagnostic challenges posed by AIHA.

Direct Antiglobulin Test

Direct antiglobulin test (DAT) is one of the first-line investigations done to evaluate suspected cases of AIHA. DAT is used to detect in vivo coating of RBCs with incomplete immunoglobulin G (IgG) antibodies or complement components. DAT is performed on freshly washed RBCs, using polyspecific antihuman globulin reagent (that can detect IgG and C3). If positive, DAT is done with monospecific antiglobulin reagents to detect the type of antibody or complement [IgG, immunoglobulinM (IgM), immunoglobulinA (IgA), C3c, and C3d)] coating the RBCs. The sensitivity of the test differs based on the testing methodology **(Table 2)**.

Sample for DAT should preferably be collected in EDTA to avoid in vitro complement activation. RBCs should be tested immediately after washing to prevent false negative results due to potential elution of IgG.

Direct antiglobulin test may be positive in up to 0.1% of healthy blood donors and 8–15% of hospitalized patients, with no evidence of hemolysis. DAT positivity without hemolysis may also be seen in several situations, like passive deposition of immunoglobulin or immune complexes associated with liver disease, malignancies, chronic infections, renal diseases, autoimmune diseases such as systemic lupus erythematosus (SLE), intravenous immunoglobulin (IVIg), or antithymocyte globulin infusion.

Further workup of positive DAT is warranted only if the patient has evidence of hemolysis. Alternative causes of DAT positivity should be ruled out, which include recent blood transfusion, delayed hemolytic transfusion reaction, solid organ or allogenic hematopoietic stem cell transplant, or hemolytic disease of newborn.

Direct antiglobulin test positivity in patients having evidence of hemolysis suggests AIHA after all alternative causes have been ruled out.

TABLE 1: Classification of autoimmune hemolytic anemia (AIHA).

	Warm		Cold		Mixed		PCH	
	Primary	**Secondary**	**Primary**	**Secondary**	**Primary**	**Secondary**	**Primary**	**Secondary**
Causes	Idiopathic	Neoplasia (CLL, lymphoma, solid organ), infections (e.g., hepatitis C, HIV, respiratory pathogens, leishmaniasis, and tuberculosis), immune dysregulation disorder (e.g., common variable immunodeficiency), and autoimmune/connective tissue disorders (e.g., SLE)	Idiopathic	Malignancy (e.g., CLL, NHL, and solid organ), infection (e.g., mycoplasma, viral infections, including IM), autoimmune disease postallogeneic HSCT	Idiopathic	Lymphoma, SLE, and infection	Idiopathic	Tertiary syphilis, upper respiratory infections of viral origin, e.g., adenovirus, influenza A, syphilis, CMV, IM, VZV, measles, mumps, *Mycoplasma pneumoniae*, *Haemophilus influenza*, etc.
Frequency	40–70%		16–32%		7–8%		1–10% (32% of AIHA in children)	
DAT	• IgG only (20–35%) • IgG + C3 (56–67%) • Rarely C3 alone (9–13%)		• C3 only • Weak positive IgG in up to 20% of cases		IgG ± C3		C3 only	
Ig	IgG; occasionally IgA or IgM		IgM		IgG and IgM		IgG	

Continued

Continued

	Warm		Cold		Mixed		PCH	
	Primary	Secondary	Primary	Secondary	Primary	Secondary	Primary	Secondary
Serum	• IAT-panreactive • Direct agglutination at room temperature in one-third of patients		• Panreactive • IgM agglutinating antibody		• Panreactive • IgG IAT-reactive antibody plus IgM direct agglutinating antibody reactive at >30°C		• IAT-nonreactive at 37°C, • IgG biphasic hemolysin in DL testing	
RBC eluate	IgG		Nonreactive		IgG		Nonreactive	
Thermal reactivity	20–37°C (optimum at 37°C)		4–32°C, rarely to 37°C (optimum 4°C)		Usually ≥30°C		4–20°C	
Antibody specificity	Broadly reactive, usually a high incidence antigen. ~3% have specificity (e.g., anti-e, anti-E or anti-c)		Usually anti-I (~90%), sometimes anti-i, rarely anti-Pr		Warm IgG usually lacks specificity. The cold antibody may be anti-I, anti-I, or lack specificity		Usually anti-P	
Titer (at 4°C)	Not applicable		Titer usually ≥500 at 4°C		Cold antibody may have a low titer ≤1:64		Usually <1:64	

(CLL: chronic lymphocytic leukemia; CMV: cytomegalovirus; HIV: human immunodeficiency virus; HSCT: hematopoietic stem cell transplantation; IAT: indirect antiglobulin test; IgA: immunoglobulin A; IgG: immunoglobulin G; IgM: immunoglobulin M; NHL: non-Hodgkin lymphoma; SLE: systemic lupus erythematosus; VZV: varicella zoster virus)

TABLE 2: Sensitivity of different laboratory tests used to diagnose autoimmune hemolytic anemia (AIHA).

Direct antiglobulin test (DAT)	Sensitivity in detecting autoantibodies
Conventional tube test	500 molecules
Column agglutination test	200–300 molecules
Solid phase red cell adherence assay	200–300 molecules
Flow cytometry (FCM)	30–40 molecules

Indirect Antiglobulin Test

Indirect antiglobulin test (IAT) is used to detect the presence of antibody/ies (Ab) in a patient's serum. The patient's serum is reacted with a panel of red cells representing clinically significant antigens to identify the presence and specificity of the antibodies. Depending on the nature of Ab, IAT can be done at different phases, using polyspecific or monospecific antiglobulin serum, at different temperatures, and with or without enhancement [enzymes, polyethylene glycol (PEG), etc.]. It is essential to put up "autocontrol" to show reactivity against self-RBCs.

Elution

Elution is the method of removing the antibody coating the RBCs to recover it in a more concentrated and usable form. Eluate is reacted with panel red cells to identify the reactivity of the antibody.

Adsorption

Adsorption removes the antibody from the serum sample by reacting with RBCs that express the corresponding antigen.

Use of sulfhydryl reagents [2-mercaptoethanol (2-ME) or dithiothreitol (DTT)—to cleave disulfide bonds], enzymes (papain, bromelin, ficin, etc.), or ZZAP treatment may be required for further immunohematological workup of AIHA cases.

The diagnostic algorithm for AIHA is provided in **Flowchart 1**.

WARM AUTOIMMUNE HEMOLYTIC ANEMIA

Warm AIHA (WAIHA) is characterized by accelerated red-cell destruction due to the presence of warm agglutinins (mostly IgG-type antibodies), which bind to autologous red-cell surfaces at 37°C.

Warm AIHA is the most common type. WAIHA is reported from all age groups, with a median age in sixth decade of life, and shows female predominance. Nearly 50% of reported WAIHAs are idiopathic, and the rest are secondary to other disorders.

Pathogenesis

The IgG autoantibody-bound RBCs are phagocytosed by binding to Fc receptors expressed by tissue macrophages in the spleen and liver. Complete phagocytosis

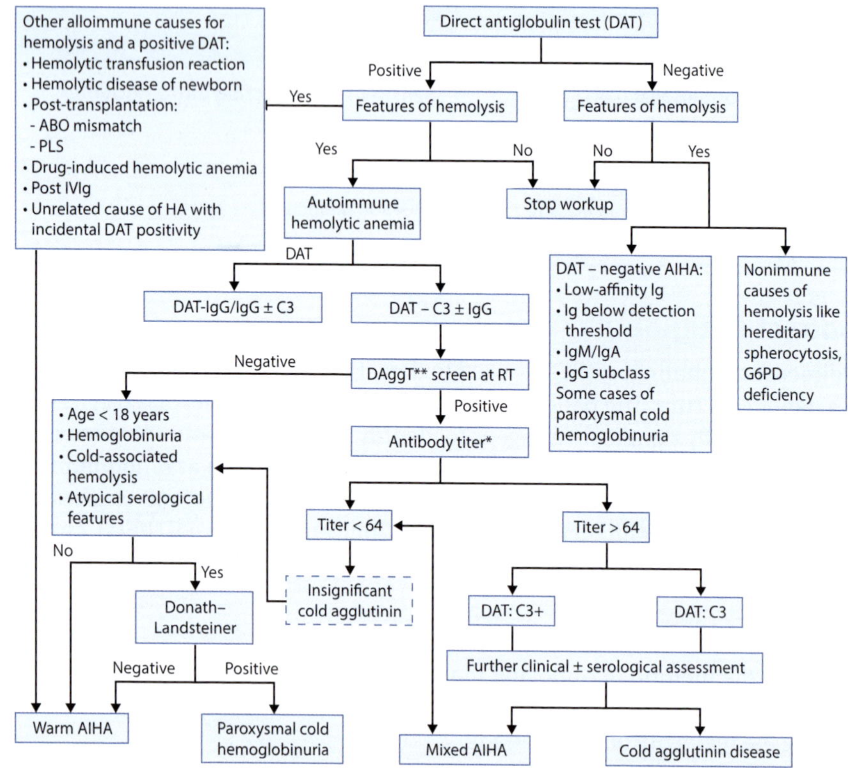

* Titer at 4°C.
** Saline suspended red cells and patient's serum at room temperature for 30–60 minutes.

FLOWCHART 1: Diagnostic flowchart for AIHA1, 2, 5

(AIHA: autoimmune hemolytic anemia; PLS: passenger lymphocyte syndrome)

results in the removal of RBCs, whereas partial phagocytosis results in the removal of a portion of the membrane, leading to microspherocyte formation. The spleen is 100 times more efficient than the liver in removing IgG-sensitized RBCs.

The extent and degree of extravascular hemolysis depend on the subclass and quantity of antibody, complement fragments, and activity of helper and suppressor T cells.

Depending on IgG subclass, splenic macrophages have the highest affinity for IgG3, followed by IgG1 (IgG3 > IgG1 > IgG4 >>> IgG2).

Though IgG antibodies are not very efficient activators of the classic complement pathway, high titers of IgG antibodies and certain subclasses such as IgG1 and IgG3 can cause intravascular hemolysis by fixing and activating complement. C3 fragment deposition on RBCs leads to subsequent removal by the liver macrophages.

Autoimmune hemolytic anemia is considered warm when DAT is positive for IgG ± C3, in a patient having a consistent clinical picture, and when clinically significant cold-reactive antibody has been excluded.

Serological Workup

Warm IgG autoantibodies have optimum thermal reactivity at 37°C, in IAT phase. They usually do not interfere with saline room temperature ABO grouping procedures. However, heavy coating of IgG on RBCs may cause spontaneous agglutination in forward grouping, particularly when high protein reagents are used. Use of monoclonal, low protein antisera and gentle heat elution may resolve the problem.

Red blood cells showing positive DAT cannot be typed correctly with blood typing reagents that require an antiglobulin phase. Use of EDTA/acid glycine (EGA) or chloroquine diphosphate (to dissociate antibodies from RBCs without altering antigen expressions and membrane integrity) permits complete phenotyping of RBCs coated with warm autoantibodies. Directly agglutinating monoclonal reagents may also be used to circumvent the problem.

Direct antiglobulin test in WAIHA is positive for IgG + C3 or only IgG; rarely with C3 alone. Initially, when the quantity of autoantibodies is small, only DAT is positive. When autoantibodies exceed RBC binding sites, they appear in the serum (DAT > IAT).

Antibody identification panels (in IAT phase, at 37°C) show a panagglutination reaction (reactivity with all donor/ reagent red cells), which is enhanced by enzyme treatment or PEG. Underlying alloantibodies are present in 12–40% of WAIHA patients. Differences in the grade of reaction or in different phases give clues to the presence of the underlying alloantibody. For alloantibody identification, adsorption studies may be performed with autologous or allogenic RBCs.

Autoadsorption is the preferred method to remove autoantibodies but can only be performed if the patient has not been transfused in the past 3 months (as transfused cells can adsorb clinically significant alloantibodies). For allogenic adsorption, cells of adsorption studies should be chosen depending on the phenotype of the patient and antigens against which the patient is likely to produce alloantibodies.

Adsorbed serum is tested for the presence of alloantibody. Eluate also reveals pan-agglutinating IgG antibody. If complement is the only protein adherent to RBCs, the eluate is negative.

Specificity of autoantibody: No specificity is identified in most of the cases, and the antibody reacts against all the donor/panel red cells. It was thought that they react with basic Rh blood group antigen, as the reaction is weaker/negative with rare Rh null or D-phenotypes. Sometimes, relative specificity against Rh antigens may be seen (apparent anti-e, anti-E, anti-c, etc.). Warm autoantibodies may also show specificity against LW, Kell, Kidd, Duffy, and Diego system.

Clinical Presentation and Management

Presentation may be insidious or with sudden, life-threatening hemolysis. Patients may present with signs and symptoms of anemia and hemolysis. Splenomegaly may be present. Secondary AIHA patients may present with complaints related to underlying illness.

Symptomatic anemia is the principal indicator of management in WAIHA. Therapy is aimed at treating the underlying pathology. Patients with mild, stable anemia may be closely monitored. Corticosteroids and rituximab have been used as the first-line and second-line therapy, respectively. Splenectomy and use of immunosuppressants are based on individual assessment of risk-benefit ratio. IVIg and plasma exchange are used as rescue therapy in severely hemolysing patients.

Blood transfusion: Decision to transfuse should be based on risk-benefit analysis, and transfusion should not be withheld on the basis of serologic incompatibility. It is significant to determine the presence of underlying alloantibodies and provide a donor unit negative for the corresponding antigen. Transfusion with phenotype-matched units is recommended. However, in critical cases, transfusion should not be delayed to complete immunohematological workup. "Best matched" or "least incompatible" unit should be provided for transfusion. In vivo compatibility tests (*biological crossmatch*) involve 20 mL of rapid infusion of RBCs, followed by 20 minutes of close observation. Only the smallest amount required to maintain oxygenation should be transfused, slowly and under close monitoring.

COLD AUTOIMMUNE HEMOLYTIC ANEMIA

Cold AIHA is characterized by agglutinins, which react preferentially in cold temperature. It is subdivided into CAD and PCH.

Cold Agglutinin Disease

Cold agglutinins are primarily IgM antibodies that can agglutinate RBCs at an optimum temperature of 3–4°C, with subsequent complement-mediated hemolysis.

Pathogenesis

Immunoglobulin M (IgM) CAs bind to RBC antigens at low temperatures in peripheral circulation and dissociate from the cells at central body temperature. CAs activate the classic complement pathway, leading to binding of C3 to the RBC surface. C3b-opsonized RBCs undergo extravascular destruction by interaction with complement receptors on liver macrophages. Formation of the membrane attack complex leads to intravascular RBC lysis. Unlike IgG-mediated extravascular destruction in WAIHA, complement-mediated phagocytosis occurs more commonly in the liver. Complement-mediated RBC lysis is inhibited by regulatory proteins, including DAF (CD 55) and MIRL (CD 59)

Definition: Patients with biochemical evidence of chronic hemolysis are diagnosed with CAD if the DAT is strongly positive for complement protein C3d and negative (or only weakly positive) for IgG, combined with a CA titer of ≥64.

Cold agglutinin disease may be:
- *Primary*: Idiopathic CAD
- *Secondary*: Cold agglutinin syndrome

Primary CAD is a well-defined clinico-pathologic entity associated with clonal B-cell lymphoproliferative disorder (LPD). It affects mainly elderly or middle-aged people (peak ~70 years). Both sexes are affected with female predominance. Antibodies have been largely found to be encoded by the IGH4-34 immunoglobulin heavy chain gene. CAs in CAD are monoclonal, usually of the IgMκ class.

Clonal CD20+, κ+ lymphocytes can usually be detected by flow cytometry (FCM) of bone marrow aspirates. All patients with suspected CAD should be evaluated for clonal B-cell disorder.

Cold Agglutinin Syndrome

Cold agglutinin syndrome, also known as secondary CAD, is a transient condition that is secondary to a bacterial or viral infection, such as *Mycoplasma pneumoniae* or Epstein–Barr virus, aggressive lymphoma, SLE, and allogenic stem cell transplant. IgM antibodies seen in CAS are generally polyclonal, with normal kappa and lambda light chain distribution.

Serological Characteristics

Cold agglutinin disease (primary) and CAS (secondary) have similar immunohematological findings.

Benign nonpathological CAs are commonly encountered and are distinguished from pathological CAs by their titer (<1:64 at 4°C) and thermal amplitude (thermal range up to 20–24°C). However, pathologic CAs typically have titers of >500 at 4°C and the thermal amplitude ≥30°C.

Pathologic CAs are reactive at room temperature, and the sample may show agglutination at room temperature. This may interfere with hematological investigations [spurious macrocytosis or increased mean corpuscular hemoglobin concentration (MCHC)], blood grouping, and compatibility testing. Collecting, transporting, and maintaining the sample at 37°C are recommended for serological workup and titer studies.

Autoagglutination can cause false-positive reactions in forward grouping. This can be resolved by warming the sample at 37°C or washing the RBCs with warm normal saline. If agglutination persists, RBCs can be treated with sulfhydryl reagent, e.g., 2-ME or DTT to denature IgM molecules. The use of low-protein monoclonal antisera is recommended for Rh typing. Prewarming the serum and eliminating the centrifugation step for serum grouping may avoid interference with cold agglutinins. Cold autoadsorption (at 4°C) may be used for high thermal amplitude or high-titer CAs.

Direct antiglobulin test profile reveals the presence of only C3d although weak positive IgG may be present. Eluate is generally nonreactive.

IAT: CAs generally do not interfere with antibody screening or compatibility testing (and hence, rarely mask clinically significant alloantibodies) if serum tests are done at 37°C and IgG-specific reagents are used for the antiglobulin phase. Potentiators such as PEG and enzymes enhance the reactivity of CAs and should be avoided. In cases of CAs reactive at 37°C, cold autoadsorption (with ZZAP or enzyme-treated RBCs) or rabbit erythrocyte stroma may be utilized to remove CAs.

To evaluate thermal amplitude and titers (at 4°C), a sample must be strictly collected and maintained at 37°C, till cells and plasma are separated, to avoid in vitro autoadsorption.

Specificity: CAs have specificity for the erythrocyte surface carbohydrate antigen termed I (90%) or i (10%), rarely for the protein antigen Pr and infrequently for Gd, Fl, Vo, Li, Sa, Lud, M, N, Me, Om, D, and Sd^a.

To determine the specificity, the patient's serum is tested against cord blood cells (possessing the i antigen) and adult RBCs (possessing the I antigen). Auto anti-i is most often associated with infectious mononucleosis, and auto anti-I with *Mycoplasma pneumoniae* infection.

Clinical Presentation

Patients with primary CAD usually present with mild chronic hemolytic anemia, which can be exacerbated by cold exposure, infections, vaccination, surgery, etc. The patient may present with acrocyanosis, Raynaud's disease, or an acute intravascular hemolytic episode. Hepatosplenomegaly is infrequent.

Treatment

Most patients suffer from mild-to-moderate anemia with intermittent exacerbations. The patient is advised to avoid cold exposure. Any febrile illness or trigger should be managed promptly. Therapeutic intervention should be considered for symptomatic anemia, severe cold-induced circulatory symptoms, or transfusion dependence.

Blood transfusions may be required in severely anemic or clinically symptomatic patients and should be given preferentially with a blood warmer. Blood transfusions, IVIG, and/or plasma exchange are used as rescue therapies in severe and life-threatening hemolysis.

Rituximab, alone or in combination with bendamustine, is the best-documented first-line treatment for chronic CAD. Role of BTK inhibitors and complement inhibitors (eculizumab inhibits C5 and sutimlimab inhibits C1) is being explored. Thromboprophylaxis is recommended in acute exacerbations or for chronic disease in risk situations (immobilization, etc.). Corticosteroids and splenectomy are usually not effective in the management of CAD.

For secondary CAS, management is based on supportive care, avoidance of cold, and treatment of the underlying condition. If indicated, transfusions can be given, preferably with blood warmers. The prognosis is good, and hemolysis is usually self-remitting.

MIXED AUTOIMMUNE HEMOLYTIC ANEMIA

Mixed AIHA is diagnosed in patients with a DAT positive for C3d and IgG, a cold antibody with a thermal amplitude ≥30°C, and evidence of a warm IgG antibody by IAT or IAT eluate. It can be primary or secondary to another disease process.

Serum shows the presence of both warm (IgG) and cold (IgM) antibodies, resulting in pan-agglutination reaction in all phases of testing. Cold antibody may have a low antibody titer (<1:64) but with a thermal amplitude up to 30–37°C. Cold IgM autoantibody has a specificity similar to CAD (anti I/i).

The eluate shows warm IgG autoantibody. To look for an underlying alloantibody, adsorption at both 37°C and 4°C may be necessary.

For blood transfusion, blood is selected as in cases of WAIHA. The least incompatible units are transfused with blood warmers. Mixed AIHA is generally characterized by a severe onset and relapse/refractoriness to several therapies. Early therapy with corticosteroids and rituximab is recommended. Splenectomy is typically not recommended.

PAROXYSMAL COLD HEMOGLOBINURIA

Paroxysmal cold hemoglobinuria is a rare form of AIHA characterized by intravascular hemolysis due to a biphasic IgG antibody that binds to RBCs at low temperatures and causes complement-mediated lysis as the temperature is raised. It was first described in 1872, and the associated antibody was first described by Dr Donath and Dr Landsteiner in 1904.

Pathophysiology

The cold-reactive IgG autoantibody binds to RBCs at temperatures <37°C. Upon warming to body temperature, the antibody activates the complement system and dissociates from the RBCs, leaving complement as the only detectable marker on the RBCs.

Serological Characteristics

- Visual inspection of a centrifuged blood sample for intravascular hemolysis
- In the majority of the patients, the DAT result will be positive with polyspecific antiglobulin reagent, and on monospecific testing, C3 is detected on the RBCs.
- *IAT*: Negative
- *Donath-Landsteiner test*: Three sets of three test tubes, containing the patient's serum, are incubated at different temperatures with group O RBCs (having the P antigen). Patient's serum and fresh normal serum as a complement source are added to the respective tubes. Hemolysis is interpreted as a positive result, and the detailed interpretation is provided in **Table 3**.

TABLE 3: Interpretation of D-L test.

Phase of reaction	• Tubes • A1, B1, and C1 • Patient serum and P antigen positive RBC	• Tubes • A2, B2, and C2 • Patient serum and donor serum and P antigen positive RBC	• Tubes • A3, B3, and C3 • Donor serum and P antigen positive RBC
Incubation at ice bath followed by warming at 37°C; A1, A2, and A3	Hemolysis	Hemolysis	No lysis
Incubate at Ice bath only B1, B2, and B3	No lysis	No lysis	No lysis
Incubate at 37°C only C1, C2, and C3	No lysis	No lysis	No lysis

Characteristic Features

Paroxysmal cold hemoglobinuria primarily affects children, often following a recent viral infection, and presents acutely. The median age of onset is around 5 years. Chronic cases in adults have been associated with syphilis. PCH is characterized by intermittent hemoglobinuria triggered by cold exposure. Patients may experience acute intravascular hemolysis with symptoms such as fever, chills, malaise, abdominal cramps, and back pain. Approximately 25% may exhibit hepatosplenomegaly.

IgG immunoglobulin commonly shows anti-P specificity, though other specificities such as anti-i33 and anti-Pr-like reactivity have been reported.

Treatment

Paroxysmal cold hemoglobinuria is mostly self-limiting, frequently managed with supportive measures and avoiding cold temperatures. The blood transfusion is required in cases with severe anemia, and warmer is used while administering the blood. In patients with refractory PCH, immunosuppressive therapy such as rituximab is considered.

DRUG-INDUCED AUTOIMMUNE HEMOLYTIC ANEMIA

Drug-induced immune hemolytic anemia (DIIHA) is due to a drug that mediates the RBC hemolysis via various immunological mechanisms. There are more than 150 drugs that have been implicated in DIIHA, with a reported incidence rate of 1 per million. However, the incidence may be higher (0.25–0.5%) with recent use of checkpoint inhibitors. This clinical entity is characterized by the presence of antibodies reacting to RBCs (neoantigen formation) either in the presence of the drug (drug dependent) or when the drug is attached to the RBCs (antibody against both drug and the RBC membrane protein) or in some cases, the antibody may be directed against the metabolites of the drug. Another category is drug-independent AIHA, where the causative drugs (e.g., α-methyldopa) induce an autoimmune reaction toward RBCs, leading to anti-RBC antibodies triggering an AIHA. Complement-mediated hemolysis is most often involved in DI-AIHA. Apart from positive DAT (IgG and C3d), the drug-dependent DIIHA can be confirmed with a reference laboratory by analyzing the elute of the patient RBCs and testing the elute in the presence of RBCs pretreated with suspected drug or its metabolites. The drug-independent DIIHA is usually indistinguishable from a typical AIHA.

The DIIHA is managed by interpreting the suspected drug. The improvement is expected in 1–2 weeks after the drug discontinuation; however, packed RBCs may be considered in case of emergencies.

ATYPICAL AUTOIMMUNE HEMOLYTIC ANEMIA

Some forms of AIHA do not fit into well-characterized types, referred to as atypical AIHA. These include DAT negative, IgA-driven, and warm-IgM AIHA.

Direct Antiglobulin Test-negative Autoimmune Hemolytic Anemia

Direct antiglobulin test may be negative in 5–10% of AIHAs. Rule out alternative causes of congenital or acquired hemolytic anemias.

Causes

- Bound antibodies are less than the threshold of detection.
- *Low-affinity autoantibodies*: Can be overcome by the use of low ionic strength saline (LISS) or cold washing
- Warm IgM autoantibodies
- IgA AIHA

Warm-IgM Autoimmune Hemolytic Anemia

This is an unusual category of WAIHA, caused by IgM autoantibodies with a thermal range close to 37°C. RBCs may show spontaneous agglutination. DAT may be negative (or weakly positive for anti-C3) with polyspecific AHG. Antibody titers at 4°C are usually low (<64). Warm-IgM AIHA is characterized by severe hemolysis and poor prognosis.

IgA-mediated Autoimmune Hemolytic Anemia

IgA antibodies are present in approximately 14% of patients with WAIHA and are almost always associated with IgG or IgM. However, WAIHA caused exclusively by IgA antibodies is a rarity. IgA antibodies react optimally at 37°C and mainly target Band 3 on the RBC membrane. DAT and IAT done by polyspecific antiglobulin serum will miss the diagnosis. DAT is positive with monoclonal antibodies specific for IgA. Case reports have shown higher binding potency of IgA, more disease severity, and refractoriness to corticosteroid treatment.

CELLULAR ASSAYS

These are used to determine the clinical significance of autoantibodies to RBCs.

Monocyte monolayer assays (MMA) can be used to assess the interaction of monocytes and red blood cells in the presence of an antibody or other factors that may lead to RBC destruction. This test evaluates the clinical relevance of antibodies and their ability to kill RBCs. MMA can also be used to decide if the red cells can be used for transfusion if the compatible units are unavailable. The major limitation of this test is that it requires trained manpower; the results may vary depending on the source of monocytes used, antibody concentration, and assay conditions.

The principles and characteristics of other cellular and functional assays are mentioned in **Table 4**.

TABLE 4: The principle and characteristics of cellular assays in AIHA.

Assay	Principle	Characteristics
Chemiluminescence	Monocyte metabolic response during erythrophagocytosis is assessed	Objective, quantitative, rapid, requires a luminometer
Antibody-dependent cellular cytotoxicity	Extracellular lysis of erythrocytes by monocytes or NK cells	Objective, quantitative, requires isotopes
Monocyte monolayer assay	Adherence and phagocytosis of erythrocytes by monocyte	• Sensitive and simple • Does not require additional equipment • Subjective

FLOW CYTOMETRY

Flow cytometry is a valuable diagnostic tool in the evaluation of AIHA. It may help detect low levels of autoantibodies or provide detailed insights into the immunological mechanisms underlying the disease.

- It can detect IgG, IgM, IgA, and C3d autoantibodies (as low as 30–40 antibody molecules per RBC).
- It can be done along with bone marrow biopsy to detect the possible underlying disease and in all CAD before therapy.

Take Home Points

- ➢ Autoimmune hemolytic anemia is a distinct clinicopathologic entity, and proper characterization and diagnosis are required for appropriate management.
- ➢ Diagnosis of AIHA requires both evidence of hemolysis and serologic evidence of autoantibodies.
- ➢ AIHA is classified as warm, cold (CAD and PCH), mixed, and DI-AIHA, depending on antibody type, thermal reactivity, and specificity.
- ➢ Treatment of AIHA is witnessing new promising developments.

SUGGESTED READINGS

1. Hill QA, Stamps R, Massey E, Grainger JD, Provan D, Hill A; British Society for Haematology. The diagnosis and management of primary autoimmune haemolytic anaemia. Br J Haematol. 2017;176(3):395-411.
2. Hill A, Hill QA. Autoimmune hemolytic anaemia. Hematology am Soc Hematol Edu Program. 2018;382-9.
3. Simon TL, Gehrie EA, McCullough J, Roback JD, Snyder EL. Rossi's Principles of Transfusion Medicine, 6th edition. John Wiley & Sons, Ltd; 2022.
4. Jäger U, Barcellini W, Broome CM, Gertz MA, Hill A, Hill QA, et al. Diagnosis and treatment of autoimmune hemolytic anaemia in adults: Recommendations from the First International Consensus Meeting. Blood Rev. 2020;41:100648.
5. Means RJ, Rodgers G, Glader B, Arber DA, Appelbaum FR, Dispenzieri A, et al. Wintrobe's Clinical Hematology. Lippincott Williams & Wilkins; 2023.
6. Harmening DM. Modern Blood Banking and Transfusion Practices, 7th edition. Philadelphia, PA: FA Davis; 2019.

7. Cohn CS, Delaney M, Johnson ST, Katz LM, Schwartz J; American Association of Blood Banks. Technical Manual, 21st edition. AABB; 2023.
8. Brodsky RA. Warm Autoimmune Hemolytic Anemia. N Engl J Med. 2019;381(7):647-54.
9. Jacobs JW, Villalba CAF, Booth GS, Woo JS, Stephens LD, Adkins BD. Clinical and epidemiological features of paroxysmal cold hemoglobinuria: a systematic review. Blood Adv. 2023;7(11):2520-7.
10. Garratty G. Drug-induced immune hemolytic anemia. Hematology Am Soc Hematol Educ Program. 2009:73-9.
11. Chadebech P, Michel M, Janvier D, Yamada K, Copie-Bergman C, Bodivit G, et al. IgA-mediated human autoimmune hemolytic anemia as a result of hemagglutination in the spleen, but independent of complement activation and FcRI. Blood. 2010;116(20):4141-7.
12. Engelfriet CP, Ouwehand WH. 6 ADCC and other cellular bioassays for predicting the clinical significance of red cell alloantibodies. Baillières Clin Haematol. 1990;3(2):321-37.

CHAPTER 38

Recent Advances in Splenic Lymphomas: Histopathology and Flow Cytometry

Surabhi Jain, Roopam Deka, Saumyaranjan Mallick

ABSTRACT

Primary splenic lymphomas (PSL) are a heterogeneous group of rare lymphomas, the diagnosis of which require comprehensive analysis of peripheral blood—counts, morphology, and flow cytometry; bone marrow examination and molecular approach. Splenic tissue, at most times is not available for the initial diagnosis. Recent advances in the molecular biology have deepened our understanding which has been reflected in the recent World Health Organization Classification of Haematolymphoid Tumours 5th edition (WHO-HAEM5) and the International Consensus Classification (ICC) classifications, with refinement of the diagnostic criteria. Though the splenic B-cell lymphomas have overlapping clinical, histomorphological, and immunophenotypic findings; pathognomonic molecular alterations and subtle differences in flow cytometry may aid their exact classification. Hairy cell leukemia-variant has been excluded from WHO-HAEM5 and is now included in splenic B-cell lymphoma/leukemia with prominent nucleoli. In this chapter, we will focus mainly on the recent advances and diagnostic approach to PSLs.

INTRODUCTION

Spleen is the largest reticuloendothelial organ which primarily acts as a site of extramedullary hematopoiesis and a clearance site for abnormal cells. It can serve as a rich reservoir and culture medium for the development of hematological malignancies. However, literature suggests that primary splenic lymphomas (PSL) are rarities with most lymphomas involving spleen arising elsewhere. Since spleen acts as blood filter, it becomes a frequent secondary site of lymphomatous/leukemia-involvement. Furthermore, PSLs were often missed due to late occurrence of symptoms, lack of distinct phenotype, and increased proportion of phagocytic cells which keeps a check on the proliferation of neoplastic cells. It is one challenging area of expertise for a pathologist wherein we attempt to make a diagnosis without doing microscopic examination of the primarily involved organ, i.e., spleen.

With the recent advancements in the understanding of pathobiology of PSLs, the diagnostics have become clear and we will focus on PSLs.

NORMAL HISTOMORPHOLOGY AND IMMUNOPHENOTYPING OF SPLEEN

In adults, the spleen weighs about 150–200 g. Its cut surface shows mainly red pulp (RP) with white specks representing the white pulp (WP) follicles. The splenic parenchyma shows a normal RP:WP ratio of 3-4:1 along with stromal and vascular components. WP comprises of germinal centers (GC) (pale) surrounded by mantle (dark) and a marginal zone (pale). The tripartite arrangement is accompanied by an adjacent arteriole. RP comprises of venous sinuses (patent and are lined by endothelial cells) and cords of Billroth (are solid and contain stromal components). An expansion of marginal zone of >10-layers is defined as marginal zone hyperplasia. Rarely, follicular hyperplasia can also occur with decreased RP:WP ratio.

In a normal spleen, the T-cells (CD3) are distributed in the periarteriolar zone known as periarteriolar lymphoid sheath (PALS). Mature B-cells are present in one end of PALS and comprises lymphoid follicle and the GCs are supported by follicular dendritic-cells. Bcl2 highlights only the mantle and marginal zones and the GC is negative. CD4 and CD8 highlight the helper T-cells (WP and RP) and littoral cells in RP respectively; hence, CD8 is a good delineating marker for RP. CD163 highlights the cords **(Figs. 1A to F)**.

LYMPHOMATOUS INVOLVEMENT OF SPLEEN

The lymphomas can involve the RP predominantly, WP predominantly or both. Involvement of WP is characterized by small pale nodules (military pattern) on cut surface of spleen, RP involvement shows beefy red cut surface and both involvement shows proportionate representation of either.

Among the T-cell lymphomas are:

- *Predominantly WP:* Anaplastic large cell lymphoma.
- *Predominantly RP:* T-cell large granular lymphocytic leukemia, T-prolymphocytic leukemia, hepatosplenic T-cell lymphoma (HSTCL), extranodal natural killer (NK)/T-cell lymphoma, other T- and NK-cell leukemia.
- *Both red and WP:* Peripheral T-cell lymphoma, not otherwise specified, nodal T follicular helper lymphoma, angioimmunoblastic type, mycosis fungoides.

Among B-cell lymphomas are:

- *Predominantly WP:* Splenic marginal zone lymphoma (SMZL), nodal MZL, chronic lymphocytic leukemia/small lymphocytic lymphoma (CLL/SLL), lymphoblastic lymphoma, Mantle cell, follicular.
- *Predominantly RP:* Hairy cell leukemia (HCL), splenic diffuse RP small B-cell lymphoma (SDRPL), lymphoplasmacytic lymphoma (LPL), HCL-variant (HCL-v) (now, splenic B-cell lymphoma/leukemia with prominent nucleoli).
- *Both RP and WP:* Burkitt lymphoma, diffuse large B-cell lymphoma, SMZL, CLL/SLL.

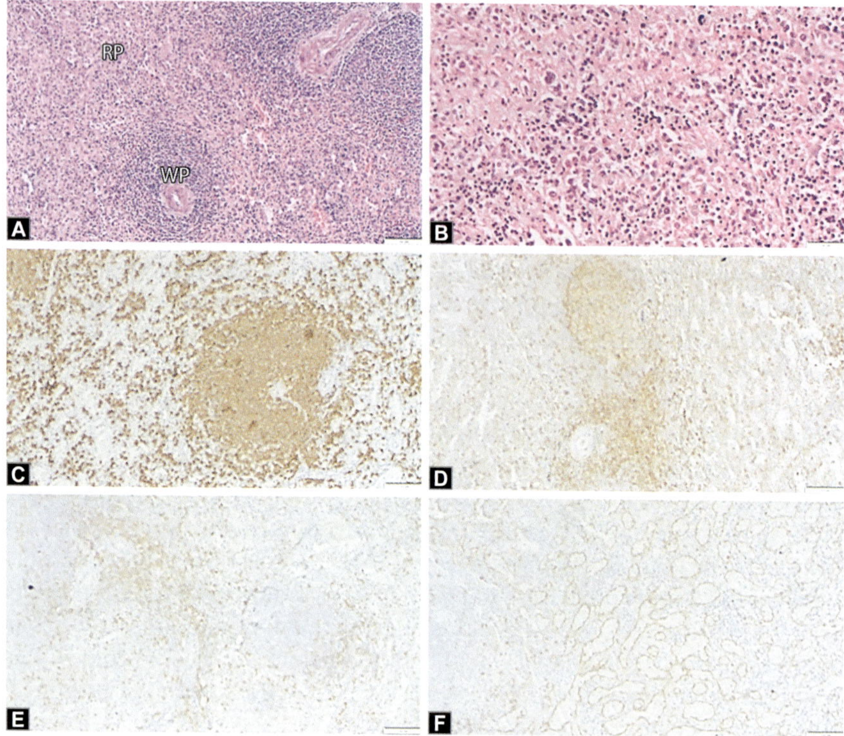

FIGS. 1A TO F: Microphotographs of normal splenic architecture and immunophenotype: (A) White pulp (WP) and red pulp (RP); (B) Extramedullary hematopoiesis; (C) CD20 highlights germinal centers (GCs); (D) CD3 highlights mature lymphoid cells in the WP and RP. (E) CD4 immunostain highlights helper T-cells in WP. (F) CD8 highlights littoral cells.

PRIMARY SPLENIC LYMPHOMA

The PSLs constitute of 1% of non-Hodgkin lymphomas and about <2% of all lymphomas. The criteria for the diagnosis of PSLs include: (1) Presence of splenomegaly documented clinically (palpable spleen), radiologically (length >12 cm in adults) or on laparotomy (weight of spleen > 400 g), (2) Lymphomas arising in spleen or primarily confined to spleen, and (3) Absence of significant or generalized lymphadenopathy (perisplenic or hilar lymph nodes are an exclusion and are found enlarged in cases). Dasgupta et al., who defined the initial criteria had an addition of at least 6 months tumor free interval postsplenectomy. Liver or bone marrow involvement can be seen in PSLs and remain an exclusion to the systemic involvement criteria.

Radiologically, splenic lymphomas may appear solitary, multinodular (small or large), or show diffuse infiltration which is often reflected in the histopathology. The lesions are hypovascular and homogeneous. Patients usually show cytopenias, which probably occurs as a result of increased sequestration and phagocytosis of the blood elements.

In view of the highly vascular nature of the organ, splenic biopsies are usually avoided and an attempt to diagnose is based on peripheral blood, flow cytometric, and bone marrow evaluation. However, splenectomies are performed to reduce the disease burden, in chemotherapy refractory cases, and where definite diagnosis in the cases of splenic B-cell lymphoma unclassifiable requires whole spleen examination.

WORLD HEALTH ORGANIZATION CLASSIFICATION AND INTERNATIONAL CONSENSUS CLASSIFICATION OF SPLENIC LYMPHOID TUMORS (TABLE 1)

WHO-HAEM5 has currently included newer entities in addition to the previous with minor revisions.

TABLE 1: Classification of splenic lymphoid tumors.

	WHO-HAEM 4R	WHO-HAEM 5	ICC 2022	Postulated cell of origin
B-cell lymphomas	Splenic marginal zone lymphoma	Same	Same	Splenic white pulp germinal centers (WP GCs) (? memory B-cell)
	Hairy cell leukemia	Same	Same	Proposed late, activated memory B-cell
	Splenic diffuse red pulp small B-cell lymphoma under "splenic B-cell lymphoma/ leukemia, unclassifiable (NOS)"	Splenic diffuse red pulp (RP) small B-cell lymphoma	Splenic diffuse RP small B-cell lymphoma	Unidentified B-cell precursor
	Hairy cell leukemia-variant under "splenic B cell lymphoma/ leukemia, unclassifiable (NOS)"	Splenic B-cell lymphoma/ leukemia with prominent nucleoli	Hairy cell leukemia-variant (HCL-v)	Unidentified B-cell precursor
T-cell lymphoma	Hepatosplenic T-cell lymphoma	Same	Same	Nonactivated cytotoxic T-cells
Stroma derived neoplasms of lymphoid tissue	Not previously included	• Littoral cell angioma • Splenic hamartoma • Sclerosing angiomatoid transformation of spleen		

(NOS: not otherwise specified)

MATURE SPLENIC B-CELL LYMPHOMAS

These neoplasms are an enigmatic yet challenging group to diagnose since they share overlapping clinical, histopathology, immunophenotypic, and molecular features. Recent advances in the genomic profiling of these tumors have aided our cause and today, to an extent we can precisely make a diagnosis. We will discuss the entities in a prototypical case-based approach.

Case 1

A 67-year-old male presented with history of fatigue, fullness of abdomen for the past 3 months. On examination, the patient was found to have splenomegaly. Imaging of abdomen revealed hypoenhancing multiple lesions in an enlarged spleen on computed tomography (CT), and there was no evidence of peripheral lymphadenopathy. Peripheral blood smear showed 40% abnormal lymphocytic population with scant cytoplasm and presence of irregular cytoplasmic borders. Flow cytometric evaluation of peripheral blood revealed an abnormal population: which was positive for CD20, PAX5, CD79a, FMC7, CD27, CD38 (dim), CD200 (dim), immunoglobulin (Ig)M, and IgD while were negative for CD3, CD103, SOX11, and LEF1. About half of the population showed dim positivity for CD5.

Markers helpful in diagnosis of splenic lymphomas by flow cytometry are discussed in **Table 2**.

A diagnosis of SMZL was made and the patient was started on rituximab therapy. Bone marrow biopsy revealed infiltration of abnormal B-lymphoid cells in nodular pattern. In view of persistent splenomegaly, splenectomy was performed.

Gross examination showed enlarged spleen with presence of multiple millet sized grey white nodules, across all spleen. Section from spleen shows expansion of WP in the form of nodules **(Figs. 2A to L)**.

Splenic Marginal Zone Lymphoma

The SMZLs are the most common PSL and higher prevalence is noted in malaria endemic region, people with autoimmune disease and hepatitis C infection. It is an indolent B-cell lymphoma, often asymptomatic in patients. SMZLs affect middle-aged adults and elderly population with a median age of seventh decade and show a slight male preponderance.

Peripheral smear shows the atypical lymphoid cells which are usually small sized, containing moderate amount of basophilic cytoplasm, condensed chromatin, and can show unevenly distributed or polar villous projections; they show plasmacytoid morphology or may resemble small lymphocytes. Histomorphology of spleen shows nodular expansion of WP. There is coalescence of WP along with many tiny small nodules of atypical cells. Small atypical lymphoid cells also involve the cords and sinuses (RP involvement). The tumor cells are often admixed with lymphoplasmacytic cells. Bone marrow shows interstitial, intrasinusoidal, or nodular involvement. Presence of large cells and sheets may indicate aggressive forms and transformation to large B-cell lymphoma (seen in 13% of cases and usually related to 7q deletion).

TABLE 2: Immunophenotypic markers useful in differential diagnosis of splenic lymphomas.

WHO category of splenic lymphoma	Usual immunophenotype (flow cytometry)
Hairy cell leukemia	• *Positive:* CD20, CD22 (bright), CD200 (bright), surface immunoglobulin (Ig) (bright), CD11c, CD25, CD103, CD123, CD26, CD43, CD81 (dim), FMC7, CD305, Annexin A1, CD72 (DBA 44), TRAP, Cyclin D1 • *Negative:* CD5, CD10 (these markers may be rarely positive in 10–20% of the cases)
Splenic marginal zone lymphoma	• *Positive:* CD20, PAX5, CD79a, FMC7, CD27, CD38 (dim), CD200 (dim), CD180, IgM, and IgD. Up to half of the cases express CD25 • Some cases express CD11c, CD123, CD5 (usually weak), CD43, rarely CD10+ • *Negative:* CD103, SOX11, Annexin A1, and LEF1
Splenic diffuse red pulp (RP) small B-cell lymphoma	• *Positive:* CD19, CD20, CD79a, IgG, PAX5, CD72 • *Negative:* CD5, CD10, CD11c, CD23, CD25, CD26, CD38, CD43, CD103, CD123, Annexin A1, and IgD. However, these markers can be rarely expressed • Role of CD180 and CD200 by flow cytometry in distinguishing SDRPL from HCL and SMZL • CD200 median fluorescence (MFI)/CD180 MFI ratio 0.5 or less favors a diagnosis of SDRPL rather than HCL, or SMZL
Splenic B-cell lymphoma/leukemia with prominent nucleoli	• *Positive:* CD19, CD20, CD22, monotypic surface immunoglobulin (most frequently IgG, either alone or with another isotype), FMC7, CD11c, CD81 (bright), CD103, CD72, PAX5, CD79a • *Negative:* CD25, CD123, CD200, TRAP
Hepatosplenic T-cell lymphoma	• *Usually positive* for CD2 and CD3 • *Express cytotoxic markers* such as TIA-1, perforin, granzyme M, and granzyme B (30–40% of cases) • *TCR expression:* ○ Nearly 75% of cases are positive for TCRγδ; nearly 20% express TCRαβ; ○ 5% lack TCRs (silent or "null"). TCRVδ expression seems to be restricted to the Vδ1 chain ○ *Usually negative* for CD4, CD5, and CD8, however, nearly 15% cases show CD5 dim expression, and nearly 20% are positive for CD8 ○ *NK-cell associated markers:* CD56 and CD16 are nearly positive in 70% and 60% cases, respectively

(WHO: World Health Organization; HCL: hairy cell leukemia; SMZL: splenic marginal zone lymphoma; SDRPL: splenic diffuse red pulp small B-cell lymphoma)

It should not be mistaken for splenic marginal zone hyperplasia which is a benign entity lacking the cytogenetic alteration and shows expansion of polyclonal lymphocytes, with minimal splenic enlargement, WP involvement and absence of clusters in the sinusoids. Ki67 immunohistochemistry (IHC) will show low proliferation within the GCs in the case of SMZL, as the proliferating GC cells are replaced by atypical lymphoid cells. Immunonegativity for CD43 helps to differentiate from nodal MZL.

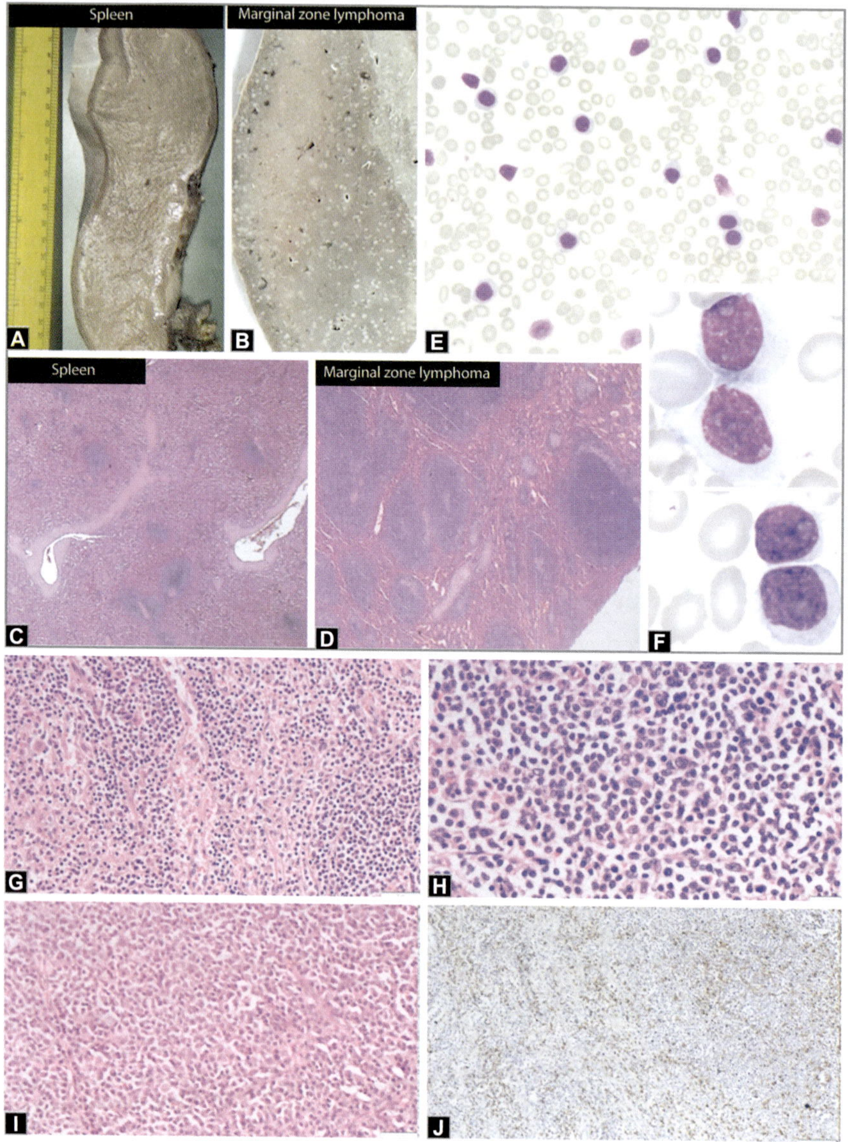

FIGS. 2A TO L: *Continued*

Continued

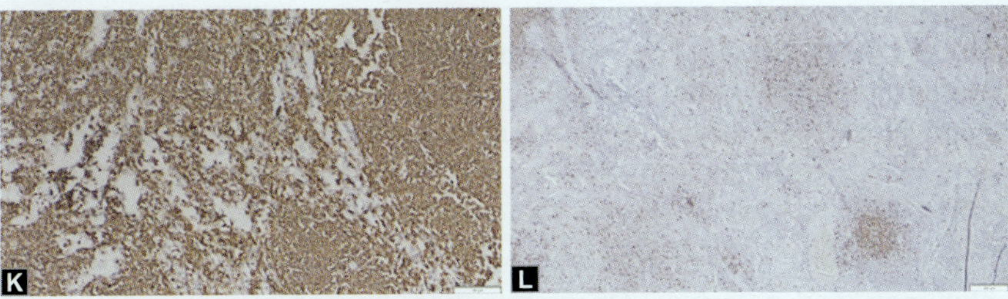

FIGS. 2A TO L: Morphology and immunophenotype of SMZL: (A) Gross photograph of congestive splenomegaly showed homogeneous surface. (B) Cut surface splenic lymphoma shows multiple small nodules varying in size 2–6 mm. (C) Microphotograph of congestive splenomegaly shows few small white pulp (WP). (D) Nodular expansion of WP with coalescences of nodule. (E and F) Atypical lymphoid cells in peripheral blood smear, which contain moderate amount of basophilic cytoplasm, condensed chromatin, and can show unevenly distributed or polar villous projections; Splenic involvement; (G and H) The infiltrate is composed of small sized lymphoid cells and involves RP; (I) Plasmacytoid morphology; (J) The atypical lymphoid cells are immunonegative for CD3; and (K) are immunopositive for CD20; (L) Mib1 labeling highlights low Ki67 in the SMZL germinal centers (GCs) in comparison to high Ki67 in a normal WP GC SMZL peripheral smear.

Courtesy: Dr Richa Chauhan, Assistant Professor, Department of Hematology, AIIMS, New Delhi, India.

Dysregulation of NOTCH and nuclear factor kappa B (NF-κB) pathways are primarily implicated in the pathogenesis. Krüppel-like factor 2 (*KLF2*) mutations (20–40%) and *KLF2* deletions (11%) can be seen. Karyotype shows loss of 7q31–32 (30%) along with trisomies chromosome 18 and 3. In rare cases, translocation of cyclin-dependent kinase 6 (CDK6) to transcriptionally active IG gene loci can be present. Mutations in genes *KLF2* (master regulator of both above pathways) (silencing) and *NOTCH 2* (activating) (15–25%) which are involved in marginal zone differentiation are usually seen and <5% of cases can harbor *BRAF*V600E mutations.

A recent study based on detailed genomic analysis developed a genomic classifier for SMZL, dividing this entity into four genetically defined groups which were found to have distinct clinical and molecular phenotype with varied clinical outcomes. Depending on the genes involves in various pathways of B-cell program, four groups were identified namely—NNK (NF-κB, NOTCH, and *KLF2* modules), DMT [DNA-damage response, mitogen-activated protein kinase (MAPK), and Toll-like receptors modules such as TP53, ATM, CBS (cytokine, B-cell receptor signaling, and spliceosome modules), and PA (PI3K/AKT module)]. The majority proportion of SMZL, about 60% belong to the NNK group followed by DMT group (30%). The NNK group showed usage of immunoglobulin heavy variable 1-2 (IGHV1-2)*04 allele and deletion of 7q with an overall poorer survival. Based on tumor microenvironment, they divided SMZLs into immune-suppressed and immune-silent groups. The immune suppressed groups showed signatures of macrophages, cytokine, chemokine, T-cell, and regulatory T-cell with an immune evasive profile. The immune silent class showed a higher expression of B-cell (tumor cell) signature. The worst overall outcome was seen in NNT-immune-suppressive cohort. Poor prognostic factors include presence of p53 and NOTCH2 mutations, complex karyotype.

The hemoglobin-platelet-LDH-extra-hilar-lymphadenopathy (HPLL) score by *splenic marginal zone lymphoma working group* (SMZL-WG) is used to stratify the SMZL patients wherein hemoglobin of less than 95 g/L, presence of extrahilum-splenic lymphadenopathy, platelets of <80 × 10^9/L and raised lactate dehydrogenase (LDH) levels were determinants of unfavorable prognosis.[5]

Case 2

A 57-year-old male presented with fatigue, chronic cough, discomfort in left side of abdomen, and petechiae. On examination, he had massive splenomegaly. Complete blood count (CBC) showed pancytopenia, monocytopenia, and peripheral smear showed intermediate sized lymphoid cells with bland "spongy" chromatin, inconspicuous nucleoli, and circumferential surface projections. Flow cytometry from the bone marrow aspirate shows 35% events with high forward scatter and low side scatter; these were positive for CD19, CD20, CD11c, CD103, CD25, CD123, IgG, CD200, and CD43. The events were negative for CD5, CD10, and CD81 **(Fig. 3)**.

Bone marrow aspiration was a dry tap and biopsy revealed interstitial infiltration by small to intermediate sized atypical lymphoid cells having pale to clear cytoplasm and an indented nucleus. Reticulin stain showed characteristic fried egg appearance. Tartrate resistant acid phosphatase (TRAP) stain and DBA.44c, CD123, Annexin A1, and cyclinD1 (weak) IHC were positive. Overall features are those of hairy cell leukemia **(Figs. 4A to F)**.

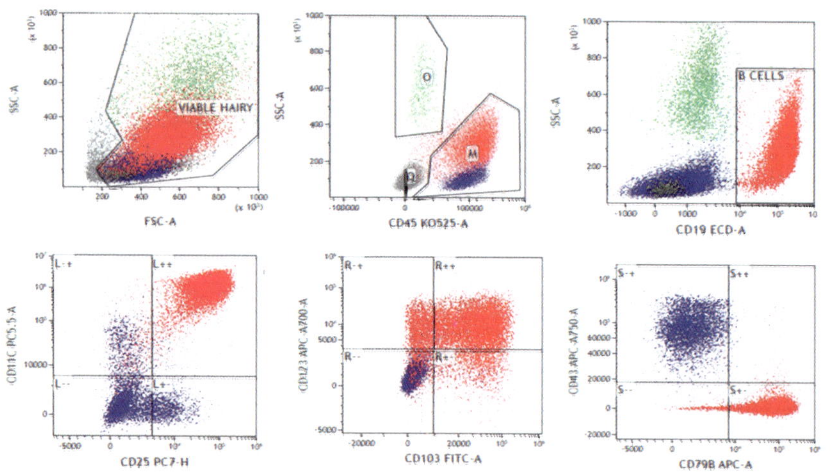

FIG. 3: Immunophenotype of hairy cell leukemia by flow cytometry. The neoplastic cells (red dots) show higher forward scatter (FSC), occupy the monocytic region in CD45/SSC plot, and express CD19, CD11c, CD25, CD123, CD103, and CD79b; the cells are negative for CD43.

Courtesy: Dr Richa Juneja, Associate Professor, Department of Pathology, AIIMS, Nagpur, Maharashtra, India.

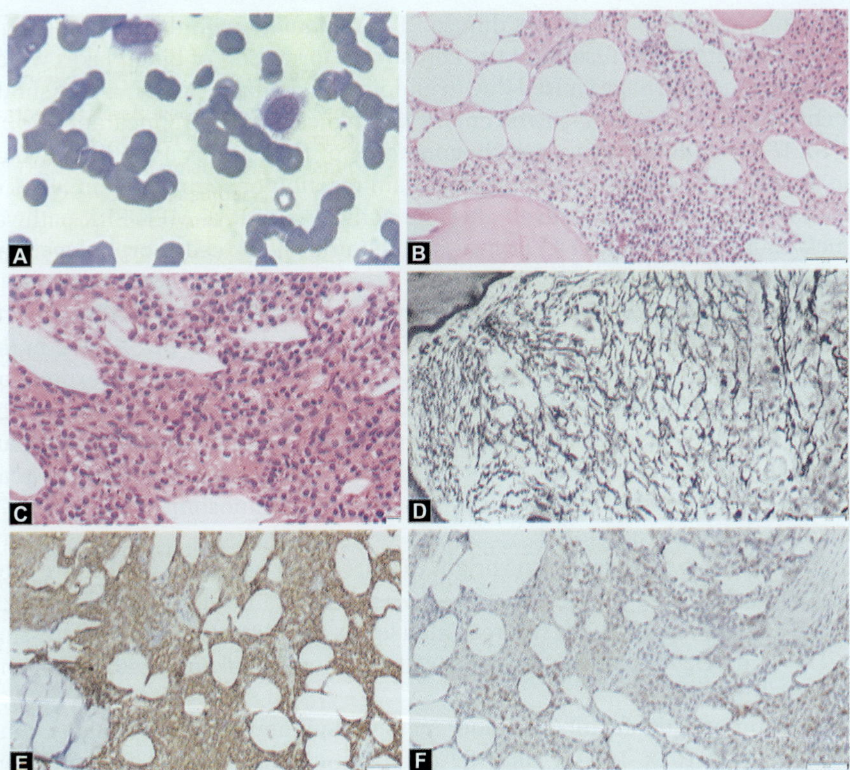

FIGS. 4A TO F: Morphology and immunophenotype of hairy cell leukemia (HCL). (A) Peripheral blood smear shows presence of atypical lymphoid cells with circumferential villi, oval to reniform nuclei, and moderate to abundant pale cytoplasm. Bone marrow biopsy of HCL. (B and C) Interstitial involvement of HCL by atypical lymphoid cells having clear cytoplasm. (D) Reticulin stain highlights typical fried egg appearance (fibrosis around each cell). (E) CD20, and (F) Annexin A1 highlights the atypical lymphoid cells.

Courtesy: HCL peripheral smear: Dr Richa Juneja, Associate professor, Department of Pathology, AIIMS, Nagpur, Maharashtra, India.

Hairy Cell Leukemia

The HCL is a mature indolent B-cell leukemia, which involves the RP commonly. It accounts for 2–3% of adult leukemias. They commonly affect the middle aged and older adults with a median age of sixth decade with male preponderance. It usually involves peripheral blood, spleen, and bone marrow. Absolute monocytopenia and pancytopenia is almost always seen. Individuals with human leukocyte antigen (HLA)-DRB*11, exposure to benzene and pesticides are associated with increased risk.

The abnormal lymphoid cells in peripheral blood show presence of circumferential villi, reniform to oval nuclei, moderate to abundant pale/clear cytoplasm, and fine granular chromatin with inconspicuous or absent nucleoli.

Histopathology of spleen shows diffuse RP involvement with the monomorphic cells infiltrating the sinuses and the cords, with formation of blood lakes which are areas of hemorrhage caused due to endothelial damage. Bone marrow shows patchy or diffuse interstitial involvement with typical fried egg appearance.

BRAF p.V600E mutation is pathognomonic of HCL and is a hallmark which can be detected with IHC, polymerase chain reaction or sequencing in >95% of the cases; The mutation leads to aberrant activation of RAF-MEK-ERK pathway which causes increased cell survival, induction of hairy cell morphology, and HCL-specific gene expression signature.

The HCL without *BRAF*V600E are reported and may harbor IGH::BRAF fusion and other activating mutations of *BRAF*; implying the role of *BRAF* gene in the pathobiology; also, in its absence, IGHV4-34 can be seen. CyclinD1 expression can be seen in about 40% cases; but lack t (11;14). Other mutations including in histone methyltransferase genes such as *CDKN1B* and *MLL3*, DNA repair, NOTCH signaling, and others such as *CEBPA*, *RUNX1*, *MED12*, and *BRD4* can be seen. Chromosomal aberrations such as gain of chromosome 5 and loss of 7q (up to 20%) and 13q are noted.

The HCL shows characteristic bright CD43, CD200, and dim CD81 expression along with the other classical markers (CD20, surface immunoglobulin, CD25, CD11c, CD103, and CD123), whereas high levels of CD81, with lower expression of CD43 and CD200 is seen in splenic B-cell lymphoma/leukemia with prominent nucleoli (SBLPN).

Poor prognostic factors include massive splenomegaly (late detection), leukocytosis (>10 × 10^9/L), high β2-microglobulin (>2N), CD38 expression, IGHV4-34, and hairy cells in blood (>5 × 10^9/L).

First line of therapy is a pruine analog (2-chloro-2'-deoxyadenosine); alternative purine analog, splenectomy, interferon-α, or monoclonal antibodies to B-cell markers (anti-CD25 antibody-LMB2, anti-CD20–rituximab, and anti-CD22-BL22) can be helpful in refractory cases.

Splenic B-cell Lymphoma/Leukemia with Prominent Nucleoli (Figs. 5A to C)

It is a new terminological addition to WHO-HAEM5 which includes the previously defined HCL-v and CD5 negative B-prolymphocytic leukemia. In contrast ICC system still uses the older terminology like WHO-HAEMR (revised 4th edition of the World Health Organization classification of tumors of hematopoietic and lymphoid tissues). It has been recognized that HCL-v was more of a morphological similar tumor to HCL, but biologically distinct.

It is important to note that this is not a definite defined entity but is a placeholder for the cases that morphologically fit into the definition; and further studies are required for the understanding of its pathobiology.

The SBLPN can either arise de novo or may represent a clonal evolution of other lymphoma and needs to be further elucidated. HCL-v still remains a provisional entity in ICC classification.

It is a rarity and affects middle aged and elderly with slight male preponderance; splenomegaly is commonly seen. Usually associated with leukocytosis (initial) and lymphocytosis; monocytopenia is usually not seen.

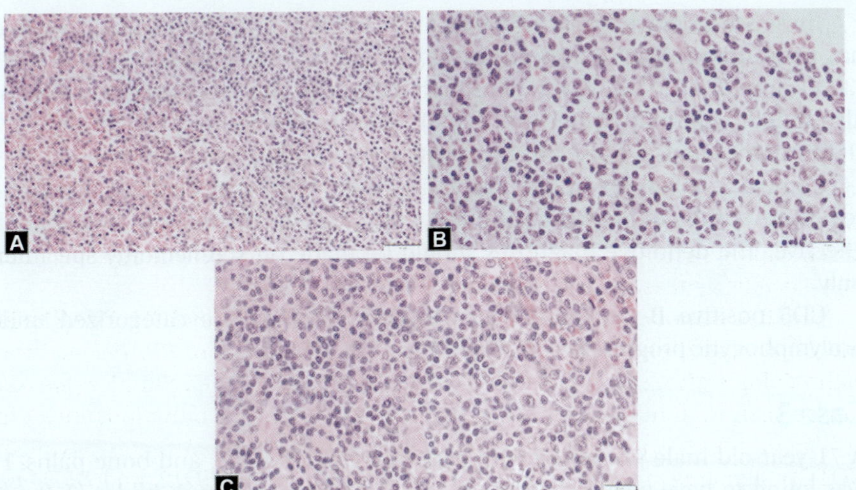

FIGS. 5A TO C: A case of splenic B-cell lymphoma, previously classified as "unclassifiable" has the presence of prominent nucleoli.

TABLE 3: Comparison of salient immunophenotypic features (by flow cytometry) helpful in differential diagnosis of splenic B-cell lymphomas.

Immunophenotype by flow cytometry	HCL	SMZL	SDRPL	SBLPN
CD11c	Bright	Moderate (70%)	Bright (~67%)	Bright (25%)
CD25	Positive (most cases)	Positive (30–50%)	Usually negative (positive in 3%)	Negative
CD43	Positive (~31%)	Variable	Negative	Dim to negative
CD103	Bright	Negative	Positive (20%)	Positive (65–100%)
CD123	Bright	Negative	Usually negative (positive in 3%)	Usually negative (positive in 9%)
CD180	Strong	Moderate (93%)	Strong	Not described
CD200	Strong	Moderate (93%)	Dim (40%)	Not described

(HCL: hairy cell leukemia; SMZL: splenic marginal zone lymphoma; SDRPL: splenic diffuse RP small B-cell lymphoma; SBLPN: splenic B-cell lymphoma/leukemia with prominent nucleoli)

Circulating tumor cells have morphology intermediate between prolymphocytes and hairy cells with circumferential hairy villous processes and characteristically contain round nuclei with prominent nucleoli. Neoplastic B cells express CD103 and CD11c but not CD25 and Annexin A1 **(Table 3)**. Histologically, it is characterized by diffuse RP splenic involvement (splenic cords and sinuses) and the lymphoid cells have prominent nucleoli. Bone marrow is aspirable and shows minimal fibrosis with sinusoidal involvement.

These are negative for *BRAF*V600E; and can harbor *MAP2K1* (p.C121S) which has been detected in 7–50% of cases. *CCND3* (21–24%), *KMT2C* (25%), *TP53* (33%), and *U2AF1* (13%) mutations with large copy number DNA variations are also noted including 7q deletion (20%). There is preferential use of IGCH4-34 (IGHV unmutated). Cases with 17p deletion may undergo transformation.

Clinically, these are more aggressive than HCL and cladribine resistant requiring combination therapies; The anti-CD22 immunotoxin is potentially effective. The definitive diagnoses should be made on splenectomy specimens only.

CD5 positive B-prolymphocytic leukemia (B-PLL) are categorized under prolymphocytic progression of CLL/SLL in WHO-HAEM5.

Case 3

A 71-year-old male presented with pain abdomen, fatigue, and bone pains. He was found to have a spleen of 21 cm with splenic hilar lymph nodes (1–2 cm). CBC revealed a hemoglobin of 12 g/dL, total leukocyte count of 4,000/dL, and a platelet count of 39,150/dL. 33% of the peripheral blood lymphocytes showed villous processes and presence of inconspicuous nucleoli. A broad diagnosis of splenic B-cell lymphoma was made on initial flow cytometric evaluation **(Fig. 6)**.

Splenectomy was performed and showed diffuse RP involvement by monotonous small to intermediate sized lymphoid cells in both the cords and sinuses **(Figs. 7A to F)**.

On further evaluation, the atypical lymphoid cells were negative for Annexin A1 (excluding HCL), CD103, CD123 (excluding HCL-v), and CD138 (excluding LPL). Bone marrow revealed intrasinusoidal pattern of involvement.

A final diagnosis of splenic diffuse RP small B-cell lymphoma was made.

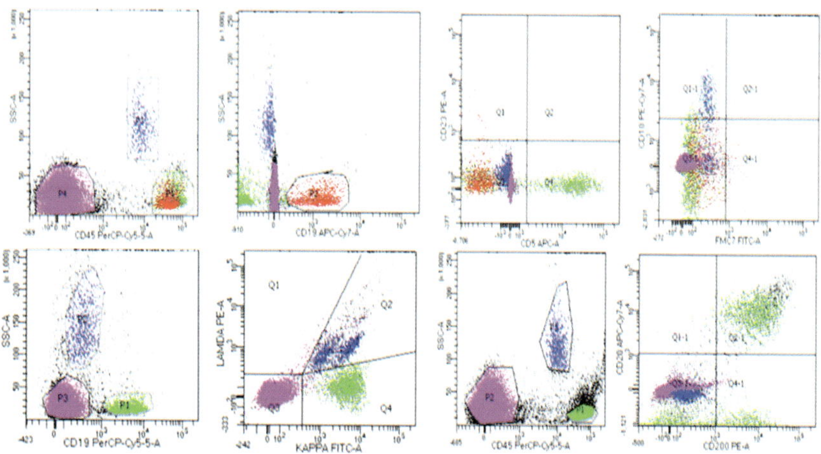

FIG. 6: Immunophenotype of splenic B-cell lymphoma by flow cytometry. The neoplastic cells (red dots) show higher forward scatter (FSC), in CD45/SSC plot, and express CD19, CD20, and CD200; the cells are negative for FMC7, CD10, CD23, and CD5.

Courtesy: Department of Hematopathology, AIIMS, Delhi, India.

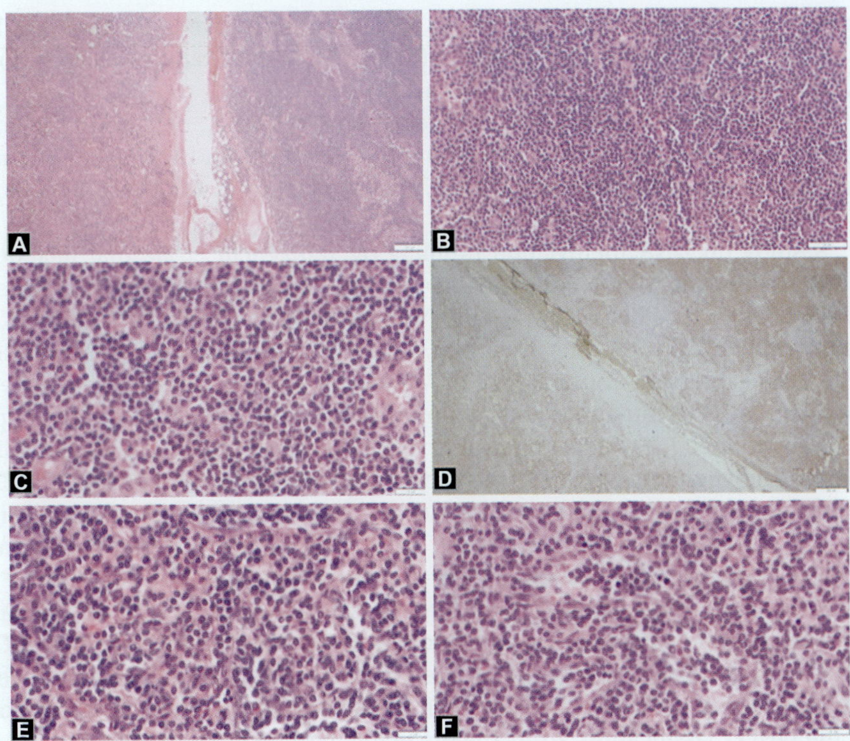

FIGS. 7A TO F: Histomorphology of SDPRL. (A) Microphotograph shows a lymphoma involving red pulp (RP) with adjacent congestive spleen. (D) CD20 highlights the atypical lymphoid cells (B, C, E, and F) The atypical lymphoid population is monomorphic with atretic lymphoid follicles.

(SDPRL: splenic diffuse RP small B-cell lymphoma)

Splenic Diffuse Red Pulp Small B-cell Lymphoma

This entity was a provisional entity in WHO-HEAM4R. In WHO-HAEM5 this has become a definitive entity; however, it is still provisional in the ICC system. In view of its overlapping clinical, histopathological and immunophenotypic features with other splenic B-cell lymphomas, especially HCL-v/SBLPN; the diagnosis is usually concluded on splenectomy specimen. Bone marrow shows a predominant intrasinusoidal pattern of infiltration unlike SMZL and SBLPN which have varied patterns of involvement and HCL shows a typical diffuse pattern with reticulin fibrosis. SDRPL commonly affects the older adults with a male preponderance.

Mild lymphocytosis is seen with the peripheral blood showing abnormal lymphoid cells which are small to intermediate sized, contain oval to round nuclei, condensed chromatin and inconspicuous nucleoli, and basophilic cytoplasm. Villous projections can be seen which are polar or unevenly distributed. Histomorphology of spleen shows marked diffuse expansion of RP by monomorphic population of small sized lymphoid cells with atretic WP lymphoid follicles. Bone marrow involvement is usually in the interstitial or sinusoidal pattern with no significant increase in mast cells (mast cells are increased in LPL with diffuse or interstitial involvement). Cyclin D3 is positive in the tumor cells. A CD200 mean fluorescence intensity (MFI)/CD180 MFI ratio of <0.5 on flow cytometry bends toward a diagnosis of SDRPL.

Chromosomal abnormalities like deletion 7q (18%), deletion 17p, and trisomy 18 can be observed. Mutations in *TP53, NOTCH1*, and *MAP2K1* (10%) are associated with an aggressive outcome. High frequency of *BCOR* (16–24%) and *CCND3* (25%) mutations are seen.

A study on DNA methylation profiling by Yamaguchi et al., that included HCL, SDRPL, and SBLPN identified five groups—M-HCL subgroup constituted of *BRAF*V600E positive HCL; M-SBPLN1 was found to enriched in MAP2K1, Telomerase (TERT) promoter mutations, and an unmutated IGHV status with wild type TP53 expression and presence of ARID1A variants; M-SBPLN2 had highest frequency of TP53 mutations and genomic instability, and SBLPN 3 and 4 groups showed mutated *IGHV* genes and spleen tyrosine kinase (SYK), immunoglobulin light like polypeptides 5 (*IGLL5*) and baculoviral IAP repeat-containing 3 (*BIRC3*) mutations. SBLPN 2, 3, and 4 showed lower frequencies of *MAP2K1* mutations with increased TP53 mutations. Except, M-HCL; all the other cohorts showed an admixture of the entities, reiterating the molecular overlap.

Until more information is available, cases that do not fit into the entities described may be classified as splenic B-cell lymphoma/leukemia in WHO-HAEM5 at the family level in the hierarchical structure, and as splenic B-cell lymphoma/leukemia, unclassifiable in ICC 2022, as per the updated 4th edition of the WHO Classification, 2017. The preferable term to be used in this regard is "splenic B-cell leukemia/lymphoma, not further classified."

OTHER LYMPHOMAS INVOLVING SPLEEN

Approximately a third of (40%) of systemic diffuse large B-cell lymphoma (DLBCL) show splenic involvement. Literature reports an incidence of 22.4–77% of DLBCLs among PSL. Transformation of low grade lymphomas to DLBCLs should always be ruled out. Splenic DLBCLs are often associated with hepatitis C virus (HCV) and human immunodeficiency virus (HIV) infections. WP is commonly involved in diffuse or nodular (macro and micronodular patterns).

Among the other B-cell lymphomas, secondary involvement of spleen by chronic lymphocytic leukemia/small lymphocytic lymphoma is common in the form of trabecular, sinusoidal, or subendothelial infiltration. It may due to higher expression of adhesion molecular such as CD11c and CD44. Mantle cell lymphoma, follicular lymphomas may also involve spleen. Non-nodal mantle cell lymphomas lack expression of CD5 and SOX11, show low proliferation indices, increased somatic hypermutation load, biased use of IGHV1-8, and less genetic complexity.

Involvement by lymphoplasmacytic lymphomas (Waldenstrom's macroglobulinemia) show RP involvement with plasmacytic morphology and immunopositivity for CD25 and CD22 (weak) combined with faint CD11c expression can be seen. The tumor cells are immunonegative for CD5, CD23, and CD10. *MYD88* L265P, a somatic mutation is noted >90% of the cases which can be determined by molecular or immunophenotypic methods. Deletion 6q is also seen.

Splenic Involvement by T-cell Lymphoma

Primary splenic NK- and T-cell lymphomas are rarer; however, have been reported in literature. They exhibit RP involvement in the periarteriolar area commonly with clonal T-cell receptor (TCR) study.

Case 4

A 36-year-old male presented with complaints of abdominal discomfort and fever for 2 months. On per abdominal examination, patient was found to have enlarged liver and spleen. Fluorodeoxyglucose (FDG) positron emission tomography (PET) showed uptake in liver, spleen, and bone marrow. Biopsy from liver and spleen showed sinusoidal infiltration by small to intermediate sized lymphoid cells with evidence of hemophagocytosis **(Figs. 8A to F)**. The atypical lymphoid cells were immunopositive for CD3, CD7, TIA1, granzyme and TCR γδ

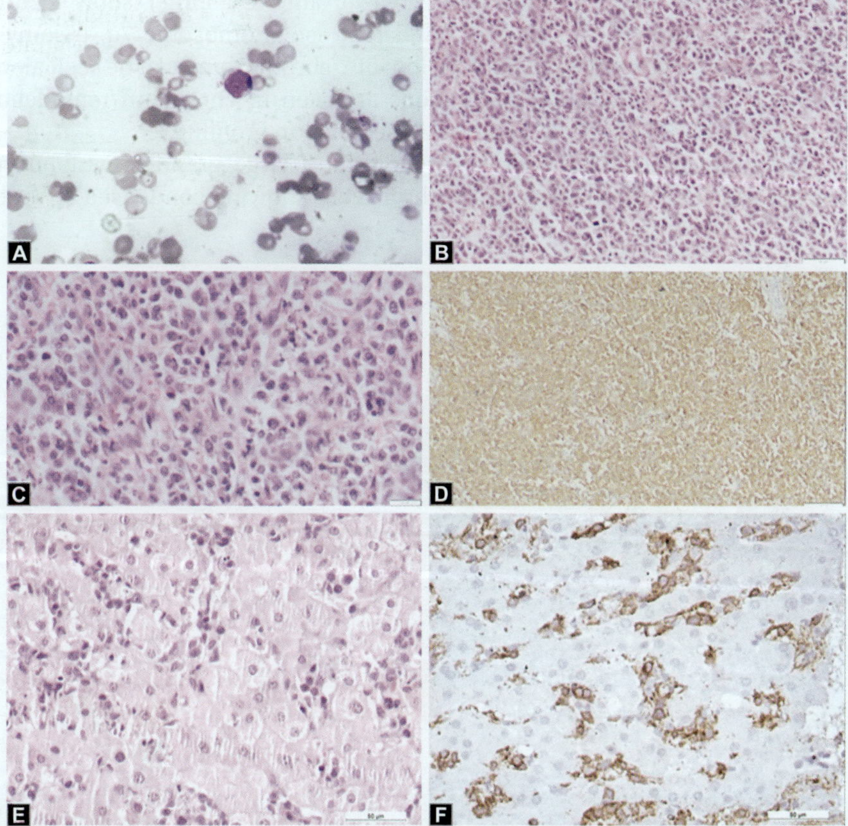

FIGS. 8A TO F: Histomorphology and immunophenotype of hepatosplenic T-cell lymphoma (HSTCL). (A) Peripheral blood smear shows an atypical lymphoid cell with blastoid morphology. (B and C) Splenic red pulp (RP) involvement by atypical lymphoid cells. (E) Sinusoidal infiltration of hepatic parenchyma by atypical lymphoid cells. (D and F) Atypical lymphoid cells immunopositive for CD3.

and were immunonegative for CD20, CD4, CD8, CD5, CD30, TCR αβ, Epstein–Barr virus latent membrane protein 1 (EBV-LMP1), and Epstein–Barr encoding region (EBER) (in situ hybridization) **(Fig. 9)**.

Hepatosplenic T-cell Lymphoma

The HSTCL is an aggressive lymphoma and is the most common T-cell lymphoma that affects spleen. Though the median age is 35-years with male preponderance; they can affect elderly with only 49% younger than 60 years. They usually arise de novo, however, 20% cases show association with immunosuppressed states.

Spleen shows characteristic RP sinusoidal involvement and the cells contain scant cytoplasm; Erythrophagocytosis can be commonly seen. In peripheral blood, the atypical lymphoid cells are monotonous and show blastic morphology, i.e., scant cytoplasm, high nucleus to cytoplasmic ratio and fine granular chromatin). Bone marrow involvement usually shows dyspoiesis of the hematopoietic cells; however, this does not have clinical relevance.

Three-fourths of the cases express TCRγδ; and rest either show TCRαβ rearrangement and 5% can also be TCR-silent. Isochromosome 7q, trisomy 8 (associated with poorer prognosis), and loss of Y chromosome can be seen along with *STAT5B/STAT3* mutations. Mutations are seen in chromatin remodeling genes *TET3*, *SMARCA2*, *SETD2*, and DNA methylation profiling.

Among the other T-cell derived neoplasm, T-large granular lymphocyte leukemia can show RP involvement with the cells showing condensed or ropey

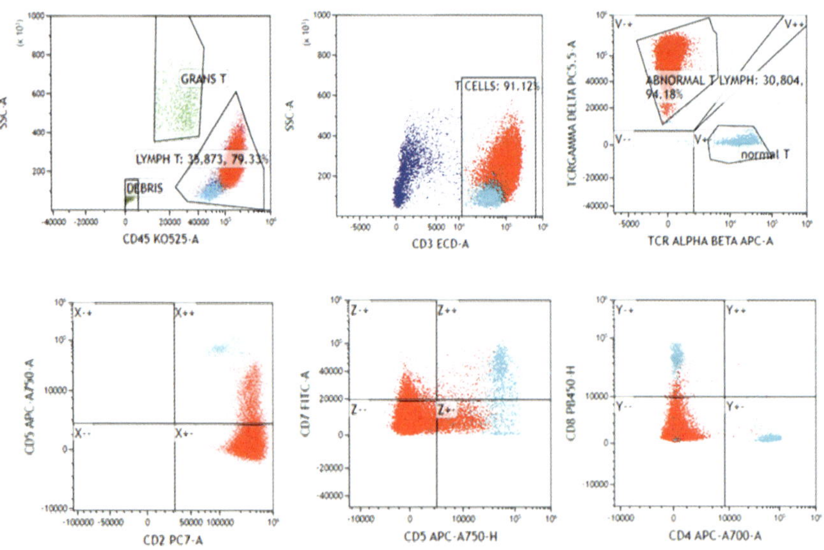

FIG. 9: Immunophenotype of hepatosplenic T-cell lymphoma by flow cytometry. The neoplastic cells (red dots) occupy the monocytic region in CD45/SSC plot, express CD3, TCRγδ, and CD2 with a subset dim positive for CD5; the cells are negative for TCRαβ, CD7, CD4, and CD8.

Courtesy: Dr Richa Juneja, Associate Professor, Department of Pathology, AIIMS, Nagpur, Maharashtra, India.

chromatin, unlike HSTCL which appear blast like. The atypical cells are immunopositive for CD3, CD8, CD16, CD57, granzyme, T-cell intracellular antigen 1 (TIA1), and αβTCR and are negative for CD4, TCRγδ, and EBV-LMP1. The expression of CD5 and CD7 is variable. T prolymphocytic leukemia (T-PLL) also involves the RP but lacks cytotoxic phenotype. Extranodal NK/T-cell lymphoma and aggressive NK-cell leukemia will show absence of sCD3 and positivity for EBER and EBV-LMP1. Patients usually have a poor prognosis, with TCRαβ having a poorer prognosis.

Hodgkin lymphomas can involve the spleen, with initial periarteriolar and Malpighian corpuscle periphery, followed by diffuse involvement with variable presence of granulomas. The involvement can mimic the primary nodal site morphology or show areas of fibrosis and lymphocyte depletion or predominance.

Take Home Points

- Primary splenic lymphomas are rare; Histologic variations and phenotypic aberrations are challenges in the precise diagnosis of splenic lymphomas.
- Needle biopsies from spleen are usually avoided; Flow cytometry from peripheral blood or bone marrow aspirate is a less invasive and widely applicable technique which can be used to diagnose splenic lymphomas. Most of splenic B-cell lymphomas are negative for CD5 and CD10, which help in broadly excluding common entities such as chronic lymphocytic leukemia and Mantle cell lymphoma involving spleen.
- Hairy cell leukemia, SMZL, SDRPL, and SBLPN are splenic B-cell lymphomas with overlapping clinical, morphologic, and immunophenotypic features. Expression and intensity of multiple markers in combination by flow cytometry (mainly CD20, CD22, surface immunoglobulins, CD11c, CD25, CD103, CD123, CD26, CD43, CD81, CD180, and CD200) helps in arriving at a diagnosis without splenectomy.

SUGGESTED READINGS

1. International Agency for Research on Cancer. (2024). WHO Classification of Tumours, 5th edition, Volume 11: Haematolymphoid tumours. [online] Available from https://www.iarc.who.int/news-events/publication-of-the-who-classification-of-tumours-5th-edition-volume-11-haematolymphoid-tumours/ [Last accessed May, 2025].
2. Campo E, Jaffe ES, Cook JR, Quintanilla-Martinez L, Swerdlow SH, Anderson KC, et al. The International Consensus Classification of mature lymphoid neoplasms: a report from the clinical advisory committee. Blood. 2022;140(11);1229-53.
3. Blombery P, de Jong D, Ferry JA, Hsi ED, Ondrejka SL, Seymour JF, et al. Closing the gap between biology and classification in splenic B-cell lymphomas. Histopathology. 2025;86(1):69-78.
4. Bonfiglio F, Bruscaggin A, Guidetti F, Terzi di Bergamo L, Faderl M, Spina V, et al. Genetic and phenotypic attributes of splenic marginal zone lymphoma. Blood. 2023;141(13):1647.
5. Montalbán C, Abraira V, Arcaini L, Domingo-Domenech E, Guisado-Vasco P, Iannitto E, et al. Risk stratification for splenic marginal zone lymphoma based on hemoglobin concentration, platelet count, high lactate dehydrogenase level and extrahilar lymphadenopathy: development and validation on 593 cases. Br J Hematol. 2012;159(2):164-71.
6. Yamaguchi K, Abdelbaky S, Arons E, Cross M, Wu YZ, Weigel C, et al. DNA methylation-based classification of hairy cell leukemia and splenic B cell lymphoma. Blood. 2023;142(1);174.

CHAPTER 39

Genetics in Hemophilia and Platelet Function Disorders

Bipin Prakash Kulkarni, Sharda Dilip Shanbhag, Nikesh Krishna Kawankar

ABSTRACT

Genetic disorders of hemostasis encompass a range of bleeding disorders caused by mutations affecting coagulation and platelet function. Understanding their molecular mechanisms and inheritance patterns is crucial for diagnosis, treatment, and genetic counseling. This chapter examines hemophilia and platelet function disorders (PFDs), highlighting their clinical implications and diagnostic approaches.

Hemophilia A and B, X-linked recessive disorders caused by F8 and F9 mutations, lead to factor VIII and IX deficiencies, impairing clot formation, and causing prolonged bleeding. Hemophilia A results from intron inversions, point mutations, deletions, and splicing defects, while hemophilia B arises from various mutations. Disease severity correlates with residual factor activity, and inhibitor development complicates treatment. Advances in genetic testing, including polymerase chain reaction (PCR), Sanger sequencing, multiplex ligation probe amplification (MLPA), and next-generation sequencing (NGS), have improved diagnosis. Gene therapy offers promising long-term solutions.

The PFDs, including von Willebrand disease (VWD), Bernard–Soulier syndrome (BSS), and Glanzmann thrombasthenia (GT), arise from mutations affecting platelet adhesion, aggregation, and secretion. Diagnosis involves coagulation tests, platelet aggregometry, and genetic analysis. Treatment varies based on severity, including platelet transfusions, recombinant factors, and emerging gene therapies.

Advancements in gene editing and personalized therapies offer new hope for managing these disorders, enhancing patient outcomes and quality of life.

INTRODUCTION

Genetic disorders of hemostasis represent a significant subset of bleeding disorders, impacting the coagulation cascade as well as platelet function. These conditions arise from mutations in genes critical to clot formation or platelet activity. Understanding their genetic basis is essential for accurate diagnosis, appropriate management, and genetic counseling **(Fig. 1)**.

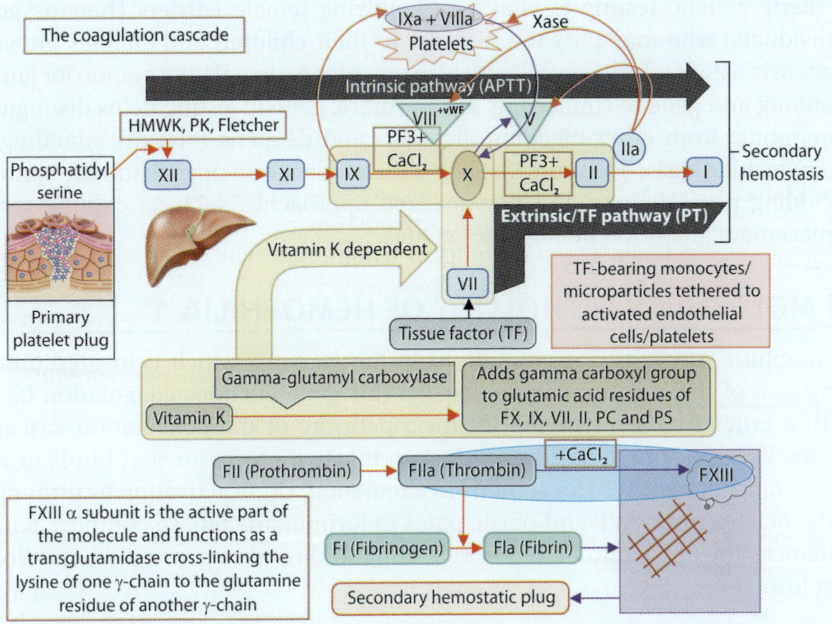

FIG. 1: The coagulation cascade.

This chapter delves into the genetic mechanisms underlying hemophilia and platelet function disorders (PFDs), exploring their molecular basis, inheritance patterns, clinical implications, and prenatal diagnosis methods.

HEMOPHILIA: GENETIC BASIS AND CLINICAL IMPLICATIONS

Hemophilia A and B are X-linked recessive bleeding disorders caused by genetic mutations that affect blood clotting. Hemophilia A results from mutations in the *F8* gene, responsible for producing coagulation factor VIII, while hemophilia B is due to mutations in the *F9* gene, which encodes coagulation factor IX. Both conditions hinder proper blood clotting, leading to prolonged bleeding after injuries or surgery, spontaneous joint bleeds, and an increased risk of internal hemorrhages.

The severity of hemophilia is determined by the level of clotting factor activity: severe cases have <1% of normal activity, moderate cases range between 1 and 5%, and mild cases fall between 5 and 40%. Genetic testing plays a crucial role in diagnosing hemophilia by identifying specific mutations in the *F8* or *F9* genes. Methods such as polymerase chain reaction (PCR), DNA sequencing, inverse and multiplex PCR, and multiplex ligation-dependent probe amplification (MLPA) detect various mutations, including point mutations, small insertion and/or deletions, intron 22 and intron 1 inversions, and large gene rearrangements respectively.

Early genetic testing is vital for identifying female carriers (heterozygous individuals) who may pass the disorder to their children and enables prenatal diagnosis within affected families. It also provides essential information for family planning and genetic counseling. Furthermore, genetic testing helps distinguish hemophilia from other bleeding disorders and deepens the understanding of its molecular basis. This knowledge is critical for advancing treatment options, including gene therapy and personalized approaches such as clotting factor replacement and novel hemostatic agents.

MOLECULAR PATHOLOGY OF HEMOPHILIA A

Hemophilia A results from mutations in the *F8* gene, which is located on the long arm of the X chromosome (Xq28). This gene encodes coagulation factor VIII, a crucial cofactor in the intrinsic pathway of the coagulation cascade. Factor VIII is normally synthesized as an inactive precursor that binds to von Willebrand factor (vWF) for stability in circulation. Upon activation by thrombin, it dissociates from vWF and participates in forming the tenase complex, which enhances the activation of factor X, leading to thrombin generation and fibrin clot formation.

Types of Mutations in *F8* Gene

- *Intron 22 inversion (~45–50% of severe cases):*
    - The most common cause of severe hemophilia A.
    - This occurs due to homologous recombination between the *F8* gene and a distal intron 22 repeat sequence (*int22h* repeats), leading to disruption of the gene and loss of factor VIII production.
    - Results in a nonfunctional truncated or absent protein.
- *Intron 1 inversion (~2–5% of severe cases):*
    - Another large structural rearrangement caused by an inversion involving homologous sequences in intron 1.
    - Leads to a complete loss of functional factor VIII production.
- *Point mutations (~20–30% of cases):*
    - Nonsense mutations introduce a premature stop codon, resulting in truncated, nonfunctional factor VIII.
    - Missense mutations cause single amino acid substitutions, potentially altering protein stability or function.
    - Some missense mutations may lead to mild or moderate hemophilia A by affecting factor VIII activity rather than completely abolishing it.
- *Small deletions/insertions (~5–10% of cases):*
    - Frameshift mutations from small insertions or deletions disrupt the open reading frame, leading to a nonfunctional protein.
    - Deletions of critical exons can cause severe hemophilia A.
- *Large gene deletions (~5% of severe cases):*
    - Complete or partial deletion of the *F8* gene results in the absence of factor VIII, leading to severe disease.

- *Splicing mutations (~5% of cases):*
    - Alterations in splicing sites lead to aberrant messenger ribonucleic acid (mRNA) splicing, resulting in exon skipping or the production of unstable transcripts.
    - The severity depends on the extent of factor VIII disruption.

MOLECULAR PATHOLOGY OF HEMOPHILIA B

Hemophilia B is caused by mutations in the *F9* gene, located on the X chromosome at Xq27.1. This gene encodes coagulation factor IX, a vitamin K-dependent serine protease that plays a critical role in the coagulation cascade. Factor IX is activated by factor XIa or the tissue factor/factor VIIa complex, and it, in turn, activates factor X, leading to thrombin generation and fibrin clot formation.

Types of Mutations in *F9* Gene

- *Missense mutations (~60–70% of cases):*
    - The most common type of mutation in hemophilia B.
    - These mutations result in single amino acid substitutions, which can affect factor IX stability, secretion, or enzymatic activity.
    - Some mutations, like *F9* p.Arg338Leu, cause severe disease by disrupting the active site of the enzyme.
- *Nonsense mutations (~10–15% of cases):*
    - Introduce premature stop codons, leading to truncated, nonfunctional factor IX proteins.
    - Generally associated with severe hemophilia B.
- *Small deletions/insertions (~10% of cases):*
    - Cause frameshift mutations that disrupt the reading frame, resulting in a nonfunctional protein.
    - Larger deletions spanning critical regions of *F9* lead to a complete loss of function.
- *Large deletions (~3–5% of cases):*
    - Rare but associated with severe disease.
    - Often result in the complete absence of factor IX protein, making patients more likely to develop inhibitors.
- *Splicing mutations (~10–15% of cases):*
    - Mutations affecting splice donor or acceptor sites lead to incorrect mRNA splicing.
    - This can result in exon skipping, frameshift mutations, or unstable transcripts, reducing or eliminating functional factor IX.
- *Promoter mutations (unique to hemophilia B leyden):*
    - Mutations in the promoter region of *F9* can lead to a condition known as hemophilia B leyden.
    - Affected individuals have severe hemophilia at birth but experience a spontaneous increase in factor IX levels after puberty, leading to mild or no bleeding symptoms in adulthood.

- These mutations disrupt transcription factor binding but are partially compensated by androgen-responsive elements that enhance gene expression after puberty.

PATHOPHYSIOLOGICAL CONSEQUENCES OF HEMOPHILIA

- *Factor deficiency and impaired coagulation cascade:*
  - Mutations in *F8* or *F9* reduce or eliminate the function of factor VIII or IX, preventing proper activation of factor X.
  - This leads to inadequate thrombin generation and impaired fibrin clot formation, causing prolonged bleeding.
- *Inhibitor development:*
  - Severe mutations, particularly large deletions or nonsense mutations, increase the risk of developing inhibitors (antibodies) against replacement therapy.
  - The immune system may recognize infused factor VIII or IX as foreign, neutralizing its effect and complicating treatment.
- *Genotype-phenotype correlation:*
  - The type of mutation often determines disease severity:
    - Large deletions, nonsense mutations, and inversions usually cause severe form of hemophilia.
    - Missense mutations can result in mild, moderate, or severe hemophilia, depending on their impact on protein function.
    - Splicing mutations may have variable effects, depending on whether alternative splicing produces some functional protein.

CLINICAL IMPLICATIONS OF MOLECULAR PATHOLOGY

- *Genetic testing and carrier screening:*
  - Molecular analysis of *F8* and *F9* genes is essential for accurate diagnosis, carrier detection, and prenatal testing.
  - Identifying specific mutations informs family planning and reproductive choices.
- *Personalized treatment approaches:*
  - Knowledge of the underlying mutation can help predict the likelihood of inhibitor development.
  - Advances in gene therapy (e.g., *F8* or *F9* gene replacement) rely on understanding the molecular basis of hemophilia.
- *Potential for gene therapy:*
  - Gene therapy using viral vectors (such as adeno-associated viruses, AAV) aims to introduce a functional copy of *F8* or *F9* into liver cells.
  - Patients with nonsense mutations or deletions may benefit most from gene therapy, as they lack endogenous protein production.

- *Tailored hemostatic agents:*
  - Novel therapies such as emicizumab (a bispecific antibody mimicking factor VIII function) are particularly beneficial for severe hemophilia A patients with inhibitors.
  - Factor IX variants with enhanced activity (e.g., *FIX-Padua*) are under investigation for hemophilia B treatment.

BLEEDING SYMPTOMS IN HEMOPHILIA

- *Prolonged bleeding from minor injuries:*
  - Individuals with hemophilia may experience excessive bleeding from small cuts, dental extractions, or surgical procedures.
  - Bleeding may persist for a longer duration than expected, even after minor trauma.
- *Spontaneous bleeding (severe hemophilia):*
  - In severe cases (clotting factor activity <1%), spontaneous bleeding episodes occur without an apparent injury.
  - Common sites of spontaneous bleeding include joints, muscles, and soft tissues.
- *Excessive bruising (ecchymosis and hematomas):*
  - Large, deep bruises (ecchymosis) form easily, even with minor bumps or pressure.
  - Internal bleeding can lead to the formation of hematomas (accumulation of blood in tissues), causing swelling and pain.
- *Joint bleeding (hemarthrosis):*
  - *Commonly affected joints:*
    - Knees, elbows, ankles, hips, shoulders, and wrists are most frequently affected.
    - Recurrent bleeding into the same joint (target joint) increases the risk of long-term damage.
  - *Symptoms of joint bleeding:*
    - *Pain and stiffness:* Initially mild, but progressively worsens.
    - *Swelling and warmth:* The joint becomes swollen, red, and warm to the touch.
    - *Limited range of motion:* Difficulty moving the affected joint due to swelling and pain.
    - *Chronic joint damage (hemophilic arthropathy):* Repeated bleeding leads to cartilage erosion and joint deformity, resulting in permanent disability over time.
- *Muscle bleeding (Intramuscular hemorrhage)*:
  - *Commonly affected muscles:* Thighs, calves, forearms, and buttocks are common sites of deep muscle bleeds.
- *Symptoms of muscle bleeding:*
  - *Swelling and tightness:* The affected muscle enlarges due to internal bleeding.
  - *Pain and tenderness:* Increased pressure causes pain, especially when moving the muscle.

    - *Compartment syndrome:* Large hematomas can compress nerves and blood vessels, leading to severe pain, numbness, weakness, and tissue damage. This is a medical emergency requiring immediate treatment.
- *Internal bleeding:*
    - *Gastrointestinal (GI) bleeding:*
        - *Blood in stool (melena or hematochezia):* Dark, tarry stools (melena) indicate bleeding from the upper GI tract, while bright red blood (hematochezia) suggests lower GI bleeding.
        - *Vomiting blood (hematemesis):* May occur if there is bleeding in the stomach or esophagus.
- *Urinary tract bleeding (hematuria):*
    - Blood in urine may appear as pink, red, or brown discoloration.
    - Can be accompanied by pain in the lower back or abdomen, indicating bleeding in the kidneys or bladder.
- *Retroperitoneal bleeding:*
    - Bleeding into the space behind the abdominal cavity (retroperitoneum) can cause severe back or abdominal pain.
    - Large-volume blood loss can lead to shock.
- *Central nervous system (CNS) bleeding (intracranial hemorrhage—ICH):*
    - *Causes and risk factors:*
        - Can occur spontaneously or after head trauma.
        - More common in severe hemophilia but can also affect moderate cases.
    - *Symptoms of CNS bleeding:*
        - *Severe headache:* Persistent and worsening pain.
        - *Vomiting:* Without relief, often associated with increased intracranial pressure.
        - *Seizures:* Indicate significant brain involvement.
        - *Weakness or paralysis:* One-sided weakness (hemiparesis) due to brain hemorrhage.
        - *Altered consciousness:* Drowsiness, confusion, or loss of consciousness.
        - *Vision problems:* Blurred or double vision due to pressure on the optic nerve.
- *Prolonged bleeding after surgery or dental procedures:*
    - Individuals with hemophilia experience excessive bleeding following medical procedures, including:
        - Tooth extractions
        - Tonsillectomy
        - Minor surgeries (e.g., biopsies)
        - Major surgeries (e.g., joint replacements)
    - Bleeding may continue for days without proper clotting factor replacement.
- *Post-traumatic bleeding:*
    - Even minor injuries can lead to excessive internal bleeding.
    - Trauma-related symptoms depend on the site of bleeding:
        - *Abdominal trauma* → Internal bleeding, swelling, and signs of shock.
        - *Head trauma* → Risk of brain hemorrhage.

  - *Fractures or deep cuts* → Persistent bleeding despite standard wound care.
- *Symptoms in female carriers (symptomatic carriers):*
  - Some female carriers of hemophilia have reduced clotting factor levels, leading to mild bleeding symptoms, including:
    - Easy bruising
    - Heavy menstrual bleeding (menorrhagia)
    - Prolonged bleeding after childbirth, surgery, or dental procedures
    - Nosebleeds (epistaxis)
- *Neonatal symptoms:*
  - Newborns with severe hemophilia may exhibit:
    - Prolonged bleeding from umbilical cord stump
    - Cephalohematoma (bleeding under the scalp after birth)
    - Excessive bleeding from circumcision
    - Intracranial hemorrhage at birth (rare but serious)

DIAGNOSIS OF HEMOPHILIA

- *Bleeding history and physical examination:*
  - *Personal bleeding history:*
    - Spontaneous bleeding episodes.
    - Prolonged bleeding after trauma or surgery.
    - Nosebleeds (epistaxis) and mucosal bleeding.
    - Easy bruising and hematomas.
    - Postpartum and menstrual bleeding (for female carriers with mild-to-moderate deficiency).
  - *Family history of bleeding disorders.*
  - *Severity and frequency of symptoms.*
- *Blood tests:*
  - Prothrombin time (PT) and activated partial thromboplastin time (aPTT) to assess clotting function.
  - Specific tests to measure levels of factor VIII, IX.

Laboratory Diagnosis of Hemophilia

Coagulation Screening Tests

Assessment of suspected bleeding disorders includes platelet count, platelet function analysis (PFA closure times), aPTT, PT, thrombin time, and plasma fibrinogen concentration.

In hemophilia, all tests except aPTT are typically normal. aPTT is prolonged in most cases, though it may appear normal in mild hemophilia.

Coagulation Factor Assays

Patients with bleeding tendencies should undergo specific coagulation factor assays, even if initial screening tests are normal. Normal factor VIII and IX clotting activity ranges from 50 to 150%. Hemophilia is characterized by factor activity below 40%, with normal vWF levels in case of hemophilia. Approximately 70% of patients are categorized as severe, though this figure may be overestimated due to the higher likelihood of severe cases seeking medical care.

Genetic Diagnosis of Hemophilia

Hemophilia A and B are X-linked recessive disorders caused by mutations in the *F8* (Factor VIII) and *F9* (Factor IX) genes, respectively. Genetic testing plays a vital role in confirming diagnoses, identifying carriers, and enabling prenatal screening. Various molecular techniques are employed to detect these mutations, each differing in sensitivity, specificity, and application. Below is an overview of the primary methods used for the genetic diagnosis of Hemophilia A and B **(Flowchart 1)**.

PCR-based Techniques

Polymerase chain reaction is a widely used molecular method for amplifying specific DNA sequences to detect mutations in the *F8* and *F9* genes. It is preferred for its high sensitivity, specificity, and cost-effectiveness.

Inversion Mutation Analysis for Hemophilia A

- *Intron 22 inversion:* This mutation accounts for approximately 45–50% of severe hemophilia A cases. It occurs when a segment of the *F8* gene inverts

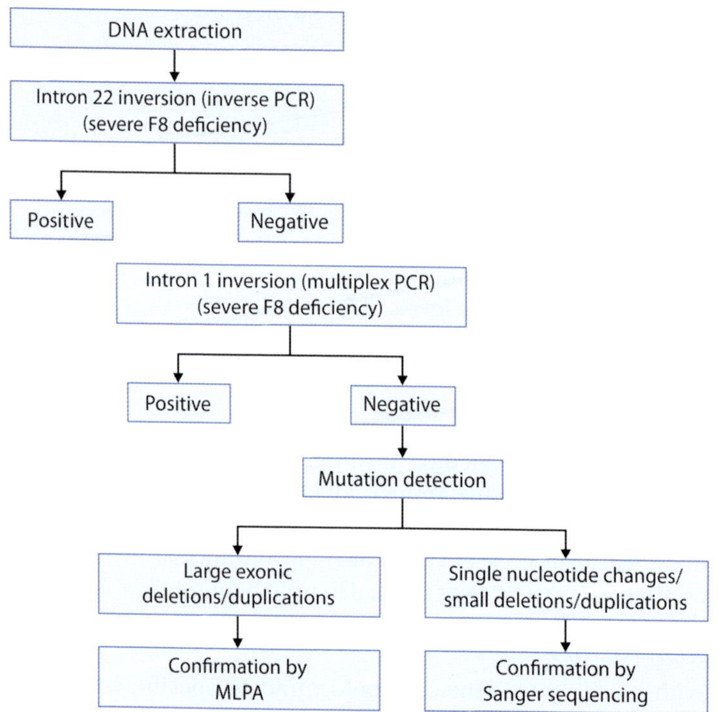

FLOWCHART 1: Genetic diagnosis of hemophilia A and B at NIIH (National Institute of Immunohematology) protocol.

(PCR: polymerase chain reaction; MLPA: multiplex ligation probe amplification) due to recombination between homologous intronic regions, leading to a deficiency of factor VIII. Inverse-shifting PCR (IS-PCR) and long-range PCR (LR-PCR) are commonly used to detect this inversion, aiding in genetic testing and family counseling.

- *Intron 1 inversion:* Representing 1–5% of severe hemophilia A cases, this inversion results from homologous recombination between intronic repeat sequences. Long-range PCR and multiplex PCR help identify this mutation, providing an accurate molecular diagnosis for cases that test negative for intron 22 inversion.

Detection of Point Mutations and Small Genetic Variations

- *Sanger sequencing:* Recognized as the gold standard for identifying point mutations, Sanger sequencing involves amplifying the exonic regions of *F8* and *F9* genes, followed by dideoxy chain termination sequencing. It effectively detects missense, nonsense, and small insertions/deletions (INDELs). This method is particularly useful for diagnosing both severe and mild-to-moderate cases when large deletions or structural mutations are absent. Additionally, it plays a critical role in carrier screening and prenatal diagnosis.
- *Multiplex ligation-dependent probe amplification:* The MLPA is designed to detect copy number variations (CNVs) such as large deletions or duplications that PCR and Sanger sequencing may miss. By employing hybridization-based probe ligation followed by PCR amplification and capillary electrophoresis, MLPA ensures comprehensive genetic analysis, particularly for hemophilia cases linked to exon deletions or duplications **(Flowchart 2)**.
- *Next-generation sequencing:* The NGS enables high-throughput sequencing of the *F8* and *F9* genes, covering both exonic and intronic regions. This technique allows for the simultaneous detection of single nucleotide variations (SNVs),

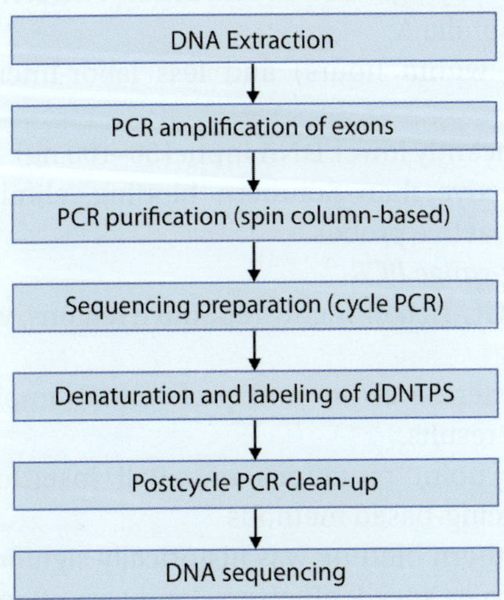

FLOWCHART 2: Gene (exons) amplification and DNA sequencing.

(dDNTPS: deoxyribonucleotides; PCR: polymerase chain reaction)

insertions/deletions (INDELs), and large structural mutations. Faster and more cost-effective than traditional sequencing, NGS is preferred for cases where conventional methods fail to identify mutations.

Southern Blotting in Hemophilia Genetic Diagnosis

Historically, Southern blotting and long-range PCR have been used to identify large-scale mutations, inversions, and structural variations in hemophilia A and B.

- *Advantages of Southern blotting:*
  - Detects large genomic rearrangements, including intron 22 inversions.
  - Effective for identifying large deletions and duplications.
  - Highly specific, directly detecting genomic alterations.
  - Unaffected by GC-rich sequences or repetitive regions, which may pose challenges for PCR-based methods.
- *Limitations of Southern blotting:*
  - Time-consuming and labor-intensive (2–3 days for results).
  - Requires high DNA concentrations (10–20 μg).
  - Cannot detect point mutations or small deletions.
  - Expensive due to the use of radioactive or chemiluminescent probes.
  - Requires technical expertise, with results varying across laboratories.

Long-range Polymerase Chain Reaction in Hemophilia Genetic Diagnosis

Long-range PCR (LR-PCR) is a modified PCR technique that amplifies large DNA fragments (>10 kb), making it ideal for detecting structural rearrangements and deletions in the *F8* and *F9* genes.

- *Advantages of long-range PCR:*
  - Effective for identifying intron 22 and intron 1 inversions, the major causes of severe hemophilia A.
  - Faster (results within hours) and less labor-intensive than Southern blotting.
  - Requires significantly lower DNA input (50–100 ng).
  - More cost-effective than Southern blotting, eliminating the need for expensive radioactive probes.
- *Limitations of long-range PCR:*
  - Struggles with GC-rich or highly repetitive regions, which may hinder full amplification.
  - Prone to polymerase errors and preferential amplification, potentially leading to false results.
  - Cannot detect point mutations or small insertions/deletions, which require sequencing-based methods.

Overall, while Southern blotting was historically significant, long-range PCR is now preferred due to its speed, efficiency, and cost-effectiveness. Meanwhile, modern techniques such as qPCR, MLPA, and NGS are increasingly used for more comprehensive genetic screening.

Linkage Analysis (Indirect Genetic Testing)

Linkage analysis is a method used to trace the inheritance of hemophilia within families. Instead of detecting the actual mutation, it tracks genetic markers [microsatellites or single-nucleotide polymorphisms (SNPs)] that are closely linked to the *F8* or *F9* genes on the X chromosome.

- *Advantages:* Useful for carrier detection and prenatal diagnosis in families with a history of hemophilia.
- *Limitations:*
  - Requires DNA samples from multiple family members.
  - Risk of recombination errors.
  - Unable to detect de novo (new) mutations.

As a result, direct mutation testing (Sanger sequencing, MLPA, or NGS) is preferred for higher accuracy, while linkage analysis is used when direct testing is not feasible.

COINHERITANCE OF THROMBOPHILIA GENES AND CLINICAL PHENOTYPE

In severe hemophilia, heterozygosity for thrombophilic genes may contribute to milder clinical presentations. Coinheritance of prothrombotic genes, such as protein C, protein S, and antithrombin deficiencies, as well as mutations such as factor V Leiden, PT20210A, and methylenetetrahydrofolate reductase (MTHFR) C677T polymorphisms, has been associated with reduced bleeding severity.

Studies have demonstrated that prothrombotic mutations, such as factor V Leiden and prothrombin G20210A, may compensate for low factor VIII levels, enhancing thrombin generation and attenuating bleeding severity. However, this association has not been consistently confirmed, suggesting that the variability in severe hemophilia phenotypes is likely multifactorial.

Conversely, the presence of prothrombotic mutations alongside other inherited or acquired thrombophilic factors may increase the risk of thrombotic complications in individuals with hemophilia.

OTHER MODIFIERS OF HEMOPHILIA A PHENOTYPE

Factor VIII Pharmacokinetics

Interindividual differences in the pharmacokinetics of factor VIII (FVIII) significantly influence the hemophilia phenotype. For instance, patients with blood group O and low vWF levels have reduced FVIII half-lives, leading to increased clotting factor consumption.

Fibrinolytic Pathway

Variability in fibrinolytic pathway activity may also affect bleeding severity. It has been hypothesized that ineffective hemostasis in response to trauma triggers prolonged stimulation of the hemostatic system, including fibrinolysis, creating a cycle that exacerbates bleeding.

Inflammatory Mediators

Inflammatory responses in the synovium may influence the severity of joint damage and partially explain variability in the extent of hemophilic arthropathy.

These findings highlight the multifaceted nature of phenotype variability in hemophilia, with contributions from genetic, environmental, and systemic factors.

PLATELET FUNCTION DISORDERS: GENETIC INSIGHTS AND CLINICAL IMPACT

Overview of Platelet Function Disorders

Platelet function disorders are a group of heterogeneous conditions caused by genetic defects that impair platelet adhesion, aggregation, secretion, or procoagulant activity. These disorders result in mucocutaneous bleeding and increased susceptibility to hemorrhage.

Diagnosis of platelet disorders requires an integrative approach that combines clinical history, laboratory testing, and genetic analysis. Genetic testing enhances diagnostic accuracy, facilitates targeted therapies, and enables family screening for hereditary conditions.

Key Steps in Primary Hemostasis (Fig. 2)

Platelet Adhesion

- Glycoprotein (GP)Ib/V/IX receptor complex binds to vWF immobilized on exposed subendothelial collagen.
- GPVI and GPIa/IIa receptors also bind to exposed subendothelial collagen.

Platelet Granule Secretion

- *Thromboxane A2 (TxA_2), adenosine triphosphate (ATP), adenosine diphosphate (ADP):* Secreted from platelet dense granules.
- *α granules contain:* Fibrinogen, vWF, and factor V.

Platelet Aggregation

- Platelet activation triggers conformational change in GPIIb/IIIa from inactive to active state.
- Fibrinogen and vWF bridge between GPIIb/IIIa receptors on adjacent platelets.

DISORDERS THAT MAY CAUSE PLATELET FUNCTION DEFECTS

Adhesion Defects

Platelet adhesion defects are a subset of inherited platelet function disorders (IPFDs) that result in impaired hemostasis, leading to excessive bleeding. Platelet

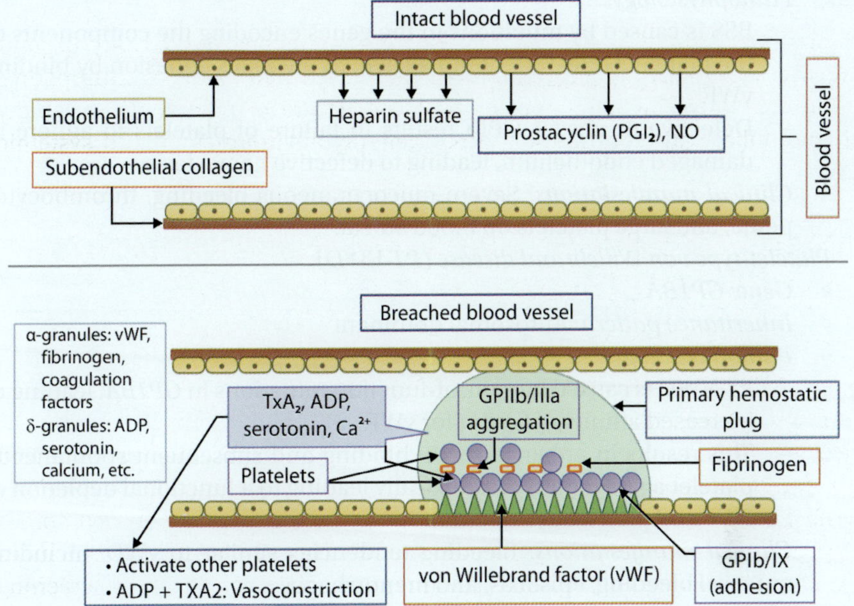

FIG. 2: Primary hemostasis.

(ADP: adenosine diphosphate; GP: glycoprotein; TxA_2: thromboxane A_2)

adhesion is a critical initial step in primary hemostasis, allowing platelets to bind to the subendothelial matrix at sites of vascular injury. This process is largely mediated by glycoprotein receptors and adhesive ligands such as vWF and collagen. Genetic mutations affecting these proteins lead to platelet adhesion defects, causing bleeding diatheses of varying severity.

Key Genetic Components of Platelet Adhesion Defects

- *Von Willebrand disease:*
  - *Gene: VWF*
  - *Inheritance pattern:* Autosomal dominant or recessive
  - *Pathophysiology:*
    - vWD is caused by mutations in the *VWF* gene, which encodes vWF, a crucial protein for platelet adhesion and aggregation.
    - Mutations result in either a quantitative deficiency (types 1 and 3) or a qualitative defect (type 2) of vWF, impairing its ability to bind to platelet glycoprotein Ib (GPIb) and collagen.
  - *Clinical manifestations:* Easy bruising, mucocutaneous bleeding, epistaxis, menorrhagia, and prolonged bleeding after injury or surgery.
- *Bernard–Soulier syndrome:*
  - *Genes: GP1BA, GP1BB, GP9*
  - *Inheritance pattern:* Autosomal recessive

- *Pathophysiology:*
  - BSS is caused by mutations in the genes encoding the components of the platelet GPIb-IX-V complex, which mediates adhesion by binding vWF.
  - Defective or absent GPIb results in failure of platelets to adhere to damaged endothelium, leading to defective hemostasis.
- *Clinical manifestations:* Severe mucocutaneous bleeding, thrombocytopenia, and large platelets on blood smear.

- *Platelet-type von Willebrand disease (PT-VWD):*
  - *Gene: GP1BA*
  - *Inheritance pattern:* Autosomal dominant
  - *Pathophysiology:*
    - PT-VWD is caused by gain-of-function mutations in *GP1BA*, leading to increased affinity of GPIbα for vWF.
    - This results in enhanced vWF binding and subsequent spontaneous platelet aggregation, paradoxically leading to a functional depletion of vWF and platelet dysfunction.
  - *Clinical manifestations:* Bleeding tendencies similar to vWD, including mucosal bleeding, epistaxis, and menorrhagia.
- *Collagen receptor defects:*
  - *Genes: GP6, ITGA2*
  - *Inheritance pattern:* Autosomal recessive or dominant (depending on the mutation)
  - *Pathophysiology:*
    - Mutations in *GP6* (encoding glycoprotein VI) or *ITGA2* (encoding integrin α2, part of α2β1) impair platelet-collagen interaction, reducing adhesion at injury sites.
    - This defect leads to poor platelet activation and defective thrombus formation.
  - *Clinical manifestations:* Mild-to-moderate bleeding diathesis, including excessive bruising and prolonged bleeding.

Diagnosis and Genetic Testing

The diagnosis of platelet adhesion defects involves:

- *Clinical evaluation:* History of bleeding episodes, family history of bleeding disorders.
- *Laboratory tests:*
  - Platelet count and morphology
  - Bleeding time and platelet function assays
  - Flow cytometry for glycoprotein expression
  - von Willebrand factor antigen and activity levels
- *Genetic testing:*
  - Next-generation sequencing panels for known platelet disorder genes.
  - Sanger sequencing for specific mutations.
  - Whole-exome sequencing (WES) in cases with unclear genetic etiology.

Treatment Approaches

- *Supportive care:*
    - Antifibrinolytics (e.g., tranexamic acid) for mild bleeding
    - Desmopressin (DDAVP) in type 1 vWD and some cases of PT-VWD
- *Platelet transfusion:* For severe cases such as BSS and GT during major bleeding or surgery.
- *Gene therapy:* Emerging experimental treatments targeting *VWF* and *ITGA2B/ITGB3* mutations.
- *Recombinant factor therapy:*
    - Recombinant vWF for severe vWD
    - Recombinant factor VIIa for GT

Platelet Aggregation Defects

Platelet aggregation is a crucial step in primary hemostasis, allowing platelets to clump together at sites of vascular injury to form a stable platelet plug. This process is primarily mediated by integrins, glycoproteins, and signaling pathways that facilitate platelet-platelet interactions via fibrinogen and vWF. Genetic mutations affecting these mechanisms can lead to platelet aggregation defects, resulting in bleeding disorders of varying severity.

Key Genetic Components of Platelet Aggregation Defects

- *Glanzmann thrombasthenia:*
    - *Genes: ITGA2B, ITGB3*
    - *Inheritance pattern:* Autosomal recessive
    - *Pathophysiology:*
        - GT is caused by mutations in *ITGA2B* and *ITGB3*, which encode the integrin αIIbβ3 (GPIIb/IIIa) complex.
        - This integrin is essential for fibrinogen binding, which bridges adjacent platelets to form aggregates.
        - Mutations lead to either a deficiency or functional impairment of αIIbβ3, preventing normal platelet aggregation.
    - *Clinical manifestations:* Severe mucocutaneous bleeding, epistaxis, menorrhagia, and spontaneous hemorrhage.
- *Defects in fibrinogen receptor binding:*
    - *Genes:* Fibrinogen alpha (*FGA*), fibrinogen beta (*FGB*), fibrinogen gamma (*FGG*)
    - *Inheritance pattern:* Autosomal recessive or dominant
    - *Pathophysiology:*
        - Fibrinogen binds to αIIbβ3, facilitating platelet aggregation.
        - Mutations in *FGA, FGB, and FGG* can lead to afibrinogenemia (complete absence), hypofibrinogenemia (reduced levels), or dysfibrinogenemia (dysfunctional fibrinogen).
    - *Clinical manifestations:* Prolonged bleeding, poor wound healing, and spontaneous soft tissue bleeding.

- *ADP receptor (P2Y12) deficiency:*
  - *Gene: P2RY12*
  - *Inheritance pattern:* Autosomal recessive
  - *Pathophysiology:*
    - P2Y12 is a G-protein coupled receptor essential for ADP-induced platelet aggregation.
    - Mutations in *P2RY12* lead to impaired ADP signaling, reducing secondary platelet aggregation.
  - *Clinical manifestations:* Mild-to-moderate bleeding, prolonged bleeding time, and poor response to ADP in platelet function tests.

Secretion Defects

Platelet secretion plays a crucial role in hemostasis by releasing granule contents that amplify platelet activation, recruit additional platelets, and stabilize clot formation. There are two major types of platelet granules: dense granules (which contain ADP, ATP, serotonin, and calcium) and α granules (which contain fibrinogen, vWF, and platelet-derived growth factors). Genetic mutations affecting platelet granule biogenesis, storage, or secretion lead to platelet secretion defects, resulting in bleeding disorders of varying severity.

Key Genetic Components of Platelet Secretion Defects

- *Dense granule deficiency (Hermansky-Pudlak syndrome, HPS):*
  - *Genes: HPS1-10*
  - *Inheritance pattern:* Autosomal recessive
  - *Pathophysiology:*
    - HPS is caused by mutations in genes involved in lysosome-related organelle biogenesis, leading to defective formation of dense granules in platelets.
    - Deficiency in dense granules impairs the release of ADP and serotonin, reducing platelet recruitment and aggregation.
- *Clinical manifestations:* Mild-to-moderate bleeding tendency, easy bruising, epistaxis, prolonged bleeding time, and oculocutaneous albinism.
- *Griscelli syndrome type 2 (GS2):*
  - *Gene: RAB27A*
  - *Inheritance pattern:* Autosomal recessive
  - *Pathophysiology:*
    - Mutations in *RAB27A* disrupt intracellular vesicle trafficking, leading to defective dense granule secretion.
    - Patients often exhibit immune dysregulation (hemophagocytic lymphohistiocytosis, HLH) in addition to platelet dysfunction.
- *Clinical manifestations:* Increased bleeding tendency, hypopigmentation, and recurrent infections due to immune system defects.
- *Chediak-Higashi syndrome (CHS):*
  - *Gene: LYST*
  - *Inheritance pattern:* Autosomal recessive

  - *Pathophysiology:*
    - *LYST* mutations result in the formation of giant granules in platelets and other cells, leading to defective secretion.
    - The disorder also affects immune cells, increasing susceptibility to infections.
- *Clinical manifestations:* Prolonged bleeding time, easy bruising, recurrent infections, and partial oculocutaneous albinism.
- *Gray platelet syndrome (GPS):*
  - *Gene: NBEAL2, GFI1b (platelet transcription factor)*
  - *Inheritance pattern:* Autosomal recessive
  - *Pathophysiology:*
    - Mutations in *NBEAL2* lead to defective α granule formation, resulting in platelets lacking critical hemostatic proteins.
    - *GFI1B* mutations affect megakaryocyte differentiation and proplatelet formation, leading to gray platelet syndrome-like characteristics with platelet α-granule deficiency and thrombocytopenia.
    - Platelets appear large and gray on blood smears due to the absence of α granules.
- *Clinical manifestations:* Moderate-to-severe bleeding tendency, thrombocytopenia, myelofibrosis, and prolonged bleeding time.

Diagnosis and Genetic Testing

- *Clinical evaluation:* History of excessive bleeding, albinism, recurrent infections, or immune dysfunction.
- *Laboratory tests:*
  - Platelet aggregometry with ADP, collagen, and epinephrine.
  - Electron microscopy to assess granule presence.
  - Flow cytometry for platelet granule markers.
- *Genetic testing:*
  - Next-generation sequencing panels for PFDs.
  - Whole-exome sequencing for complex cases.

Treatment Approaches

- *Supportive care:*
  - Antifibrinolytics (e.g., tranexamic acid) to reduce bleeding
  - Desmopressin for mild bleeding episodes
- *Platelet transfusion:* For severe cases, particularly during surgery or major bleeding events
- *Bone marrow transplantation:* Potential cure for syndromic disorders affecting both platelets and the immune system (e.g., Griscelli syndrome, CHS)
- *Gene therapy:* Investigational approaches targeting *NBEAL2, HPS1-10*, and *LYST*

Signal Transduction Defects

Platelet signal transduction is a critical process in hemostasis, enabling platelets to respond to vascular injury by activating, adhering, and aggregating to form a stable clot. This process is mediated by a complex network of receptors, intracellular signaling molecules, and secondary messengers that regulate platelet function. Genetic mutations affecting these pathways lead to platelet signal transduction defects, resulting in impaired clot formation and increased bleeding risk.

Key Genetic Components of Platelet Signal Transduction Defects

- *Thromboxane A_2 signaling defects:*
  - *Genes: TBXA2R, PTGS1*
  - *Inheritance pattern:* Autosomal dominant or recessive
  - *Pathophysiology:*
    - TXA_2 is a key platelet agonist that enhances platelet activation and aggregation via the thromboxane receptor (*TBXA2R*).
    - Mutations in *TBXA2R* lead to impaired receptor function, reducing platelet response to TXA_2.
    - *PTGS1* mutations affect cyclooxygenase-1 (COX-1), leading to decreased TXA_2 synthesis.
  - *Clinical manifestations:* Mild-to-moderate bleeding tendencies, prolonged bleeding time, and reduced platelet aggregation in response to arachidonic acid.
- *ADP receptor (P2Y12) deficiency:*
  - *Gene: P2RY12*
  - *Inheritance pattern:* Autosomal recessive
  - *Pathophysiology:*
    - The P2Y12 receptor is crucial for ADP-mediated platelet activation and aggregation.
    - Mutations in *P2RY12* lead to defective ADP signaling, reducing platelet recruitment and sustained aggregation.
  - *Clinical manifestations:* Mild-to-moderate bleeding diathesis, prolonged bleeding time, and poor response to ADP in platelet function tests.
- *Calcium signaling defects:*
  - *Genes: STIM1, ORAI1, RASGRP2*
  - *Inheritance pattern:* Autosomal recessive
  - *Pathophysiology:*
    - Calcium influx is critical for platelet activation and integrin activation.
    - Mutations in *STIM1* and *ORAI1* disrupt store-operated calcium entry (SOCE), impairing platelet responses to activation signals.
    - *RASGRP2* is a calcium and diacylglycerol-regulated guanine nucleotide exchange factor I (CalDAG-GEFI) that leads to activation of Rap1, an essential signaling-knot in the "inside-out" αIIbβ3 integrin activation in platelets.
  - *Clinical manifestations:* Bleeding diathesis, reduced platelet aggregation, and impaired clot formation.
- *Defective platelet signal transduction:*
  - *Genes: STXBP2, UNC13D*
  - *Inheritance pattern:* Autosomal recessive

- *Pathophysiology:*
  - Mutations in these genes impair platelet granule exocytosis by affecting SNARE complex interactions, essential for vesicle fusion.
  - These defects can also lead to immune disorders, including familial hemophagocytic lymphohistiocytosis (FHL).
- *Clinical manifestations:* Increased bleeding tendency, recurrent infections, and immune dysfunction.

- *G-protein signaling defects:*
  - *Genes: GNAQ, GNA11*
  - *Inheritance pattern:* Autosomal dominant or recessive
  - *Pathophysiology:*
    - G-proteins mediate signal transduction from platelet receptors to intracellular effectors.
    - Mutations in *GNAQ* or *GNA11* can impair platelet activation and aggregation.
  - *Clinical manifestations:* Mild bleeding symptoms and reduced response to platelet agonists.
- *Defects in protein tyrosine kinases and phosphatases:*
  - *Genes: FERMT3, SRC, PTPN6*
  - *Inheritance pattern:* Autosomal recessive or dominant (depending on the mutation)
  - *Pathophysiology:*
    - *FERMT3* mutations cause leukocyte adhesion deficiency type III (LAD-III), affecting integrin activation.
    - *SRC* and *PTPN6* mutations impair phosphorylation events crucial for platelet activation.
  - *Clinical manifestations:* Severe bleeding disorder in LAD-III, impaired clot formation, and prolonged bleeding time.

Diagnosis and Genetic Testing

- *Clinical evaluation:* History of excessive bleeding, poor wound healing, and prolonged bleeding time.
- *Laboratory tests:*
  - Platelet aggregometry to assess response to ADP, thromboxane, and other agonists.
  - Flow cytometry for receptor expression.
  - Thromboelastography to evaluate clot strength.
- *Genetic testing:*
  - Next-generation sequencing panels for PFDs.
  - Whole-exome sequencing for complex cases.

Treatment Approaches

- *Supportive care:*
  - Antifibrinolytics (e.g., tranexamic acid) to reduce bleeding.
  - Desmopressin for mild platelet function defects.

- *Platelet transfusion:* For severe cases, particularly during surgery or major bleeding events.
- *Targeted therapies:* Investigational approaches targeting signal transduction pathways for potential treatments.

Platelet Procoagulant Activity Defects

Platelet procoagulant activity plays a crucial role in secondary hemostasis by promoting the assembly of coagulation factor complexes on the platelet surface, leading to thrombin generation and fibrin clot formation. This process is regulated by the exposure of phosphatidylserine (PS) on the outer membrane, calcium signaling, and interactions with clotting factors. Genetic mutations affecting these mechanisms can lead to platelet procoagulant activity defects, resulting in impaired thrombin generation and a bleeding tendency.

Key Genetic Components of Platelet Procoagulant Activity Defects

- *Scott syndrome:*
    - *Gene: ANO6* (TMEM16F)
    - *Inheritance pattern:* Autosomal recessive
    - *Pathophysiology:*
        - *ANO6* encodes anoctamin-6, a calcium-activated phospholipid scramblase essential for PS exposure on the platelet membrane.
        - Mutations in *ANO6* impair the translocation of PS to the outer leaflet, reducing the surface available for coagulation factor assembly.
    - *Clinical manifestations:* Mild-to-moderate bleeding tendency, prolonged clotting time, and reduced thrombin generation.
- *Stormorken syndrome*:
    - *Gene: STIM1*
    - *Inheritance pattern:* Autosomal dominant
    - *Pathophysiology:*
        - *STIM1* mutations cause abnormal calcium homeostasis, leading to defective platelet procoagulant activity and aberrant platelet activation.
        - This results in both bleeding and thrombotic complications.
    - *Clinical manifestations:* Thrombocytopenia, muscle fatigue, miosis, asplenia, and bleeding diathesis.

Diagnosis and Genetic Testing

- *Clinical evaluation:* History of excessive bleeding, prolonged clotting times, and abnormal platelet function tests.
- *Laboratory tests:*
    - Flow cytometry to assess PS exposure on activated platelets.
    - Thrombin generation assays.
    - Platelet function tests, including light transmission aggregometry.
- *Genetic testing:*
    - Next-generation sequencing panels for PFDs.
    - Whole-exome sequencing for complex cases.

Treatment Approaches

- *Supportive care:*
    - Antifibrinolytics (e.g., tranexamic acid) to reduce bleeding episodes.
    - Desmopressin for mild cases.
- *Platelet transfusion:* For severe bleeding episodes or surgical interventions.
- *Gene therapy:* Investigational approaches targeting *ANO6* and calcium signaling pathways.

Inheritance Patterns

- *Autosomal recessive:* Most severe PFDs (e.g., GT, BSS).
- *Autosomal dominant:* Some mild PFDs (e.g., mild vWD).
- *X-linked:* Rare, as seen in some forms of Wiskott–Aldrich syndrome.

Clinical Manifestations

The PFDs commonly present with:

- Easy bruising
- Prolonged bleeding from cuts or minor surgeries
- Mucocutaneous bleeding (e.g., epistaxis, menorrhagia)
- Hematomas or petechiae

  The severity varies based on the specific defect and gene involved.

Diagnosis and Genetic Testing in Platelet Disorders

The diagnostic approach to platelet disorders involves a combination of clinical assessment, laboratory testing, and genetic analysis.

Clinical Assessment

A detailed patient history and physical examination are essential in diagnosing platelet disorders. Key aspects include:

- Personal and family history of bleeding disorders.
- Symptoms such as easy bruising, prolonged bleeding, epistaxis, menorrhagia, and excessive bleeding postsurgery.
- History of thrombosis or stroke in cases of platelet hyperfunction disorders.
- Medication use, infections, or underlying systemic conditions.

Laboratory Testing

- *Complete blood count (CBC):* Evaluates platelet count; thrombocytopenia (low count) or thrombocytosis (high count) suggests underlying pathology.
- *Peripheral blood smear:* Assesses platelet morphology for conditions like BSS (giant platelets) or May–Hegglin anomaly.
- *Platelet function tests:*
    - *Platelet aggregometry:* Measures platelet response to agonists (e.g., ADP, collagen, ristocetin) to detect functional defects like GT.
    - *PFA-100 (platelet function analyzer):* Screens for primary hemostatic defects.

- *Flow cytometry:* Detects deficiencies in surface glycoproteins (e.g., GPIb in BSS, GPIIb/IIIa in GT).
- *Clot retraction assay:* Evaluates platelet contractility in GT.

- *Coagulation studies:* Rule out clotting factor deficiencies.
- *Bone marrow examination:* Considered in cases of suspected bone marrow failure syndromes or inherited thrombocytopenias.

Genetic Testing in Platelet Disorders

Genetic testing plays a crucial role in confirming hereditary platelet disorders, differentiating them from acquired conditions, and identifying at-risk family members.

Indications for genetic testing are:

- Unexplained inherited thrombocytopenia.
- Persistent platelet dysfunction with normal coagulation studies.
- Family history suggestive of a hereditary platelet disorder.
- To guide treatment and preventive strategies.

Methods of Genetic Testing

- *Targeted gene sequencing:* Used when a specific disorder is suspected, such as *ITGA2B* or *ITGB3* mutations in GT or GP1BA mutations in BSS.
- *Next-generation sequencing panels:* Allows simultaneous screening of multiple genes associated with inherited platelet disorders.
- *Whole exome sequencing or whole genome sequencing (WGS):* Useful for diagnosing rare or novel platelet disorders when targeted panels are inconclusive.
- *Cytogenetic and CNV analysis:* Detects larger chromosomal alterations associated with syndromic platelet disorders, such as 22q11.2 deletion syndrome.

Challenges and Considerations

- *Genetic variability:* Some platelet disorders exhibit variable expressivity and incomplete penetrance.
- *Variants of uncertain significance (VUS):* Interpretation challenges in genetic sequencing results.
- *Cost and accessibility:* Advanced genetic testing may not be widely available in all clinical settings.
- *Ethical considerations:* Genetic counseling is essential to discuss implications for patients and family members.

Treatment Approaches

- *Supportive care:*
  - Antifibrinolytics (e.g., tranexamic acid) to control bleeding.
  - Desmopressin in mild cases.
- *Platelet transfusion:* For severe cases like GT during major bleeding or surgery.

- *Gene therapy:* Investigational approaches targeting *ITGA2B* and *ITGB3.*
- *Recombinant factor therapy:* Recombinant factor VIIa for severe platelet aggregation defects.

Intersection of Hemophilia and Platelet Function Disorders in Clinical Practice

Differential Diagnosis

Accurate differentiation between hemophilia and PFDs is essential for appropriate management. Key distinctions include:

- *Bleeding pattern:*
  - *Hemophilia:* Deep tissue bleeding (e.g., joints, muscles).
  - *PFDs:* Mucocutaneous bleeding (e.g., nosebleeds, gum bleeding).
- *Laboratory findings:*
  - *Hemophilia:* Prolonged aPTT.
  - *PFDs:* Normal coagulation tests with abnormal platelet function assays.
- *Coexisting disorders:* Rarely, patients may exhibit overlapping features due to combined defects in coagulation and platelet function, necessitating a comprehensive genetic workup.

Future Directions in Genetic Research and Therapy

- *Whole-genome sequencing:* Enhances the discovery of novel mutations and modifier genes.
- *Epigenetics:* Investigates how nongenetic factors influence disease expression.
- *Gene editing:* Advances in CRISPR-based approaches hold promise for curative therapies.
- *Personalized medicine:* Tailored treatments based on individual genetic profiles.

Ethical Considerations in Genetic Diagnosis

Pursuing genetic diagnosis for hereditary blood disorders involves several ethical considerations that require careful assessment by both parents and healthcare professionals.

Informed Consent

Securing informed consent is vital for prenatal testing. Parents must have a comprehensive understanding of the procedure's risks, benefits, and limitations, including possible outcomes and their implications. Additionally, they should reflect on the emotional, psychological, and social impacts of discovering a potential genetic disorder.

Reproductive Choices

Prenatal diagnosis can present parents with significant decisions regarding their pregnancy, such as whether to continue or terminate it. This introduces ethical debates concerning reproductive rights, potential discrimination against disabilities, and societal perceptions of individuals with genetic conditions.

Use of Genetic Information

The management of genetic data in reproductive decision-making must be handled with caution to ensure privacy and prevent misuse. Employing genetic testing for nonmedical purposes, like selecting a child's gender or other social preferences, also raises ethical dilemmas.

CONCLUSION

Genetic disorders of hemostasis significantly impact blood clotting and platelet function, leading to severe bleeding disorders. Understanding the genetic mechanisms underlying these conditions is crucial for accurate diagnosis, management, and genetic counseling. This chapter explores the molecular basis, inheritance patterns, clinical implications, and diagnostic methods related to hemophilia and PFDs.

Hemophilia A and B are X-linked recessive disorders caused by mutations in the *F8* and *F9* genes, respectively. These mutations result in deficiencies of coagulation factors VIII and IX, leading to prolonged bleeding, spontaneous joint bleeds, and internal hemorrhages. Diagnosis involves bleeding history, coagulation tests, and genetic testing, including PCR-based techniques, sequencing, and MLPA. Treatment includes factor replacement therapy, gene therapy, and tailored hemostatic agents.

PFDs result from defects in platelet adhesion, aggregation, granule secretion, and signal transduction. Key disorders include vWD, BSS, and GT, caused by mutations in genes such as *VWF*, *GP1BA*, *ITGA2B*, and *ITGB3*. Diagnosis includes platelet function tests, flow cytometry, and genetic sequencing. Treatment involves platelet transfusion, recombinant factor therapy, and emerging gene therapies.

A comprehensive understanding of hemophilia and PFDs aid in differential diagnosis, guiding targeted treatments, and improving patient outcomes.

The genetics of hemophilia and PFDs provide a critical framework for understanding their pathophysiology, diagnosis, and treatment. Advances in molecular biology and gene therapy continue to transform patient care, offering hope for improved outcomes and potential cures. Future research will likely uncover new genetic pathways and therapeutic strategies, further enhancing our ability to manage these complex disorders effectively.

Take Home Points

- *Genetic basis of hemostasis disorders:* Hemophilia and PFDs arise from genetic mutations affecting coagulation factors and platelet activity. Understanding these genetic mechanisms is crucial for accurate diagnosis and treatment.
- *Molecular pathology of hemophilia:* Hemophilia A and B are X-linked recessive disorders caused by mutations in the *F8* and *F9* genes, respectively. These mutations disrupt clotting factor production, leading to prolonged bleeding and severe clinical manifestations.

- *Platelet function disorders:* Platelet adhesion, aggregation, and secretion defects result from mutations in key genes such as *VWF, GP1BA, ITGA2B*, and *NBEAL2*. These disorders lead to mucocutaneous bleeding, prolonged clotting times, and varying degrees of severity.
- *Advancements in diagnosis and treatment:* Genetic testing, including PCR, NGS, and linkage analysis, enhance diagnosis accuracy. Emerging therapies such as gene therapy and recombinant factor replacement hold promise for personalized treatment approaches.

SUGGESTED READINGS

1. Liu Y, Li D, Yu D, Liang Q, Chen G, Li F, et al. Comprehensive analysis of hemophilia A (CAHEA): Towards full characterization of the F8 gene variants by long-read sequencing. Thromb Haemost. 2023;123(12):1151-64.
2. Srivastava A, Santagostino E, Dougall A, Kitchen S, Sutherland M, Pipe SW, et al.; WFH Guidelines for the Management of Hemophilia panelists and co-authors. WFH Guidelines for the management of hemophilia, 3rd edition. Haemophilia. 2021;27(4):699.
3. Hayward CPM. How I investigate for bleeding disorders. Int J Lab Hematol. 2018;40(Suppl 1): 6-14.
4. Zegers SAM, Smit Y, Saes JL, van Duren C, Schuijt TJ, van Heerde WL, et al. Diagnostic work up of patients with increased bleeding tendency. Haemophilia. 2020;26(2):269-77.
5. Greaves M, Watson HG. Approach to the diagnosis and management of mild bleeding disorders. J Thromb Haemost. 2007;5(Suppl 1):167-74.
6. Dutta D, Gunasekera D, Ragni MV, Pratt KP. Accurate, simple, and inexpensive assays to diagnose *F8* gene inversion mutations in hemophilia A patients and carriers. Blood Adv. 2016;1(3):231-9.
7. Manderstedt E, Lind-Halldén C, Ljung R, Astermark J, Halldén C. Detection of F8 int22h inversions using digital droplet PCR and mile-post assays. J Thromb Haemost. 2020; 18(5):1039-49.
8. Shetty S, Ghosh K, Bhide A, Mohanty D. Carrier detection and prenatal diagnosis in families with haemophilia. Natl Med J India. 2001;14(2):81-3.
9. Jayandharan G, Shaji RV, George B, Chandy M, Srivastava A. Informativeness of linkage analysis for genetic diagnosis of haemophilia A in India. Haemophilia. 2004;10(5):553-9.
10. Tantawy AAG. Molecular genetics of hemophilia A: Clinical perspectives. Egypt J Med Hum Genet. 2010;11(2):105-14.
11. Pezeshkpoor B, Fischer R, Preisler B, Hartlieb K, Rühl H, Müller J, et al. Modulation of haemostatic balance in combined von Willebrand disease and antithrombin deficiency: A comprehensive family study. Haemophilia. 2025;31(1):140-7.
12. Acharyya S, Acharyya K, Parasar A, Pramanik S. Attenuation of phenotypical expression of severe hemophilia A in presence of simultaneous prothrombotic Factor V mutation: The debate continues. J Family Med Prim Care. 2019;8(9):3051-3.
13. van den Berg HM, De Groot PH, Fischer K. Phenotypic heterogeneity in severe hemophilia. J Thromb Haemost. 2007;5(Suppl 1):151-6.
14. Franchini M, Lippi G. Factor V Leiden and hemophilia. Thromb Res. 2010;125(2):119-23.
15. Gallinaro L, Cattini MG, Sztukowska M, Padrini R, Sartorello F, Pontara E, et al. A shorter von Willebrand factor survival in O blood group subjects explains how ABO determinants influence plasma von Willebrand factor. Blood. 2008;111(7):3540-5.
16. Moore EE, Moore HB, Kornblith LZ, Neal MD, Hoffman M, Mutch NJ, et al. Trauma-induced coagulopathy. Nat Rev Dis Primers. 2022;8(1):25.
17. Kornblith LZ, Moore HB, Cohen MJ. Trauma-induced coagulopathy: The past, present, and future. J Thromb Haemost. 2019;17(6):852-62.

18. Pasta G, Annunziata S, Polizzi A, Caliogna L, Jannelli E, Minen A, et al. The progression of hemophilic arthropathy: The role of biomarkers. Int J Mol Sci. 2020;21(19):7292.
19. Favaloro EJ. Classification of von Willebrand disease in the context of modern contemporary von Willebrand factor testing methodologies. Res Pract Thromb Haemost. 2020;4(6):952-7.
20. Sharathkumar AA, Shapiro A. Treatment of Hemophilia. Platelet Function Disorders, 2nd edition. Montréal, Canada: World Federation of Hemophilia (WFH); 1999; revised 2008.
21. Othman M. Platelet-type von Willebrand disease: a rare, often misdiagnosed and underdiagnosed bleeding disorder. Semin Thromb Hemost. 2011;37(5):464-9.
22. Nurden A, Nurden P. Advances in our understanding of the molecular basis of disorders of platelet function. J Thromb Haemost. 2011;9(Suppl 1):76-91.
23. Nurden P, Stritt S, Favier R, Nurden AT. Inherited platelet diseases with normal platelet count: phenotypes, genotypes and diagnostic strategy. Haematologica. 2021;106(2):337-50.
24. Smith N, Bornikova L, Noetzli L, Guglielmone H, Minoldo S, Backos DS, et al. Identification and characterization of novel mutations implicated in congenital fibrinogen disorders. Res Pract Thromb Haemost. 2018;2(4):800-11.
25. Wei ML. Hermansky-Pudlak syndrome: a disease of protein trafficking and organelle function. Pigment Cell Res. 2006;19(1):19-42.
26. Mishra K, Singla S, Sharma S, Saxena R, Batra VV. Griscelli syndrome type 2: a novel mutation in RAB27A gene with different clinical features in 2 siblings: a diagnostic conundrum. Korean J Pediatr. 2014;57(2):91-5.
27. Turner ME, Che J, Mirhaidari GJM, Kennedy CC, Blum KM, Rajesh S, et al. The lysosomal trafficking regulator "LYST": an 80-year traffic jam. Front Immunol. 2024;15:1404846.
28. Kawankar N, Shanmukhaiah C, Kulkarni B. Identification of a GFI1B variant associated with abnormal platelet function and normal platelet count. Br J Haematol. 2025;206(2):777-80.
29. Deppermann C, Cherpokova D, Nurden P, Schulz JN, Thielmann I, Kraft P, et al. Gray platelet syndrome and defective thrombo-inflammation in Nbeal2-deficient mice. J Clin Invest. 2013;123(8):3331-42.
30. Rucker D, Dhamoon AS. Physiology, Thromboxane A2. In: StatPearls. Treasure Island (FL): StatPearls Publishing; 2025.
31. Gachet C. P2Y(12) receptors in platelets and other hematopoietic and non-hematopoietic cells. Purinergic Signal. 2012;8(3):609-19.
32. Kawankar N, Shetty S, Kulkarni B. Novel RASGRP2 variants in platelet function defects: Indian study. Br J Haematol. 2022;197(3):377-80.
33. Canault M, Alessi MC. RASGRP2 structure, function and genetic variants in platelet pathophysiology. Int J Mol Sci. 2020;21(3):1075.
34. Al Hawas R, Ren Q, Ye S, Karim ZA, Filipovich AH, Whiteheart SW. Munc18b/STXBP2 is required for platelet secretion. Blood. 2012;120(12):2493-500.
35. Tuteja N. Signaling through G protein coupled receptors. Plant Signal Behav. 2009;4(10):942-7.
36. Senis YA. Protein-tyrosine phosphatases: a new frontier in platelet signal transduction. J Thromb Haemost. 2013;11(10):1800-13.
37. Millington-Burgess SL, Harper MT. Gene of the issue: *ANO6* and Scott Syndrome. Platelets. 2020;31(7):964-7.
38. Silva-Rojas R, Laporte J, Böhm J. *STIM1/ORAI1* Loss-of-function and gain-of-function mutations inversely impact on SOCE and calcium homeostasis and cause multi-systemic mirror diseases. Front Physiol. 2020;11:604941.

CHAPTER 40

Neonatal Transfusion

Anil Kumar Gupta, Kailash Chander Aggarwal

ABSTRACT

The majority of hospitalized neonates receive one or more transfusion during their stay. Transfusions are typically based on the hemoglobin concentration, platelet count, and coagulation screening. Newer randomized controlled trial has provided evidence-based guidelines and recommendation for components transfusion in neonates. Transfusions are life-saving, however, pose inherent risk and predispose neonates for transfusion associated complications. Alternative approaches have been advocated in neonates to minimize transfusions and thereof complications. Special considerations are also employed to prevent metabolic complications unique for this age group.

INTRODUCTION

Transfusions of red blood cells (RBCs), platelets, and plasma are critical therapies in a neonatal intensive care unit (NICU). Transfusions are typically based on the hemoglobin concentration, platelet count, and coagulation screening. Transfusion guidelines in neonates are predominantly based on studies in "very low birth weight" (VLBW) weighing < 1,500 g and "extremely low birth weight" (ELBW) neonates weighing < 1,000 g. In general, all term or preterm neonates will tend to receive transfusions using the same guidelines with minor variations. In this article, our objective is to provide recent transfusion issues for different blood component especially related to neonates.

Standard definitions of neonates (up to 28 days of postnatal age), infants (>28 days to <1 year), and preterm neonates (born before 37 completed weeks of gestation) are used. Transfusions in fetuses and infants are not included as they have different consideration due to their unique characterization.

RED CELL TRANSFUSION IN NEONATE

RBCs are the most commonly transfused blood component in neonates. 90% ELBW and 60% VLBW received one or more RBC transfusions. Transfusion thresholds in neonates are variable. Despite numerous attempts to establish clinical guidelines for RBC transfusion in neonates, transfusion decisions currently consider hemoglobin level and the cardiorespiratory compensatory mechanism.

Transfusion Threshold for Red Blood Cells in Neonate

A hemoglobin threshold for RBC transfusion vary according to the cardio-respiratory status, gestational age, and postnatal age. Two randomized clinical trials (RCT) comparing transfusion practices in preterm neonates have been published in 2020; first was an European RCT—"Effect of Transfusion Thresholds on Neurocognitive Outcomes (ETTNO)" trial, and second was "transfusion of prematures (TOP)" trial conducted in USA. Both studies found statistically significant correlation between birth weight and transfusion; found more transfusions in low birth weight (LBW) neonates. Associated comorbidities such as neonatal sepsis, disseminated intravascular coagulopathy (DIC), respiratory distress, and unconjugated hyperbilirubinemia increase the requirement of RBCs transfusion.

Recent systematic review of six RCTs in year 2024 involving 3,483 neonates recommends transfusion thresholds based on postnatal age and need of respiratory support. Respiratory support is defined as ventilator support, or continuous positive airway pressure or noninvasive intermittent positive pressure ventilation or nasal cannula O_2 flow rate ≥ 1 L/min **(Table 1)**.

Small Volume Transfusion

The majority of neonates received small volume (10–20 mL/kg) "top up" transfusions for correction of "anemia of prematurity"; usually transfused in 4 hours, typically given at a rate of 15 mL/kg, which is sufficient to raise the hemoglobin by 2–3 g/dL. A higher transfusion volumes of 20 mL/kg is advocated to reduce the transfusion need. Transfusion volume exceeding 20 mL/kg may lead to volume overload in neonates with no bleeding. Small volume transfusions owing to small amount of plasma in it, does not pose threat for post-transfusion hyperkalemia.

TABLE 1: Recommendations in neonates.

Neonatal age	Hct% with respiratory support	Hct% with no respiratory support
Postnatal week 1	33	30
Postnatal week 2	30	25
≥Postnatal week 3	27	21

Large Volume Transfusion

Large volume transfusion is defined as transfusion of a single circulating blood volume (80 mL/kg for neonates) over 24 hours or 50% of the blood volume within 3 hours. Large volume transfusion have risk for post-transfusion hyperkalemia, particularly if infused rapidly. A large volume transfusion through central venous line deliver large amount of K^+ directly to the heart, may lead to cardiac arrest, thus necessitate close monitoring of potassium.

Irradiation also causes hemolysis and releases K^+. Transfusion of irradiated blood beyond 24 hours of storage should be avoided to prevent hyperkalemia. Serum electrolytes should be monitored during transfusion including potassium and calcium (to prevent hypocalcemia secondary to calcium chelation by citrate). Fast infusion, use of radiant warmers and phototherapy during transfusion may cause hemolysis and increases plasma potassium in blood unit. This can be prevented by shielding transfusion tubing. Inline potassium adsorption filters have been implied for removing extracellular K^+ from blood, its routine feasibility probably will require time.

Exchange Transfusion in Neonates

Aim of exchange transfusion (ET) is to manage a high or rapidly rising plasma bilirubin not responding to phototherapy or intravenous immunoglobulin, or for correction of severe anemia. Cord blood showing hemoglobin level ≤ 8 g/dL; or total bilirubin > 5.0–5.5 mg/dL or rapidly increasing total bilirubin levels ≥ 0.5–1.0 mg/dL/hour, despite phototherapy are indication for ET. ET is mainly used in the treatment of hemolytic disease of newborn (HDN) to prevent bilirubin encephalopathy by removing the antibody-coated red cells and excess plasma bilirubin. ET is also used for neonatal hyperbilirubinemia due to glucose-6-phosphate dehydrogenase (G6PD) deficiency.

The ET should be performed with "O cells" or antigen compatible RBCs suspended in antibody negative AB plasma. A single blood volume (80 mL/kg) ET will remove 75% of the neonatal red cells, and a double volume (160–200 mL/kg) up to 85–90% red cells, and up to 50% of circulating bilirubin. A double-volume exchange transfusion is more effective in removing antibody coated red cells and reduce the need for a subsequent ET.

Adverse Outcomes from Red Blood Cells Transfusions

The RBC transfusions are life-saving, however, pose inherent immunologic risk associated with transfusion. In addition, RBC transfusions, itself has shown increased risk for morbidity and mortality in preterm neonates, including necrotizing enterocolitis (NEC) and intraventricular hemorrhage (IVH).

Red Blood Cell Transfusion and Necrotizing Enterocolitis

The NEC is closely associated with RBC transfusion and is responsible for about 10% mortality in NICU. Studies showed that severe anemia (≤8 g/dL) rather RBC transfusion have increased risk of NEC in VLBW neonates. Ischemia followed by reperfusion was suggested for transfusion-related injury to the intestine in NEC. Increase production of cytokine gamma interferon was postulated as underlying cause for NEC.

Red Blood Cells Transfusion and Intraventricular Hemorrhage

Association between blood transfusions and IVH has been established. IVH is the most common complication in neonates, occurring during the first 3 days of life and is associated with poor neurodevelopmental outcomes. VLBW have higher risk of neurological sequelae than term neonates. The worsening of IVH from grade 1 to grade 4, noted following RBC transfusion. Cardiorespiratory alterations rather than hematological abnormalities is postulated for IVH.

Other Adverse Outcomes

Association between RBC transfusion and development of bronchopulmonary dysplasia (BPD) has been reported. Iron and free radical injury were possible mechanisms for development of BPD. Association also exists for the development of retinopathy of prematurity (ROP) and RBC transfusion. The association was dose dependent and related to the frequency of RBC transfusion.

Alternative Approaches to Minimize Red Blood Cell Transfusion

Overall transfusions are safe in neonates, however, neonates, are prone for transfusion complications, e.g., transfusion-associated circulatory overload (TACO), transfusion-associated acute lung injury (TRALI), in addition to transfusion-transmitted infections (TTI). Therefore, alternative strategies to minimize RBC transfusions have been developed and include prevention of iatrogenic anemia, placental transfusion through delayed cord clamping, and use of erythropoietin.

Minimize Iatrogenic Blood Loss

There is hidden loss of blood which is concealed in dead spaces of cannula, syringes, intravenous (IV) tubings, cotton swabs, as well direct loss due to frequent blood sampling for various investigations. This is known as iatrogenic blood loss, estimated to be 40–50 mL/kg in a neonate which corresponds a blood loos of 600–700 mL in an adult. This is major cause for transfusions in 90% preterm neonates.

This iatrogenic anemia and thereof transfusions can be minimized by changes in neonatal practice, and include use of micromethods testing and point-of-care testing devices, minimizing unnecessary investigations, delaying the investigation if not urgent, and optimizing frequency and volume of blood draws to avoid waste or repeat testing. Cord blood can be implied for blood group and screen, blood counts, and blood culture which significantly decreases iatrogenic loss and decreases the need for RBC transfusion.

Improve Hemoglobin Concentration by Delayed Cord Clamping

Delayed cord clamping results in transfer of placental blood to neonate and thus decreases the need of RBC transfusions. Delayed cord clamping have a favorable effect on developmental outcomes in neonates and decreases incidence of IVH, NEC, as well morbidity and mortality. The World Health Organization recommends delaying of cord clamping for 1–3 minutes after birth, which increases hemoglobin level by 1–2 g/dL. American College of Obstetricians and Gynecologists also recommend delayed cord clamping.

Recombinant Human Erythropoietin

Recombinant human erythropoietin (rEPO) has been found effective in stimulating erythropoiesis in premature neonates. It decreases frequency and amount of RBC transfusions; and improves cognitive outcome at 18–22 months of age. Extremely premature infants in PENUT clinical trial found no statistical significant difference in mortality or neurodevelopmental outcome at 2 years of age that were randomized to receive placebo. Neonates who received rEPO, require lesser volume for RBCs transfusion compared to placebo group. Also, rEPO decreases the need of frequent RBC transfusion in neonates.

Specific Consideration for Red Blood Cell Transfusion in Neonates

Use of Fresh versus Stored Red Blood Cells in Neonates

Studies found no difference in outcome when utilizing fresh (≤7 days old RBCs) or stored RBCs for transfusion in neonates. The American Association of Blood Banks (AABB) recommend blood from standard RBC units instead of blood from fresh RBC units (<10 days) for small volume "top up" transfusions in neonates. However, need of large volume transfusion necessitate fresher, washed RBCs to prevent hyperkalemia. In study, two groups of preterm neonates were compared receiving either fresh RBCs stored for <7 days or standard stored RBCs and found no differences in mortality and major morbidities such as NEC, severe IVH, severe ROP, and BPD between two groups.

RBCs are usually stored in citrate, phosphate, dextrose, adenine solution (CPDA1), or in saline, adenine, glucose, mannitol (SAGM), to diminish RBC lysis. Many blood centers collect RBC in AS-1 (Adsol preservative) to extend RBCs shelf life (42 days). The use of AS-1 RBCs is concerning in neonates because of high exposure to dextrose, adenine, and mannitol; however, use of small volume AS-1 preserved RBCs are safe and well tolerated in neonates. The question of large volume transfusion of Adsol preserved RBCs (≥20 mL/kg) especially in premature neonates need to be justified.

Group and Compatibility

Neonatal blood grouping differ from adults as ABO antigen over red cells are poorly expressed and corresponding antibodies are usually not developed in plasma. Lastly neonatal plasma also possess maternal antibodies [immunoglobulin G (IgG)], transferred through placenta as well any prophylactic anti-D administered during pregnancy. Due to these factors, antibody screening of a neonate represents the maternal antibody rather than the neonates own antibody.

RBC must be compatible to both neonate and mother. ABO-specific blood or group O RBCs suspended in AB plasma can be transfused if no antibodies is detected toward the neonatal RBCs. For antibody screen, maternal blood should be used, as any antibodies present in neonates originated from mother. A negative antibody screen need not to be repeated until 4 months of age, as neonate's immature immune system rarely produces antibodies to RBC transfusion. If antibody screening is positive, antigen-negative units should be transfused.

In case where multiple aliquots or multiple pediatric packs are used from dedicated single unit, only first aliquot be tested for compatibility procedure, as this will be representative of all satellite units from dedicated blood unit. Subsequent aliquot from same blood unit will be issued for transfusion with no further compatibility testing until the unit expires or infant aged 4 months.

Irradiated Products

Premature neonates are at higher risk for transfusion associated graft versus host disease (TAGvHD), especially those receiving ETs. Blood components in VLBW neonates especially from first or second degree relative donors should receive irradiated components, to prevent fatal TAGvHD. Irradiation, also effectively decreases the risk of transfusion transmitted cytomegalovirus (TT-CMV) and should be used in VLBW neonates.

Blood Warming

Neonates are vulnerable for hypothermia due to their low body fat and large surface area. Hypothermia is common with large volume transfusion. ET should not be undertaken with red cells direct from 4°C storage. Transfusions at room temperature further contribute to a decrease in core body temperature of neonate by 0.7–2.5°C. Use of blood warmers during transfusion is recommended. The counter-current technology has been found most effective way for safe and efficient blood warming during transfusions in neonates.

Limiting Multiple Donor Exposure

Premature neonates with need of frequent transfusions should be identified at early stage. Frequent RBCs are usually given as small-volume transfusions, to maintain the hemoglobin. RBC transfusion from fresh blood unit against blood requirement will make prone for multiple donor exposure. This can be prevented either by using "pediatric packs" (which are multiple aliquots from a single blood bag); or dedicated blood bag from which small aliquots withdrawn using sterile connecting device for transfusion in neonate as and when needed, till expiry of blood. The blood from an adult blood unit (350/450 mL) can be transferred into several small satellite bags through a closed system, using a sterile connecting device. Such system is found safe and can prevent blood waste. In addition, it can reduce the donor exposure by increasing the number of transfusions from a single blood unit.

PLATELET TRANSFUSION IN NEONATES

Platelets transfusion is the second most commonly transfused component in neonates. Thrombocytopenia is common in NICU and affects 20–35% of admitted neonates. About 70% of VLBW neonates experienced thrombocytopenia and results in platelet transfusion.

Platelet Transfusion Thresholds

Premature newborns have lower normal platelet counts, compared to adult ranging from 100,000 to 150,000/μl. The incidence of thrombocytopenia in neonates is extremely variable and inversely related with gestational age. Thrombocytopenia is more in LBW as a result of accelerated destruction of platelets, and also more in neonates with intrauterine infection, placental insufficiency, neonatal sepsis, and immune mediated thrombocytopenia. Moderate thrombocytopenia resolve with treatment of underlying cause; 20–25% neonates receive one or more platelet transfusion. Neonates with thrombocytopenia are, therefore clinically evaluated for platelet transfusion.

Two RCTs, evaluated platelet transfusion threshold in the premature neonates. *PlaNeT-1 trial* evaluated bleeding episodes in preterm neonates with severe thrombocytopenia (platelet count < 60 × 10^9/μl). Study revealed that severe thrombocytopenia with NEC are strong predictors for bleeding episodes; and necessitate prophylactic platelet transfusion. In addition to thrombocytopenia, the incidence of bleeding increases with decreasing gestational age.

The PlaNeT-2 trial, compared platelet transfusion in two different groups of platelet thresholds (25,000/μL vs. 50,000/μL) in premature neonates and yielded surprising results. Low platelet threshold of 25,000/μL was associated with a significant reduction in mortality and major bleeding compared to platelet threshold of ≥50,000/μL. Lower platelet threshold was associated with absolute risk reduction and is currently advocated for clinical practice.

Platelet Transfusions Threshold and Current Practices

Most platelet transfusions are given therapeutically for thrombocytopenia (<50,000/μl) with active bleeding and is considered appropriate, but there is uncertainty about prophylactic use of platelet in the absence of bleeding. Platelet count and bleeding risk is not directly correlated. A prophylactic platelet transfusion at 25,000/μL was found effective in preterm neonates regardless of their predicted risk for major bleeding and/or mortality. A little higher platelet threshold (<30,000/μl) is indicated with active bleeding, or with an increased risk of IVH.

Platelet Product Selection in the Neonate

ABO identical/compatible platelets are ideal to avoid the transfer of incompatible isohemagglutinins (anti-A, anti-B, or anti-A, B antibodies) with donor plasma to prevent risk of hemolysis. Neonates, owing to their small plasma volume are unable to dilute these isohemagglutination. Platelets are usually given in a dose of 10–15 mL/kg in neonate. Volume reduced ABO-mismatched platelets can be given if identical platelets are not available. ABO-compatible, apheresis platelets may improve platelet increment with platelet refractoriness.

Adverse Effect of Platelet Transfusions

Platelet transfusions have been implied usual risks inherent to any other blood component, including clinical or transfusion errors, and have higher risks of bacterial or septic infection owing to its storage at 22–24°C.

FRESH FROZEN PLASMA TRANSFUSION IN NEONATES

A very few studies for evidence-based guidelines for transfusion of fresh frozen plasma (FFP) are available. FFP unit should be ABO compatible, however, Rh typing is not required as it contains no red cells. Alternatively, AB plasma can be transfused if group is not known.

Prophylactic use of FFP in sepsis, DIC, liver disease, vitamin K deficiency, trauma, and correction of dilutional effects of massive transfusion are indicated to prevent coagulopathy.

Therapeutic plasma exchange is indicated with FFP as replacement fluid. Plasma is also used for reconstitution of whole blood for exchange transfusion, and to prime cardiothoracic circuits or extracorporeal membrane oxygenation (ECMO) circuits. However, data are conflicting for optimal combination for reconstitution of products for priming a circuit.

Coagulation Factor Deficiencies in Neonates

The hemostatic system in neonates is immature at birth, the "normal" reference ranges in neonates are quite different from those in adults. Plasma transfusion in neonate is based on "cutoffs" used to define coagulopathy in adult. Prothrombin time (PT) and activated partial thromboplastin time (aPTT) are prolonged in premature neonates due to the decreased synthesis in hepatocytes; however, prematurity itself is not an indication for FFP transfusion. FFP should not be used to correct prolonged international normalized ratio (INR) in absence of bleeding. DIC without active bleeding does not justify the use of FFP. In absence of commercially availability of specific factor concentrates, FFP is transfused alternatively at a rate of 10–15 mL/kg particularly factors V and X deficiency, in bleeding neonates with congenital bleeding disorder while awaiting for a definite diagnosis.

Adverse Outcomes from Plasma Transfusions

Plasma have inherent risks ranging from mild allergic reaction secondary to plasma proteins to severe life-threatening reactions. Most of these reactions in neonates are under-recognized or under-reported. Plasma is usually transfused for its hemostatic properties, but also have been reported to cause venous thrombosis in neonates, due to platelet-derived microparticles in plasma.

Cryoprecipitate (Factor VIII)

Volume of cryoprecipitate is usually 15–20 mL/unit containing at least 80 IU of factor VIII and >150 mg of fibrinogen/unit. Grouping is not required for cryoprecipitate and is transfused across the groups. Severe congenital hypofibrinogenemia may present in the neonatal period but neonatal hypofibrinogenemia is most likely to be acquired, secondary to DIC, or liver dysfunction. The management of hypofibrinogenemia necessitate use of cryoprecipitate.

Take Home Point

Transfusion in neonates requires careful balancing of benefits depending upon gestational age, birth weight, hematological parameters, comorbidities, and possible adverse effects. Delayed cord clamping and minimizing iatrogenic blood loss are very effective in preventing anemia and reducing transfusion need. When transfusing neonates, particularly preterm infants, efforts should be made to reduce allogenic donor exposure. Although small volume transfusion pose no or minimal risk, it is large volume which should follow special consideration to prevent post-transfusion hyperkalemia, hypothermia, and hypocalcemia. Use of platelets transfusion and plasma transfusion are increasing, their need to be specialized according to patient need.

SUGGESTED READINGS

1. Venkatesh V, Khan R, Curley A, New H, Stanworth S. How we decide when a neonate needs a transfusion. Br J Haematol. 2013;160(4):421-33.
2. New HV, Berryman J, Bolton-Maggs PHB, Cantwell C, Chalmers EA, Davies T, et al. Guidelines on transfusion for fetuses, neonates and older children. Br J Haematol. 2016;175(5):784-828.
3. Wang YC, Chan OW, Chiang MC, Yang PH, Chu SM, Hsu JF, et al. Red blood cell transfusion and clinical outcomes in extremely low birth weight preterm infants. Pediatr Neonatol. 2017;58(3):216-22.
4. Fasano RM, Said M, Luban NL. Blood component therapy for the neonate. In: Martin RJ, Fanaroff AV, Walsh MC (Eds). Fanaroff and Martin's neonatal perinatal medicine: diseases of the fetus and infant, 10th edition. Philadelphia (PA): Elsevier Saunders; 2015.
5. Markham C, Small S, Hovmand P, Doctor A. Transfusion decision making in pediatric critical illness. Pediatr Clin North Am. 2017;64(5):991-1015.
6. Fredrickson LK, Bell EF, Cress GA, Johnson KJ, Zimmerman MB, Mahoney LT, et al. Acute physiological effects of packed red blood cell transfusion in pre term infants with different degrees of anaemia. Arch Dis Child Fetal Neonatal Ed. 2011;96:F249-53.
7. Franz AR, Engel C, Bassler D, Rüdiger M, Thome UH, Maier RF, et al. Effects of liberal vs restrictive transfusion thresholds on survival and neurocognitive outcomes in extremely low-birth-weight infants: The ETTNO Randomized Clinical Trial. JAMA. 2020;324(6):560-70.
8. Kirpalani H, Bell EF, Hintz SR, Tan S, Schimdt B, Chaudhary AS, et al.; Eunice Kennedy Shriver NICHD Neonatal Research Network. Higher or lower hemoglobin transfusion thresholds for preterm infants. N Engl J Med. 2020;383(27):2639-51.
9. Amrutiya RJ, Mungala BM, Patel VT, Ganjiwale JD, Nimbalkar SM. Blood component transfusion in tertiary care neonatal intensive care unit and neonatal intermediate care unit: An audit. Cureus. 2020;12(8):e9952.
10. Deschmann E, Dame C, Sola-Visner MC, Fustolo-Gunnink SF, Guyatt GH, Patel RM, et al. Clinical practice guideline for red blood cell transfusion thresholds in very preterm neonates. JAMA Network Open. 2024;7(6):e2417431.
11. Strauss RG, Sacher RA, Blazina JF, Blanchette VS, Schloz LM, Butch SH, et al. Commentary on small volume red cell transfusions for neonatal patients. Transfusion. 1990;30:565-70.
12. Hensch LA, Indrikovs AJ, Shattuck KE. Transfusion in extremely low birth weight premature neonates: current practices trends, risks, and early interventions to decrease the need for transfusion. Neo Reviews. 2015;16(5):e287-96.

13. Kim DH. Transfusion practice in neonates. Korean J Pediatr. 2018;61:265-70.
14. Strauss RG. RBC storage and avoiding hyperkalemia from transfusions to neonates and infants. Transfusion. 2010;50(9):1862-5.
15. Vraets A, Lin Y, Callum JL. Transfusion-associated hyperkalemia. Transfus Medi Rev. 2011;25(3):184-96.
16. Lee AC, Reduque LL, Luban NL, Ness PM, Anton B, Heitmiller ES. Transfusion associated hyperkalaemic cardiac arrest in paediatric patients receiving massive transfusion. Transfusion. 2014;54(1):244-54.
17. Shafique MA, Abbas SO, Habiba U, Mughal A, Ahmad TKF, Chaudhary AM. A transfusion strategies for neonates: current perspectives. Ann Med Surg. 2024;86(3):1550-62.
18. Eshghifar N, Maghsudlu M, Amini Kafi-Abad S. The effect of pre-storage irradiation blood on quality of red blood cells. Int J Hematol Oncol Stem Cell Res. 2021;15(1):1-6.
19. Balasubramanyam P, Basavarajegowda A, Hanumanthappa N, Negi VS, Harichandrakumar KT. Irradiating stored blood and storing irradiated blood: is it different? A study of serial changes in biochemical parameters of red blood cell units. Asian J Transfus Sci. 2021;15(2):172-8.
20. Laptook AR, SalhabW, Bhaskar B. Admission temperature of low birth weight infants: predictors and associated morbidities. Pediatrics. 2007;119(3):e643-9.
21. National Institute for Health and Clinical Excellence (NICE). (2010). CG 98 Neonatal Jaundice. [online] Available from www.nice.org.uk/ guidance/CG98 [Last accessed May, 2025].
22. Lathe GH. Exchange transfusion as a means of removing bilirubin in haemolytic disease of newborn. Br Med J. 1955;1(4907):192-6.
23. Forfar JO, Keay AJ, Elliott WD, Cumming RA. Exchange transfusion in neonatal hyper-bilirubinemia. Lancet. 1958;2(7057):1131-7.
24. Ghirardello S, Dusi E, Cortinovis I, Villa S, Fumagalli M, Agosti M, et al. Effects of red blood cell transfusions on the risk of developing complications or death: an observational study of a cohort of very low birth weight infants. Am J Perinatol. 2017;34(1):88-95.
25. Keir A, Pal S, Trivella M, Lieberman L, Callum J, Shehata N, et al. Adverse effects of red blood cell transfusions in neonates: a systematic review and meta-analysis. Transfusion. 2016;56(11):2773-80.
26. Mally P, Golombek SG, Mishra R, Nigam S, Mohandas K, Depalhma H, et al. Association of necrotizing enterocolitis with elective packed red blood cell transfusions in stable, growing, premature neonates. Am J Perinatol. 2006;23(8):4518.
27. Jacob J, Kamitsuka M, Clark RH, Kelleher AS, Spitzer AR. Etiologies of NICU deaths. Pediatrics. 2015;135(1):e59-65.
28. Blau J, Calo JM, Dozor D, Sutton M, Alpan G, La Gamma EF. Transfusion related acute gut injury: necrotizing enterocolitis in very low birth weight neonates after packed red blood cell transfusion. J Pediatr. 2011;158(3):403-9.
29. Patel RM, Knezevic A, Shenvi N, Hinkes M, Keene S, Roback JD, et al. Association of red blood cell transfusion, anemia, and necrotizing enterocolitis in very low-birth-weight infants. JAMA. 2016;315(9):889-97.
30. Le VT, Klebanoff MA, Talavera MM, Slaughter JL. Transient effects of transfusion and feeding advances (volumetric and caloric) on necrotizing enterocolitis development: A case-crossover study. PLoS One. 2017;12(6):e0179724.
31. De Plaen IG. Inflammatory signaling in necrotizing enterocolitis. Clin Perinatol. 2013;40(1): 109-24.
32. Maheshwari A, Schelonka RL, Dimmitt RA, Carlo WA, Munoz-Hernandez B, Das A, et al. Cytokines associated with necrotizing enterocolitis in extremely-low-birth-weight infants. Pediatr Res. 2014;76(1):100-8.
33. Baer VL, Lambert DK, Henry E, Snow GL, Butler A, Christensen RD. Among very-low-birth weight neonates is red blood cell transfusion an independent risk factor for subsequently developing a severe intraventricular hemorrhage? Transfusion. 2011;51(6):1170-8.
34. Baer VL, Lambert DK, Henry E, Snow GL, Christensen RD. Red blood cell transfusion of preterm neonates with a Grade 1 intraventricular hemorrhage is associated with extension to a Grade 3 or 4 hemorrhage. Transfusion. 2011;51(9):1933-9.

35. Franz AP, Bolat GU, Bolat H, Matijasevich A, Santos IS, Silveira RC, et al. Attention-deficit/hyperactivity disorder and very preterm/very low birth weight: A meta-analysis. Pediatrics. 2018;141(1):e20171645.
36. Bassan H. Intracranial hemorrhage in the preterm infant: understanding it, preventing it. Clin Perinatol. 2009;36(4):737-62.
37. Reddy PA, Sreenivasulu H, Shokrolahi M, Muppalla SK, Abdilov N, Ramar R, et al. Navigating the complexities of intraventricular hemorrhage in preterm infants: an updated review. Cureus. 2023;15(5):e38985.
38. Joseph RM, O'Shea TM, Allred EN, Heeren T, Hirtz D, Paneth N, et al. Prevalence and associated features of autism spectrum disorder in extremely low gestational age newborns at age 10 years. Autism Res. 2017;10(2):224-32.
39. Treyvaud K, Ure A, Doyle LW, Lee KJ, Rogers CE, Kidokoro H, et al. Psychiatric outcomes at age seven for very preterm children: rates and predictors. J Child Psychol Psychiatry. 2013;54(7):772-9.
40. Ballabh P. Intraventricular hemorrhage in premature infants: mechanism of disease. Pediatr Res. 2010;67(1):1-8.
41. Sharp M, French N, McMichael J, Campbell C. Survival and neurodevelopmental outcomes in extremely preterm infants 22–24 weeks of gestation born in Western Australia. J Paediatr Child Health. 2018;54(2):188-93.
42. Maier RF, Sonntag J, Walka MM, Liu G, Metze BC, Obladen M. Changing practices of red blood cell transfusions in infants with birth weights less than 1000 g. J Pediatr. 2000;136(2):220-4.
43. Inder TE, Clemett RS, Austin NC, Graham P, Darlow BA. High iron status in very low birth weight infants is associated with an increased risk of retinopathy of prematurity. J Pediatr. 1997;31(4):541-4.
44. Dani C, Reali MF, Bertini G, Martelli E, Pezzati M, Rubaltelli FF. The role of blood transfusions and iron intake on retinopathy of prema turity. Early Hum Dev. 2001;62(1):57-63.
45. Lieberman L, Petraszko T, Yi Q, Hannach B, Skeate R. Transfusion-related lung injury in children: a case series and review of the literature. Transfusion. 2014;54(1):57-64.
46. Stainsby D, Jones H, Wells AW, Gibson B, Cohen H; SHOT Steering Group. Adverse outcomes of blood transfusion in children: analysis of UK reports to the serious hazards of transfusion scheme 1996–2005. Br J Haematol. 2008;141(1):73-9.
47. Kumar P, Marshall BC, deBlois G, Koch WC. A cluster of transfusion-associated babesiosis in extremely low birth weight premature infants. J Perinatol. 2012;32(9):731-3.
48. Glanternik JR, Baine IL, Rychalsky MR, Shapiro E, Baltimore R. A cluster of cases of babesia microti among neonates traced to a single unit of donor blood. Pediatr Infect Dis J. 2018;37(3):269-71.
49. Aher SM, Ohlsson A. Early versus late erythropoietin for preventing red blood cell transfusion in preterm and/or low birth weight infants. Cochrane Database Syst Rev. 2020;2(2):CD004865.
50. Lemyre B, Sample M, Lacaze-Masmonteil T; Canadian Paediatric Society, Fetus and Newborn Committee. Minimizing blood loss and the need for transfusions in very premature infants. Paediatr Child Health. 2015;20(8):451-62.
51. Yu VY. Blood transfusion in the neonate. In: Gupta S (Ed). Recent advances in Pediatrics, Special Volume 5, Neonatology 2. New Delhi: Jaypee Brothers Medical Publishers; 2000. pp. 230-218-253.
52. Yu VYH, Zaho SM, Bajuk B. Results of intensive care for 375 very low birthweight infants. Aus Pediatr J. 1982;18:188-92.
53. ObladenM, Sachsenweger M, Stahnke M. Blood sampling in very low birthweight infants receiving different levels of intensive care. Eur J Pediatr. 1988;147:399-404.
54. Lenes BA, Sacher RA. Blood component therapy in neonatal medicine. Clin Lab Med. 198;1(2):285-309.

55. Carroll PD, Livingston E, Baer VL, Karkula K, Christensen RD. Evaluating otherwise-discarded umbilical cord blood as a source for a neonate's complete blood cell count at various time points. Neonatology. 2018;114(1):82-6.
56. Christensen RD, Carroll PD, Josephson CD. Evidence-based advances in transfusion practice in neonatal intensive care units. Neonatology. 2014;106(3):245-53.
57. Rabe H, Gyte GM, Diaz-Rossello JL, Duley L. Effect of timing of umbilical cord clamping and other strategies to influence placental transfusion at preterm birth on maternal and infant outcomes. Cochrane Database Syst Rev. 2019;9:CD003248.
58. Committee on Obstetric P. Committee Opinion No. 684: Delayed Umbilical Cord Clamping after Birth. Obstet Gynecol. 2017;129(1):e5-e10.
59. Andersson O, Domellof M, Andersson D, Hellstrom-Westas L. Effect of delayed vs early umbilical cord clamping on iron status and neurodevelopment at age 12 months: a randomized clinical trial. JAMA Pediatr. 2014;168(6):547-54.
60. WHO. Guideline: Delayed umbilical cord clamping for improved maternal and infant health and nutrition outcomes. Geneva: World Health Organization; 2014.
61. Leslie MS, Greene J, Schulkin J, Jelin AC. Umbilical cord clamping practices of US obstetricians. J Neonatal Perinatal Med. 2018;11(1):51-60.
62. Ohls RK, Kamath-Rayne BD, Christensen RD, Wiedmeier SE, Rosenberg A, Fuller J, et al. Cognitive outcomes of preterm infants randomized to darbepoetin, erythropoietin, or placebo. Pediatrics. 2014;133(6):1023-30.
63. Juul SE, Comstock BA, Wadhawan R, Mayock DE, Courtney SE, Robinson T, et al. A randomized trial of erythropoietin for neuroprotection in preterm infants. New Engl J Med. 2020; 382(3):233-43.
64. Juul SE, Vu PT, Comstock BA, Wadhawan R, Mayock DE, Courtney SE, et al. Effect of high-dose erythropoietin on blood transfusions in extremely low gestational age neonates: Post hoc analysis of a randomized clinical trial. JAMA Pediatr. 2020;174(10):933-43.
65. Zerra PE, Josephson C. Transfusion in the neonatal patient: Review of evidence based guidelines. Clin Lab Med. 2021;41(1):15-34.
66. Spinella PC, Dressler A, Tucci M, Carroll CL, Rosen RS, Hume H, et al. Survey of transfusion policies at US and Canadian children's hospitals in 2008 and 2009. Transfusion. 2010;50(11): 2328-35.
67. Fergusson DA, Hébert P, Hogan DL, LeBel L, Rouvinez-Bouali N, Smyth JA, et al. Effect of fresh red blood cell transfusions on clinical outcomes in premature, very low-birth-weight infants: the ARIPI randomized trial. JAMA. 2012;308:1443-51.
68. Carson JL, Guyatt G, Heddle NM, Grossman BJ, Cohn CS, Fung MK, et al. Clinical practice guidelines from the AABB: Red blood cell transfusion thresholds and storage. JAMA. 2016; 316(19):2025-35.
69. Opoku-Okrah C, Acquah BK, Dogbe EE. Changes in potassium and sodium concentrations in stored blood. Pan Afr Med J. 2015;20:236.
70. Sesok-Pizzini D, Pizzini MA. Hyperkalemic cardiac arrest in pediatric patients undergoing massive transfusion: unplanned emergencies. Transfusion. 2014;54(1):4-7.
71. Pyles R, Lowery J, Delaney M. The use of red cell units containing additives in large volume neonatal transfusion in neonatology units in the USA. ISBT Science Series. 2017;12:322-3.
72. Liu EA, Mannino FL, Lane TA. Prospective, randomized trial of the safety and efficacy of a limited donor exposure transfusion program for premature neonates. J Pediatr. 1994; 125(1):92-6.
73. Lee DA, Slagel TA, Jackson TM, Evan CS. Reducing blood donor exposures in low birth weight infants by the use of older, unwashed packed red blood cells. J Pediatr. 1995;126:280-6.
74. Wood A, Wilson N, Skacel P, Thomas R, Tidmarsh E, Yale C, et al. Reducing donor exposures in preterm infants requiring multiple blood transfusions. Arch Dis Child Fetal Neonatal Ed. 1995;72(1):F29-33.
75. Fung MK, Roseff SD, Vermoch KL. Blood component preference of transfusion services supporting infant transfusions: A university health system consortium benchmarking study. Transfusion. 2010;50(9):1921-5.

76. Cohn CDM, Johnson S, Katz L. Technical Manual, 20th edition. Bethesda, MD: AABB; 2020.
77. Dender MR, Graeber JE. Post transfusion graft versus host disease in infancy. J Pediatr. 1990;117(1):159-63.
78. Strauss RG. Leukocyte-reduction to prevent transfusion-transmitted cytomegalovirus infections. Pediatr Transplant. 1999;3 (Suppl 1):19-22.
79. Vamvakas EC. Is white blood cell reduction equivalent to antibody screening in preventing transmission of cytomegalovirus by transfusion? A review of the literature and meta-analysis. Transfus Med Rev. 2005;19(3):181-99.
80. Kekre N, Tokessy M, Mallick R, McDiarmid S, Huebsch L, Bredeson C, et al. Is cytomegalovirus testing of blood products still needed for hematopoietic stem cell transplant recipients in the era of universal leukoreduction? Biol Blood Marrow Transplant. 2013;19(12):1719-24.
81. Fergusson D, Hébert PC, Lee SK, et al. Clinical outcomes following institution of universal leukoreduction of blood transfusions for premature infants. JAMA-2003;289:1950-6.
82. Jackson JC. Adverse events associated with exchange transfusion in healthy and ill newborns. Pediatrics. 1997;99(5):e7.
83. Uhl L, Pacini D, Kruskall MS. A comparative study of blood warmer performance. Anesthesiology. 1992;77(5):1022-8.
84. Fabres J, Wehrli G, Marques MB, Phillips V, Dimmitt RA, Westfall AO, et al. Estimating blood needs for very-low-birth-weight infants. Transfusion. 2006;46(11):1915-20.
85. Cook S, Gunter J, Wissel M. Effective use of a strategy using assigned red cell units to limit donor exposure for neonatal patients. Transfusion. 1993;33(5):379-83.
86. Wang-Rodriguez J, Mannino FL, Liu E, Lane TA. A novel strategy to limit blood donor exposure and blood waste in multiply transfused premature infants. Transfusion. 1996;36(1):64-70.
87. Dos Santos AM, Trindade CE. Red blood cell transfusions on the neonate. Neo Reviews. 2011;12:c139.
88. Gupta AK, Kumari S, Singhal A, Bahl A. Neonatal thrombocytopenia and platelets transfusion. Asian J of Transf Sci. 2012;6:161-4.
89. Castle V, Andrew M, Kelton J, Giron D, Johnston M, Carter C. Frequency and mechanism of neonatal thrombocytopenia. J Pediatr. 1986;108(5 Pt 1):749-55.
90. Christensen RD, Henry E, Wiedmeier SE, Stoddard RA, Sola-Visner MC, Lambert DK, et al. Thrombocytopenia among extremely low birth weight neonates: data from a multihospital healthcare system. J Perinatol. 2006;26(6):348-53.
91. Sola-Visner M, Bercovitz RS. Neonatal platelet transfusions and future areas of research. Transfus Med Rev. 2016;30(4):183-8.
92. Guida JD, Kunig AM, Leef KH, McKenzie SE, Paul DA. Platelet count and sepsis in very low birth weight neonates: is there an organism-specific response? Pediatrics. 2003;111(6 Pt 1): 1411-5.
93. Aballi AJ, Puapondh Y, Desposito F. Platelet counts in thriving premature infants. Pediatrics-1968;42(4):685-9.
94. Roberts IA, Murray NA. Thrombocytopenia in the newborn. Curr Opin Pediatr. 2003;15(1): 17-23.
95. Estcourt LJ. Platelet transfusion thresholds in premature neonates (PlaNeT-2 trial). Transfus Med. 2019;29(1):20-2.
96. Marret S, Ancel PY, Marpeau L, Marchand L, Pierrat V, Larroque B, et al. Neonatal and 5-year outcomes after birth at 30–34 weeks of gestation. Obstet Gynecol. 2007;110(1): 1171-2.
97. Josephson CD. Neonatal and pediatric transfusion practice. In: Roback JD, Combs MR, Grossman BJ, Hillyer CD (Eds). AABB technical manual, 18th edition. Bethesda: AABB Press; 2014. pp. 580-3.
98. Patel RM, Knezevic A, Yang J, Shenvi N, Hinkes M, Roback JD, et al. Enteral iron supplementation, red blood cell transfusion, and risk of bronchopulmonary dysplasia in very-low-birth-weight infants. Transfusion. 2019;59(5):1675-82.

99. Fustolo-Gunnink SF, Fijnvandraat K, van Klaveren D, Stanworth SJ, Curley A, Onland W, et al. Preterm neonates benefit from low prophylactic platelet transfusion threshold despite varying risk of bleeding or death. Blood. 2019;134(26):2354-60.
100. Josephson CD, Castillejo MI, Grima K, Hillyer CD. ABO-mismatched platelet transfusions: strategies to mitigate patient exposure to naturally occurring hemolytic antibodies. Transfus Apher Sci. 2010;42(1):83-8.
101. Davoren A, Curtis BR, Aster RH, McFarland JG. Human platelet antigen-specific alloantibodies implicated in 1162 cases of neonatal alloimmune thrombocytopenia. Transfusion. 2004;44(8):1220-5.
102. Motta M, Del Vecchio A, Perrone B, Ghirardello S, Radicioni M. Fresh frozen plasma use in the NICU: a prospective, observational, multicentred study. Arch Dis Child Fetal Neonatal Ed. 2014;99(4):F303-8.
103. Doyle JJ. The role of erythropoietin in the anemia of prematurity. Semin Perinatol. 1997;21(1):20-7.
104. Padmanabhan A, Connelly-Smith L, Aqui N, Balogun RA, Klingel R, Meyer E, et al. Guidelines on the use of therapeutic apheresis in clinical practice: Evidence-Based Approach from the Writing Committee of the American Society for Apheresis: The Eighth Special Issue. J Clin Apher. 2019;34(3):171-354.
105. Williams MD, Chalmers EA, Gibson BE; Haemostasis and Thrombosis Task Force, British Committee for Standards in Haematology. The investigation and management of neonatal haemostasis and thrombosis. Br J Haematol. 2002;119(2):295-309.
106. Maruyama H, Kitajima H, Yonemoto N, Fujimura M. Frequent use of fresh frozen plasma is a risk factor for venous thrombosis in extremely low birth weight infants: a matched case-control study. Acta Med Okayama. 2012;66(1):61-6.
107. DGHS, National aids control organization, GOI New Delhi. (2022). National standards for blood centres and blood transfusion services, 2nd edition. [online] Available from https://mohfw.gov.in/sites/default/files/National%20Standards%20for%20Blood%20Centres.pdf [Last accessed May, 2025].
108. Murray NA, Roberts IA. Neonatal transfusion practice. Arch Dis Child Fetal Neonatal Ed. 2004;89:F101-7.

CHAPTER 41

Newer Parameters in Cell Counters

Mrinalini Kotru, Anil Handoo

ABSTRACT

Advancements in automated hematology analyzers have introduced a suite of new parameters that significantly enhance the diagnostic and monitoring capabilities of the most widely used complete blood count (CBC). Parameters such as reticulocyte hemoglobin content, immature granulocyte count, monocyte distribution width, and immature platelet fraction provide *real-time insights* into bone marrow function, iron status, infection, and platelet kinetics that were previously unavailable without specialized tests. Meanwhile, artificial intelligence is beginning to transform hematology by analyzing complex data patterns and images to yield novel diagnostic indicators and improve workflow efficiency. The *clinical relevance* of these innovations is evidenced by their ability to detect conditions earlier (e.g., sepsis or iron deficiency before overt laboratory changes), differentiate similar presentations (e.g., types of anemia or thrombocytopenia) with greater confidence, and guide therapy in a timely manner. The algorithms presented in this chapter illustrate how incorporating these new parameters can streamline patient management and improve outcomes. In summary, the newer parameters in cell counters represent a leap forward in hematologic diagnostics, turning the CBC into a richer source of diagnostic intelligence.

INTRODUCTION

Modern automated hematology analyzers have evolved far beyond simple cell counts. They now report a plethora of *new parameters* that provide deeper insights into red blood cells (RBCs), white blood cells (WBCs), and platelets. These extended indices, made possible by advances in flow cytometry, optical analysis, and computational algorithms, allow better characterization of blood cell abnormalities and can facilitate more accurate differential diagnoses.

This chapter reviews the newly developed hematology parameters for RBCs, WBCs, and platelets, as well as artificial intelligence (AI)-driven parameters, highlighting their clinical relevance. Practical diagnostic algorithms are provided in a stepwise format to demonstrate the application of these new parameters in everyday clinical decision-making. The goal is to provide an evidence-based, in-depth insight into these recent advances in hematology, tailored for hematopathology and clinical hematology professionals.

RATIONALE FOR NEW PARAMETERS

Conventional CBCs provide limited information, often requiring additional tests. New parameters fill these gaps by assessing size distribution, maturity, and morphology. Novel erythrocyte and reticulocyte indices detect iron-restricted erythropoiesis earlier than traditional iron studies, while advanced leukocyte parameters flag infection or sepsis sooner, and platelet indices help differentiate peripheral destruction from marrow failure. Many of these automated CBC innovations are rapid, cost-effective, and clinically useful. AI-based tools further enhance hematology by analyzing complex data patterns, detecting subtle abnormalities, and automating differential counts with high accuracy. The following sections explore these advancements by cell lineage.

NEW RED BLOOD CELL PARAMETERS

Modern analyzers report extended red blood cell (RBC) indices that include reticulocyte hemoglobin content, percentages of hypochromic and microcytic RBCs, immature reticulocyte fraction (IRF), and fragmented RBC counts that go beyond the traditional hemoglobin, mean corpuscular volume (MCV), mean corpuscular hemoglobin (MCH), and red cell distribution width (RDW). These new parameters enhance the evaluation of anemia by assessing the hemoglobin content of cells, the variation in RBC size/hemoglobinization, and the output of young red cells from the bone marrow.

Reticulocyte Hemoglobin Content (Ret-He/R-He or CHr)

Ret-He measures the hemoglobin content of reticulocytes, reflecting real-time iron availability for erythropoiesis. With a lifespan of ~1–2 days, reticulocytes provide an immediate snapshot of marrow iron utilization. A low Ret-He (<28–29 pg) indicates iron-deficient erythropoiesis, even before anemia manifests. Unlike serum iron or ferritin, Ret-He is unaffected by acute-phase inflammation and responds rapidly to therapy, rising within ~2–3 days of iron supplementation if marrow function improves. Ret-He is available on many analyzers (e.g., Sysmex Ret-He, Siemens/Advia CHr, Mindray RHE, and Horiba RHC) and is highly concordant across platforms. Clinically, a low Ret-He suggests iron deficiency or inflammatory blockade, while a normal Ret-He in anemia makes iron deficiency less likely. Its integration into anemia workups improves diagnostic accuracy, distinguishing iron deficiency anemia from anemia of chronic disease or thalassemia trait.

Clinical relevance: Ret-He is included in anemia management guidelines, particularly in chronic kidney disease (CKD) and oncology, where functional iron deficiency is common. Dialysis protocols use Ret-He (or %hypochromic cells) to guide IV iron therapy. A persistently low Ret-He (<29 pg) in erythropoietin-treated patients signals inadequate iron supply, prompting supplementation, while a rising Ret-He confirms effective repletion. As a dynamic marker, Ret-He allows more precise therapy adjustments than ferritin or transferrin saturation.

Percentage of Hypochromic and Microcytic Red Cells (%Hypo, %Micro)

Advanced analyzers quantify hypochromic (%Hypo) and microcytic (%Micro) RBCs, aiding in anemia differentiation. %Hypo (~<280 g/L or <28 pg per cell) reflects iron-restricted erythropoiesis over ~2–3 months, with >10% suggesting iron deficiency, particularly in dialysis patients. Ret-He indicates immediate iron status, while %Hypo reflects cumulative effects. %Micro (<60 fL) quantifies microcytosis, elevated in iron deficiency and thalassemia but lower in anemia of chronic disease. Iron deficiency raises both %Micro and %Hypo, while thalassemia primarily increases %Micro with less impact on %Hypo. These parameters improve anemia classification, monitor therapy response, and reduce interobserver variability.

Immature Reticulocyte Fraction and Reticulocyte Indices

Immature reticulocyte fraction represents the proportion of reticulocytes that are "immature," usually defined by high RNA content/fluorescence. Analyzers (Sysmex XN series, Beckman Coulter DxH series, Mindray CAL series, Horiba Helo series, etc.) categorize reticulocytes by maturity [low fluorescence reticulocytes (LFR), medium fluorescence reticulocytes (MFR), high fluorescence reticulocytes (HFR)]. IRF, representing HFR% among total reticulocytes, is a marker of marrow regeneration. A high IRF indicates increased young reticulocyte release, seen in hemolysis, anemia recovery, or postchemotherapy marrow engraftment, often rising before neutrophil or platelet recovery. It aids in anemia classification: Low IRF with low reticulocyte count suggests marrow hypoproliferation, while high IRF with adequate reticulocytes indicates hemolysis or hemorrhage recovery. Automated refinements such as the Immature Reticulocyte Index (IRI) or Reticulocyte Production Index (RPI) enhance assessment. IRF is valuable in engraftment monitoring and may help predict marrow failure, prompting earlier bone marrow evaluation.

Fragmented Red Cells and Other RBC Morphologic Flags

Fragmented red cells (FRC), available on advanced analyzers (e.g., Sysmex XN), quantify schistocytes, aiding in diagnosing thrombotic microangiopathy (TMA), disseminated intravascular coagulation (DIC), and mechanical hemolysis. Automated FRC correlates with manual schistocyte counts, supporting TMA diagnosis and prompting urgent smear review in suspected thrombotic thrombocytopenic purpura (TTP)/hemolytic uremic syndrome (HUS) **(Figs. 1A and B)**. Serial FRC monitoring helps track treatment response (e.g., decreasing FRC% as TMA resolves). Additional RBC-focused new parameters (Ret-He, %Hypo, IRF, FRC, etc.) enrich anemia diagnostics, enabling earlier detection, reducing unnecessary tests, and improving treatment monitoring.

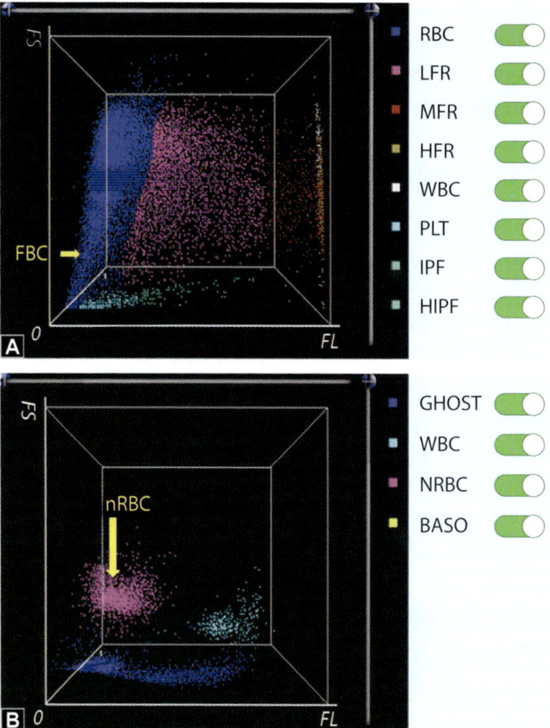

FIGS. 1A AND B: (A) Showing fragmented RBCs (FRC) and (B) showing nucleated RBCs (nRBC) in a case of microangiopathic hemolytic anemia.

(HFR: high fluorescence reticulocytes; IPF: immature platelet fraction; LFR: low fluorescence reticulocytes; MFR: medium fluorescence reticulocytes; NRBC: nucleated-red-blood cells; RBC: red blood cells; WBC: white blood cells)

NEW WHITE BLOOD CELL PARAMETERS

Leukocyte differential technology has also advanced, yielding new parameters that reflect the presence of immature cells or activation changes in WBCs. Traditional 5-part differentials classify neutrophils, lymphocytes, monocytes, eosinophils, and basophils. New parameters add *quantitative measures of early granulocyte release*, WBC morphological changes during infection, and even progenitor cell counts. Key innovations include the *Immature Granulocyte count (IG# and IG%), monocyte distribution width (MDW), Delta Neutrophil Index (DNI)*, automated *hematopoietic progenitor cell (HPC) counts*, and *high fluorescence lymphocyte count (HFLC)/high fluorescence cell count (HFC)*. These parameters have significant clinical relevance in infection diagnosis (especially sepsis), leukemia/left shift detection, stem cell transplantation, and viral illnesses, especially dengue.

Immature Granulocyte Count (IG% and IG#)

IGs (promyelocytes, myelocytes, metamyelocytes) are typically absent or in low numbers in peripheral blood, with elevated levels indicating bone marrow stress or myeloid activation (e.g., infection, inflammation, and malignancy). Historically detected manually, modern analyzers (e.g., Sysmex XE/XN, Coulter DxH) now quantify IG% and IG#, providing an objective measure of a neutrophil left shift. A high IG% serves as an early marker for infection or sepsis, often rising before WBC or neutrophils. Studies confirm its role in sepsis screening, with higher IG% linked to positive blood cultures. Fast, cost-effective, and easily integrated into early warning systems, IG% aids infection detection and reduces false alarms. Beyond infection, an elevated IG% can appear in *leukemoid reactions, chronic myeloproliferative neoplasms, or steroid use*—any scenario with marrow granulocytic stimulation. Modern laboratories often set an *IG reference range (e.g. 0–1%)* and will flag IG% above normal.

Monocyte Distribution Width

Monocyte distribution width, an FDA-cleared parameter on select analyzers (e.g., Beckman Coulter DxH 800/900), measures monocyte size variation, serving as a monocyte analogue of RDW. In acute infections and sepsis, activated monocytes show increased size heterogeneity. MDW is an early sepsis biomarker, automatically calculated with no extra cost, making it useful in emergency settings. A high MDW indicates a strong immune response, even if WBC count is normal. Studies show MDW >20 distinguishes sepsis from noninfectious systemic inflammatory response syndrome (SIRS), with a negative predictive value of ~94% and improved detection when combined with WBC [area under curve (AUC) ~0.85]. Patients with normal WBC and MDW have significantly lower sepsis risk, while an elevated MDW (e.g., 23) in a febrile emergency patient can prompt early intervention.

DELTA NEUTROPHIL INDEX

Delta Neutrophil Index (DNI) quantifies circulating immature neutrophils by measuring the difference between leukocyte subfractions in specific analyzers (e.g., Coulter LH and Advia). It is similar to IG% but calculated differently. DNI rises in sepsis and severe infections, correlating with severity and prognosis. Studies show that a DNI cutoff of ~6–7% has high sensitivity for sepsis, outperforming C-reactive protein (CRP) and procalcitonin. Extremely high DNI (>10%) may indicate worsening infection or risk of septic shock. DNI trends help monitor treatment response, with rising values suggesting progression and falling values indicating improvement. Though also elevated in inflammatory conditions and postsurgery, DNI serves as a rapid, objective measure of neutrophil immaturity, aiding early sepsis diagnosis and risk stratification in ICU protocols.

Hematopoietic Progenitor Cell Counts

Hematopoietic progenitor cell counts (HPC) are an automated count of circulating CD34-positive stem and progenitor cells, available on advanced analyzers such as the Sysmex XN series. It serves as a rapid surrogate for CD34 flow cytometry in stem cell transplantation, aiding in timing apheresis during peripheral blood stem cell mobilization. Studies show a strong correlation

($r > 0.83$) between HPC and CD34 counts, with an AUC ~0.93 for predicting poor mobilization. Clinicians use HPC# to assess collection readiness, potentially reducing unnecessary apheresis. Rising HPC may also indicate marrow recovery post-transplant or chemotherapy, while elevated HPC in leukemia could signal relapse. Though still developing, HPC enhances hematology automation, streamlining stem cell transplant workflows and integrating progenitor cell assessment into routine CBC analysis.

High Fluorescence Lymphocyte Count/High Fluorescence Cell Count

High fluorescence lymphocyte count (HFLC) or high fluorescence cell (HFC) count identifies a cell population with higher intensity of their fluorescent signals clearly distinguishable from monocytes and lymphocytes in a 5-part differential channel (HFLC on Sysmex XN analyzer and HFC count on Mindray BC series) of the newer hematology analyzers with fluorescence flow cytometry. While the cells in this area can be blasts/plasma cells or other cells with high fluorescence, studies have established that in the dengue season, the cells in this region represent the activated lymphocytes associated with dengue viral illness. Their patterns on the scatter have a characteristic figure of "8" appearance, and their numbers have an inverse correlation with platelet counts as depicted in **Figures 2 and 3**.

NEW PLATELET PARAMETERS

Platelet counts and indices have also benefited from technological advances. Beyond the platelet count and mean platelet volume (MPV), we now have parameters that gauge platelet production and functionality. Chief among them is the *immature platelet fraction (IPF)*, sometimes called reticulated platelets. Other extended platelet indices include the *platelet distribution width (PDW),*

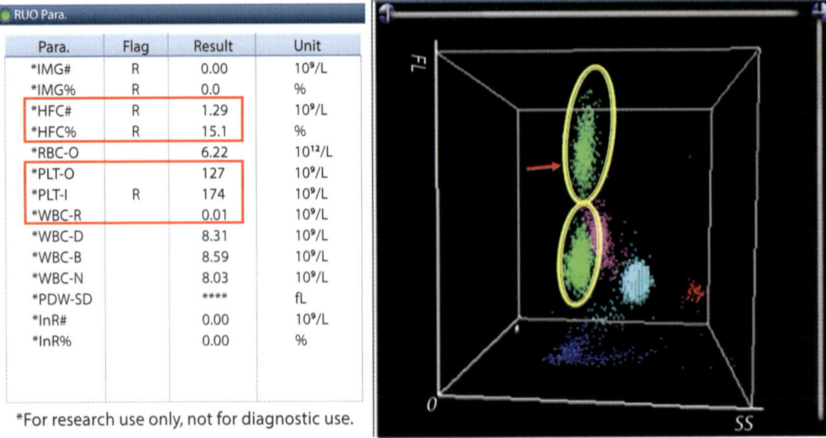

RUO Para.

Para.	Flag	Result	Unit
*IMG#	R	0.00	10^9/L
*IMG%	R	0.0	%
*HFC#	R	1.29	10^9/L
*HFC%	R	15.1	%
*RBC-O		6.22	10^{12}/L
*PLT-O		127	10^9/L
*PLT-I	R	174	10^9/L
*WBC-R		0.01	10^9/L
*WBC-D		8.31	10^9/L
*WBC-B		8.59	10^9/L
*WBC-N		8.03	10^9/L
*PDW-SD		****	fL
*InR#		0.00	10^9/L
*InR%		0.00	%

*For research use only, not for diagnostic use.

FIG. 2: Figure of "8" arrangement for high fluorescence cells with lymphocytes in dengue patients.

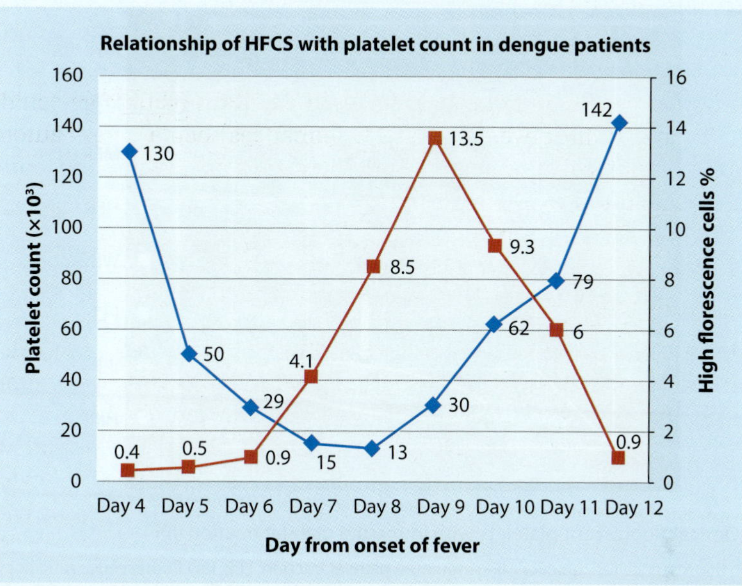

FIG. 3: An inverse relationship of high fluorescence cells with platelet counts in dengue patients.

plateletcrit (PCT), and even novel measures such as the *mean platelet component (MPC)*, which reflects platelet internal composition. These parameters are particularly useful in evaluating thrombocytopenia (low platelets) and platelet function or recovery.

Immature Platelet Fraction/Reticulated Platelet Fraction/ Large Platelet Fraction

Immature platelet fraction (IPF) measures the percentage of larger and younger, RNA-containing platelets, indicating bone marrow platelet production. It is assumed to be akin to reticulocytes for RBCs. While the normal IPF ranges from 1 to 5%, it, however, is instrument dependent. Clinical significance of higher values (>7–8%) suggests peripheral destruction (e.g., ITP, DIC, TTP), while low or normal IPF in thrombocytopenia indicates reduced production (e.g., aplastic anemia and marrow infiltration). Studies show IPF effectively differentiates these conditions, with a ~6% cutoff yielding 88% sensitivity and 76% specificity. Clinically, IPF aids in diagnosis, guiding workup, and reducing unnecessary bone marrow biopsies. It also predicts recovery, as rising IPF precedes platelet count increases in ITP and postchemotherapy. Now widely automated, IPF is routinely reported with CBCs, enhancing thrombocytopenia management without added cost **(Fig. 4)**. **Figure 5** also shows utility in predicting platelet count recovery.

Other Platelet Indices

Other platelet parameters are either older but underutilized, or newly emerging in research/advanced analyzers:

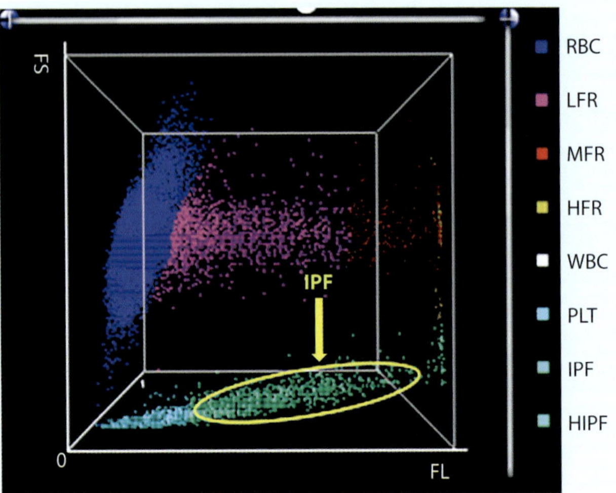

FIG. 4: Optical/fluorescent platelets with immature platelet fraction (IPF).

(HFR: high fluorescence reticulocytes; IPF: immature platelet fraction; LFR: low fluorescence reticulocytes; MFR: medium fluorescence reticulocytes; NRBC: nucleated-red-blood cells; RBC: red blood cells; WBC: white blood cells)

Days	1	2	3	4	5	6
Platelets	89	54	39	47	70	123
IPF	7.8	11.2	13.9	13.3	7.7	6.5

FIG. 5: An inverse relationship of IPF with platelet counts in dengue patients.

- *Platelet distribution width*: This measures the variability in platelet size (analogous to RDW for RBC). A high PDW indicates heterogeneity in platelet size, which can occur in myeloproliferative disorders or during active platelet production (large young platelets mixed with small older ones). PDW is often elevated in ITP (since marrow puts out very large young platelets) and lower in aplastic states. However, PDW has not gained as much clinical traction as IPF, partly due to overlap and lack of standardization.

- *Platelet large cell ratio (P-LCR)*: This gives the percentage of platelets above a certain size (e.g., >12 fL). It is another way to quantify large platelets. A high P-LCR can parallel IPF in indicating increased turnover. It is used more in research than routine practice.
- *PCT*: This is simply the volume occupied by platelets in blood (analogous to hematocrit). It is calculated as platelet count × MPV. PCT can indicate total platelet mass; for instance, in dengue fever management, some suggest PCT might correlate with bleeding risk better than platelet count alone. But in practice, PCT is rarely acted upon clinically.
- *MPC*: This is a newer research parameter reflecting the refractive index or composition of platelets (measured in g/dL, indicating the mean physical/chemical density of platelets). It is available on certain analyzers such as Abbott. In sepsis studies, a decrease in MPC (meaning platelets become less dense, perhaps due to degranulation or swelling) was observed, and a negative correlation with DNI was noted. While not yet in routine use, MPC could emerge as a marker of platelet activation (since activated platelets might lose granule content and thus have lower component concentration). Another parameter called *mean platelet mass* or *opacity* has been discussed similarly. For now, these are of academic interest but show how platelet measurement is evolving beyond just size and count.

ADVANCES IN ARTIFICIAL INTELLIGENCE-BASED HEMATOLOGY PARAMETERS

Artificial intelligence and machine learning are increasingly being integrated into hematology to create smarter analyzers and novel diagnostic indices. AI in hematology can take several forms: Image-based AI (for examining blood smear images or cell images), pattern recognition in multidimensional analyzer data [scatterplots and cell population data (CPD)], and predictive modeling using routine parameters. These approaches yield *AI-derived parameters or flags* that can augment traditional results. In this section, we discuss a few of these key advances.

Artificial Intelligence-powered Digital Morphology (Fig. 6)

Artificial intelligence-driven hematology analyzers, such as the FDA-approved Sight OLO, perform CBCs using digital microscopy and AI, enabling portable, reagent-free blood testing. Validation studies show high concordance with standard analyzers, highlighting AI's potential for near-patient testing. AI also enhances laboratory differentials through digital cell morphology systems (e.g., CellaVision), which preclassify WBCs, RBC morphology, and platelets, improving efficiency and consistency. These systems quantify new morphological features (e.g., neutrophil lobularity and blast counts in bone marrow), creating digital parameters that enrich hematology reports and trend data, revolutionizing blood analysis.

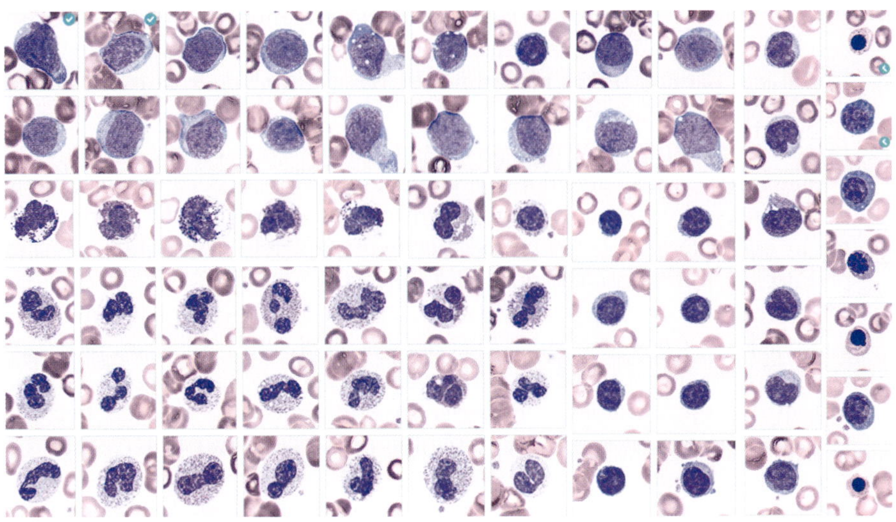

FIG. 6: Digital morphology classified by artificial intelligence.

Machine Learning Models on CBC Data

Artificial intelligence is being applied to *CPD* and CBC parameters to detect disease patterns. Machine learning models analyze multidimensional data on cell size, complexity, and fluorescence, enabling early disease detection. An *artificial neural network (ANN)* using 26 blood parameters distinguished hematologic malignancies with ~85% accuracy, detecting subtle CBC shifts suggestive of leukemia or lymphoma before human recognition.

Applications:
- Improved anemia classification, outperforming traditional indices in distinguishing *iron deficiency from thalassemia trait.*
- *Early sepsis detection* and ICU mortality prediction through AI-augmented CBC reports can integrate markers such as MDW, IG count, and DNI into a "sepsis indicator."
- Enable automated detection of malaria parasites and sickle cells, effectively adding parasitemia% or hemoglobin S% as reportable parameters.

Though still in early adoption, AI-based hematology tools are set to enhance precision, speed, and personalization in diagnostics as validation continues.

DIAGNOSTIC ALGORITHMS INCORPORATING NEW PARAMETERS

To translate these innovations into practice, clinicians can incorporate new hematology parameters into diagnostic algorithms. Here are stepwise approaches for common clinical scenarios, demonstrating how the inclusion of these parameters enhances decision-making.

Algorithm: Workup of Microcytic Anemia with New RBC Indices

Goal: Iron deficiency anemia (IDA) is *very prevalent in our country* and needs to be differentiated from other causes of microcytic hypochromic anemia in a cost-effective way. Initial CBC evaluation is done to confirm low MCV and low MCH, indicating microcytic, hypochromic indices. Further evaluation with Ret-He and % hypochromic cells is able to guide the further as follows:

- *Reticulocyte hemoglobin content (Ret-He/CHr):*
    - If *Ret-He is low* (<28–30 pg) then proceed as likely IDA or ACD with functional iron deficiency.
    - If *Ret-He is normal/high* then iron supply is adequate; consider thalassemia trait or other causes.
- *%Hypochromic RBC (%Hypo)*: *%Hypo > 10%* supports iron deficiency (absolute or functional). In IDA, %Hypo is often very high; in ACD, moderate; in thalassemia, typically normal or mildly elevated (thalassemia RBCs are microcytic but not all severely hypochromic).

Algorithm: Early Sepsis Screening Using CBC Parameters

Goal: Early diagnosis in sepsis is critical and determines the patient's outcome. Triage of a patient for possible sepsis using information available from the CBC and differential is an easy, quick, and cost-effective. While a *high or low WBC* can indicate infection, it is unreliable on its own. New WBC parameters (IG, MDW, DNI) have improved this clinical challenge using the following algorithm:

- *Immature granulocyte (IG) count:*
    - *IG% >1% (or IG# elevated)* is abnormal. This suggests a left shift (possible bacterial infection or inflammation). The higher the IG%, the more likely an acute infection (IG >3–5% would be strongly suggestive of sepsis or severe bacterial infection).
    - If IG% is normal (0%) and the patient is not on growth factors, severe bacterial infection is less likely (though not impossible). Look for other signs of immunosuppression.
- *MDW:*
    - *MDW ≥ 20* is a red flag for sepsis; combined with clinical judgment should prompt considering sepsis.
    - If MDW is normal (<20) and WBC is normal, the chance of sepsis is quite low.
- *DNI:*
    - *DNI elevated* (>3–5%) indicates a significant fraction of immature neutrophils, supporting infection/sepsis diagnosis. Very high DNI (>10%) may indicate severe sepsis or septic shock risk.
    - *DNI normal (≈0%)* in a febrile patient would argue against bacterial sepsis (unless very early or localized infection).

Hence, if *signs point to sepsis* (e.g., fever, tachycardia, possible source) *and* any of *IG%, MDW, or DNI is abnormal*, treat as sepsis (early antibiotics, fluid).

These parameters bolster the decision to treat early. A falling IG%, normalizing MDW and DNI indicate response to treatment. If they stay high or rise, it may signal treatment failure or new complications. This algorithm effectively creates a quick *"CBC-based sepsis screen."*

Algorithm: Evaluation of Thrombocytopenia with IPF

Goal: Diagnosing true thrombocytopenia with cell counters and determining if it is due to decreased production or increased destruction is a challenge. Confirming low platelets by repeat testing and alternate techniques using the inbuilt software has greatly improved accuracy. Moreover, newer parameters such as immature platelet fraction (IPF) are extremely useful in ascertaining the cause and monitoring recovery as discussed here.

- *High IPF (>7–10%)* suggests young platelets as seen in peripheral destruction or consumption. Common causes are: ITP, DIC, TTP, hypersplenism, and massive bleeding recovery (presence of *FRC* flag along with high IPF would signal thrombotic microangiopathies).
- *Normal or low IPF* suggests that the marrow failure in production of platelets such as in aplastic anemia, bone marrow infiltration (leukemia and MDS), B12/folate deficiency (once severe, platelets drop), and chemotherapy effect. Interpretation with WBC flags, if any, would further narrow down the causes, e.g., the presence of a blast flag would suggest leukemia.
- *Monitor IPF trend:* Regardless of the cause, once intervention is done, follow IPF. In ITP treatment, for example, a high IPF should gradually normalize as platelet count recovers (persistently very high IPF could mean ongoing peripheral destruction despite therapy). In aplastic anemia treated with immunosuppression, an eventual rise in IPF would be an early sign of recovery even before platelet count improves and optimize platelet transfusion therapy.
- *Concurrent IPF and reticulocyte count:* Sometimes, both platelets and RBCs are low. If IPF is low and reticulocyte count is also low, this strongly points to global bone marrow failure (production issue). If IPF is low but reticulocytes are high, consider combined processes (or a specific lineage issue affecting megakaryocytes).

By integrating IPF early, this algorithm efficiently triages patients: Those likely with ITP/consumption get appropriate therapy quickly, while those likely with production issues get a marrow examination without unnecessary delay or empiric treatments. This targeted approach reduces both undertreatment and overtreatment in thrombocytopenia.

Take Home Points

- ➢ The automated hematology analyzers provide a wide array of parameters in the RBC, WBC, and platelet assessment.
- ➢ The older red cell indices combined with the newer RBC indices, such as % Micro, %Hypo, and reticulocyte parameters such as Ret-He/CHr, can help detect and monitor hematinic therapy in IDA and accurately differentiate it from other causes of microcytic hypochromic anemia.

- The parameters such as DNI, MDW, and %IG can be used as quick, early CBC sepsis screen to guide early and lifesaving clinical intervention.
- Newer platelet parameters can effectively differentiate between causes of platelet destruction and hypoproduction. Further, IPF can be used as a marker for platelet recovery and aide in optimizing transfusion requirements.

ACKNOWLEDGMENT

We acknowledge the contribution of Shubham Varshney, Senior Resident, Department of Pathology, UCMS and GTBH, Delhi, who played a very important part in writing the manuscript.

SUGGESTED READINGS

1. Daves M, Roccaforte V, Lombardi F, Panella R, Pastori S, Spreafico M, et al. Modern hematology analyzers: beyond the simple blood cells count (with focus on the red blood cells). J Lab Precis Med. 2023;8:32.
2. Hoenemann C, Ostendorf N, Zarbock A, Doll D, Hagemann O, Zimmermann M, et al. Reticulocyte and erythrocyte hemoglobin parameters for iron deficiency and anemia diagnostics in patient blood management: a narrative review. J Clin Med. 2021;10(18): 4250.
3. Urrechaga E, Borque L, Escanero JF. Biomarkers of hypochromia: the contemporary assessment of iron status and erythropoiesis. Biomed Res Int. 2013;2013:603786.
4. Jo SJ, Kim SW, Choi J-H, Choi SP, Lee J, Lim J. Monocyte distribution width (MDW) as a useful indicator for early screening of sepsis and discriminating false positive blood cultures. PLoS ONE. 2022;17(12):e0279374.
5. Goel G, Semwal S, Khare A, Joshi D, Amerneni CK, Pakhare A, et al. Immature platelet fraction: its clinical utility in thrombocytopenia patients. J Lab Physicians. 2021;13(3):214-8.
6. Jekarl DW, Kim Y, Lim J, Kim M, Han K, Cho B, et al. Fragmented red cell as a possible favorable prognostic marker of hematopoietic stem cell transplantation associated thrombotic microangiopathy. J Clin Lab Anal. 2015;29(6):444-50.
7. Lakshmipriya V, Kavitha K, Yogalakshmi E, Sridevi M. The clinical utility of automated immature granulocyte measurement in the early diagnosis of bacteremia. Cureus. 2024; 16(2):e53660.
8. Crouser ED, Parrillo JE, Seymour CW, Angus DC, Bicking K, Esguerra VG, et al. Monocyte distribution width: a novel indicator of sepsis-2 and sepsis-3 in high-risk emergency patients. Crit Care Med. 2019;47(8):1018-25.
9. Lee T, Lee J, Shin DH, Lee H, Kim SK. Prognostic and diagnostic power of delta neutrophil index and mean platelet component in febrile patients with suspected sepsis. Biomedicines. 2023;11(12):3190.
10. Villa CH, Porturas T, Sell M, Wall M, DeLeo G, Fetters J, et al. Rapid prediction of stem cell mobilization using volume and conductivity data from automated hematology analyzers. Transfusion. 2018;58(2):330-8.
11. Jayaram A, Mathews NS, Nair SC, Geevar T, Rose W, Verghese VP, et al. High fluorescent lymphocyte cell count and scattergram patterns on the Sysmex XN series cell counters-Novel parameters in early and reliable diagnosis of dengue on a background of acute febrile illness. Int J Lab Hematol. 2021;43(4):O156-60.
12. Yang TH, Tsai CK, Wang HY, Ko PS, Chien SH, Lin TA, et al. Early prediction of platelet recovery with immature platelet fraction in patients receiving hematopoietic stem cell transplantation. Ann Hematol. 2024;103(11):4661-70.

13. Bachar N, Benbassat D, Brailovsky D, Eshel Y, Glück D, Levner D, et al. An artificial intelligence–assisted diagnostic platform for rapid near-patient hematology. Am J Hematol. 2021;96(10):1264-74.
14. Sun D, Chen W, He J, He Y, Jiang H, Jiang H, et al. A novel method for screening malignant hematological diseases by constructing an optimal machine learning model based on blood cell parameters. BMC Med Inform Decis Mak. 2025;25(1):72.
15. Uçucu S, Azik F. AI-driven diagnosis of β-thalassemia minor and iron deficiency anemia using machine learning models. J Med Biochem. 2024;43(1):39-47.

INDEX

Page numbers followed by *b* refer to box, *f* refer to figure, *fc* refer to flowchart, and *t* refer to table.

A

B

C

F

G

H

J

K

L

M

T

W

X

Z